To Lauren Berry, RPT, for his generosity in selflessly passing on his wealth of knowledge, and to my parents, Bill and Jean Hendrickson, for their love and encouragement.

To Lauren Berry, RPT, for his generosity in
selflessly passing on his wealth of knowledge, and to
my parents, Bill and Jean Hendrickson, for their love
and encouragement.

Preface to the Second Edition

I have been very gratified that the first edition of this book was well received and that Lippincott Williams & Wilkins asked me to write a second edition. This new edition allows me the opportunity to update the text with the latest research in the effects of massage and manual therapy on the functional rehabilitation of the musculoskeletal system. I added extensive new information on the treatment protocol for acute and chronic injuries as well as the scientific rationale for choosing the appropriate technique for each stage of healing. I have chosen to retain the preface to the first edition, as it provides important information about the history and development of the method of treatment described in this text.

A NEW TITLE FOR THE SECOND EDITION

I have chosen to change the title of the first edition from *Massage for Orthopedic Conditions* to *Massage and Manual Therapy for Orthopedic Conditions.* This new title more accurately reflects the contents of the book. The term *manual therapy* is typically used to describe mobilization of the joints and soft tissue and also refers to other techniques, including muscle energy technique. Because these techniques are included in the method of treatment described in this text, I elected to include the term in the title.

NEW CONTENT FOR THIS EDITION

The second edition has been extensively rewritten on the basis of the latest research and my experience in clinical practice and input from students, the teaching staff at the Hendrickson Method Institute, and colleagues in the field. The only exception to this is the description of the techniques, which has withstood the test of time and remains essentially unchanged.

■ The first chapter has been extensively rewritten and reorganized for clarity. The chapter is divided into four sections: General Overview, Overview of Theory and Technique, Essentials of Anatomy and Physiology for Orthopedic Conditions, and Injury and Repair.

■ A completely new section, General Overview, has been added to the first chapter. This section provides a clear and concise overview of the more detailed information that follows in each chapter.

■ I have added a greatly expanded section on an exciting new paradigm in biology and medicine, which hypothesizes that electromagnetic signaling controls cellular processes, including repair. This new paradigm also hypohesizes that the biomagnetic field emanating from the hands of the therapist can be focused for healing. This is an exciting time for massage and manual therapy because the science of rehabilitation and that of energy medicine are confirming our clinical experience that soft tissues are highly responsive to touch.

■ Extensive new information on the treatment protocol for acute and chronic injuries has been carefully delineated. In the second edition, each orthopedic condition now has clear guidelines on how to apply soft tissue mobilization, joint mobilization, and muscle energy technique for each stage of healing.

■ The section in Chapter 2 entitled "Treatment Guidelines" has been rewritten and greatly expanded. New sections have been added that describe the scientific rationale for each technique in each phase of healing and repair, the factors that indicate which phase of repair the condition is in, the treatment goals, and guidelines for treatment.

■ A new, expanded "Clinical Examples" section in each chapter describes how I applied the three treatment techniques on patients who were in acute and and chronic pain for each area of the body. This section provides examples on ways to integrate the theory and techniques in the clinical setting.

■ Each chapter has been rewritten to reflect the latest research in musculoskeletal rehabilitation, with updated references.

CLARIFICATION OF THE TERMS *MASSAGE, ORTHOPEDIC MASSAGE, AND SOFT TISSUE MOBILIZATION*

Because massage therapy has become more widely utilized in the clinical setting, it is important to define certain terms. The classical meaning of the term *massage* describes three principle techniques: effleurage, or stroking; petrissage, or kneading; and tapotement, or percussion. While these techniques are very effective in the spa environment and can induce relaxation, promote circulation, reduce stress, and provide many other benefits, they are not specifically designed to treat acute injuries, nor are they the most effective style of soft tissue therapy to help resolve injuries and induce the optimum functional improvement in the musculoskeletal system. Many terms are used in the literature to describe more "clinical" massage therapy, such as *orthopedic massage*;, *soft tissue therapy*, *medical massage*, *soft tissue mobilization*, *soft tissue manipulation*, *neuromuscular therapy*, *trigger point therapy*, *clinical massage*, and *myofascial manipulation*, to name a few.

In the first edition, I used the term *orthopedic massage* to describe the more clinically oriented method of treatment in the text. Since the publication of the first edition, *orthopedic massage* has become widely used as a term that defines a field of massage rather than a specific technique. With this in mind, in this second edition, I have elected to use the term *soft tissue mobilization* to describe the "massage" portion of the technique. All references to *orthopedic massage* have been removed.

Soft tissue mobilization is simply defined as the manual manipulation of soft tissues. This term is more accurate for the soft tissue techniques that are described in this text because they are not classical massage strokes. After decades of clinical practice, I developed a new way to mobilize the soft tissue that I named *wave mobilization*. Modeled on ocean waves, this is completely different from classical massage techniques. The strokes are precise, rounded scooping motions, perpendicular to the fiber, performed rhythmically, in precise directions.

It is my hope that this expanded and revised edition will inspire massage and manual therapists to learn a new way of working that is not only clinically effective, but also relaxing for the client to receive and energizing for the therapist to perform. The treatments become a moving meditation that creates stillness and deepened awareness in the therapist as well profound relaxation in the client. For too long, clinical musculoskeletal therapy has been painful to receive and straining for the therapist to perform. This new way of working will provide an opportunity of looking forward to a long and healthy career in the healing arts.

Preface to the First Edition

This book was written to fulfill the need for advanced training in massage and manual therapy specializing in the management of musculoskeletal pain and dysfunction. It is intended as a textbook for massage therapists as well as for chiropractors, physical therapists, osteopaths, physical therapy and orthopedic assistants, athletic trainers, and other health care providers.

The demand for safe and effective treatment of pain and disability is growing rapidly as the population seeks alternatives to drugs and surgery. In addition, an increasing number of people are experiencing musculoskeletal pain and dysfunction. Many factors can be cited for this, such as a more active elderly population, the popularity of recreational sports, the increased number of people using computers, and the growing numbers of people involved in car accidents.

The medical community has recognized that much of the pain and disability suffered by their patients involves soft tissue injury and dysfunction. Yet at a 1987 symposium of the American Academy of Orthopedic Surgeons entitled "The Mechanisms of Injury and Repair of the Musculoskeletal Soft Tissue," experts addressed the limitations of orthopedic medicine in treating soft tissue injuries. They concluded that strains and sprains of the musculoskeletal soft tissue not only cause significant pain and impairment, but also are often poorly diagnosed and inadequately managed. Most massage schools have not provided adequate training in the assessment and management of soft tissue injuries, and chiropractors, osteopaths, and physical therapists often have had little or no training in advanced massage techniques for musculoskeletal pain and dysfunction in their degree programs.

Massage and Manual Therapy for Orthopedic Conditions provides a scientific basis for massage and manual resistive techniques and a rational, step-by-step guide to the assessment and management of the most common orthopedic conditions. The therapeutic protocol that is described in this text includes soft tissue mobilization, joint mobilization, and manual resistive techniques.

These techniques are based on 30 years of clinical experience and the latest scientific developments in the management of soft tissue injuries and dysfunction. This book began as a training manual for the 200-hour certification program at the Hendrickson Method Institute in Kensington, California. The techniques have been refined each year for the past 20 years of teaching and have been clinically tested with tens of thousands of patients.

THE THERAPEUTIC CONTRIBUTIONS OF SOFT TISSUE MOBILIZATION

The therapeutic protocols described in this text can provide reproducible results of functional improvement for most orthopedic conditions, including increased range of motion and decreased pain. In line with the modern goals of rehabilitation, these techniques help normalize musculoskeletal function rather than merely provide symptomatic relief.

These techniques are designed to manage conditions related to orthopedics, such as low back pain, neck stiffness and pain, rotator cuff and knee injuries, and many other conditions, such as arthritis, frozen shoulder, and tennis elbow. The techniques are applicable whether the pain or dysfunction is acute or chronic and whether the condition arose from an injury, cumulative stress, or degenerative condition.

These techniques also enhance the performance of dancers and athletes and assist anyone wishing to achieve optimum health. In addition to providing the benefits of traditional massage, such as relaxation and increased circulation, these techniques have several other treatment goals: They dissolve adhesions and lengthen the connective tissue; help to normalize muscle function by reducing hypertonicity in the muscles and strengthening inhibited and weak muscles; normalize the position of the soft tissue and release its torsion; help to restore normal joint function by restoring natural lubrication, range of motion, and normal biomechanics; release entrapped peripheral nerves; and facilitate normal neurological function through reeducation of the nervous system through muscle energy technique (MET), a system of manual therapy that uses active participation of the client.

THE UNIQUE ASPECTS OF HENDRICKSON METHOD

This text introduces a new theoretical model of soft tissue alignment developed by my mentor, Lauren Berry, RPT. Berry was a mechanical engineer and physical therapist who theorized that muscles, tendons, ligaments, and all soft tissues have a normal position relative to the joint that they affect. He taught manipulations in very specific directions, transverse to the line of the fiber, to realign the soft tissue and help normalize the function of the soft tissue and its associated joint.

Massage and Manual Therapy for Orthopedic Conditions also introduces a new style of massage therapy that I developed called *wave mobilization*. This unique style of performing the massage strokes is based on both the science of ergonomics and the practice of tai chi, a Chinese internal martial art. In this book, I describe the ergonomics of giving a treatment, including the functional position of the hand and the resting position of each joint, to teach the therapist how to use his or her body most efficiently. This text also describes the rational basis and provides step-by-step instructions for how to develop and use this internal energy, or "chi," in your massage strokes instead of relying only on muscular effort.

This method is not only an efficient and remarkably effective technique for the management of the majority of orthopedic conditions, it is also deeply relaxing for both the client and the therapist. It allows the therapist to use minimal muscular effort and solves the problem of overuse injuries within the field of massage therapy. The Chinese call this use of minimal effort the "wu wei," the path of effortless effort. For the therapist, the effort of giving a massage is refreshing and energizing, akin to taking a walk. Tai chi emphasizes internal strength, postulating that we can develop our inner life force, or chi, and learn to transmit it to others. It teaches that softness will dissolve hardness. After nearly 30 years of performing soft tissue therapy, I am using dramatically less physical effort in my treatments and achieving more profound results.

This method of therapy is also unique because the treatment can be given through clothing. This has allowed me to provide treatments to a diverse patient population, including Tibetan lamas and elderly patients in third-world countries where it would be inappropriate to have clothing removed for their therapy. Dramatic clinical results can be achieved even across ethnic, cultural, and language barriers.

In addition to describing a new method of massage, this book describes the fundamentals of taking a history and performing an assessment. To gain their rightful place as a member of the health care team, massage therapists must know how to gather objective information, properly assess an injury or dysfunction, determine whether massage is contraindicated, communicate that information to other health-care providers and insurance companies, and know when to refer.

THE DEVELOPMENT OF HENDRICKSON METHOD

The development of this method was influenced by many practitioners over a 30-year period. I began studying massage in 1972 as part of a teacher's training course in yoga and immediately began to appreciate the healing power of touch. In 1974, I completed a year-long training in shiatsu massage with Riuho Yamada, a Zen priest and shiatsu master. Master Yamada's treatments had tremendous power, which I believe resulted not only from his technical skill, but also from his lifelong practice of meditation. I realized that his effectiveness was related not to how hard he worked, but to the way he combined his internal energy with outward movements. This insight has been reinforced throughout my years of training and practice.

In 1976, I participated in an intensive, four-month residential training program in Lomi work. Lomi work was developed by Robert Hall, MD, et al., and synthesizes the work of Ida Rolf (Rolfing), Fritz Perls (Gestalt therapy), and Randolph Stone (polarity therapy). Lifelong postural habits and emotional patterns are often dramatically changed. The deep tissue and shiatsu approaches are limited, however, in treating soft tissue injuries.

The greatest influence in my career came in 1978 when I met Lauren Berry, RPT. By then, Lauren had been a healer for more than 50 years. He began his training with a Finnish doctor who taught him massage and manipulation. As a physical therapist and mechanical engineer, Lauren traveled all over the world studying healing. Lauren had a very pragmatic "nuts-and-bolts" approach. He used manipulation of the soft tissue and joints to correct mechanical dysfunctions in the body. People traveled from all over the country to be treated by this legendary healer. I trained with Lauren for four years. My last year was an apprenticeship, in which I assisted him in treating thousands of people. His work had not been previously documented, and I felt deeply honored when he permitted me to record his method of manipulating the joints. *The Berry Method, Volume I: The Joints* was published in 1981. Unfortunately, Lauren died shortly after completing the first volume, so the planned second volume on soft tissue was never realized.

Lauren's contributions to the treatment of soft tissue injuries were original and invaluable. He theorized that all of the soft tissues in the body have a specific position relative to the neighboring soft tissue and its associated joints and that massage must be applied in specific directions to correct its positional dysfunction. Lauren observed predictable patterns of soft tissue misalignment over the entire body and developed a system of manipulation to correct those dysfunctional positions.

I began a four-year chiropractic training program in 1982, concurrently training massage therapists in methods of advanced soft tissue therapy. Training massage therapists in Lauren's techniques presented me with two challenges. First, much of Lauren's method involved high-speed joint manipulation, which is not within the scope of practice for massage therapists. His techniques also involved quick manipulations of the soft tissue, which is incompatible with a relaxing massage. I realized that my work was to change the joint manipulations into gentle mobilizations and to transform his quick soft tissue manipulations into massage strokes while maintaining their therapeutic effectiveness.

The second challenge was to create a treatment that was as relaxing as it was therapeutic. Lauren's students debated about how hard one needed to work to be effective. Some students believed that a very deep, often painful touch was necessary to be effective, while others believed that a gentle touch was more effective. It was my personal goal to be as gentle as possible without sacrificing therapeutic results.

Over years of clinical practice and teaching, I developed the concept of "interfascicular torsion" to describe the microscopic adhesions and abnormal twists that I could feel with my hands. I observed that these torsional dysfunctions in the soft tissue were winding the body into abnormal spirals, and I developed techniques to unwind these segments.

As I developed my techniques for working on the spine, I placed my patients in a side-lying fetal position. This position was comfortable even for the patient with acute low back pain and it also allowed me to stand upright during the treatment rather than leaning over the table. As tai chi teaches that water will dissolve stone, I began experimenting with a rounded, wavelike stroke, transverse to the fiber. I also applied the principles of tai chi and moved my whole body into each stroke and practiced keeping my body relaxed and supple. Rocking my patients in rhythmic oscillations created subtle wavelike movements in the patient's entire body. These rocking movements had a quieting and calming effect. I began to explore different frequencies of applying the wave mobilization strokes and found that performing the strokes to the rhythm of the resting heartbeat, about 60 cycles per minute, had the most profound effect on the nervous system. I realized that this is the same rhythm that each of us felt as developing babies in our mother's womb from our mother's heartbeat. As I was performing these rhythmic oscillations, I too became more relaxed internally and began to notice an expansion of my own energy field. The therapy that I was giving became a method to develop my own internal energy.

My chiropractic education emphasized the role of the nervous system in both health and dysfunction or injury and focused on the vast reflex connections between the soft tissue, joints, and central nervous system. I also gained an appreciation of the profound neurophysiological effects of mobilization of the spine and joints of the extremities. As I began to incorporate joint mobilization techniques into my soft tissue work, I achieved better results with less effort. These were not the high-speed, low-amplitude thrusting techniques associated with the chiropractic adjustment; rather, they were techniques that involved gentle, rhythmic, oscillating movements of the joints.

Moving the joint while massaging the surrounding soft tissue has several effects: It helps to reduce hypertonicity in the muscles; it helps to normalize joint function by stimulating the normal lubrication of the synovial membrane, articular cartilage, and discs within the joint; it helps in pain management by stimulating the mechanoreceptors; and it creates a profound relaxation response.

My work has also been influenced by the insights of James Cyriax, MD, the modern developer of transverse friction massage. Cyriax's work has many parallels with Berry's, as both approaches work transverse to the line of the fiber. Cyriax theorized that brisk, transverse strokes at sites of injury restore the normal parallel alignment of the collagen fibers, which can become distorted after an injury. He focused his soft tissue therapy on critical junction sites, that is, where a muscle interweaves with its tendon (myotendinous junction), where the tendon interweaves with the periosteum of the bone (tenoperiosteal junction), and at the attachment sites of ligaments, but he did not address the function of the entire soft tissue complex. For example, transverse massage techniques on a lesion in the supraspinatus help to resolve that lesion but do not address postural distortions, muscle weakness or hypertonicity, and positional dysfunctions in the neighboring soft tissue. I incorporate some of Cyriax's friction techniques but in a unique style by mobilizing the associated joint with the friction strokes, which dramatically reduces the discomfort associated with transverse friction massage.

Another tremendous influence in the evolution of my work came from Vladimir Janda, MD, and Karel Lewit, MD, two physicians from the Czech Republic. These remarkable pioneers in manual therapy have made major contributions to the assessment and treatment of soft tissue injury and dysfunction. Janda discovered predictable patterns of muscle dysfunction, in which some muscles become weak and inhibited and others become short and tight in response to pain or joint dysfunction. Lewit and Janda also developed methods of treatment in the tradition of proprioceptive neuromuscular facilitation (PNF), which requires the client's resistance to pressures applied by the therapist. Some texts, including this one, call these techniques muscle energy techniques (MET). I have incorporated Janda's insights into each chapter, and I use MET within the massage session to reduce muscle hypertonicity, facilitate or strengthen weak or inhibited muscles, reeducate muscles in their normal firing patterns, help to normalize joint function, and help to restore normal neurological function. MET can change chronic pain patterns and has proved extremely effective clinically.

Revelations have also come from my study of healing with Muriel Chapman, DO, and Rosalyn Bruyere. I learned from each that gentle touch itself is healing. I noticed in my clinical practice that with patients who are in severe pain, effective clinical results could be achieved even if I used very light pressure. I have come to realize that one of the most important goals of the therapist in the clinical setting is to create an experience with touch in which the client feels completely safe and completely comfortable. This induces a state of relaxation and trust in the client that not only allows for the healing of the physical pain, but also provides an environment for the healing of the emotional and psychological components.

The method of treatment that I describe in this text is intended to be a nurturing experience for both the therapist and the client. One of the hallmarks of this method is that the client should be able to completely relax into the massage strokes. In the healthy individual, all of the massage strokes described in this text should feel comfortable to receive. If the massage stroke is painful, it indicates that the area is injured or dysfunctional and requires that the therapist adjust the pressure of the massage strokes to ensure the client's comfort.

Each session is also an opportunity for the therapist to create an environment of kindness for the client. It is important to realize that anyone who is experiencing pain or dysfunction is emotionally vulnerable, perhaps worried, depressed, or anxious. Whether the client is out of shape, noncompliant, or irritable, the therapist should aspire to be nonjudgmental. The massage session gives us an opportunity to practice loving kindness. There is no greater calling.

ORGANIZATION AND FEATURES

The book is divided into four sections. The first section should be read before performing the massage techniques described in the other sections. The first section has two chapters. Chapter 1 describes the scientific and theoretical foundations for treatment. It reviews the fundamentals of neuromusculoskeletal anatomy, describing the structure and function of all the soft tissues in the body, the mechanics of dysfunction and injury, the mechanical and neurological consequences of these dysfunctions and injuries, and, finally, how this information can guide the therapist in the most effective therapy.

Chapter 2 is divided into two parts. The first part provides an overview of clinical assessment, including taking a history and how to perform a fundamental orthopedic examination. The process of performing an objective examination is given in detail, including the assessment of active and passive range of motion, isometric testing, special tests, and palpation. This is followed by a summary of examination findings for the most common categories of orthopedic dysfunctions and injuries.

The second part of Chapter 2 is an overview of the techniques used in this book. The essential massage stroke, called *wave mobilization*, is described in detail, and exercises are provided to practice this stroke on a client or fellow student. A description of MET follows. The neurological basis of MET is described, as are exercises to practice the six different styles of MET used in this text. The third modality of treatment, joint mobilization, is described next. A summary of the clinical effects of soft tissue mobilization, joint mobilization, and MET are described. Finally, guidelines for the treatment of clients in acute or chronic pain are described in detail, as well as contraindications for massage therapy and when to refer your client to another provider.

The next sections of the book are divided into eight chapters and describe specific techniques for particular regions of the body. Each chapter provides an overview of the anatomy of the region, the structure and function of all the soft tissues, the most common orthopedic injuries and dysfunctions, and the protocol for the treatment of each of these conditions. Each chapter also describes a basic assessment of the region for the massage therapist and provides a step-by step guide for how to perform the massage strokes, MET and joint mobilization for that area of the body. The strokes are divided into Level I and Level II. Level I strokes are massage strokes that can be performed on anyone, whether the client is symptomatic or not. These strokes bring the area to its highest level of functioning. Level II strokes are used as needed to supplement Level I strokes if pain or dysfunction is present in the region. They are typically deeper strokes and often work on sensitive attachment points, which is unnecessary for most clients.

Each technique chapter has a variety of features that were specifically designed to enhance the reader's learning experience:

- The easy-to-reference bulleted format allows students to "keep their place" in the text and encourages students to practice the techniques with a partner as they read.

- Muscle anatomy and kinesiology are organized into tables for easy reference.

- Consistent organization reinforces basic concepts and fosters retention of fundamental information. For example, anatomy sections are divided into *structure, function, dysfunction and injury,* and *treatment implications* subsections. Similarly, muscle energy technique sections are divided into *intention, position,* and *action* subsections.

- A "Caution" icon (**!**) highlights contraindi-cations and precautions that the massage therapist should be aware of before performing a particular technique.

- The Study Guide section at the end of each chapter lists concepts and objectives that the reader should master for both the Level I and Level II techniques.

- References and Suggested Readings point the reader to articles and books that provide more information about anatomy, kinesiology, assessment, and the science of injury and repair.

- Clinical examples describing the assessment and management of an orthopedic condition using an actual patient are included in each technique section.

HOW TO USE THIS BOOK

It is essential that the student read Chapters 1 and 2 first and practice the exercises described in Chapter 2 before attempting the techniques described in Chapters 3–10. In the training program at the Hendrickson Method Institute, the MET and Level I strokes are learned in the first semester, and the assessment and Level II strokes are learned in the second semester. The MET is listed in the section before the massage strokes for convenience and easy reference, but in clinical practice, the MET and massage strokes are interspersed throughout the massage session. The massage strokes are described very precisely and in a specific sequence. The student is encouraged to "follow the recipe" exactly as it is described. It is natural to feel insecure when you are learning something new. Be patient and kind with yourself. As you master the techniques over time, you will naturally create your own unique style of performing this method. It is akin to learning to play the guitar. First, learn the exact way to form the chords and the sequence of how the chords change in familiar songs. Then use these skills to create your own music. Enjoy the rewards of learning something new, and have faith that with dedication and practice, you will help relieve the suffering of all whom you touch.

Feedback from clinicians, students, or schools with constructive ideas about how to improve this text is appreciated. For instructional DVDs and information regarding training programs in Hendrickson Method, go to www.hendricksonmethod.com.

Thomas Hendrickson, DC
Hendrickson Method Institute
388 Colusa Circle
Kensington, CA 94707
Online at www.hendricksonmethod.com
E-mail: school@hendricksonmethod.com
Phone: (510) 524-3107
Fax: (510) 524-8242

strokes are divided into Level I and Level II. Level I strokes are massage strokes that can be performed on anyone, whether the client is symptomatic or not. ...-tic strokes bring the area to its highest level of functioning. Level II strokes are used as needed to supplement Level I strokes if pain or dysfunction is prevalent in the region. They are typically deeper strokes that often work on sensitive attachment points. It is unnecessary for most clients.

Each technique chapter has a variety of features that were specifically designed to enhance the reader's learning experience.

The easy-to-reference build...

Acknowledgments

I am very grateful to the students and teaching staff at the Hendrickson Method Institute (formerly Institute of Orthopedic Massage) who have helped to craft this text for nearly 28 years. During the 200-hour training sessions offered each year at the Institute, they have carefully read the text year after year and made thoughtful suggestions about how to best describe and teach these techniques. In the preparation of the second edition, I would especially like to thank Jennifer Lane and Candace Palmerlee. Jennifer edited my revisions with meticulous attention and offered many helpful suggestions. Candace carefully reviewed the technique section and helped to clarify the instructions. I would also like to thank Rachel McMullin for running the Hendrickson Method Institute with great skill and ease and Claudia Moore for managing my clinic with such grace and good humor.

I would also like to thank my managing editor Laura Horowitz, whose careful attention to every detail I greatly appreciated; Lippincott Williams & Wilkins, especially Andrea Klinger and Jennifer Clements; the copyeditor Barbara Willette; and Kim Battista for her beautiful illustrations.

I owe many thanks to my angel Margaret, for teaching me about service to those in need and for being a sanctuary of love, and to Luke for expanding my faith in healing.

Finally, this book would never have been created if not for the inspiration and teaching of my mentor, Lauren Berry, RPT.

Contents

The Theory and Science of Massage and Manual Therapy

Part One: General Overview

This first part provides a brief summary of the key concepts in the first two chapters. This will allow the reader to have an overview of the theory, science, and rationale for treatment before reading the more detailed material that follows.

MUSCULOSKELETAL COMPLAINTS ARE DUE TO FUNCTIONAL PROBLEMS

Musculoskeletal complaints are the most common reason for patients to visit primary care physicians and emergency departments in the United States and account for 10% to 28% of all primary care visits.[1] These conditions become "the most common cause of disability and severe long-term pain in the industrialized world".[2] The vast majority of these complaints are due not to pathology and disease, but to soft tissue injuries and functional problems. Yet, according to the American Academy of Orthopedic Surgeons, soft tissue injuries are often poorly diagnosed and inadequately managed.[3] The premise of manual therapy and massage is that loss of mobility in the soft tissue and joints creates pain and disability, and *restoration of mobility becomes the primary treatment objective.*[4]

SCIENTIFICALLY BASED PRACTICE IS ESSENTIAL FOR OPTIMUM TREATMENT

To provide the most effective treatment for our client's condition requires an understanding of normal musculoskeletal structure and function, the science of injury and repair, and the scientific basis for each technique. The therapist needs to understand the rationale for the choice of technique to create specific treatment goals that match the client's condition. The intention of treatment is to promote optimum function rather than merely to reduce symptoms.

MUSCULOSKELETAL TISSUE IS HIGHLY RESPONSIVE TO STIMULI

Research has shown that musculoskeletal tissues, including muscles, tendons, ligaments, bone, and cartilage are highly responsive to mechanical stimuli.[5] The body's tissues are "adaptable", that is, they change in response to stimulus (or lack of stimulus), and every structure in the body can improve its structure and function if given the proper stimulus.[6] Even older clients with chronic conditions can experience functional improvement because the body still contains cells (undifferentiated mesenchymal cells) that will respond to appropriate stimuli by "migrating, proliferating, and differentiating into mature cells of bone, cartilage, and dense fibrous tissue . . . including chondrocytes (cartilage cells)".[7] This is very good news for "touch" therapists because we can stimulate profound changes in the body with the appropriate treatment.

A NEW PARADIGM IN SOFT TISSUE THERAPY

The current model or paradigm in biology and medicine, which has been dominant for over 100 years and holds that the body is regulated by biochemistry, is the "lock-and-key" model, according to which molecules move randomly throughout the body to find the right receptor site. An exciting new electromagnetic paradigm is emerging that holds that these biochemical process are controlled by electromagnetic forces.[8] Research has shown that molecular and intermolecular forces are electromagnetic. Every heartbeat, muscle contraction, gland secretion, bodily movement, thought, and emotion generates an electromagnetic signal. It has also been discovered that the human body radiates a potent electromagnetic field that extends 12 to 15 feet beyond the body, and a new hypothesis is that this field can be focused for healing.[9] This has profound implications for manual therapy because touch transmits a focused electromagnetic signal that is carried throughout the entire body. This electromagnetic signal influences cellular regulation, including repair and regeneration.

FOUNDATIONS OF THE ELECTROMAGNETIC PARADIGM

TENSEGRITY

From an architectural perspective, the body is called a *tensegrity structure* because it is a continuous, interconnected system of connective tissue and muscles that provides the force that holds the body upright, rather than the bones. Buckminster Fuller[10] coined the word *tensegrity* to describe this type of structure. Recent research has discovered a class of molecules called integrins, connecting every cell to neighboring cells and to the connective tissue throughout the body.[11] The cytoskeleton and extracellular connective tissue matrix combined with water is what Oschman calls the "living matrix."[9] The living matrix is not only structurally continuous, but also energetically continuous, as it regulates growth, form, and repair and regeneration. The connective tissue network is considered a second "nervous system" because of its ability to communicate electromechanical and electromagnetic signals.

WATER CARRIES ELECTROMAGNETIC WAVES

Water surrounds every molecule in the body and provides the energetic and structural framework for the body. Water holds the molecules of the body together. It forms an essential part of the "second nervous system," transmitting energy throughout the body. The conductivity of any tissue is highly dependent on its water content.[12] Indeed, there are 15,000 molecules of water for every molecule of protein.[9] Like protein molecules, water is highly ordered and exhibits coherence, much like a laser, in which water in the body becomes coupled to carry the electromagnetic waves. Because water is polar molecule, it greatly increases electromagnetic conductivity in the transmission of energy throughout the body.

SOFT TISSUE IS A LIQUID CRYSTAL

Soft tissue may be described as a liquid crystal, that is, a material that is a combination of a liquid and a solid. Soft tissue is composed of regularly arranged, parallel protein fibers, mostly collagen, embedded in water. Cell membranes, ligaments, tendons, muscles, bones, nerve, and the filaments that provide structure to the cells (cytoskeleton) are all crystalline lattices, meaning that the water and protein molecules are in a regularly ordered, repeating pattern. The collagen and the water are polar molecules, similar to a magnet with a north and a south pole. Because the soft tissue is electrically charged and has a tremendous degree of structural order, there is a coupling between molecules that gives them the ability to vibrate together, called *coherence*. Research has shown that these electrically polarized molecular arrays are extremely sensitive to energy fields, acting like molecular antennae, sending and receiving signals.[9,12] The new paradigm suggests that every movement, every touch, every thought and feeling is transmitted to every cell in the body at the speed of light.

MECHANOTRANSDUCTION

Mechanotransduction is a property of the soft tissue by which cells and the extracellular matrix (fibers and ground substance) convert mechanical stimuli into chemical, electrical, and electromagnetic signals. The tensions and compressions of massage and manual therapy induce mechanical signals that are transformed into electromagnetic waves, stimulating all cellular functions, including repair and regeneration.[13]

PIEZOELECTRICITY

One form of mechanotransduction is piezoelectricity ("pressure electricity"), the phenomenon in which soft tissue converts mechanical energy into electrical energy. Massage and manual therapy compress and stretch the soft tissue, creating waves of mechanical vibration that are transformed into electric currents. By their very nature, electric currents create magnetic fields. Because of the structural order or coherence of the soft tissue, these electromagnetic forces cause the molecules to vibrate together, hypothetically transmitting the energy of touch to every cell in the body.

OVERVIEW OF SOFT TISSUE INJURY AND REPAIR

Soft tissue includes muscles, tendons, ligaments, joint capsules, cartilage, bursa, skin, and fascia, as well as the body's fluids, including blood, lymph, synovial fluid, cerebrospinal fluid, cellular water, and interstitial fluids (the fluids surrounding the cells). These tissues may be broadly divided into fibers and fluids (see Part Two). Most of the fibers consist of parallel fibers of collagen, wrapped in bundles called *fascicles*. These fibers and fascicles are able to slide freely relative to each other in the healthy state. The body's fluids are a medium for the transport of cells, oxygen, and nutrition and for the removal of waste. After injury or repetitive strain, the fibers are pulled apart (torn). Tissue disruption creates inflammation, swelling, and congestion of fluids. Swelling increases pressure in the tissue, not only causing pain, but also decreasing movement of cells, nutrition, and oxygen needed for repair. Repair of the injury starts immediately. If the area is not mobilized in the early stages of healing, the body lays down a random mesh of fibers that develop into thick adhesions, leading to loss of motion and degeneration of the soft tissue. *Therefore, early mobilization of the soft tissue and joints is now recommended immediately after injury.*[14] Chronic musculoskeletal complaints are characterized by loss of normal motion due to adhesions of the fibers, myofascial shortening, restricted joint motion, joint misalignment, and potential degeneration. Massage and manual therapy induce normal movement in the soft tissue and joints to reduce adhesions, lengthen myofascia, and mobilize joints.

ACUTE AND CHRONIC COMPLAINTS: INJURY AND DYSFUNCTION

Musculoskeletal complaints can be divided into two broad categories: acute/injury and chronic/dysfunction. These are artificial categories, used to distinguish between inflammatory and noninflammatory conditions. In clinical practice, musculoskeletal complaints manifest on a wide spectrum between acute/inflammatory and chronic/noninflammatory in their stage of healing. This topic is discussed fully in Chapter 2. Throughout the text, the terms *acute* and *injury* will be used to describe an inflammatory condition. Inflammation may manifest with the classic signs of redness, heat, and pain, but it may also manifest subclinically with the only sign being pain at rest. The term **injury** may apply to a specific traumatic event to healthy tissue, such as a sports injury, household accident, or motor vehicle accident, or may apply to the result of a cumulative or repetitive stress in which the tissue eventually fatigues and weakens, resulting in an acute onset of inflammation, such as carpal tunnel syndrome from keyboard work, tennis elbow, or foot pain in runners. Injury to the soft tissue includes the sprains and strains of ligaments and muscles and means that the tissue is disrupted (torn), even if microscopically, resulting in swelling and pain.

The term **dysfunction** implies a chronic condition and indicates that the body is not functioning normally. The client might or might not be in pain. Loss of normal function may be due to prior injury, emotional and psychological stress, or faulty posture. It is characterized by limited joint motion, muscular weakness, sustained muscle tightness, adhesions, and shortened tissue. Examples of dysfunction include inability to elevate the arm overhead, a limp, chronic low back stiffness, chronic neck tension, and poor posture.

CHARACTERISTICS OF SOFT TISSUE INJURY

- **Pain:** Injury creates pain from damaged tissue, swelling, and inflammatory chemicals.

- **Swelling:** Injury creates swelling, which decreases the normal movement of fluids. Swelling reduces the tissue's ability to repair itself, owing to decreased cellular activity, decreased nutrition, and the accumulation of waste products.

- **Neurological dysfunction:** A vast network of nerves is embedded within the soft tissue and joints. Swelling from inflammation creates abnormal function in the nerves, leading to muscular inhibition (weakness) or spasms (guarding, splinting) and decreased coordination, balance, and muscular control.

- **Fibers lose parallel alignment:** Injury of the soft tissue on the microscopic level is a tearing apart of the fibers. The fibers are repaired in a random orientation and lose their normal parallel orientation.

- **Soft tissue misalignment:** Injury creates soft tissue misalignment relative to the neighboring soft tissue and joint (see "Soft Tissue Alignment Theory" below). This introduces an abnormal twist into the tissue and an abnormal position of the tissue.

- **Restricted joint motion:** Injury may involve soft tissue surrounding the joint, such as ligaments and joint capsules, or soft tissue within the joint itself, including the cartilage. Swelling, pain, and muscle spasms prevent normal movement, reducing joint lubrication and nutrition, which are dependent on movement.

- **Emotional distress:** Injury leads to pain that affects the emotional centers of the brain (limbic region). Pain is both a physical and an emotional experience. Depression, anxiety, and fear are common emotions associated with pain.

- **Biomagnetic field disturbance:** Electronic signaling depends on the organized structure of the system.[15] In acute injuries, the normal parallel alignment of the fibers is disrupted, which decreases the ability of the tissue to carry an electromagnetic signal, disturbing normal cellular communication. With the excessive water due to swelling, there is a decrease in the electronic transmission.

CHARACTERISTICS OF SOFT TISSUE DYSFUNCTION

▪ **Soft tissue misalignment:** Soft tissue dysfunction creates misalignment relative to the neighboring soft tissue or joint.

▪ **Soft tissue torsion:** Misaligned soft tissue introduces an abnormal torsion or twist into the tissue. The abnormal twist decreases the water content of the tissue, leading to adhesions and abnormal function in the soft tissue and associated joint.

▪ **Adhesions:** Abnormal crosslinks may develop between the fibers, creating adhesions. Adhesions develop if the soft tissue and joints were not adequately mobilized after an injury, if the area adapted to the shortened position to avoid pain, or because of poor posture. The fibers stick together, losing their ability to glide. This limits normal extensibility (length) in the tissue and creates dysfunction in the muscles, joints, and nerves. Adhesions also prevent the normal broadening of the muscle fibers that occurs during muscle contraction, decreasing their function.

▪ **Fluid stagnation:** Sustained muscle contraction and adhesions in chronic dysfunction create fluid stagnation, disrupting the rhythmic waves of fluids that normally circulate through every region of the body. Stagnation causes decreased cellular activity, decreased nutrition, and the accumulation of waste products, reducing the tissue's ability to function normally and slowing down the body's constant cellular regeneration.

▪ **Neurological dysfunction:** Adhesions and fluid stagnation create abnormal neurological function, leading to muscle hypertonicity or inhibition and loss of coordination, balance, and postural stability.

▪ **Altered muscle performance:** Optimum function in the body for good posture and movement requires that the muscles crossing the joints are balanced in strength, extensibility (length), and normal neurological function. This is necessary for fine motor control, balance, and coordination. Dysfunction leads to patterns of sustained hypertonicity or sustained weakness (inhibition) in the muscles.

▪ **Joint restrictions and misalignment:** Loss of normal joint mobility is due to internal or external restrictions. Internal restrictions may be due to loss of glide between the joint surfaces. This is called *loss of joint play*. External restrictions may be due to shortened or tightened tissue surrounding the joint, such as adhesions in the ligaments and joint capsule or short and tight muscles. Joint restrictions and misalignment lead to impaired movement.

▪ **Emotional and psychological distress:** Clients in chronic pain are often afraid of moving, a condition called *pain avoidance behavior*, which leads to disuse, deconditioning, and abnormal function in the muscles and joints, predisposing the area to degeneration.

▪ **Biomagnetic disturbance:** In chronic conditions, the tissue becomes dehydrated because of the increased fiber content of the adhesions, which conduct electrical charge very poorly, owing to the decreased water content.[15]

THREE TREATMENT MODALITIES

This text introduces a unique combination of three modalities, performed in a specific protocol or "recipe" that has been found in 30 years of clinical practice to achieve the most efficient and effective success in the treatment of soft tissue conditions. How to apply these modalities varies dramatically depending on many factors, such as whether the client has an acute or chronic condition and the client's age, conditioning, and level of pain. The goal of massage and manual therapy is to provide the appropriate treatment specific to the client's condition to optimize the body's own healing potential. The underlying goal of this method of therapy is to induce profound relaxation while performing the techniques. This has been found to optimize the healing potential of the body and create the most successful outcome. The three modalities are as follows:

▪ **Soft tissue mobilization (STM):** This text introduces a new style of massage (soft tissue mobilization) called *wave mobilization*, which mobilizes the soft tissue transverse to the fiber in a rounded, scooping motion. These strokes are performed rhythmically and are modeled on ocean waves.

▪ **Muscle energy technique (MET):** MET is a method of manual therapy in which the client provides active resistance to the therapist's pressure. This technique provides rehabilitation for the nervous system.

▪ **Joint mobilization (JM):** The joints are the source of most of the pain and disability in chronic conditions. Passive movement induced to the joints helps to ensure their optimum function.

FOUR DIMENSIONS OF TREATMENT

The goal of massage and manual therapy is to induce change in the structure and function of the musculoskeletal soft tissue to promote optimum function and healing of the whole person. The goals of treatment can be artificially divided into four categories that are based on which dimension of the client we are primarily affecting: **structural, neurological, psychological** and **emotional**, and **energetic**.[16]

TREATMENT GOALS: STRUCTURAL

- **Mobility:** The loss of mobility applies to the fluids, muscles, tendons, joint capsules and ligaments, and joints. In **acute** injuries the loss of mobility is due to swelling, pain, and muscular guarding. *Our treatment goal in acute conditons is to assist repair and regeneration of the soft tissue by inducing movement in the fluids and fibers.* In **chronic** dysfunction, the loss of normal mobility may be due to adhesions, tight muscles, or degenerated joints. This loss of mobility leads to alterations of normal movement, compensations in related joints, and pain avoidance behavior. *Our treatment goals in chronic conditions are to restore mobility in the soft tissue and to restore normal range of motion in the joints.*

- **Alignment:** Injury pulls apart (tears) the collagen fibers and disrupts their normal parallel alignment. The collagen fibers are repaired in a random weave. Loss of parallel alignment not only weakens the tissue, but also decreases the electrical charge in the tissue.[9] In **acute** conditions, misalignment may also develop macroscopically in the muscles, tendons, and ligaments because of swelling, pain, and muscular guarding. *Our treament goals in acute conditons are to help align the healing fibers, realign the soft tissue crossing the joint, and provide passive motion to the joint to help maintain normal alignment.* In **chronic** conditions, misalignment describes an abnormal torsion or twist in the soft tissue and faulty alignment of the soft tissue relative to the surrounding soft tissue structures and the joint. Misalignment may be due to adhesions from prior injury, cumulative strain, poor posture, muscular imbalances, or abnormal movement patterns. *Our treament goals are to educate the client in good posture, dissolve adhesions, balance muscular forces, and mobilize restricted joints.*

- **Extensibility (length):** In **chronic** conditions, clients may complain of stiffness, loss of motion, slumped posture, or chronic pain. Over time, the body will adapt to limited motion by developing contractures; short, tight muscles; and loss of normal joint motion. *Our treatment goal is to lengthen shortened tissue.* It is contraindicated to stretch or lengthen tissue in the acute phase of repair, because the fibers are fragile and easily torn.

TREATMENT GOALS: NEUROLOGICAL

- **Neuromuscular reeducation:** The initial response of muscle to **acute** injury is either spasm or muscular inhibition. The spasms can protect the muscle and joint by preventing further movement, but they also prevent normal movement of the fluids and joint, limiting repair. Over time, swelling and pain inhibit and weaken muscles. *The treatment goals in acute conditions are to reduce muscular spasms, and minimize muscular inhibition.* In **chronic** dysfunction, muscles develop predictable patterns of muscular tightness or muscular weakness (inhibition). *The goals of treatment in chronic conditions are to identify which muscles are tight and which are weak through isometric testing and to correct those muscular dysfunctions.*

- **Proprioception reeducation:** Sensory nerves provide information about position and movement, and their normal function is essential for balance, coordination, posture, and fine motor control. The swelling of an **acute** condition prevents normal proprioception. *The treatment goal in acute conditions is to provide active stimulation to these nerves though muscle energy technique to help maintain optimum function.* **Chronic** dysfunction leads to an atrophy of sensory nerves and a decreased sense of balance, coordination, and fine muscle control. *The treatment goals in chronic conditions are to educate the client in balance exercises and posture and to use MET to bring conscious awareness to muscle action, providing effective rehabilitation for the proprioceptors.*

- **Sensory awareness:** This goal is for **chronic** conditions. Chronic pain and dysfunction often lead to the inability of the clients to feel if they are tight or weak or how to contract specific muscles. Bringing the client's attention to these areas through touch and conscious contraction (MET) reeducates the client's sensory awareness.

- **Pain management:** Pain information is conducted into the brain through a "gate." For example, the nerves that carry mechanoreceptor information about pressure and movement "close the gate," reducing pain. Compressing the tissue during massage and mobilizing the joint through rhythmic oscillations will help to reduce pain. *In acute conditions, the therapist can reduce pain by applying gentle touch, slow rocking movements of the body, gentle MET, and mobilization to the soft tissue and joints.* In chronic dysfunction, pain can develop from degeneration, sustained muscle contration leading to ischemia (low oxygen), or abnormal function of the nervous system. The goals of treatment are to reduce muscle contraction by reeducating the muscles, improve joint function by restoring lubrication and nutrition to the cartilage, and reeducate the nervous system by reducing aberrant nerve signals.

- **Relaxation:** A primary goal of therapy is relaxation. Relaxation engages the parasympathetic nervous system, lowering blood pressure and heart rate, and promotes repair and rejuvenation in the body. *The goal of treatment described in this text for both acute and chronic conditions is to bring the client into a state of profound relaxation* while the other goals of therapy are being accomplished. This is achieved by gentle touch and rhythmic rocking, which engages both the central and parasympathetic nervous systems.

TREATMENT GOALS: PSYCHOLOGICAL, EMOTIONAL

It is important for the therapist to remember that the painful knee or frozen shoulder is one small part of a human being. A client's injury and pain lead to negative thoughts, such as "I'm always going to be in pain," which can lead to anxiety, depression, or irritability. In chronic conditions, pain or disability often leads to pain avoidance behavior, in which the person limits activities and movements. Negative thinking, such as "my life is ruined," and negative emotions, such as depression, can develop. Our role as therapists is to encourage the client to become proactive in taking responsibility for their rehabilitation and to help create an image of healing. Our touch can provide comfort and emotional support.

- **Healing words:** It is important for the therapist to create a mental image of healing for the client through healing words. An important aspect of therapy is to give positive feedback while working with a client. For example, when a tight musle relaxes, say to the client, "Your body is responding beautifully." When better range of motion is achieved in a restricted knee, say to the client, "Your knee is really moving better." Encourage chronic pain patients by telling them that recovery takes a long

time, to be patient, and just try to move a little bit more each week. When they show slight improvement or try to move a little more, praise their efforts.

- **Nurturing touch:** A gentle, nurturing touch decreases blood pressure, decreases stress, and improves mood. One of the hallmarks of the therapy that is described in this text is that the therapist attempts to provide comfort during treatment. Working deeply does not mean working hard. Deep touch can be achieved with gentle hands and sensitivity.

TREATMENT GOALS: ENERGETIC

- **Induce electrical flow:** Areas of injury or dysfunction have disruptions in normal electrical signaling due to swelling or adhesions. Massage and manual therapy create currents of electricity (streaming potentials) by the phenomenon of piezoelectricity (see "Piezoelectricity" above). These currents are generated from the pressure of touch, from stretching and the contractions of soft tissue during MET.

- **Improve vitality:** Injury and dysfunction create loss of mobility, which leads to stasis or sluggishness in the body. Movement induces electromagnetic waves, which improve cellular communication, cellular synthesis, and energy.

- **Create inner calmness (coherence):** Therapists can be trained to establish a state of coherence within themselves before working with their client by taking a few minutes to focus on the breath or to practice prayer, meditation, or other centering practices. The therapist can entrain (couple) the client to this inner calmness.

- **Healing:** Medical research has shown that the pulsing magnetic fields that emanate from the hands of therapists (biomagnetic fields) stimulate healing. It has also been demonstrated that this biomagnetic field can be focused for healing.

Part Two: Overview of Theory and Technique

BODY COMPOSITION: MAINLY FIBERS AND FLUIDS

The soft tissues are mainly composed of fibers and fluids; even the bones are mineralized fibers. These

fibers give the body its form and are akin to the steel cables that hold up a bridge. They provide the tension to keep the body upright and transmit the forces that create movement. Most of the fibers run parallel to each other and are arranged in a spiral at both the microscopic and macroscopic levels. A hypothesis that is developed in this text is that the spiral orientation of the fibers has a specific direction for each joint and that the normal spiral can wind into an abnormal torsion or twist.

The human body is approximately 70% water, which is contained in the fluids of the body. These fluids include the blood, lymph, synovial fluid, cerebrospinal fluid, and interstitial fluids (the fluids that surround the cells). Like the earth's oceans, water moves within the body in waves. This is due to the rhythmic contractions of the heart, respiratory diaphragm, and muscles, which form the three pumps that move the fluids through the body. There are also waves of electromagnetic energy moving throughout the body from the heartbeat, muscle contraction, compression of the bones, and other cellular functions. Unlike fluid waves, which lose strength as they travel, the waves of electromagnetic energy are propagated throughout the body because collagen and water are an "excitable medium," which means that they are a source of energy to carry the waves of energy.[9]

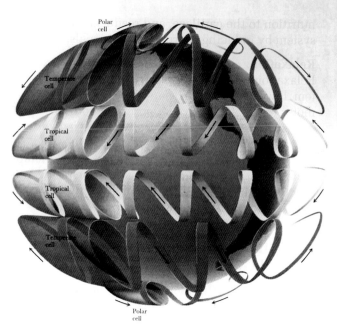

Figure 1-2. Spiraling circulation patterns of the air currents of the earth's atmosphere. (Reprinted with permission from Kaufman W. Universe, 3rd ed. New York: WH Freeman, 1991.)

SPIRALS, WAVES, AND THE HUMAN BODY

We live in a spiral universe. Our local galaxy, the Milky Way, forms a spiral (Fig. 1-1). The spiral is a fundamental shape in the movement of air currents over the surface of the earth (Fig. 1-2). Water, which covers 70% of the earth's surface, moves in a spiral

pattern, not only as it snakes its way across the land, but also as it spirals internally in the form of secondary currents within the moving water (Fig. 1-3).

The spiral is also an essential pattern in the body and is present at many levels. Tendons, ligaments, joint capsules, and the fascia of muscles are composed of parallel fibers of collagen, which resemble the spiral weave of a rope. Each collagen molecule is a triple helix spiral (Fig. 1-4). Visually, the gross structure of a tendon is also a spiral (Fig. 1-5).

Many muscles such as the teres major, latissimus dorsi, pectoralis major, and levator scapula, form a spiral twist from origin to insertion (Fig. 1-6). Muscles are composed of parallel fibers organized in spirals. Actin and myosin are the two basic contractile proteins that

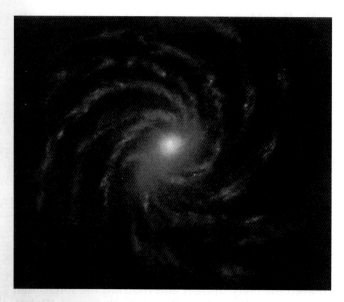

Figure 1-1. The galaxy we live in has a spiral shape. (Reprinted with permission from Kaufman W. Universe, 3rd ed. New York: WH Freeman, 1991.)

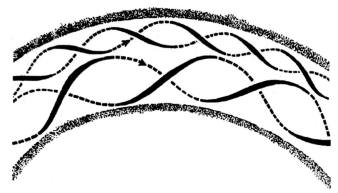

Figure 1-3. Spiraling movements within moving water. (Reprinted with permission from Schwenk T. Sensitive Chaos. New York: Schocken Books, 1976.)

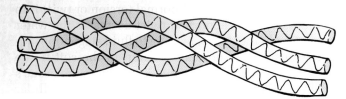

Figure 1-4. Triple helix spiral structure of collagen.

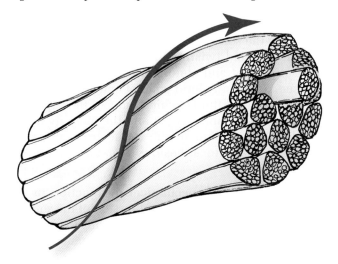

Figure 1-5. Arrangement of collagen fibers in a tendon shows its spiral orientation.

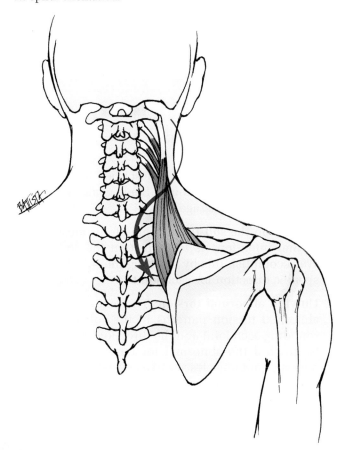

Figure 1-6. Levator scapula muscle shows the spiral orientation of the muscle from its origin to its insertion.

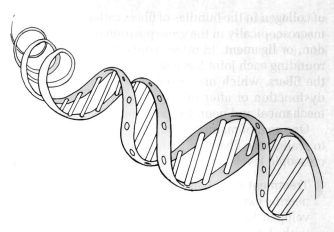

Figure 1-7. Spiral structure of DNA.

compose the functional unit of muscle contraction and form the myofibrils (literally, "muscle threads"), which are woven together in a spiral like a rope.[6] Each actin filament is a double helix that is composed of two strands that spiral around each other during muscle contraction, and myosin contains globular heads that are arranged in a spiral. DNA, the code of instructions for cellular reproduction, is also a double helix spiral (Fig. 1-7). The advantage of the spiral weave of soft tissue is that it increases the ability of the tissue to withstand stress. The twist pulls the fibers together, "preloading" the soft tissue by creating tension at the attachment points.[17] This allows the structure to withstand greater pulling forces (tensile loads).

SOFT TISSUE ALIGNMENT THEORY

This book introduces a new theoretical model of massage therapy: *Muscles, tendons, and ligaments have a normal position or alignment relative to the neighboring soft tissue and to the joint that they affect.* The author's mentor, Lauren Berry, RPT, a physical therapist and mechanical engineer, introduced this concept and also theorized that dysfunction and injury to a joint create abnormal positions or misalignment in the soft tissue surrounding the joint. The soft tissues are like guy wires holding up a tower. The bones represent the tower. In normal function, the guy wires are balanced in length and strength. Injury and dysfunction create abnormal positions for the guy wires and place excessive tension on some of the guy wires while others are slack and not functioning properly. This is analogous to joint dysfunction in which some muscles become too tight while others become too weak.

Berry's model hypothesizes that these soft tissues become misaligned and twisted. This misalignment occurs microscopically in the normal spiral alignment of collagen in the bundles of fibers called fascicles and macroscopically in the gross position of a muscle, tendon, or ligament. In other words, the soft tissue surrounding each joint has a normal spiral orientation of the fibers, which may wind into a torsion (twist) in dysfunction or after injury. Abnormal alignment has mechanical and neurological consequences.

One goal of manual therapy is to unwind the tissue to realign the fibers on both the macroscopic and microscopic levels.

■ **Treatment implications:** From Lauren Berry's engineering experience, he discovered that if a twist developed in one of the steel cables he was working with, he could "unwind" it by rocking the cable back and forth perpendicular to the cable and reestablish the normal alignment of the steel strands. Berry discovered predictable patterns of misalignment of the soft tissue, which are described throughout this text. To correct the misalignment of the soft tissue, it is mobilized in a specific direction. Because muscles, tendons, ligaments, and other soft tissue are structured like steel cables (or ropes), our fundamental method of mobilizing the soft tissue is stroking perpendicular to the line of the fiber.

EXAMPLE OF SOFT TISSUE MISALIGNMENT

An example of the mechanisms of soft tissue misalignment can be illustrated with an injury to the knee. An injury causes swelling. To accommodate the excess fluid, the joint is held in a sustained flexion. This position pulls the soft tissue on the medial and lateral aspects of the knee into an abnormal posterior alignment. This misalignment also creates an abnormal torsion in the muscles, tendons, and ligaments on the medial and lateral aspects of the knee. The increased torsion causes a decreased flow of cells and fluids in the area, leading to a decreased ability for repair. The torsion adds excessive compression to the nerves traveling through the soft tissue, leading to potential dysfunction of muscle function, coordination, and balance. The treatment of the soft tissue on the medial and lateral sides of the knee is performed in a specific direction. The therapist mobilizes the soft tissue in a posterior-to-anterior direction to restore the normal alignment and to unwind the tissue to remove the abnormal torsion in the fascicles and fibers.

MECHANICAL AND NEUROLOGICAL CONSEQUENCES OF SOFT TISSUE MISALIGNMENT

■ **Abnormal torsion (twist):** If the soft tissue develops an abnormal position owing to dysfunction or in-

jury, it introduces an abnormal torsion or twist into the tissue. The abnormal twist decreases the water content of the tissue, leading to fluid stagnation, adhesions, and abnormal function in the soft tissue and associated joint. Stagnation reduces the tissue's ability to repair itself owing to decreased cellular activity, decreased nutrition, and the accumulation of waste products.

■ **Dehydration of soft tissue:** Placing an excessive twist to the soft tissue is analogous to taking a wet washcloth and twisting it, wringing out the water. Misalignment and abnormal torsion compress the tissue, decreasing fluid content and decreasing the normal flow of fluids, which reduces the supply of vital nutrients and oxygen and the mobility of the cells. Compression to the tissue from abnormal torsions leads to adhesions and loss of normal extensibility.

■ **Neurological and mechanical dysfunction in the joint:** Abnormal position and torsion of the soft tissue also create abnormal forces moving through the joint, creating joint dysfunction and potential degeneration. Joint dysfunction and degeneration cause irritation to the sensory nerve receptors in the soft tissue surrounding the joint. This irritation can create neurological reflexes that inhibit (weaken) or create hypertonicity in the surrounding muscles, leading to abnormalities of coordination and balance.

TREATMENT GOALS FOR SOFT TISSUE MISALIGNMENT

The treatment goals are fully described in Chapter 2, "Assessment and Technique." Some goals are unique to this method of massage:

■ **Reposition the soft tissue:** One of our most fundamental intentions is to reposition the soft tissue. We accomplish this by resetting the soft tissue in a specific direction for each joint.

■ **Unwind abnormal torsion:** The text describes the abnormal torsion patterns in the soft tissue surrounding each joint and the direction of the strokes to unwind the abnormal torsion. The ligaments, tendons, and muscles are like braided ropes or long phone cables, with tubes within tubes of fibers. The normal spiral alignment is reintroduced by "unwinding" the tissue, stroking the fibers perpendicular to their longitudinal axis.

■ **Reestablish the normal parallel alignment of soft tissue fibers:** The ligaments, tendons, and muscles are composed of collagen fibers that pull apart after injury and repair themselves in a random weave, losing their normal parallel alignment. Chronic dysfunction is characterized by adhesions, which prevent normal alignment of the fibers. This method of treatment restores alignment.

▨ **Restore the ability of the bundles of fibers (fascicles) to slide relative to each other:** STM applied perpendicular (transverse) to the line of the fibers dissolves abnormal adhesions, increases lubrication, and promotes mobility of the tissue.

▨ **Restore the movement of fluids:** STM strokes are applied in rhythmic cycles of compression and decompression while rocking the body in oscillating waves. This technique restores the natural rhythmic movement of the body's fluids.

A NEW METHOD OF MASSAGE: WAVE MOBILIZATION

To help accomplish successful treatment, the author has created a new method of massage called *wave mobilization*. This method is based on 30 years of clinical experience and the author's 30 years of practice of tai chi. Tai chi was developed by the Taoists, who observed nature and especially water as embodying the essence of their spiritual path. Water is so yielding that it takes the shape of whatever container it is in yet so powerful that it dissolves rocks and forms canyons. The massage stroke that is used in wave mobilization is patterned after an ocean wave and is performed most effectively if the therapist is relaxed and supple, using energy (chi) rather than muscular strength. Through disciplined practice of energy exercises (see Chapter 2) and focused attention, the therapist can learn to develop a strong biomagnetic field (chi) for healing.

The energy pattern of an ocean wave is circular. The direction of the waves is perpendicular to the coastline (Fig. 1-8). The waves are repeated in rhythmic cycles, ebbing and flowing on the shore. Just as strong waves can dissolve a shoreline, massage applied in specific rhythmic cycles, perpendicular to the line of the fiber can dissolve adhesions and reintroduce normal motion in the tissue.

The wave mobilization strokes are performed while mobilizing the body in rhythmic oscillations, like the ebb and flow of the ocean. For much of the session, the client is put in a fetal position and is rocked in rhythmic oscillations at a frequency of about 60 cycles per minute, which mimics the mother's heartbeat that we all felt as waves of energy and fluids pulsating in her womb. This form of mobi-

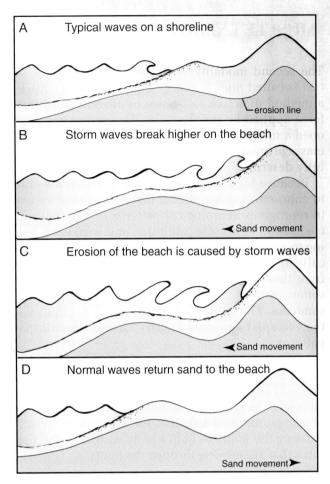

Figure 1-8. Wave mobilization stroke is modeled after the pattern of ocean waves. The ocean wave moves a molecule of water in a circular pattern. The waves move perpendicular to the shoreline, creating a digging motion.

lization may be described as *heart-wave resonance*. Resonance is a coupling of systems to the same frequency. Rocking the body in rhythmic oscillations to the rhythm of the heartbeat sends waves of energy throughout the entire body. It is profoundly relaxing and profoundly healing.

The massage strokes are applied in a specific direction to reposition the soft tissue to its normal alignment and to remove the abnormal twist or torsion from the tissue. The strokes are applied perpendicular (transverse) to the line of the fiber to dissolve abnormal crosslinks and microscopic adhesions between the fibers and the fascicles. Dissolving these adhesions allows the fibers and fascicles to slide relative to each other, promotes the normal broadening of the muscle fibers, and helps to realign the normal parallel orientation of the fibers. We perform the strokes in cycles of compression and decompression to restore the normal waves of movement of the fluids within the body.

MUSCLE ENERGY TECHNIQUE

The second modality of treatment described in this text is called *muscle energy technique* (MET). MET is a method of active resistance by the client against a force applied by the therapist. The author has developed a unique method of incorporating MET into the massage treatment. The clinical effects of MET are fully described in Chapter 2.

Because MET uses voluntary effort from the client to contract muscles, higher brain functions are used to reprogram neurological patterns of habitual muscle tension or muscle inhibition and weakness, helping to restore normal muscle function. MET dramatically transforms the role of the massage therapist from that of a practitioner who gives a treatment *to* someone to that of a practitioner who works *with* someone. The active participation of the client with the therapist can dramatically change chronic pain patterns.

MET also stimulates the synthesis of new cells to repair injured tissue, helps to realign and strengthen connective tissue fibers, lengthens shortened tissue, increases the range of motion of the joints, eliminates trigger points, and balances the strength of muscles crossing the joints to help evenly distribute the pressures that are moving through the joints.

Active contraction and relaxation of the muscles create a spiral winding and unwinding of the soft tissue surrounding the joint. This process of tightening and relaxation of the soft tissue promotes the movement of cells and fluids deep within the body to disperse stagnation and promotes the reoxygenation of tissue and the elimination of waste products.

JOINT MOBILIZATION

The third modality that is used in this form of treatment is joint mobilization. Joint mobilization can be defined as any form of passive movement at a joint.[18] A unique feature of wave mobilization is that STM and joint mobilization are performed with the same movement. Some techniques that are described in this text focus on specific joint mobilization. These movements are within the scope of practice for the massage therapist. The intentions of joint mobilization are to restore the normal joint play, promote the exchange of cells and fluids into and out of the joint for joint repair and regeneration, stimulate lubrication in the joint by stimulating the synovial membrane, normalize neurological function by stimulating sensory nerves of the joint, decrease swelling, and reduce pain.

Part Three: Essentials of Anatomy and Physiology for Orthopedic Conditions

The body's tissues are composed of three basic elements: cells, fibers, and body fluids. On the structural level, massage and manual therapy affect these elements in a very profound way, because they are "mechanotransducers," that is, they take mechanical information, such as touch, movement, and stretch, and translate that mechanical information into chemical energy, electrical energy, and electromagnetic energy, which promote cellular communication for optimum health. To achieve clinical success, the therapist needs to understand the structure and function of these tissues, understand the mechanisms of injury and repair, be able to perform a thorough assessment (see Chapter 2), and develop treatment goals based on which structures are being addressed and their stage of healing.

BASIC ORGANIZATION OF THE BODY

BODY, MIND, AND EMOTIONS FORM A UNIFIED WHOLE

■ It is important to realize that all of the tissues form an interrelated whole and that each tissue not only influences other tissues, but also affects a person's emotions and psychology. For example, when you massage a tight muscle, you are touching skin, connective tissue, blood vessels, muscles, and nerve endings that communicate with every other part of the body. The touch stimulates sensory nerves that communicate to other muscles; to the neighboring joint, to the spinal cord, to the area of the highest centers of the brain that receives sensory information, and to the limbic area of the brain, which is the emotional center of the body. Touch also communicates with the autonomic nervous system, which regulates blood flow, heart rate, and respiration.

- **Treatment implications:** When you touch a person, you not only influence the local tissue that you are touching, but also influence every other aspect of the physical body, as well as the client's emotions and psychology. A nurturing and gentle touch can lower the blood pressure, slow the heart rate, relax muscle tone, and reduce anxiety, allowing for emotional and psychological healing as well as inducing the body's repair functions. An aggressive or hard touch has the opposite effect, inducing a state of anxiety, muscle guarding, and distress.

FOUR PRIMARY TYPES OF TISSUE

There are four primary types of tissue in adults:

- **Epithelium:** The epithelium consists of the skin, called the *external epithelium*, and the tissue that lines the internal organs and glands, called the *internal epithelium*.

- **Connective tissue:** The connective tissue forms the structural framework of the body. It is the basic building block of soft tissue, including ligaments, tendons, joint capsules, and fascia (forms the structural framework of muscles). These are generalized types of connective tissue, and this category also includes superficial and deep fascia, nerve and muscle sheaths, tissue covering the bones (periosteum), and the coverings and support framework of most organs. There are also specialized types of connective tissue, including cartilage, bone, blood, and lymph.

- **Muscle:** The muscles are classified into three types: skeletal (also called *voluntary muscle*), smooth (intestinal tract and blood vessels), and cardiac (heart).

- **Nerve:** The nerves consist of long cells grouped in bundles. The nervous system includes the brain, spinal cord, peripheral nerves, and autonomic nervous system.

External Epithelial Tissue (Skin)

- **Structure:** The skin consists of a superficial cellular layer called the *epidermis* and an underlying connective tissue layer called the *dermis*. The epithelium and the nervous system are derived from the same embryological tissue, the ectoderm. In a

manner of speaking, we are wearing our nervous system.
  - ☐ The skin is the body's largest organ and contains blood vessels, glands, muscles, connective tissue, and nerve endings.
  - ☐ The skin contains four types of sensory nerve receptors called *mechanoreceptors*, which communicate with every other part of the body. The mechanoreceptors are sensitive to touch, pressure, movement, superficial proprioception (positional changes), pain, and temperature.

- **Function:** The skin provides sensation and protection, helps to regulate water balance, and regulates temperature. The sense of touch is the first of the senses to become functional in embryonic life, followed by proprioception.
  - ☐ Sensory information from the skin communicates to the spinal cord, where reflex (automatic, unconscious) connections are made to muscles, internal organs, and blood vessels. Skin pain can cause a contraction in the skeletal muscles or internal organs. A calming touch applied to the skin can reflexively relax muscles and internal organs.[19]

- **Dysfunction and injury:** Adhesions in the skin can develop after a blunt injury, cut, or surgery. Because the superficial fascia in the dermis is connected to the underlying deep fascia covering the muscles, these adhesions decrease the ability of the tissue to stretch and thus limit joint function. Adhesions in the superficial fascia can also entrap cutaneous nerves, leading to pain, numbing, and tingling. A potential outcome of joint or muscle dysfunction is reflex changes in the skin. The most common example is an area of increased sensitivity called the *hyperalgesic skin zone*.[18] In this condition, an area of skin becomes painful to light touch, and the skin and underlying fascia become tight and resistant to stretch.

- **Treatment implications:** Treatment of skin zones of increased sensitivity requires assessment and treatment of the neighboring joints. STM, MET, and joint mobilization release the nerves and fascia of the skin. Although most of the massage strokes are applied with a gentle, touch, the exception to this is treatment of adhesions in the skin or deep connective tissues, which require deeper pressures and typically elicit discomfort. Perform skin rolling to treat adhesions in the skin or entrapped cutaneous nerves. Using thumbs and the first two fingers, pull the skin and subcutaneous tissue in front of the thumb, and then the thumb rolls the skin toward the fingers in a wavelike motion. The cardinal rule in applying techniques that could be uncomfortable is that the client needs to be able to completely relax into the treatment to achieve the greatest success.

Connective Tissue

Connective tissue is composed of cells, fibers, and ground substance. As the name implies, connective tissue connects all the parts of the body. It forms the structural walls for the heart, lungs, and blood vessels, and it binds joints together through ligaments and joint capsules. It gives shape to the body through broad sheets of fascia and compartments, called *septa*, which contain the muscles. It forms the structural framework within muscles and transmits the pull of the muscles through the tendons. Connective tissue plays an important defense and immunological role in response to injury and infection.[18] As we will see, it is the connective tissue that is primarily injured in the strains and sprains of muscles, tendons, and ligaments. Therefore, it is one of the primary tissues to be addressed in massage and manual therapy.

COMPONENTS OF CONNECTIVE TISSUE

CELLS

▨ The cells are responsible for maintenance and repair and are essential for healing. The cells remove damaged or aged structures and synthesize new cells, fibers, and ground substance to remodel and repair the body. There are six different types of cells in ordinary connective tissue, but only the fibroblast is important for our consideration. Important cells of specialized connective tissue are the chondrocyte and the synoviocyte.

   ☐ **Fibroblasts:** Fibroblasts produce all of the components of connective tissue, including fibers and ground substance, and are active in inflammation and repair. These cells are found in ligaments, tendons, joint capsules, and fascia.

   ☐ **Chondrocytes:** Chondrocytes or cartilage cells are found in the collagen matrix of cartilage. Chondrocytes synthesize new cartilage in the normal turnover of cells and in the repair of damaged cartilage.

   ☐ **Synoviocytes:** Synoviocytes form the lining of the joint capsule, which is in contact with the joint cavity.[20] They synthesize the lubricant (synovium) for the joint cartilage, supply nutrition to the chondrocytes, and remove waste products.

▨ **Function:** The normal function of cells and the creation of new cells (synthesis) are stimulated by

movement. Cellular activity is also increased by the inflammatory process after an injury.

▨ **Dysfunction and injury:** Swelling decreases cellular movement and the ability of cells to synthesize new cells, fibers, and ground substance necessary for repair. In chronic conditions, decreased movement from adhesions or immobilization causes cells to break down tissue (lysis); creates atrophy in the muscles, tendons, and ligaments; and leads to osteoporosis in the bones.

▨ **Treatment implications:** In acute conditions, it is critical to reduce swelling as quickly as possible to promote cellular movement. Gentle, passive motion, especially in the flexion-extension planes, MET, and gentle STM provide mechanical stimulation to increase movement of fluids and to stimulate cellular activity. Chronic conditions require the same techniques but for different goals: to dissolve adhesions and tissue stagnation and to improve joint movement to promote cellular synthesis and cellular movement, which help to remodel and regenerate new tissue.

FIBERS

The three types of connective tissue fibers are reticulin, elastin, and collagen. Reticulin is a meshlike network for support of organs and glands. Elastin is more elastic and is found in ligaments and the linings of arteries. Collagen is the main component of the tendons, ligaments, joint capsules, and fascia (the framework for the shape and function of the muscles). Connective tissue is classified by the arrangement and density of the fibers. Ordinary connective tissue is divided into loose and dense. Dense connective tissue is further divided into regular and irregular, based on the alignment of the fibers.

THREE GENERALIZED TYPES OF CONNECTIVE TISSUE

Loose Irregular

▨ **Structure:** Loose, irregular connective tissue consists of a meshwork, similar to a spiderweb, of collagen and elastin fibers interlacing in all directions and an abundance of ground substance and cells.

▨ **Function:** Loose, irregular connective tissue is found in superficial and deep fascia; forms sheaths around muscles, arteries, veins, nerves, and organs; and also forms between these structures, suspending them and connecting them to each other. This tissue has enough extensibility to allow mobility in the healthy state.

- **Dysfunction and injury:** Inflammation, irritation, or immobilization can create adhesions between the fibers. If the area is not adequately mobilized, the tissue becomes dense and hard.[21] This inhibits the ability of these structures to slide freely within their connective tissue spaces. Excessive tension can tether (pull) the nerve, leading to parathesias (altered sensations).

- **Treatment implications:** Perform STM perpendicular to the line of the muscle or nerve. In the acute condition, these strokes provide the necessary mobility to the healing fibers to help induce normal alignment and mobility. In chronic conditions, these scooping strokes dissolve adhesions with the heat caused by tissue compression and friction and by the mechanical pressure of stretching the tissue perpendicular to the line of the fiber. By taking the tissue into tension and then releasing it with the stroke, abnormal crosslinks are reduced, and the mobility and resilience increase, allowing greater range of motion and increasing the ability of the tissue to slide relative to neighboring tissue.

Dense Irregular

- **Structure:** Dense, irregular connective tissue forms thick bundles of collagen interweaving in three dimensions. There are few cells, and there is little ground substance. This type of tissue is found in the joint capsules, periosteum, fascial sheaths, flattened tendons called *aponeuroses*, synovial tendon sheaths, connective tissue covering of muscles, and dermis of the skin. (See below for further discussion of the joint capsule, periosteum, and fascia.)

- **Function:** Because of the three-dimensional interweaving of the collagen, this tissue has considerable strength and can withstand forces from various angles.

- **Dysfunction and injury:** This type of tissue forms scars from persistent swelling or immobilization.[21]

- **Treatment implications:** Mobility must be maintained during healing. In the acute phase, edema must be reduced quickly, and pain-free motion must be introduced into the area as soon as possible. A dense, contracted scar forms with inadequate mobilization.

Dense Regular

- **Structure:** Dense, regular connective tissue primarily consists of parallel bundles of collagen fibers that form tendons and ligaments (see below). Tendons and ligaments are mostly fibers, which gives them great tensile strength (resistance to pulling). This type of tissue also has a limited blood supply, limiting its ability to repair, unlike bone, which has an extensive blood supply and a remarkable ability to repair.

- **Function:** Tendons transmit the contractile force of the muscle to the joint. Ligaments connect the joints, providing stability and a profound neurosensory function.

- **Dysfunction and injury:** Because dense regular connective tissue has a limited blood supply, it requires motion to stimulate healing.

- **Treatment implications:** Tendons and ligaments require movement to stimulate blood supply to the tissue, bringing needed cells, oxygen, and nutrition to the area (see below).

COLLAGEN

On the structural level, massage and manual therapy are primarily concerned with how to affect deep, connective tissue, which is mostly collagen. Collagen makes up one-third of all the protein in the body and forms not only the tendons and ligaments, but also adhesions and scars. Understanding its structure and function is essential to achieving effective clinical outcomes.

- **Structure:** Collagen forms approximately 80% to 99% of the dry weight of tendons, ligaments, and joint capsules and 50% to 90% of the dry weight of cartilage and bone. It is the fascia that forms the shape and structural support for muscles; blood vessels; nerve fibers, including those of the brain; skin; and internal organs. The collagen fibers are long, soft, white, tough fibers synthesized from fibroblasts, which make tropocollagen, a triple helical (spiral) structure (Fig. 1-9). Mature collagen resembles the structure of a rope, with small strands forming larger strands, all wound together in a spiral.
  - ☐ Tropocollagen molecules line up side by side, overlapping, and are chemically bound together in a parallel arrangement by intermolecular crosslinks to form fibrils. These crosslinks give collagen great strength and stability.
  - ☐ The fibrils are wound in a spiral structure like short threads. These threads are wound together in a spiral like a rope to form a fiber.[22] The fibers are generally collected into bundles called *fascicles*.
  - ☐ The collagen fibers are normally aligned in a parallel and longitudinal orientation. The fibers have a slightly wavy appearance in the relaxed state called **crimp**. This is the slack in the tissue.

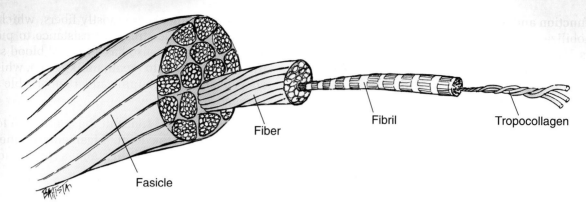

Figure 1-9. Collagen structure. Collagen fibers are organized in bundles called fascicles, which are designed to slide relative to each other in the healthy state.

The greatest strength is found when the fibers and fascicles are oriented in this parallel and longitudinal alignment along the lines of mechanical stress.

☐ The individual fibers and the fascicle bundles normally slide freely past one another.[23] The normal gliding of the collagen fibers is maintained by movement and the lubrication from the ground substance (see below).

☐ Collagen has been described as a "liquid crystal"[9] because of the ordered spatial relationship of its molecules.

Function: Collagen is a dynamic tissue, synthesized in response to "stress," such as movement; and broken down (lysis) from lack of adequate stress, such as immobilization following injury. **Wolff's law** states that bone is laid down along lines of stress. This same law applies to soft tissue. Normal stresses, in the form of exercise and the activities of daily living, increase collagen synthesis and strengthen connective tissue.

☐ Collagen stabilizes joints through ligaments, joint capsules, and periosteum.

☐ Collagen transmits the pulling force of muscle contraction through the fascia within the muscle and through the tendon.

☐ Collagen provides support in articular cartilage to resist compressive forces when the joint is loaded.

Dysfunction and injury: Injuries to collagen can be artificially divided into acute, inflammatory conditions (injury) and chronic, noninflammatory conditions (dysfunction). As was mentioned previously, these categories do not reflect the fact that in the clinical setting there are many stages of injury and repair.

☐ **Injury:** An injury to collagen is a tearing apart of the collagen fibers microscopically or a complete disruption of the structure (see "Mechanics of Soft Tissue Injury," p. 45). Injury can be de-scribed as an inflammatory condition that is the result of a macrotruama, that is, a specific event, such as whiplash, or a repetitive microtrauma that creates tissue disruption and inflammation over time, such as tennis elbow. Most soft tissue injuries are injuries to collagen.

• **Traumatic injury:** Tissue disruption creates an immediate inflammatory response. The torn collagen fibers initially clot into a weak, random mesh. During the repair phase of the inflammatory cycle, the fibrils and fibers are laid down in a random orientation instead of in the normal parallel and longitudinal arrangement. This random weave decreases the strength of collagen. Eventually, the fibers pack closer together, forming abnormal crosslinks and adhesions, thus preventing the normal gliding characteristics of the collagen.[23]

• **Cumulative or repetitive stress:** Collagen is also disrupted through repetitive mechanical stress. Low-grade irritation-inflammation signals the body to lay down more collagen in a random arrangement in the entire area of stress. These deposits of collagen contain abnormal crosslinks, forming adhesions. As with traumatic injury, the fibers pack closer together, and the lubrication is decreased, which decreases the ability of the fibers and fascicles to slide relative to each other. Cumulative stress is caused by four main factors:

• **Posture:** Abnormal postural stress, such as a forward-head posture, creates an excessive tension or pulling force on the soft tissues around the cervicothoracic junction. The client complains of stiffness and lack of full range of motion. To palpation, the area feels thick and lacks normal tissue mobility due to excessive deposits of collagen (adhesions).

• **Dynamic stress:** The stress of repetitive gripping of a tennis racquet and the reactive force of hitting the ball causes a thickening of the collagen within the muscles of the elbow, wrist, and hand and at their attachment sites.

- **Static stress:** Excessive sitting or standing, such as working as a retail clerk, places abnormal forces on the tissue and leads to excessive deposits of collagen.
- **Misalignment:** An example of misalignment is patellar-tracking dysfunction. The kneecap (patella) is typically pulled laterally due to pronation or other postural dysfunctions, and rubs against the lateral side of the femur. This chronic irritation creates excessive deposits of collagen, leading to loss of normal mobility and function of the patellofemoral joint, and eventual degeneration.

☐ **Dysfunction:** Chronic irritation to collagen creates excessive deposits, leading to adhesions. Collagen can also weaken and atrophy due to lack of adequate stress. Sedentary lifestyle and immobilization are two examples.

- **Adhesions:** Adhesions are abnormal crosslinks of connective tissue between gliding surfaces. These adhesions can occur at every level of the soft tissue, from the ligament or tendon adhering to the bone to adhesions between the fascicles or between the fibers themselves. Adhesions decrease tissue pliability (mobility) and extensibility (length). The tissue becomes less elastic, thicker, and shorter. The client will often feel stiff in the area of adhesions.
- **Atrophy:** Loss of collagen may be due to immobilization from injury or lack of use from a sedentary lifestyle. Lack of stress on the tissue causes a decrease in collagen production, leading to atrophy in the connective tissue and to osteoporosis in the bone. Without movement, the body begins to break down the tissue, in a process called *lysis*. New collagen is laid down in a random orientation without adequate stress, packing the fibers close together, forming adhesions. Atrophy and randomly oriented fibers create weakness in the tissue and instability in the associated joint.

▨ **Treatment implications:** Collagen is extremely sensitive to mechanical load, that is, the touch, movement, contractions, and stretching of manual therapy. The manual therapist can guide how the newly synthesized collagen is laid down by stimulating the tissue appropriately. The stimulus must be dosed correctly: In the acute phase, the stimulus to the tissue must be very gentle; in chronic conditions, the stimulus can be more vigorous. The guiding principle of treatment is that motion must be maintained throughout the process of repair and rehabilitation.[24] Treatment goals are determined by the stage of healing and repair. In the early phase of healing, collagen is easily influenced because weak, unstable bonds are holding the tissue together.[18] In the later phases of healing, it takes more stimulus over a greater period of time to influence the tissue. The details of assessment to determine the stage of healing and further discussion of treatment goals are found in Chapter 2.

☐ For injury and inflammatory conditions the goals of treatment for collagen are as follows:

- To reduce the swelling as quickly as possible to allow the exchange of cells, oxygen, and nutrients to the healing tissue.
- To stimulate the cells, including the fibroblasts, which will synthesize new collagen and the other elements of connective tissue to repair the injured tissue.
- To provide mechanical stimulation to realign the new collagen fibrils along their lines of stress and to their normal parallel alignment.

☐ For chronic dysfunction, the treament goals are as follows:

- To dissolve abnormal crosslinks (adhesions).
- To lengthen shortened tissue.
- To stimulate the fluids to promote the movement of nutrition, oxygenation, and elimination of waste products. Stimulate the fibroblasts to synthesize ground substance and thus increase the lubrication between the fibers and the fascicles, promoting normal gliding.
- It is essential to maintain motion for the collagen to align itself properly. Movement also promotes the normal sliding of the fascicles and helps to maintain the normal interfiber distance. If the movements of daily life are inadequate to restore function, then the abnormal crosslinks in the collagen can be reduced through STM, joint mobilization, and MET.

> ❗ **CAUTION:** *The treatment of injuries requires special precautions: In the early stages after an injury, the therapist must exercise great care to use only gentle massage, MET, and joint mobilization so as not to disturb the newly forming crosslinks. These normal crosslinks are essential to maintaining the strength of the tissue. Gentle isometric MET is used to help realign the developing fibrils, but excessive force of stretching is contraindicated in the first two weeks after an injury (see Chapter 2).*

GROUND SUBSTANCE

▦ **Definition:** Ground substance is a transparent, viscous (thick) fluid—much like raw egg whites in appearance and consistency—that surrounds all the structures in the body and binds them together.

▦ **Structure:** The primary components of ground substance are water and glycoaminoglycans, which look like bottle brushes at the molecular level. Glycoaminoglycans draw water into the tissue and bind it and are electrostatically bound to the collagen fibers, increasing their strength.[18] Because glycoaminoglycans hold water, this causes the tissue to swell, giving healthy tissue the feeling of a water balloon. Water makes up approximately 70% of ground substance.

▦ **Function:** Ground substance acts as the medium for the transport of nutrition and removal of waste products. It also acts as a lubricant and spacer between the collagen, elastin, and reticular fibers, preventing the fibers from adhering to each other.[25] Because of the high water content, ground substance also acts as a shock absorber. Ground substance has a thixotropic quality. **Thixotropy** is the quality by which a substance becomes more fluid when stirred and more solid when undisturbed.[19]

▦ **Dysfunction and injury:** Injury leads to inflammation and swelling, which decrease the function of the fibroblasts, which synthesize ground substance. This causes a decrease of the glycoaminoglycans, which decreases the lubrication and spacing provided by the ground substance. The fibrils and fibers pack more closely together, leading to abnormal crosslinks and adhesions. This decreases the normal gliding of the fibers, fascicles, tendons, ligaments, joint capsules, and muscles relative to the neighboring soft tissues and bone. In chronic dysfunction and immobilization, tissue fluids stagnate and nutrition is decreased, which inhibits repair. There is a decrease in glycoaminoglycan and water content, decreasing the interfiber distance, leading to adhesions. The tissues tend to cool, and the ground substance becomes thicker and more gel-like, leading to greater stiffness and decreased circulation, nutrition, and lubrication.

▦ **Treatment implications:** STM, joint mobilization, and MET reintroduce motion into the tissue. Movement stimulates the synthesis of ground substance and glycoaminoglycans, and promotes the circulation of blood, lymph, and ground substance, which contains a high percentage of water. This water can then bind to the glycoaminoglycans, creating greater lubrication to the tissue. Movement also transports nutrients and promotes the exchange of waste products. As was mentioned above, heat creates a change in the ground substance from being sluggish and thick to a more fluid state. MET creates heat through muscle contraction and the pulling and release of the fascial components. MET also promotes circulation deep within the body by means of the pumping action of muscle contraction, which affects the lymph and blood flow.

EXAMPLES OF CONNECTIVE TISSUE STRUCTURES

TENDONS

▦ **Structure:** Tendons are a continuation of the connective tissue (fascia) of the muscle (myofascia), so the entire connective tissue of the muscle transmits the force of contraction. This fascia is called a tendon after the muscle fibers end. The muscle and tendon are therefore best described as a unit, the **musculotendinous** unit. The tendon has three distinct sections: the **myotendinous junction,** where the muscle fibers end and the connective tissue forming the tendon continues; the **tenoperiosteal junction,** where the tendon attaches to the bone by interweaving to the connective tissue (periosteum) covering of the bone; and the mid-portion or **body of the tendon.**

▦ Tendons are composed of long, spiraling bundles of parallel collagen fibers, oriented in a longitudinal pattern along the line of stress and embedded in a matrix of ground substance and a small number of fibroblasts. The ground substance binds with water, which forms two-thirds of the total weight of the tendon.

▦ Collagen molecules combine to form ordered units of microfibrils, fibrils, and fibers (Fig. 1-10). These fibers run parallel to each other and are contained in a bundle called a *fascicle.* Each fascicle is normally capable of sliding past the other fascicles in the healthy state.[3] Fascicles are bound together by loose connective tissue called the **endotenon,** which supports the blood vessels, lymphatics, and nerves. A group of fascicles together forms the gross tendon.

▦ Tendons and ligaments have a microscopic crimp or wavelike structure that acts like a spring and can withstand large internal forces. The crimp in the tendon imparts an elastic quality to the structure. When you stretch a muscle and "take the slack out," you are straightening out the crimp in the tissue.

 ☐ Tendons may be a cordlike structure, such as the Achilles tendon; a flattened band of tissue, such

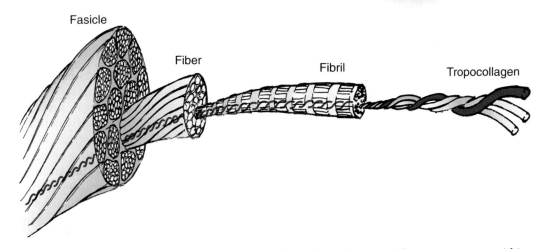

Figure 1-10. Longitudinal and parallel alignment of the collagen fibers and the crimp or wave within the fibers of a tendon and ligament.

as the rotator cuff; or a broad sheet of tissue called an aponeurosis, such as the origin of the latissimus dorsi.

☐ In areas of high pressure or friction, such as where tendons rub over the bones of the wrist and ankle, the tendon is enclosed within a sheath called the **epitenon**, which is lined with a synovial layer that secretes synovial fluid to facilitate gliding of the tendon (Fig. 1-11). Tendons that are not enclosed within a sheath and move in a straight line are surrounded by a loose connective tissue sheath called a **paratenon**.

■ **Function:** Tendons attach muscle to bone and transmit the force of muscle contraction to the bone, thereby producing motion of the joint. The musculotendinous unit also helps to dynamically stabilize the joint by providing strength and support to the joint. Tendons act as "shock absorbers" by lengthening to absorb tension during high-

impact motions.[6] The tendon also acts as a sensory receptor through Golgi tendon organs (GTOs), which sense the level of tension in the tendon. (See "The Nervous System" for more information on GTOs.)

■ **Dysfunction and injury:** An injury to the tendon is called a **strain** and typically represents a tearing of the collagen fibers, primarily at the musculotendinous junction and secondarily at the tenoperiosteal junction. Tendon ruptures are rare within the body of the tendon itself except in chronic, weakened tendons, because tendons can withstand much higher pulling (tensile) stresses than muscle or bone. The term ***tendinitis*** is used to describe inflammation to the tendon. Inflammation may be due to a specific event; cumulative or repetitive strain; friction irritation, such as iliotibial band friction syndrome; or compression, such as impingement of the supraspinatous of the shoulder. As was previously described, injury and inflammation disrupt the normal parallel alignment of the collagen. Repair creates random weaves of collagen and abnormal crosslinks (adhesions), leading to stiffness, weakness, and loss of range of motion.

☐ Reid has categorized tendinitis into five functional grades, depending on the symptoms reported by the patient:[21]

• **Grade I:** Pain only after activity.
• **Grade II:** Minimal pain with activity.
• **Grade III:** Pain interferes with activity but disappears with rest.
• **Grade IV:** Pain with rest, significant pain and swelling.
• **Grade V:** Pain interferes with activities of daily living; chronic and recurrent pain; significant pain and swelling, signs of soft tissue changes, and altered muscle function.

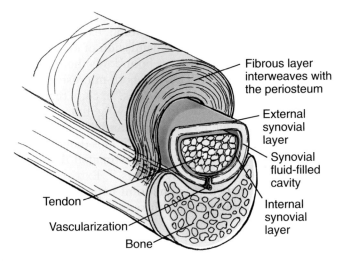

Figure 1-11. Tendon sheath structure.

☐ Tendinitis is also categorized on the basis of the structures affected. **Tenosynovitis** is an inflammation of the synovial lining of the tendon sheath caused by irritation of the sheath from roughened surfaces of the tendon, and **tenovaginitis** is an inflammation with a thickening of the tendon sheath and/or an enlargement of the tendon that jams in the sheath (commonly called "trigger finger"). An injury to the tendon has neurological consequences, which are described further in the section "The Nervous System."

▨ Chronic overuse injuries are the result of repetitive stresses that cause disruption and disorganization of the collagen but do not necessarily lead to inflammation. The tendon can become degenerated because it has failed to heal properly through lack of inflammation and repair. Degenerated tendons are susceptible to fatigue, leading to weakness and dysfunction, a condition called **tendinosis** or **tendinopathy.** Currently, these two terms are favored over *chronic tendinitis* because surgical examination of chronic tendon lesions often reveals degenerative tissue rather than inflamed tissue.[26] The tendon might be painful, but the pain is due to ischemia and lactic acid rather than inflammation. A chronic tendon dysfunction is susceptible to reinjury, due to atrophy of the tendon.[27] Loss of normal motion and inadequate exercise in a tendon from a prior injury or immobilization create loss of collagen fibers (atrophy) and adhesions between the tendon and the surrounding structures, including the tendon sheath. This decreases the strength of the tendon.

▨ **Treatment implications:** Inflammation should be limited, so rest from excessive activities, ice, compression, and elevation are recommended. As with other collagen injuries, studies show that immediate, pain-free mobilization promotes tendon healing.[28] In acute tendinitis, STM in the early phases of repair stimulates collagen synthesis, improves the strength of the tendon, reduces the number of adhesions, and helps to realign the developing collagen fiber in the early stages of repair.[23] Increased DNA and cells are found in mobilized tendons compared with immobilized tendons, signifying increased repair.[16] MET helps to reduce swelling, promotes nutritional exchange, and prevents muscular inhibition. As with other collagen structures, great care must be taken in the early stages after an injury, because the collagen is fragile. Too much manual pressure can disturb the newly forming tissue, and stretching is contraindicated. Examination includes isometric contraction of the involved musculotendinous structures, which typically will be painful at the site of the lesion. The structure may also be weak, owing to either pain or muscular weakness or inhibition. Palpable tenderness at the site of the injury is also typical.

▨ Chronic tendon conditions are the result of failed tendon healing and are characterized by disorganized and immature collagen and degenerated tissue.[23] Although tendinopathy can be painful to the client and painful to isometric challenge, the tissue is not hot, swollen, or tender before tissue tension, so it is not inflamed. Because of this, treatment involves deep pressure, transverse to the fiber, to intentionally create a microinflammatory response to stimulate collagen synthesis, reorganize the collagen to its normal parallel alignment, and stimulate cellular synthesis to repair the degenerated tissue. The therapeutic goals are also to dissolve abnormal crosslinks and adhesions; realign the fibers and fascicles to their normal parallel alignment; restore the ability of the tendon to glide relative to the surrounding soft tissue and bone; unwind and reposition the tendon as necessary; increase the lubrication and nutrition by improving movement of the fluids in areas of thickened or congested tissue; lengthen the tissue if indicated; and help to restore neurological function with MET. If a chronic tendon lesion is reinjured and shows signs of inflammation, it is treated as an acute injury. If the musculotendonous unit has weakened through injury, immobilization, aging, or disuse, exercise is necessary to strengthen the tissue. If the therapist is not trained in exercise rehabilitation, referral to a physical therapist or personal trainer is necessary.

LIGAMENTS

▨ **Structure:** Ligaments are composed of dense, white, short bands of nearly parallel bundles of collagen fibers embedded in a matrix of ground substance and a small number of fibroblasts. Ligaments are two-thirds water, which is a critical component for cellular function, nutritional exchange, mechanical behavior, and transmission of electromagnetic waves. The fibers are bound together in a fascicle (see Fig. 1-10). They are both microscopically and grossly similar to tendons, except that they contain some elastic fibers, giving them greater elasticity. Ligaments are pliable and flexible. Given that there are over 120 movable bones that make up the major synovial joints, it is estimated that there are several hundred ligaments.[29] Extrinsic ligaments are located over the joint capsule, whereas intrinsic ligaments are thickened portions of the capsule itself.

☐ There is a normal parallel sliding of fibers, and the fascicles are free to slide relative to each other in the healthy state.[23] They have a crimp or wavelike structure that acts like a spring, withstanding large internal forces and giving the ligaments a small amount of slack (see Fig. 1-11).

☐ All ligaments contain specialized nerve endings, including mechanoreceptors and nociceptors (pain fibers).

☐ Ligaments have a rich vascular supply, which must be constantly maintained for synthesis and repair. Swelling or immobilization leads to ligament atrophy and risk of rupture.[26]

■ **Function:** Ligaments attach one bone to another, help to stabilize the joint, help to guide joint motion, and prevent excessive motion. They also play an important neurological role as sensory receptors. Mechanoreceptors give information about posture, movement, and joint position; have reflex connections to the surrounding muscles; and play an important role in joint function. They help to coordinate muscular activity for stability, protection, and efficient movement of the joint. A reflex connection exists between the ligaments of a joint and the surrounding muscles, which has instantaneous effects on muscle tone.[30] Nociceptors send pain information in reaction to inflammation and harmful stimuli.

■ **Dysfunction and injury:** Ligament injuries are called **sprains** and are a tearing of the collagen fibers.

☐ Sprains are categorized into three grades, depending on the extent of the injury:
  • **Grade I:** Microscopic tearing of a few fibers. There is some pain but no loss of stability.
  • **Grade II:** Gross tears and some loss of structural integrity.
  • **Grade III:** Complete tearing through the body of the ligament or at its attachment. Frequently requires surgery.

☐ Because of their functions to help stabilize the joint and as potent neurosensory structures, injuries to the ligaments can create profound disturbances to joint function.

☐ Similar to the joint capsule, the ligaments might respond to an injury by becoming excessively stretched, creating joint instability; or they may become shortened, contributing to joint stiffness and loss of normal range of motion in the joint. Immobilization causes ligaments to atrophy and weaken, owing to decreased collagen content.

☐ Irritation or injury of the ligaments can cause a reflexive contraction or inhibition in the surrounding muscles caused by reflexive connections between the ligaments and the musculature.[31] Injured ligaments, even without laxity, lead to to muscle dysfunction, loss of proprioception, and instability.[32]

☐ Ligaments can twist into abnormal torsion, a concept contributed by Lauren Berry, RPT. For example, after a finger injury, the finger typically assumes a position of sustained flexion. The ligaments on the medial and lateral sides of the finger are pulled toward the palm with this sustained flexion, winding them into abnormal torsion.

■ **Treatment implications:** Clinical assessment of ligaments involves passive joint motion that stretches the ligament and palpation. Passive testing will reveal excessive joint motion with Grade II and III injuries. It is important for the therapist to distinguish ligament involvement from musculotendinous conditions because ligaments take much longer to heal. If ligaments are part of the injury, the therapist needs to tell the client that ligaments might take many months to heal. This will help to avoid frustration or impatience. The goals in treating acute ligament injuries include providing pain relief, reducing swelling, preserving as much mobility as possible, and maintaining neurosensory function.[14] STM is performed to help realign the healing fibrils; passive joint motion maintains range of motion and promotes adequate circulation; and MET provides neurosensory stimulation, reduces swelling, and promotes nutritional exchange. There might be mild discomfort with the STM strokes but no pain. Stretching after acute injury is contraindicated.

☐ In chronic conditions, thorough assessment is critical to differentiate whether the ligament is thick and fibrous, owing to increased collagen, abnormal crosslinks, and adhesions, or whether the ligament is too lax (atrophied), owing to degeneration from immobilization, disuse, or lack of adequate repair from a prior injury or repetitive stresses.

☐ For ligaments that have developed adhesions, perform gentle scooping strokes transverse to the line of the fiber. If you palpate thickened, fibrous tissue in the chronic state, transverse friction massage, as described by Cyriax,[33] is effective in dissolving these adhesions and rehydrating the tissue.[33] The author has contributed a new method of applying transverse friction massage that dramatically reduces the pain associated with transverse friction massage.

☐ If ligaments are too lax and degenerated, transverse STM can stimulate collagen synthesis and help to realign disorganized fibers. Exercise rehabilitation is recommended to stimulate the production of new collagen and to help restore normal integrity to the ligament.

□ Abnormal torsion in the ligaments is corrected with STM strokes applied transverse to the fiber in a specific direction for each ligament.

□ To help restore the neurological function of the ligament, MET is used. Because the muscle is connected to the ligaments with a neurological reflex, isometric contractions to the muscles surrounding the ligaments can help to restore neurological communication.

PERIOSTEUM

■ **Structure:** Periosteum is a dense, irregular connective tissue sheath covering the bones. The outer layer consists of collagen fibers parallel to the bone and contains arteries, veins, lymphatics, and a rich supply of sensory nerves. The inner layer, called the *osteogenic layer*, contains osteoblasts—cells responsible for new bone formation.

■ **Function:**

□ The bone cells in the periosteum generate new bone during growth and repair when the periosteum is stimulated.

□ The periosteum interweaves with the joint capsule and ligaments, and stretching of the periosteum gives mechanoreceptor information regarding movement and position of the joint.

□ The periosteum blends with the tendons, forming the tenoperiosteal junction, which is the site where the muscle pulls on the bone for joint movement.

□ The sensory nerves in periosteum include pain fibers and nerves that are extremely sensitive to tension (i.e., a pulling force).[34]

■ **Dysfunction and injury:**

□ Because the myofascia interweaves with the periosteum, repetitive stress can excessively stimulate the osteogenic layer to create bone spurs, a common problem in runners, who develop heel spurs from excessive or repetitive stress to the plantar fascia that interweaves with the periosteum of the heel.

□ Excessive tension on the periosteum caused by an abnormal position of the joint increases collagen deposition, creating abnormal crosslinks and adhesions. For example, as a result of forward-head posture, the excessive tension leads to the development of fibrous thickening at the lower cervical and upper thoracic vertebrae, contributing to a "dowager's hump." Increased collagen deposition leads to stiffness and loss of normal motion in the joint and diminished function of the mechanoreceptors, potentially causing problems with balance and coordination.

□ A common site of soft tissue injury is at the tenoperiosteal junction. An acute tear or cumulative microtearing of the periosteum can cause the orientation of the collagen in the area to become random, leading to the development of the abnormal crosslinks and adhesions described above. Discomfort or pain can result when the muscle contracts and pulls on the adhesions in the periosteum.

■ **Treatment implications:** The periosteum should feel smooth and glistening to the touch. If adhesions are palpated, first perform MET to the muscles that attach to the involved site. This increases the extensibility of the periosteum at the tenoperiosteal attachment. Adhesions are treated manually with transverse STM strokes or brisk transverse friction strokes for chronic conditions. Although the primary direction of the strokes is perpendicular to the shaft of the bone and therefore perpendicular to the periosteum, strokes are performed in all directions because the interweaving tendons and ligaments form oblique angles to the bone. The therapist "looks" with his or her hands to feel for a line of adhesions in order to stroke perpendicular to that line, akin to stroking across a guitar string. Performing strokes perpendicular to the fiber will dissolve all but the most thickened nodules.

FASCIA

■ **Structure:** Fascia is a fibrous connective tissue that is arranged as sheets or tubes. There are several types of fascia: thick, dense regular connective tissues; thin, loose irregular, connective tissue; and thin, filmy membranes. Fascia is an uninterrupted, three-dimensional web that interweaves with every structure in every region of the body.

□ Superficial fascia lies under the dermis of the skin and is composed of loose, irregular connective tissue.

□ Deep fascia is a dense connective tissue that surrounds muscles, bones, nerves, and blood vessels and forms fascial compartments called **septa,** which contain muscles with similar functions (Fig. 1-12). These compartments are well lubricated in the healthy state, allowing the muscles inside to move freely past each other and relative to the fascial envelope.

■ **Function:** The superficial fascia gives shape to the body, surrounds the organs and glands, and acts as a packing material throughout the body, facilitating movement between structures. The deep fascia

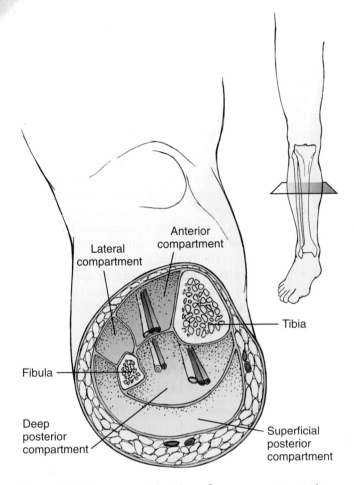

Figure 1-12. Deep connective tissue forms compartments in the body to organize muscle groups. This upward view is of the compartments of the right leg.

forms aponeurosis, ligaments, tendons, retinacula, joint capsules, and septa. It also forms the periosteum that covers bone, cartilage (perichondrium), and blood vessels; and forms the structural support of muscles (epimysium, perimysium, endomysium) and nerves. Fascia maintains structural integrity and assists in stabilization, provides support and protection, and acts as a shock absorber. It is richly endowed with nerves, reporting changes in movement, stretch, tension, and pressure through mechanoreceptors and reporting pain through nociceptors.

▨ **Dysfunction and injury:** Inflammation or repetitive stresses lead to abnormal crosslinks (adhesions), and structures begin to adhere to each other, decreasing their ability to glide. The ground substance becomes more dense, decreasing venous and lymphatic return. Adhesions also affect the nerves, creating disturbances of coordination and balance.[18]

▨ **Treatment implications:** As with other connective tissues, fascia is very responsive to mechanical

stimulation, including STM, MET, and joint mobilization (see the treatment implications for collagen, above).

PROPERTIES OF CONNECTIVE TISSUE

VISCOELASTICITY

Viscoelasticity describes the mechanical behavior of soft tissue, which contains both elastic fibers and ground substance.

▨ **Elasticity** is the ability of a tissue to be stretched and to return to its previous length. This is like a spring. Collagen has a wavelike crimp in it that lengthens when it is stretched a small amount and that springs back to its original length.

▨ **Viscosity** is the resistance of fluids to movement. The ground substance of soft tissue has the viscosity of egg whites. The degree of viscosity of a fluid depends on how quickly or how slowly it is moved. For example, if you move your hand slowly through water, little resistance is encountered. If you move your hand rapidly, greater "fluid friction" is encountered.

▨ **Treatment implications:** If the ground substance of the soft tissue is thick, the massage strokes need to be slowed down. It is helpful to perform MET to thick tissue, which increases the heat in the tissue and helps to make the ground substance less viscous (more liquid), which, in turn, decreases the friction of your strokes. If soft tissue is stretched slowly, it will lengthen more easily. When a more rapid force is applied, soft tissues become stiff and more easily injured. This helps to explain why rapid acceleration in a car accident is damaging to the soft tissue.

PIEZOELECTRICITY

▨ **Definition:** As was mentioned in the first section, piezoelectricity is the ability of a tissue to generate electrical potentials in response to mechanical deformation. Piezoelectricity is a property of most, if not all, living tissue.

▨ **Dysfunction and injury:** Adhesions create a resistance to normal electrical flow.[35] This decrease in electrical currents conducted in the connective tissues interferes with the normal repair and rejuvenation process.

▨ **Treatment implications:** Massage strokes mechanically deform the collagen fibers by compressing and crossing the fibers. This creates electric potentials, which help to realign the collagen fibers in their normal parallel array. Massage also increases the negative charge in the soft tissue, which has a strong proliferative effect, stimulating the creation of new cells to repair the injured site.[36] MET provides mechanical stimulus that also generates piezoelectric currents.

MUSCLE STRUCTURE AND FUNCTION

GENERAL OVERVIEW

Muscle Structure

▨ There are more than 600 skeletal muscles making up 40% to 45% of the total body weight, and they are responsible for all of the body movements (Fig. 1-13).[37] There are two distinct elements of the muscle's structure: the muscle fiber and the connective tissue. We will address each of these separately.

▨ **Structure of muscle fiber:** The structural unit of skeletal muscle is the muscle fiber, which is a long, thin, threadlike, cylindrical cell, less than the diameter of a human hair. Unlike other musculoskeletal tissues, muscle consists primarily of cells, contained within a highly organized matrix of connective tissue.

☐ The fibers are arranged in tightly packed, highly ordered parallel arrays, like collagen, and are collected in bundles called **fascicles.**

☐ Each fiber is composed of thousands of myofibrils (literally, "muscle threads"), which are wound in a spiral like the weave of a rope.

☐ The myofibril is subdivided into functional units known as the sarcomeres, composed of thousands of strands of proteins, also arranged in parallel, called *myofilaments.* The myofilaments are composed of actin and myosin, the proteins of contraction.

☐ Microscopically, the actin is arranged in a spiral, and recent studies show that muscle fibers and the associated connected tissue rotate (spiral) during contraction.[6]

☐ There are two types of skeletal muscle fibers:
  • The **extrafusal fiber** is under voluntary control. This is the typical muscle fiber.
  • The **intrafusal fiber,** or **muscle spindle,** lies embedded within the other fibers. This fiber functions as a sensory nerve receptor and operates without conscious control.

☐ In addition to the muscle fiber, every muscle contains **satellite cells**, which are stem cells, able to regenerate new muscle fibers in the event of injury to the muscle fiber.

▨ **Structure of connective tissue:** The muscle fibers are so interwoven with connective tissue that a more accurate term for muscle is ***myofascia.*** Three layers of connective tissue surround and support a muscle (see Fig. 1-13):

☐ Epimysium, a fascia of fibrous connective tissue that surrounds the entire muscle.

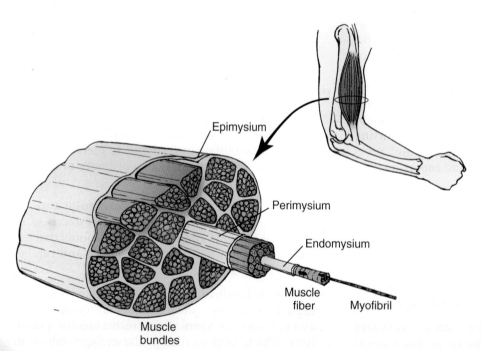

Epimysium

Perimysium

Endomysium

Muscle fiber   Myofibril

Muscle bundles

Figure 1-13. Anatomy of a muscle showing the layers of the connective tissue.

☐ Perimysium, a dense connective tissue, arranged in a spiral that surrounds each fascicle, a major component of the elastic quality of muscle. The perimysium is essential in maintaining the proper position of the muscle bundles.[37]

☐ Endomysium, a delicate, meshlike sheath that surrounds each individual fiber, providing mechanical support and acting as an elastic device, adding to the springy quality of muscle.

▨ **Function of connective tissue:**

☐ The connective tissue of muscle transmits the pull of the contracting muscle cells and gives the muscle fibers organization and support.

☐ The collagen fibers of these three layers of connective tissue form the tendon, which attaches the muscle to the bone. The tendon fibers interweave with the connective tissue of the periosteum, joint capsule, and ligaments.

☐ All of these connective tissue layers are lubricated in the healthy state. Muscles as a whole are designed to slide relative to each other, and each fascicle within the muscle is also capable of sliding relative to the other fascicles in the healthy state.

Muscle Function

▨ **Movement:** Muscles are responsible for all the movements of the body.

▨ **Proprioception:** There are three types of sensory nerve receptors in muscles (see below) that give the central nervous system information about the length, tension, pressure, movement, and sense of joint and body position in space.

▨ **Protection:** Muscles are connected to the nerves in the skin and to the nerves in the neighboring joint's capsule and ligaments through neurological reflexes; therefore, if the skin or joint is irritated or injured, the muscle can go into a reflexive spasm (called *splinting*) or into inhibition (weakness).

▨ **Pump:** The muscles are called a *musculovenous pump* because the contracting skeletal muscle compresses the veins and moves blood toward the heart.[34] This process of contraction and relaxation of the muscles is essential to normal health in that it is used to eliminate the body's waste products and to bring in nutrition, including oxygen.

▨ **Pain receptors:** Muscles have pain receptors (nociceptors) that fire with chemical or mechanical irritation.

▨ **Posture and stability:** Muscles are called *dynamic stabilizers* of the joints because they actively hold the joints in a stable position for posture and movement.

▨ **Signal transduction:** Muscle fibers and the associated connective tissue are highly ordered, tightly packed, parallel arrays. This arrangement can be described as a "liquid crystal," an ideal arrangement for the transmission of mechanical, electrical, and electromagnetic energy throughout the body.

Viscoelastic Property of a Muscle and Its Fascia

▨ Tension in a muscle and its fascia is created by active and passive elements. The passive elements include the collagen fibers and ground substance, and the active components include the contractile proteins—actin and myosin—and the nerves.

▨ The ability of a muscle to lengthen is termed *flexibility*, and the term *stiffness* describes resistance to lengthening. The limitation of a muscle's ability to stretch (lengthen) is primarily dependent on the connective tissue.[38]

▨ The connective tissue fibers of the muscle compose the **elastic** component. As was described previously, the connective tissue (fascia) of the muscle becomes the tendon. This fascia has a crimp or wavelike structure, similar to a spring. The tissue can be stretched within its normal limit and return to its resting length, in much the way that a spring can be pulled and released. When you stretch the fascia or pull on the fascia as you contract a muscle, energy is being stored, as in pulling a spring. The stored energy is released to create mechanical work or heat when the stretch or muscle contraction is released.

▨ Because muscle contains ground substance, it demonstrates **viscous** behavior. It becomes thicker and stiff when it is stretched quickly, is cold, or is immobilized. It becomes more fluid if the myofascia is stretched slowly or is warmed up.

The Muscle as Part of a Tensegrity Structure

Muscle is the tension member of the body that transmits the force of muscle contraction to the connective tissue to move the body and dynamically stabilize its posture. The bones are the compression members and cannot keep the body upright without the muscles and connective tissue. In other words, it is the tension members of the structure, not the bones, that hold the body upright. Buckminster Fuller[10] coined the word *tensegrity* to describe this type of structure. The strength and stability of a tensegrity structure, such as the human body, depend on the soft tissues, including muscles, fascia, tendons, ligaments, and joint capsules.

Role of Muscle in Movement and Stability

▨ **Agonist:** The muscle(s) that contracts to perform a certain movement is called the *agonist(s)*. This muscle is also called the prime mover. For example, the biceps is an agonist for elbow flexion. Keep in mind that all movements in the body are accomplished by more than one muscle.

▨ **Antagonist:** The muscle(s) that performs the opposite movement of the agonist is called the *antagonist(s)*. The triceps is the antagonist for the biceps, because the triceps extends the elbow.

▨ **Co-contraction:** When the agonist and antagonist are working simultaneously, they are co-contracting. For example, when you make a fist, the flexors and extensors of the wrist are co-contracting to keep the wrist in a position that ensures the greatest strength of the fingers. Typically, however, when the agonist is working, the antagonist is relaxing.
　□ **Sherrington's law of reciprocal inhibition** states that there is a neurologic inhibition of the antagonist when the agonist is working. When we contract the biceps to flex the elbow, the triceps is being neurologically inhibited (relaxed), which allows it to lengthen during elbow flexion. Co-contraction is an exception to this rule.

▨ **Synergist:** The muscle(s) that works with another muscle to accomplish a certain motion is called a *synergist(s)*. The term includes *stabilizers* (i.e., muscles that support a joint to allow the prime mover to work more efficiently) and *neutralizers* (i.e., muscles that prevent a certain motion as the agonist is working).

Tonic and Phasic Muscles

▨ **Structure:** Muscles can also be divided on the basis of which muscles have primarily a stabilizing role and which muscles have primarily a dynamic role. These categories are controversial because most muscles can function in both roles. However, it has been proved clinically useful because muscles react to pain in predictable ways, which are discussed below in the section "Dysfunction Due to Impaired Muscle Function."
　□ **Tonic (postural):** Muscles that play a primary role in maintaining posture and therefore function essentially as stabilizers are called *tonic muscles* or *postural muscles*.
　□ **Phasic:** Muscles whose primary roles are to perform quick movements are called *phasic muscles*.

▨ **Dysfunction and injury:** It has been found that tonic (postural) muscles react to stress by becoming short and tight and that phasic muscles react to stress by becoming inhibited and weak.[39] Janda and colleagues[40] have discovered that there are predictable patterns in which muscles tend to become tight and which muscles tend to become weak. His insights are incorporated throughout this text.

▨ **Treatment implications:** See the treatment implications discussed in the section "Muscle Dysfunction."

Innervation

▨ Two types of motor (efferent) nerves supply each muscle:
　□ **Alpha nerves:** The alpha nerves fire for voluntary and involuntary muscle contraction.
　□ **Gamma nerves:** The gamma nerves have voluntary and involuntary functions. They unconsciously help to set the muscle's tone in addition to its resting length, and they function during voluntary activities for fine muscular control.

▨ Three types of sensory (afferent) nerve receptors supply each muscle: two types of mechanoreceptors and nociceptors (pain receptors). The two specialized mechanoreceptors are called **muscle spindles** and **golgi tendon organs (GTOs)**, which detect muscle length and changes in length and muscle tension and changes in muscle tension, respectively (see "The Nervous System" and Figure 1-20 for further discussion).

Three Types of Voluntary Muscle Contraction

▨ **Isometric:** In an isometric contraction, the muscle contracts, but its length does not change. If, while sitting, you place your hand under the seat of your chair and attempt to lift the chair, your biceps isometrically contracts, but the origin and insertion do not move toward each other.

▨ **Concentric:** Concentric contraction is when a muscle shortens while it contracts (i.e., the origin and insertion move toward each other). As you bring a glass of water to your mouth, your biceps is shortening while it contracts.

▨ **Eccentric:** Eccentric contraction is when the origin and insertion move apart while a muscle contracts. As you lower the glass back to the table, your biceps is lengthening while it maintains some contraction. The muscle generates maximum strength during eccentric contraction, but it is more susceptible to injury. Another example is the hamstrings, which contract eccentrically at the end of the swing phase, just before heel strike, to decelerate the lower leg and control the extension of the knee during running.

Relationship Between Muscle Length and Tension

A muscle develops its maximum strength or tension at its resting length or just short of its resting length because the actin and myosin filaments have the maximum contact (crossbridges). When a muscle is excessively shortened or lengthened, it loses its ability to perform a strong contraction. A muscle can develop only moderate tension in the lengthened position and minimum tension in the shortened position. For example, if the wrist is maximally flexed, the ability to make a fist is diminished because the finger flexors are in a shortened position.

Involuntary Muscle Contraction By Voluntary Muscles

- Withdrawal reflexes, such as pulling away from a hot stove, involve instantaneous muscle contraction.

- Righting reflexes from the ligaments and joint capsule communicate to the muscle and stimulate instantaneous muscle contraction for protection of the joint and associated soft tissue.

- Arthrokinetic reflexes create unconscious muscle contraction (or inhibition) of muscles surrounding a joint caused by irritation in the joint (see "Function of the Joint Receptors").

- Splinting or involuntary muscle contraction can be caused by muscle, bone, or joint injury.

- Emotional or psychological stress creates excessive and sustained muscle tension.

- The maintenance of posture involves unconscious muscle contraction.

MUSCLE INJURY

- A muscle injury is called a **strain** or "pulled muscle" and is usually a tear within the fibers themselves, disrupting the sarcolemma, the membrane that covers the muscle fiber.[38] More extensive injuries disrupt the connective tissue layers surrounding and imbedded within the muscle. Muscle strains typically involve excessive active muscle stretching, or eccentric contraction, especially in two-joint muscles, such a hamstrings, gastrocnemius, and rectus femoris.

- Muscle strains are classified in three grades, although it is difficult to assess the severity:[21]

- ☐ **Grade I:** Mild injury, with minimal structural damage.
- ☐ **Grade II:** Moderate injury, with significant functional loss.
- ☐ **Grade III:** Severe injury, a complete tear with complete loss of function that might require surgery.

- **Areas of injury:** Injury usually occurs at the junction where the muscle and tendon meet, called the **myotendinous junction,** and secondarily where the tendon attaches to the periosteum of the bone, called the **tenoperiosteal junction.** There are two reasons why muscles are likely to fail at these sites:
  - ☐ The myotendinous junction is stiffer than other areas of the muscle, making it the weakest link. For all muscles, failure consistently occurs near the myotendinous junction.[23]
  - ☐ Junction sites of ligament, tendon, and joint capsules are relatively avascular and have an increased stiffness. These junctions, therefore, are more prone to injury.[23]

- Tearing of muscle initiates an inflammatory reaction, and the typical stages of healing (see, "Stages of Inflammation and Repair" below). Two processes are initiated: the regeneration of new muscle fibers and the repair of connective tissue.

- Within days of injury, satellite cells become activated and are transformed into new muscle fibers. At the same time, fibroblasts increase the production of collagen and ground substance to generate a new connective tissue framework. Because of the development of abnormal crosslinks in the collagen and adhesions within the muscle's fascia, a muscle typically shortens and loses some of its extensibility after an injury. Without adequate movement, adhesions form between the connective tissue layers, leading to decreased function. With severe injuries involving large ruptures, formation of excessive collagen results in contractures or dense, nodular scars, severely limiting motion.

- Symptoms vary from severe loss of function, such as the inability to bear weight with a severe gastrocnemius tear, to a mild soreness. If a muscle injury is painful at rest, the area is inflamed. There may be swelling, bruising, and spasm. Examination reveals pain with isometric challenge of the involved muscle and pain to palpation.

- **Treatment implications:** The key to treatment is to promote pain-free mobility. Early mobilization promotes rapid capillary ingrowth, regeneration of muscle fibers, and a more parallel orientation of the fibers compared with immobilization.[26] For **acute** injuries, the first treatment goal is to reduce the swelling. If circulation is decreased because of swelling, the repair process is compromised. Gentle passive motion in flexion-extension planes and very light contract-relax (CR) or reciprocal inhibition(RI) MET help to pump excess fluid out of the site of injury. STM, joint mobilization, and MET minimize adhesion formation, promote circulation for the delivery of oxygen and removal of waste products, increase lubrication for the normal gliding of the structures, and promote proper parallel alignment of the collagen and muscle fibers. Movement also stimulates the regeneration of new connective tissue and muscle fibers. MET promotes muscle regeneration that is stimulated by the longitudinal pulling force of muscle contraction.[16] As with all acute injuries, care must be taken in the first few days after injury that excessive motion is not applied, because it can result in further disruption and excessive scar formation. For **chronic** muscle conditions, the treatment goals are to use STM, joint mobilization, and MET to restore flexibility by dissolving adhesions and lengthening connective tissue, eliminating muscle hypertonicity, restoring normal muscle firing patterns, restoring strength, and promoting neurological function through sensory awareness and reeducating proprioception (See Chapter 2, "Assessment and Technique"). Immobilization causes decreased cellular activity, decreased collagen in the fascia, and loss of muscle fibers (atrophy).

MUSCLE DYSFUNCTION

Muscle Dysfunction: A New Concept in Orthopedics

- **Definition:** Muscle dysfunction is defined as loss of normal function of the muscle. There are many types of dysfunction: sustained hypertonicity, sustained inhibition (neurological), sustained weakness (deconditioning or atrophy), adaptive shortening (contractures of connective tissue elements), myofascial trigger points (hypersensitive palpable nodules), abnormal position, and abnormal torsion.

Causes of Muscle Dysfunction

- **Poor posture:** Sitting or standing with poor posture creates cumulative stress. Because of the viscoelastic properties of muscle and connective tissue, they will remodel (adapt) to the stresses that are placed on them. For example, rounded-shoulders posture leads to a shortening of the fascia of the anterior chest and tightening of the pectoralis minor. There are also lengthening and weakness of the posterior fascia and muscles.

- **Static stress:** Sitting or standing for long periods is fatiguing. As with poor posture, muscles and fascia adapt to stress by depositing excessive connective tissue in areas of excessive stress and creating atrophy of the muscle and soft tissue in areas of reduced stress.

- **Muscle injury:** A muscle can become hypertonic owing to injury (strain), leading to involunatry guarding or reflex spasms; or it can become weak from injury or posttraumatic atrophy.

- **Joint dysfunction or injury:** Injury or dysfunction to the joint can lead to a reflexive increase in tone (hypertonicity) or decrease in tone (hypotonicity) depending on the specific muscles around the joint, called the *arthrokinetic reflex* by Wyke.[41] Predictable patterns of hypertonicity and inhibition are fully described by Janda (see below).

- **Emotional or psychological stress:** Anxiety and anger can create sustained muscle contraction, and depression can cause sustained weakness in the muscles.

- **Chronic overuse:** A muscle fails to relax after intense use, leading to ischemia and tension myositis (pain in the muscle caused by sustained contraction).

- **Disuse:** Deconditioned syndrome is a phenomenon in which a muscle is weakened owing to lack of use. This phenomenon precedes muscle atrophy.

- **Viscerosomatic reflexes:** An irritation or inflammation in a visceral organ can cause a muscle spasm. For example, a kidney infection can cause a spasm of the lumbar muscles.

Three Common Types of Muscle Dysfunction

Myofascial Pain Syndrome (Trigger Points)
- Myofascial pain syndrome is a chronic, regional pain syndrome, characterized by myofascial trigger points. The trigger point is a hypersensitive palpable nodule in a tight band of muscle, which is painful on compression. Trigger points are associated with decreased ROM, decreased muscular strength, and increased pain with stretching.

- **Treatment implications:** The method of treatment that is described in this text based on the author's clinical experience supports studies that show that trigger points are effectively and painlessly treated with postisometric relaxation (PIR) MET.[42]

Dysfunction Caused by Abnormal Position and Abnormal Torsion

▨ As has been mentioned, Lauren Berry, RPT, contributed a revolutionary concept in manual therapy. He theorized that all soft tissue has a specific position relative to the neighboring soft tissues and the joint that they affect and that muscles, tendons, ligaments, bursae, and nerves can become malpositioned. This text describes the patterns of the abnormal position in the soft tissue and the treatment to correct positional dysfunction.

    ☐ Abnormal position in the anterior deltoid provides an example of positional dysfunction. In the rounded-shoulders posture, the anterior deltoid rolls or winds into a more anterior-inferior position relative to the shoulder joint (the glenohumeral joint). This abnormal position decreases the function of the muscle and contributes to the dysfunction of the shoulder (Fig. 1-14).

▨ The author has developed this concept further and theorizes that this malposition creates an abnormal torsion or twist in the muscle and fascia, including the fascicles and fibers, down to the microscopic level, creating *interfascicular torsion.*

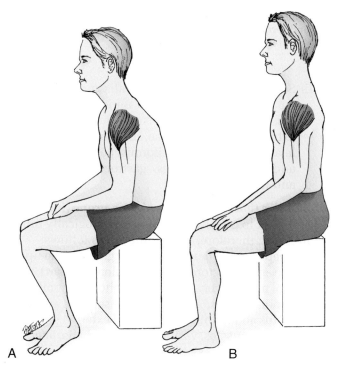

Figure 1-14. A. In a slumped, rounded-shoulder posture, the fascicles of the anterior deltoid roll into an abnormal position and abnormal torsion. The muscle twists into an internally rotated position. **B.** In the normal upright posture, the fascicles of the deltoid are aligned in a superior direction.

▨ **Treatment implications:** The muscle and fascia need to be stroked in a specific direction. In the case of the anterior deltoid, it needs to be stroked superiorly and posteriorly to restore its normal position and function and to release the torsion within the fascicles. This text describes each muscle's positional dysfunction and the direction of the massage strokes necessary to correct it.

Dysfunction Caused by Impaired Muscle Function

▨ Janda and colleagues[40] and Lewit[43] use the expression *functional pathology of the motor system* to describe unconscious reflexes from the central or the peripheral nervous system that cause sustained hypertonicity or sustained inhibition (weakness) in the muscles. Pain always creates impaired function, but impaired function can take years to develop into pain.

▨ The most important signs of impaired muscle function according to Janda[44] are as follows:

    ☐ **Increased muscle tone (muscle hypertonicity):** Muscles that are held in a sustained contraction are an important factor in the genesis of pain. Hypertonicity has many causes (see "Patterns of Inhibition [Weakness] and Hypertonicity").

    ☐ **Muscle inhibition/muscle weakness:** *Inhibition* refers to a decreased capacity of a muscle to neurologically respond to stimuli.[18] *Weakness* refers to an inability of a muscle to generate force. A short and tight muscle may be functionally weak as well as inhibited. The inhibition and weakness create joint instability and cause other muscles to become hypertonic in compensation.

    ☐ **Muscle imbalance:** Muscle imbalance is a change in function in the muscles crossing a joint, in which certain muscles react to stress by getting short and tight and others become weak. This is an important factor in chronic pain syndromes because this imbalance alters the movement pattern of the joint.

    ☐ **Joint dysfunction:** Muscle dysfunction creates an uneven distribution of forces on the weight-bearing surfaces of the joint, predisposing it to degeneration and dysfunction of the sensory nerves that provide critical information about the position and movement characteristics of the joint.

    ☐ **Abnormal muscle firing pattern:** Muscle dysfunction is often expressed by abnormal patterns of contraction. For example, hip abduction should typically be performed by the gluteus medius, but the tensor fascia lata often substitutes for this action because of a weak gluteus medius.

▓ **Treatment implications:** Impaired muscle function is best treated with MET. Having the client actively contract muscles in a precise and controlled way engages the higher brain centers, the sensory-motor cortex, to override unconscious patterns in the lower brain, and reeducates the reflexes between the muscle, joint, and spinal cord. For example, it is typical for the gluteus maximus to be weak and inhibited in clients with chronic low back pain. It is important to "recruit" the muscle by having the client consciously contract the muscle to reeducate the neuromuscular connection. Refer to "The Nervous System" below and to Chapter 2 for further discussion.

Patterns of Inhibition (Weakness) and Hypertonicity

▓ Janda and colleagues[40] discovered clinically that muscles react to pain or excessive stress in two opposite ways in predictable patterns. He found that certain muscles tend to become overactive, short, and tight, and he described these muscles as having a postural or stabilizing function, similar to tonic muscles. He found that other muscles tend to become inhibited and weak. He noticed that most of these muscles were concerned with movement rather than stability; therefore, he grouped inhibited and weak muscles as phasic muscles. An example of muscle imbalance is what Janda and colleagues[40] calls the **upper crossed syndrome** (Fig. 1-15). The terms *postural* and *phasic* have led to some confusion among clinicians and researchers, and more accurate terms have been suggested for these two groups: **tightness-prone** and **inhibition (weakness)-prone** muscles.[45]

▓ In addition to the causes of muscle dysfunction listed previously, soft tissue injury, chronic pain, and inflammation create disturbances in normal muscle function and can stimulate a neurological-based tightness or weakness in a muscle.

▓ An important difference between the two muscle groups is that a small reduction of strength in an inhibition-prone muscle initiates a disproportionately larger contraction of the antagonist tightness-prone muscle.[43] Janda and colleagues[40] notes that many of our work and recreational activities favor tightness-prone muscles getting stronger, tighter, and shorter as the inhibition-prone muscles become weaker and more inhibited. It is important, however, to realize that some muscles, such as the quadratus lumborum and the scalenes, can react with either tightness or weakness.

▓ **Muscles that tend to be tightness-prone** and react to pain or excessive stress with hypertonicity and eventual shortening are as follows:

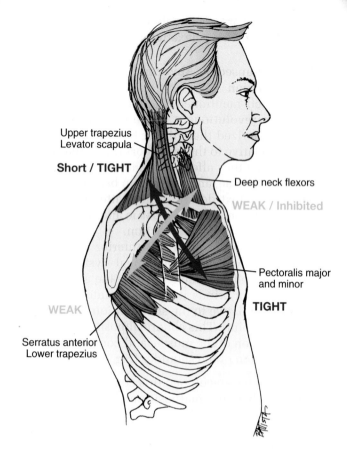

Figure 1-15. Upper crossed syndrome, a typical pattern of muscle imbalance. The upper trapezius and pectoralis major and minor are usually short and tight, and the deep neck flexors and serratus anterior and lower trapezius are typically weak and inhibited.

☐ Sternocleidomastoid, pectoralis major (clavicular and sternal parts), and minor, upper trapezius, levator scapulae, flexor groups of the upper extremity, erector spinae, iliopsoas, tensor fascia lata, rectus femoris, piriformis, pectineus, gracilis, adductors, hamstrings, gastrocnemius, soleus, and tibialis posterior.

▓ **Muscles that tend to be weakness-prone (inhibited)** and react to pain by becoming neurologically inhibited and, therefore, weakening are as follows:
☐ Deep cervical flexors, extensor group of the upper extremity, pectoralis major (abdominal part), middle and lower trapezius, deltoid, rhomboids, supraspinatus, infraspinatus, serratus anterior, rectus abdominus, internal and external obliques, gluteal muscles, vasti muscles (medialis, lateralis, and intermedius), tibialis anterior, and peroneals.

Consequences of a Hypertonic Muscle

▓ **Definition:** A muscle that is held in a sustained contraction is also called a *hypertonic muscle.*

This means that the muscle is constantly working. The most common causes of hypertonicity are stress, overuse, injury (pain), and joint dysfunction. This constant contraction has several effects.

☐ The muscle consumes more oxygen and energy than a muscle at rest and therefore contains more lactic-acid waste products, which irritate the nerves.

☐ Circulation is decreased because the muscle is not performing its normal function as a pump. This leads to ischemia, which is decreased oxygen, causing pain.

☐ The sustained tension in the muscle pulls on its attachments to the periosteum, joint capsule, and ligaments, creating increased pressure in the joint and loading the cartilage unevenly, which creates excessive wear in the joint and accelerated degeneration.

☐ Hypertonic muscles can compress the nerves that travel between the muscles or, in some cases, through the muscle. This leads to decreased nerve function and to paresthesias or altered sensations, typically, a "pins and needles" feeling. A common example is the compression of the sciatic nerve by a hypertonic piriformis muscle.

Consequences of an Inhibited (Weak) Muscle

▨ A healthy muscle functions to dynamically stabilize the joint. A weak muscle creates instability, which excessively stresses the passive stabilizers, which are the ligaments, and joint capsule. This leads to imbalanced forces moving through the joint and accelerates degeneration.

▨ Weakness contributes to poor posture, which creates areas of excessive tension and compression.

▨ Inhibition leads to loss of adequate motor control and to abnormal firing patterns in the muscle, leading to substitution of other muscles and abnormal joint movements.

▨ An inhibited muscle does not have adequate cycles of contraction; therefore, the pumping of the vascular system and lymphatics is diminished.

JOINT STRUCTURE AND FUNCTION

JOINT TYPES

▨ **Definition:** A joint is the connection (articulation) between two bones or cartilage elements. The body consists of over 150 joints, and they are classified by the type of tissue that unites the two bones.

▨ **Fibrous joint (synarthrodial):** A fibrous joint is united by fibrous tissue (e.g., sutures of the skull) that has little movement.

▨ **Cartilaginous joint (amphiarthrosis):** A cartilaginous joint is united by fibrocartilage (e.g., symphysis pubis) and the intervertebral discs of the spine and have slight movement.

▨ **Synovial joint (diarthrosis):** The most common joint in the body is the synovial joint. The joint has a joint cavity filled with synovial fluid, and the two bones are surrounded by a joint capsule and are characterized by having free mobility.

COMPONENTS OF SYNOVIAL JOINT

There are seven structures that are common to all synovial joints: (1) synovial membrane, (2) synovial fluid, (3) joint capsule, (4) capsular ligaments, (5) articular cartilage, (6) blood vessels, and (7) sensory nerves.[22] We will describe each of these below. Other structures that may form part of the joint are the intra-articular discs or menisci; labrum, which is a fibrocartilage rim found in the hip and shoulder; and fat pads, found between the synovial membrane and fibrous capsule in some joints, such as the knee and elbow.

Joint Capsule

▨ **Structure:** The joint capsule forms a fibrous cuff around synovial joints. The attachment encircles the bones that form the joint, usually at the border of the articular cartilage. It is composed of two layers (Fig. 1-16). The outer layer is fibrous connective tissue organized in parallel bundles, and the inner layer is synovial tissue. The outer layer is reinforced with intrinsic and extrinsic ligaments. Intrinsic or capsular ligaments are thickenings within the body of the capsule, whereas extrinsic ligaments lie superficial to the capsule. Many of the tendinous insertions of muscles interweave with the joint capsule. For example, the multifidus, rectus femoris (reflected head), vastus medialis and lateralis, pectoralis major, teres major, biceps, triceps, tendons of the rotator cuff, and most of the forearm flexors all interweave directly with the capsule. The inner layer is also called the *synovial membrane* and covers all the intra-articular structures except the load-bearing articular cartilage and meniscus. It has a rich network of blood vessels and lymphatics and is lined with cells called **synoviocytes**. The synovial layer also has small projections, called *villi*, which secrete synovial fluid when they are stimulated through joint movement.

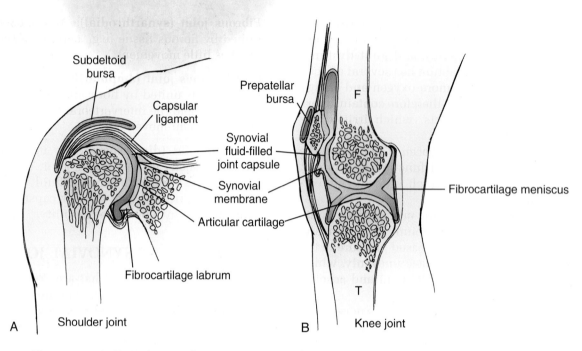

Figure 1-16. A. Typical synovial joint. **B.** Knee joint showing the fibrocartilage meniscus and bursae, which are additional features of a synovial joint.

Function:

□ The outer layer helps to stabilize the joint, helps to guide joint motion, and prevents excessive motion. It is innervated with a rich supply of nerves, including mechanoreceptors and pain fibers. The mechanoreceptors sense the rate and speed of motion, position sense (proprioception), and have reflex connections to the muscles (see "Innervation" below). Irritation or injury to the capsule can create muscle contractions, designed to protect the joint.

□ The inner layer of the joint capsule is a synovial membrane that secretes synovial fluid when it is stimulated by joint motion. Maintaining joint motion is critical, because the joint dries out and degenerates if it is not moved.

Dysfunction and injury:

□ **Outer fibrous layer:** Injury to the joint capsule may result from acute trauma or repetitive stress. Fibrosis or thickening of the joint capsule is caused by an increased production of collagen and by a decrease in ground substance. It occurs in three conditions: acute inflammation, chronic irritation or inflammation caused by repetitive stresses or imbalanced forces moving through the joint, and immobilization.[46] A tight, fibrotic joint capsule results in abnormal movement between the joint surfaces, leading to excessive compression in certain areas of the cartilage and to accelerated degeneration of the joint. The capsule and supporting ligaments may also be

excessively stretched because of injury. If there is a loss of adequate motion owing to immobilization, the fibrous layer of the joint capsule atrophies because of a loss of collagen. This creates joint instability.

□ **Inner synovial layer:** The synovial membrane can become injured or dysfunctional because of acute trauma to the joint, cumulative stresses from chronic irritation caused by imbalanced forces moving through the joint, or immobilization. Joint swelling occurs during inflammation. The swelling typically causes abnormal muscle function controlling the joint. Immobilization, on the other hand, thickens the synovial fluid with disuse and causes an eventual decrease in the amount of synovial fluid. This leads to adhesions between the capsule and the articular cartilage, tendon sheaths, and bursae, contributing to stiffness and consequent degeneration in the joint.

Treatment implications:

□ **For outer fibrous layer:** The initial treatment goal for acute injury to the capsule is to help manage the inflammation by reducing the swelling. Gentle, low force CR and RI MET and gentle, pain-free passive motion are used to pump the swelling out of the joint and promote the circulation of cells, oxygen, and nutrition and the removal of waste products. Gentle STM is begun immediately to help realign the healing fibers and to prevent adhesions. For chronic conditions, PIR MET is performed on the muscles of the associated joint. As the muscle's fascia interweaves with the joint capsule at the tenoperiosteal junction, isometric muscle contractions pull on the capsule and increase its extensibility. STM and joint mobilization are used to reduce adhesions. The massage strokes are directed in all directions, owing to the irregular alignment of the collagen. This stroke process is analogous to removing a tuck from a sheet: You spread it in all directions to smooth it out.

☐ PIR MET is performed to help restore length in the shortened capsule. Because myofascia interweaves with the joint capsule, a lengthening response of the capsule can be induced with muscle contractions. This has proved very effective clinically. For example, osteoarthritis of the hip is associated with loss of internal rotation due to shortening of the joint capsule. By performing MET to increase internal rotation, the capsule is lengthened, and the range of motion is improved, often with dramatic functional improvement.

☐ **For an atrophied or excessively stretched capsule:** A capsule that is too loose needs exercise rehabilitation to help lay down new collagen fibers, restore normal length, and stimulate the synthesis of chondrocytes and synviocytes and needs coordination and proprioception exercises to help restore neurological function.

☐ **For an acute, swollen synovial layer:** A swollen capsule is called *synovitis* and is treated with CR MET to use the muscle contractions to help pump the excess fluid out of the capsule. Pain-free, passive range of motion is also used in the flexion-extension plane to act as a mechanical pump. If there is too little fluid in the joint, the MET and passive mobilizations of the joint help to stimulate the synovial membrane, increasing synovial fluid and therefore increasing lubrication and nutrition in the joint. STM is used to disperse the excess fluid.

Ligaments

Dense connective tissue surrounds every joint and is called **periarticular soft tissue**. It is composed of fascia, periosteum, tendons, the external layer of the capsule, and ligaments. *Extrinsic ligaments* lie over the joint capsule and attach to the bones that form the joint, and *intrinsic ligaments* (capsular ligaments) are thickenings of the joint capsule. The ligaments are fully described in "Connective Tissue" above.

Cartilage

■ **Definition:** Cartilage is a dense, fibrous connective tissue composed of collagen, ground substance, a high percentage of water, and chondrocytes or cartilage cells. Synovial joints have two types of cartilage: articular or hyaline cartilage and fibrocartilage.

Articular Cartilage (Hyaline Cartilage)

■ **Structure:** Articular cartilage is composed of cells, including chondrocytes and fibroblasts, and extracellular matrix, including collagen and ground substance. Articular cartilage is 70% to 80% water. Cartilage has no nerve or blood supply. The subchondral bone (the bone under the cartilage) also provides oxygen and nutrition through blood vessels.

■ **Function:** Hyaline or articular cartilage covers the ends of bones and provides a smooth gliding surface for opposing joint surfaces. It also distributes loads and protects the underlying bone. It is elastic and porous and functions like a sponge, in that it has the capacity to absorb and bind synovial fluid. Intermittent compression and decompression creates a pumping action, which causes the movement of synovial fluid in and out of the cartilage. Cartilage is self-lubricating as long as it moves. As in other connective tissues, water plays a significant role in normal function. It is a medium for nutritional exchange and for lubrication and gives cartilage its rigidity to resist compressive forces. Water is also a medium for carrying mechanical, electrical, and electromagnetic energy. Even though cartilage has no nerve or blood supply, the chondrocytes and matrix of collagen and water are very sensitive to mechanical stimuli and act as mechanical signal transducers.[5] With a mechanical stimulus, such as the compression to the cartilage during walking, the stimulus is transformed (transduced) from a mechanical signal to chemical, electrical, and electromagnetic signals. With stimulation, cells synthesize new cells and matrix to maintain and repair the cartilage, whereas with immobilization and disuse, the cells and matrix atrophy and deteriorate.[47]

There are three normal ways in which the synovial joint goes through cycles of compression and decompression: locomotion (walking, running), intermittent contraction of the muscles, and twisting and untwisting of the joint capsule.[48]

Fibrocartilage

■ **Structure:** Consists of dense, white fibrous connective tissue, mostly collagen, arranged in dense bundles or layered sheets with chondrocytes, glycoaminoglycans, and about 70% to 80% water. It is innervated only at the periphery and has a rich blood supply at the outer portion where it attaches to ligaments and joint capsule. Nutrition is largely dependent on diffusion through the synovial fluid created by movement. As in articular cartilage, the subchondral bone (the bone under the cartilage) also provides oxygen and nutrition through blood vessels.

▥ **Function:** The fibrocartilage absorbs shock, lubricates the joint, distributes load, and stabilizes the joint. It has great tensile strength combined with considerable elasticity. Fibrocartilage deepens a joint space, such as the cartilage labrum or lip of the hip and shoulder; allows two bones to fit together better, such as the menisci of the knee; acts as a shock absorber, such as the intervertebral discs of the spine; and lines body grooves for tendons, such as in the bicipital groove for the long head of biceps.

▥ **Dysfunction and injury:** Damage to cartilage may be caused by many factors: acute trauma; cumulative stresses, either dynamic stresses, such as running, or static stresses, such as prolonged standing; obesity; immobilization; joint instability; or abnormal forces moving through the joint. Acute blunt trauma, such as falling on the knees, can damage the articular cartilage even without fracture. It is akin to a "bruise" with swelling of the cartilage and pain. The internal structure is disrupted; and without proper rehabilitation, the joint can degenerate, becoming stiff and painful, a condition called *post-traumatic arthritis*.[48] Abnormal forces are often the result of imbalances in the muscles surrounding the joint, a tight joint capsule, or joint instability due to atrophied ligaments and capsular tissues. A tight capsule creates a high-contact area in the cartilage and decreased lubrication. Imbalanced muscles create altered weight distribution through the joint, causing excessive pressures on the cartilage and fatigue in the cartilage. Atrophied ligaments and capsular tissues allow excessive joint motion, causing abrasion of the cartilage. The highly vascular synovial tissue responds with inflammation, leading to swelling and pain. Because there is a blood supply in the outer third of the cartilage, repair can occur in this region through the normal inflammatory response. But the inner portion of cartilage lacks blood vessels, and damage does not initiate an inflammatory response as is the case for other musculoskeletal tissues. The cartilage degenerates, beginning with fracturing of the collagen fibers (fibrillation) and depletion of the ground substance. The cartilage then develops cracks and loses its shock absorbing function. Eventually, it wears down, and the capsule become thickened and dried out. **Osteoarthritis** is degeneration of the cartilage of a joint.

▥ **Treatment implications:** It has been assumed that cartilage cannot repair itself, but as Hertling and Kessler[18] point out, recent studies show that cartilage cells (chondrocytes) can stay active and lay down new cartilage and that arthritis is "somewhat reversible if managed correctly." The joint must be moved to stimulate the synthesis of chondrocytes and the secretion of synovial fluid. Joint mobilization in flexion and extension pumps synovial fluid into and out of the joint. Rhythmic oscillations and MET wind and unwind the joint capsule to pump the fluid into and out of the cartilage, rehydrating the cartilage. During STM, we wind and unwind the joint capsule and compress and decompress the area we are working on to promote fluid exchange.

Bursa

▥ **Structure:** Bursae are synovial-filled sacs lined with a synovial membrane that are found in areas of increased friction. Examples include the subdeltoid bursa between the deltoid muscle and the acromion process and the trochanteric bursa on the side of the hip. There are over 150 bursae in the body.

▥ **Function:** The function of a bursa is to secrete synovial fluid between muscles, tendons, and bones, which decreases friction.

▥ **Dysfunction and injury:** A bursa is susceptible to acute trauma or repetitive stress. Bursitis is typically caused by excessive friction between the muscles, tendons, and fascia, the bursa, and the bones that lie underneath. Because there are pressure receptors in the bursa, a swollen bursa can be extremely painful. A chronic bursa can remain swollen or dry out, creating adhesions within the sac. In acute bursitis, symptoms appear suddenly. There is deep, throbbing pain, and the person has difficulty moving the affected joint. Chronic bursitis manifests as pain and limited active movement and also as painful passive motion.

▥ **Treatment implications:** Lauren Berry, RPT, contributed an effective treatment for bursitis. The method involves a gentle, slow, continuous stroke over the bursa to help massage the excess fluid out. If a bursa has dried out, the same strokes are applied more deeply to help stimulate the synovial membrane to secrete fluid.

Innervation of the Joints

▥ **Structure:** Embedded within the joint capsule, ligaments, and periosteum surrounding each joint are specialized sensory nerves called *mechanoreceptors*, which transduce or transform mechanical stimuli into electrical, electromagnetic, and chemical signals. They are named *Ruffini endings*, *Pacinian corpuscles*, *Golgi organ-like receptors*, and *free nerve endings*.[49] They can be categorized into four types:[41]

☐ **Type I:** Type I receptors, also called *Ruffini endings*, are mechanoreceptors that provide information concerning the static and dynamic position of the joint. They are sensitive to tension or stretch on ligaments and capsule, including stretch due to swelling. They have a very low threshold, so they respond to very small increases in tension.[30] Type I receptors are located in the superficial layers of the joint capsule and in ligaments.

☐ **Type II:** Type II receptors, also called *Pacinian corpuscles*, are dynamic mechanoreceptors that provide information on acceleration and deceleration of movement. They are sensitive to changes in joint position and to compression of the joint capsule. Type II receptors are found in the deep layers of the fibrous joint capsule.

☐ **Type III:** Type III receptors, also known as *Golgi-type receptors*, are dynamic mechanoreceptors monitoring the direction of movement, are sensitive to mechanical stress and have reflex effects on muscle tone to provide a "breaking effect." They respond only when high tensions are generated. Type III receptors are found in the intrinsic and extrinsic joint ligaments.

☐ **Type IV:** Type IV receptors are free-nerve endings that serve as pain receptors (nociceptors) when the tissue surrounding the joint senses excessive mechanical stress, when the tissue is irritated by inflammatory chemicals, or when the nerve is damaged. Nociceptors are inactive under normal conditions. They have increased sensitivity and fire more easily when the joint is inflamed or swollen. Type IV receptors are found in capsules, ligaments, and periosteum.

■ **Function:** Sensory nerves innervating the ligaments, capsule, and periosteum surrounding the joint convey instantaneous information on the functional status of the joint to the surrounding muscles. They also communicate automatically with the central nervous system. The functions of the sensory nerves are as follows:

☐ Control posture, coordination, and balance.
☐ Control the direction and speed of movement.
☐ Give information about the position of the joint and body image.
☐ Report pain in the joint when the joint is irritated or inflamed.
☐ Provide instantaneous reflex control of the muscles surrounding the joint. This is called the **arthrokinetic reflex**.[40] The arthrokinetic reflex

facilitates (strengthens) or inhibits muscles and coordinates agonists, antagonists, and synergists around the joint for posture, movement, reflexive guarding, and fine muscular control. Joint stability is dependent on the normal function of the mechanoreceptors.

■ **Dysfunction and Injury of Joint Receptors**
☐ Musculoskeletal injuries can lead to swelling or damage to the mechanoreceptors, which decreases arthrokinetic reflex activity. This leads to decreased proprioception (position sense); balance disturbances; abnormalities in posture, muscle coordination, and movement control; loss of fine motor control; slowed reaction times; altered movement patterns; altered muscle firing patterns; and muscle weakness. Pain from injury also causes some muscles to become weak (inhibited) and other muscles to become short and tight (facilitated) in predictable patterns. As was mentioned previously, Janda and colleagues[40] have described these patterns of muscle dysfunctions (see "Muscle Dysfunction"). Each chapter in this text will describe the patterns for each joint.

☐ Chronic dysfunction of the mechanoreceptors from adhesions (prior injury), immobilization, aging, or deconditioning can lead to mechanoreceptor atrophy.[49] If the dysfunction in sensory nerve function is not rehabilitated, it can lead to muscle atrophy, instability, and recurrent injuries and can contribute to degeneration of the joint.[16]

☐ Irritation of the pain receptors and mechanoreceptors typically causes the flexors of the joint to become facilitated or hypertonic and the extensors of the joint to become inhibited or weak.[50]

■ **Treatment implications:** Neuromuscular reeducation is also called sensory-motor rehabilitation and describes therapy to improve functional communication between the nervous system and the muscles and periarticular soft tissue. STM, joint mobilization, and MET stimulate mechanoreceptors and improve their function.[30] The clinical effects of sensorimotor rehabilitation are as follows: It induces muscle relaxation, increases muscle strength, improves posture (proprioception), improves muscle firing patterns and movement (kinesthesia), decreases pain, and increases range of motion.[30] Because MET is performed using the focused attention of the client, the higher brain centers are engaged, which helps to establish better communication from the central nervous system to the muscles and articular nerves. MET also provides feedback and guidance from the therapist that improves proprioception. Balance training is recommended not only for injuries to the lower extremeties, but also for injuries to the lumbosacral spine.

JOINT MOVEMENT: FUNCTION, DYSFUNCTION, AND TREATMENT

JOINT STABILITY AND MOVEMENT

▨ For a joint to perform a full and painless range of motion, it must be stable. Otherwise, abnormal forces move through the joint, leading to excessive wear and tear on the articular surfaces. This stability is determined by several factors:

- ☐ The **shape of the bones** that make up the joint affect stability. The hip joint sits deeply within the socket (acetabulum) of the pelvis; therefore, it is much more stable than is the glenohumeral joint of the shoulder, because the fossa of the glenoid cavity is shallow.

- ☐ **Passive stability** is provided by the ligaments and joint capsule. Because the ligaments and joint capsule do not have contractile fibers, their role is passive.

- ☐ **Dynamic stability** is provided by the muscles. As has been mentioned, it is important for the muscles that cross a joint to be balanced, or the forces that move through the joint will create uneven stresses, leading to dysfunction and eventual degeneration of the cartilage.

NORMAL JOINT MOVEMENTS

▨ Movement of the body can be described as movement between the two bones, called *osteokinematics*, or between the joint surfaces, called *arthrokinematics*. Elevation of the arm describes the motion of the humerus relative to the glenoid fossa, an osteokinematic movement. During elevation, the head of the humerus is rolling and sliding on the glenoid fossa, an arthrokinematic movement. The three fundamental motions between joint surfaces are roll, slide, and spin.[22]

▨ Normal joint movements open and close the joint surfaces, which wind and unwind the joint capsule and ligaments, keeping the ligaments and joint in a relatively open and relaxed position, or creating compression of the joint surfaces and tightening the capsule. Most of the manual therapy that is described in this text is performed with the joint in the open or resting position, so it is important for the therapist to know when a joint is in the open or closed position.

- ☐ When a joint is in the **close-packed position,** the joint surfaces are most compressed, and the joint capsule and ligaments are tightest.

- ☐ When a joint is in the **loose (open)-packed position,** the joint is most open, and the joint capsule and ligaments are somewhat lax. Generally, extension closes the joint, and flexion opens the joint surfaces.

▨ John Mennell, MD,[51] has introduced the concept of **joint play,** which describes arthrokinematic movements that can be produced passively (i.e., by the therapist) but not voluntarily. In most joint positions, a joint has some "play" that is essential for normal joint function. For example, you can move the distal part of your index finger from side to side, a movement that cannot be accomplished actively.

▨ Arthrokinematic movements are also called **accessory movements**, and are essential for normal range of motion. As discussed below, an essential goal of joint mobilization is to restore passive, accessory joint motion (joint play).

JOINT DYSFUNCTION

▨ Mennell[51] also introduced the concept of **joint dysfunction** as a cause of pain and disability. He defines *joint dysfunction* as "a loss of joint play movements." This definition is the same as the chiropractic concept of **joint fixation.** Joint dysfunction has many causes, but may be divided into two broad categories:

- ☐ From within the joint, including intra-articular adhesions, roughened surfaces of the joint cartilage, meniscoidal entrapment in the facet joints of the spine, and degenerative joint disease.

- ☐ From the surrounding soft tissue, including adhesions or shortening of the joint capsule or ligaments (periarticular adhesions), sustained muscle contraction, strength/weakness imbalances of the muscles crossing the joint, and abnormal firing patterns of the muscles moving the joint. Korr[52] hypothesized that sustained muscle contraction could be the major factor in decreased mobility of the dysfunctioning joint.

▨ **Treatment implications:** Therapists need to be able to distinguish between pain and dysfunction arising from within the joint and pain and dysfunction arising from the surrounding soft tissue. For dysfunction that arises within the joint, MET and joint mobilization are performed (see below). For soft tissue restrictions surrounding the joint, STM and MET are applied. Short and tight muscles must be lengthened and relaxed, and muscles that are weak and inhibited need to be reeducated to regain their normal firing pattern and strength. Muscles cannot be restored to normal if the joints they move are restricted, and the joints will not regain their normal movement characteristics if the muscles that move the joint are not relaxed and strong and if the ligaments and joint capsule are not normalized. It is important to realize that a joint can have too much play, owing to a loss of stability in the ligaments or muscles. These conditions are treated with exercise rehabilitation to strengthen and stabilize the area.

JOINT DEGENERATION

▨ Joint degeneration refers to the degeneration of the cartilage but affects all of the structures of the joint, including the capsule, ligaments, muscles, blood vessels, and nerves. The fibrous capsule, ligaments, and synovium become thickened, leading to capsular tightness. Muscles become either inhibited (weakened) or facilitated (hypertonic), and blood vessels and sensory nerves atrophy. Degeneration is caused by trauma; cumulative stress, including joint dysfunction and posture; and muscular and movement imbalances.

▨ Most conditions that are called *arthritis* are in fact noninflammatory and should be referred to as **arthrosis**, meaning "joint degeneration." The terms *osteoarthritis* and *degenerative joint disease* are typically used interchangeably to describe a chronic degeneration of a joint.

▨ One common cause of joint degeneration is joint dysfunction, a loss of normal movement of the joint. This altered movement can occur as a result of a prior trauma or cumulative stress on the joint, leading to restrictions within the joint, or from the surrounding soft tissue, described above.

▨ **Treatment implications:** Therapists can improve the function of most cases of joint degeneration. The primary goals of treatment are to rehydrate the cartilage, lengthen capsular tissues, reduce excessive muscular tension, facilitate inhibited muscles, and improve function of the sensory nerves. STM is performed to dissolve adhesions, and MET is used to lengthen capsular tissues, wind and unwind the capsule to stimulate the movement of synovial fluid within the joint, and improve the range of motion. Joint mobilization is used to remove restrictive barriers within the joint to improve accessory motion. Clients with degenerated joints need instruction in exercises to improve muscle strength and balance.

JOINT MOBILIZATION

▨ **Definition:** Joint mobilization is any form of passive movement at a joint.[18] Passive mobilization techniques are graded from I to IV and are usually performed as rhythmic oscillations. These movements

are within the scope of practice for the massage therapist. Grade V is a high-velocity, low-amplitude thrust and is not within the scope of the massage therapist. The grades of joint mobilization are:[53]

☐ **Grade I:** Small-amplitude rhythmic oscillations performed at the beginning of the range.

☐ **Grade II:** Large-amplitude rhythmic oscillations perfomed within the free range and not moving into any resistance.

☐ **Grade III:** Large-amplitude rhythmic oscillations perfomed up to the limit of the range and into tissue resistance.

☐ **Grade IV:** Small-amplitude rhythmic oscillations performed at the limit of the range and into tissue resistance.

☐ **Grade V:** A small amplitude, high-velocity thrust.

▨ **The goals of joint mobilization are as follows:**

☐ To restore the normal joint play. Accessory motion must be normalized to allow for full range of motion and to prevent degeneration.

☐ To promote the exchange of cells and fluids in and out of the joint to promote joint repair and regeneration.

☐ To stimulate normal lubrication in the joint by stimulating the synovial membrane and promoting rehydration of the articular cartilage.

☐ To normalize neurological function by firing type III joint receptors and GTOs, resulting in a relaxation of the muscles surrounding the joint[54] (see "The Nervous System").

☐ To decrease swelling, which can cause pain, decreased motion, and tissue stagnation.

☐ To reduce pain. Mechanoreceptor stimulation overrides pain information in the brain, and studies suggests that joint mobilization in pain-free ranges can have an analgesic effect.[30]

THE NERVOUS SYSTEM

GENERAL OVERVIEW

The nervous system could be described as having two parallel and distinct systems: the connective tissue–water system, which carries electric and electromagnetic waves, and the "classic" nervous system, which carries chemical (ionic) currents.[10] As was described previously, the new paradigm in biology proposes that the electromagnetic signals are the primary way in which the cells communicate and control biochemical reactions. We have previously described the connective tissue–water "nervous system"; we will now discuss the "classic" nervous system.

The nervous system is anatomically and functionally connected throughout the entire body, but it can be structurally divided into the central nervous system and the peripheral nervous system and can be functionally divided into the somatic nervous system and the autonomic nervous system.[34] Massage and manual therapy affect every part of the nervous system, thus inducing profound changes in every other system in the body. One guiding principle of this method of therapy is that *it is essential that the treatment promote relaxation*, even though areas of pain and disability are being treated. By focusing on relaxation during treatment, the therapist creates positive systemic changes by lowering blood pressure, reducing stress, and promoting the repair and rejuvenation functions of the nervous system. For clients who present with pain and disability in the musculoskeletal system, treatment is focused on the somatic nervous system (see below) (Fig. 1-17).

CENTRAL NERVOUS SYSTEM

The central nervous system consists of the brain and spinal cord.

The Brain

▨ **Structure and function:** The brain has 100 billion neurons, each of which has 10,000 to 15,000 connections (synapses). Three million synapses can fit on a pinhead![55] The brain is divided into three sections: the cerebrum, brainstem, and cerebellum.

  □ The cerebrum is the largest portion and the most recently developed part of the brain. It is responsible for higher mental functions, such as thinking, learning, and personality. The frontal lobe area of the cerebrum also contains the **motor cortex,** which controls voluntary movements.

  □ Another area of the cerebrum, the parietal lobe, contains the **sensory cortex,** which receives information about touch and proprioception. Some proprioceptive signals, however, go only to the spinal cord.

  □ The limbic system and hypothalamus integrate emotional states, visceral responses, and the muscular system.[16] Emotions can alter muscular tone. States of anxiety create sustained increased tone (hypertonicity), and depression creates loss of muscle tone (hypotonicity).

  □ The brainstem is the center for the automatic control of respiration, heart rate, posture, balance, and many automatic movements of the body.

  □ The cerebellum functions to control muscle coordination, muscle tone, and posture.

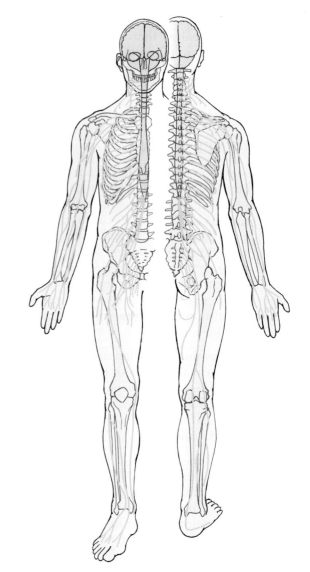

Figure 1-17. Overview of the somatic or motor nervous system, which includes the central nervous system and the peripheral nervous system. The central nervous system includes the brain and spinal cord, and the peripheral nervous system includes the cranial nerves (not shown) and the 31 pairs of spinal nerves that extend into the arms and legs. **Left.** Anterior view. **Right.** Posterior view.

The Spinal Cord

▨ **Structure and function:** The spinal cord is a continuation of the medulla portion of the brain and travels within the vertebral canal from the opening in the skull, called the *foramen magnum*, to the lumbar spine. After the cord ends at approximately the second lumbar vertebra, it continues as a collection of nerve roots called the *cauda equina*.

  □ The spinal cord is divided into gray matter, which contains the neuron cell bodies, and white matter, which contains the nerve fibers. One portion of the cord receives information from the sensory receptors, and another portion transmits motor information from the muscles. An interneuron communicates and amplifies information between the sensory and motor portions of the cord.

☐ A reflex arc is the simplest communication between the sensory and the motor nerves. The classic example is the deep tendon reflex that occurs when you tap the quadriceps tendon. When the tendon is tapped, the quadriceps automatically contracts. However, information from all four classes of sensory receptors—the mechanoreceptors, proprioceptors, thermoreceptors, and nociceptors—unconsciously send information to the cord, which stimulates countless automatic (reflexive) adjustments in the muscular system. Irritation of the sensory receptors can cause reflexive hypertonicity or reflexive inhibition (weakness) in the muscles (Fig. 1-18).

☐ The spinal cord becomes individual spinal nerves as they exit the vertebral column through openings between the sides of the vertebra called the intervertebral foramen. (See Chapters 3 to 5 for more information on the spinal nerves.)

Dysfunction and injury: When a person is under excessive or ongoing stress, the central nervous system may send unconscious signals to the muscular system, causing sustained muscular contraction. It is a common clinical experience that a client who is under chronic stress has habitually contracted muscles without any awareness that those muscles are tight. This condition is commonly experienced in the upper trapezius. When the therapist touches this muscle, the client is often surprised that it is tight and tender. Unconscious hypertonicity represents a loss of sensory awareness.

☐ Another common clinical experience is to find that the client has lost the ability to voluntarily contract a muscle that is held in an involuntary contraction. The therapist asks the client to contract a muscle against resistance, and the client is unaware of how to engage that muscle. These conditions describe what Thomas Hanna[56] calls "sensory motor amnesia."

☐ The muscles may be held in sustained tension because of overuse, poor posture, or psychological or emotional stress. States of anxiety and anger, for example, can create sustained muscular hypertonicity. Emotional stress, such as depression, can also create a decrease in muscular tone and a loss of sensory motor communication.

Treatment implications:

☐ MET is used to bring sensory awareness to the muscles, guiding the client to feel the muscles working. MET also educates the client to bring conscious awareness to the muscles through voluntary contraction. Using the higher brain by having the client actively participate in muscle movement through MET can alter unconscious habits of muscle tension and help normalize muscle function. Facilitating sensory-motor integration helps to correct sensory-motor amnesia.

☐ Studies show that stroking an animal's back stimulates the limbic system and leads to muscular

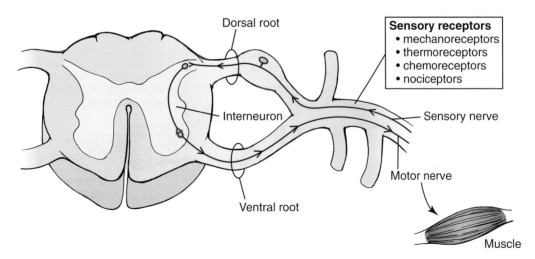

Figure 1-18. Reflex arc. The afferent or sensory nerves receive information from four broad classes of receptors: mechanoreceptors, proprioceptors, chemoreceptors, and nociceptors (pain receptors). The information is sent to the spinal cord and stimulates an interneuron and then the efferent or motor nerves. One motor nerve, the alpha nerve, innervates the extrafusal muscle fiber. Sustained sensory stimulation from mechanical irritation (muscle or joint dysfunction), injury, or emotional tension can create increased alpha stimulation and reflex muscle hypertonicity or inhibit the alpha nerve activity and cause muscle inhibition and weakness.

relaxation.[16] Massage can calm anxiety, and MET can engage the muscles to increase their tone in depressed clients.

☐ Because the brain can alter muscle function, it is important that the therapist give the client an image of healing. To create a positive image of healing, you might say, "I think you will feel a lot better after your massage" if this is a reasonable possibility. This principle of treatment is discussed in Chapter 2.

PERIPHERAL NERVOUS SYSTEM

The peripheral nervous system consists of 12 pairs of cranial nerves and 31 pairs of spinal nerves that convey information from the central nervous system to muscles, joints, skin, and sense organs and from sensory receptors in those same structures back to the spinal cord and brain.

▨ **Structure:** The structure of a peripheral nerve is similar to that of tendons and muscles and consists of long parallel fibers, arranged in bundles called fascicles (Fig. 1-19). The nerves are fluid-filled cells with three connective tissue coverings: the epineurium, perineurium, and endoneurium. Unlike tough electrical wires, they are soft structures that can be injured by compression, excessive stretching (tethering), and mechanical irritation.

☐ The nerves are lubricated, and the fibers, fascicles, and gross nerves are designed to slide within the connective tissue spaces. When a muscle contracts and a joint moves, the nerve slides in the healthy state.

☐ The spinal nerves begin from expansions of the spinal cord that form two nerve roots: the motor (anterior) root and the sensory (posterior) root. All sensory nerves merge at the dorsal root ganglion, where they are processed. See Chapter 3 for further discussion.

▨ **Function:** The spinal and cranial nerves of the peripheral nervous system have four main functional divisions.

☐ **Somatic sensory nerves (afferent):** There are four types of somatic sensory nerves: mechanoreceptors, thermoreceptors, chemoreceptors, and nociceptors. See "Somatic Nervous System" below for further discussion.

☐ **Somatic motor nerves (efferent):** The somatic motor nerves relay information from the brain, through the spinal cord, and then to the skeletal muscles.

☐ **Visceral sensory:** These nerves are part of the autonomic nervous system and send pain and pressure information from the internal organs to the central nervous system (see "Autonomic Nervous System" below).

☐ **Visceral motor:** The visceral motor nerves transmit impulses from the autonomic nervous system to the involuntary muscles, such as those found in internal organs and glandular tissue.

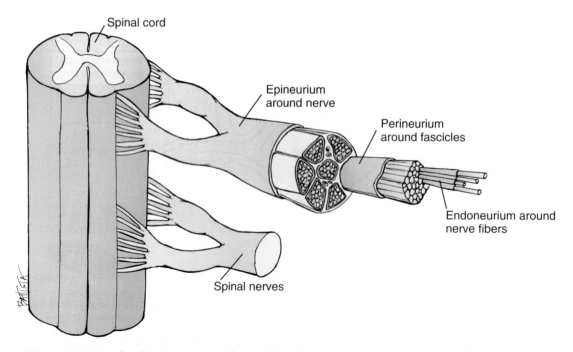

Figure 1-19. Peripheral nerve anatomy. The peripheral nerves begin as 31 pairs of spinal nerves, which then travel throughout the body. They are structured similarly to tendons, ligaments, and muscles, with long parallel fibers contained in bundles surrounded by connective tissue.

▨ **Dysfunction and injury:** Information regarding dysfunction and injury to the sensory nerves was previously discussed in the sections entitled "Ligaments," "Tendons," "Muscles," and "Joint." In this section, we will describe how peripheral nerves can become entrapped as they travel through the extremities. The peripheral nerves are susceptible to irritation because of compression or tethering (pulling) at the nerve roots in the area of the intervertebral foramen. They are also susceptible to compression and irritation in the extremities:

☐ Nerves can become restricted or entrapped by adhesions in the connective tissue spaces through which the nerves travel. This restriction prevents the normal gliding of the nerve.

☐ Nerves can become restricted or entrapped in the connective tissue spaces of hypertonic muscles.

☐ Nerves can become compressed in fibro-osseous tunnels such as the carpal tunnel.

☐ Nerves can become compressed, restricted, or irritated because of compression from the swelling or inflammation caused by overuse or injury.

▨ **Treatment implication:** Peripheral nerves are strong and resilient,[34] and they can be gently massaged without damage. Lauren Berry, RPT, insisted that all massage strokes on the peripheral nerves should be transverse (perpendicular) to the line of the nerve. This releases the adhesions in the connective tissue of the nerve itself and also releases the adhesions in the loose connective tissue that suspends the nerve. This method has proved a safe and comfortable treatment with excellent clinical results. The treatment to decompress the area of the nerve roots of the spine is addressed in each of Chapters 3 to 5, and the manual release of peripheral entrapment of the nerves in the extremities is addressed in the subsequent chapters.

AUTONOMIC NERVOUS SYSTEM

▨ **Structure:** The autonomic nervous system is the part of the nervous system that innervates the heart, blood vessels, diaphragm, internal organs, and glands and influences every other part of the body, including the muscular system. It unconsciously, automatically regulates the heartbeat, respiration, digestion, and many other functions . Although it functions unconsciously. it is also affected by conscious awareness, such as consciously slowing the breath. There are two main divisions: the sympathetic and the parasympathetic.

Sympathetic Nervous System

▨ **Structure:** The cell bodies form a cord called the *sympathetic trunk*, which borders the vertebral column on both sides and extends from the base of the skull to the coccyx.

▨ **Function and dysfunction:** The sympathetic nervous system is responsible for the "fight-or-flight" response and is active when a person is under stress. It releases adrenaline into the blood, causes constriction of the peripheral blood vessels, increases the heart rate, and inhibits the normal movement of the intestines (peristalsis) so that blood is available to the skeletal muscles.[34] When a person is experiencing chronic stress or chronic pain, there is an increased level of adrenaline, which causes sustained tension in the muscles and magnifies pain signals from the nociceptors.[55]

Parasympathetic Nervous System

▨ **Structure:** The cell bodies are located in the cranial and sacral regions.

▨ **Function and dysfunction:** The parasympathetic nervous system is responsible for energy conservation, cellular rebuilding, and rejuvenation. It slows the body down and is active when the body is at rest and during recuperation. It decreases the heart rate, stimulates the normal movement of the intestines (peristalsis), and promotes the secretion of all digestive juices. A person can be in parasympathetic override, which would contribute to lethargy and loss of normal drives. Most people in Western cultures have an underactive parasympathetic nervous system and an overactive sympathetic nervous system.

▨ **Treatment implications:** The method of treatment described in this text is given in a relaxing, calm manner to stimulate a parasympathetic state. It can be described as a moving meditation. This induces a state of relaxation in the client and therapist and promotes the healing and rejuvenation functions of the parasympathetic nervous system. To induce a relaxing, parasympathetic treatment, the therapist needs to have soft hands and a calming voice. Although the STM strokes may be deep, the therapist's hands are kept soft, and the strokes are applied rhythmically so that the client can relax into the treatment. The therapist's emotions and attitudes also play a role in the relaxation of the client. Acceptance and support for the client enhance treatment outcome.

SOMATIC (SENSORIMOTOR) NERVOUS SYSTEM

▨ **Structure:** The somatic nervous system is composed of sensory and motor nerves that convey information back and forth between the skin, muscles, and joints and the spinal cord and brain.[34] The somatic senses are distinguished from the special senses of vision, hearing, taste, smell, and equilibrium. The sensory information enters the spinal cord and goes in two directions: (1) back to the muscles during unconscious, automatic activity, such as posture, and (2) to higher centers, including the brain, where sensory information is evaluated.[57] The motor part of the somatic nervous system innervates only skeletal muscles, controls both voluntary movement and reflexive movement, and contributes to dynamic joint stability, coordination, posture, and balance. There are two motor nerves: the alpha and gamma nerves. Sensory nerves relay information to the central nervous system from **four types of receptors**: *mechanoreceptors, thermoreceptors, chemoreceptors,* and *nociceptors.* Mechanoreceptors are specialized sensory receptors that convert physical stimulus into chemical, electrical, and electromagnetic energy. They convey proprioceptive information to the spinal cord and brain. Mechanoreceptors are located in the skin, muscles, tendons, and soft tissue surrounding the joints. These receptors are stimulated by some action, such as stretching, pressure, and contraction. In addition to providing information about joint position and movement, they transmit length and tension information from muscles and tendons. (See below for more information, and refer to the section, "Joint Structure and Function.") Thousands of impulses are processed each second.[49] Sensory information from the *somatic senses* concerns **four categories of information**: *touch, proprioception, temperature,* and *pain.*

☐ **Touch:** Mechanoreceptors are located in the superficial and deep layers of the skin and communicate light touch as well as deep pressure.

☐ **Proprioception:** There are multiple definitions of proprioception in the literature.[58] This text uses the term *proprioception* in the broader sense of awareness of body position and joint movement. The sense of proprioception comes from the mechanoreceptors and from the special sense of equilibrium.

☐ **Temperature:** Sensory nerves detect hot and cold (thermoreceptors).

☐ **Pain:** The sensation of pain comes from the brain, which decides whether information from specialized receptors called nociceptors is harmful or potentially harmful. There are three categories of nociception: thermal, chemical, and mechanical. This topic is discussed on page 48 ("Cause of Soft Tissue Pain").

SENSORY RECEPTORS (MECHANORECEPTORS) IN MUSCLE

▦ Muscles are highly innervated with sensory receptors, including pain fibers and mechanoreceptors. The two types of mechanoreceptors are **muscle spindles** and **GTOs**, which function as sensory organs. Information from the receptors has a profound influence on muscle activity (Fig. 1-20). They detect the length and tension in the muscle and tendon, and they set the resting tone of the muscle.

Muscle Spindles

▦ **Structure:** Muscle spindles are specialized muscle fibers called *intrafusal fibers,* located in a fluid-filled capsule embedded within each muscle. The body has about 25,000 to 30,000 muscle spindles, with about 4000 in each arm and 7000 in each leg.[49] Spindles respond to slow and rapid changes of muscle length and to deep pressure. Unlike other mechanoreceptors, muscle spindles contain both contractile and sensory elements.

▦ **Function:** Muscle spindles detect changes in muscle *length,* so stretching a muscle will increase the rate of discharge. The spindles play an essential role in joint position, coordination, balance, fine muscular control, and proprioception.[59] Muscle spindles also help to set the tone of a muscle. The more refined the function, the greater is the concentration of muscle spindles. The greatest concentration of spindles is found in the lumbrical muscles of the hand,[60] in the suboccipital muscles, and in the muscles that move the eyes.

Golgi Tendon Organs

▦ **Structure:** GTOs are sensory receptors in the form of a slender capsule located along the muscle fiber at the musculotendinous junction.

▦ **Function:** GTOs are sensitive to changes in muscle *tension.* Originally, they were thought to have only a protective function to prevent damage to a muscle being forcefully contracted. Current research, however, suggests that the GTOs fire during minute changes in muscle tension.[57] Even a single motor unit will discharge the GTO. With excessive tension in the muscle, the GTO stimulates nerves at the spinal cord, called *inhibitory interneurons,* causing the muscle to relax.[57] Inhibitory interneurons communicate through the spinal cord to the brainstem and therefore do not

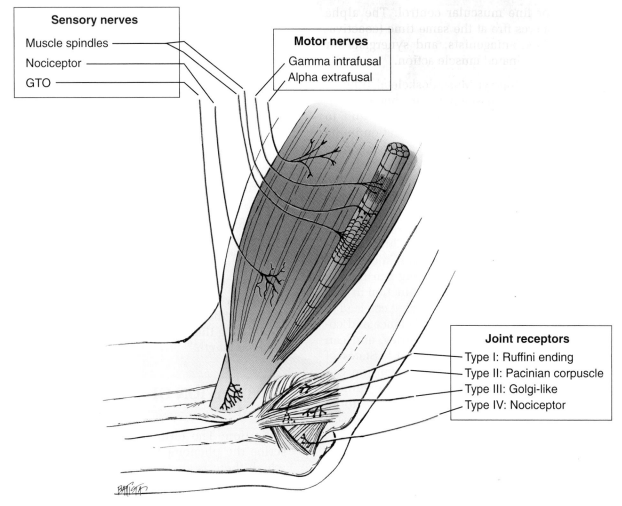

Figure 1-20. Muscle and joint receptors. The extrafusal muscle fibers are innervated by alpha motor neurons, and the intrafusal fibers (muscle spindles) are innervated by gamma motor neurons. There are three classes of sensory nerves in a muscle: the muscle spindle, GTO, and free nerve endings (nociceptors or pain fibers). Muscle spindles are sensitive to muscle length and changes in length, and the GTOs are sensitive to muscle tension. Spindle cells and GTOs also give proprioceptive information regarding position of the body. There are four classes of mechanoreceptors that innervate each joint.

reach conscious awareness. As with spindle cells, GTOs are essential for fine muscular control, because they equalize the contractile forces of agonists, antagonists and synergists. They help to adjust the tension in a muscle for joint stability, balance, and coordination. They also protect the muscle and joint through reflexes that contract or inhibit the muscle automatically. Through practice, these receptors help to adjust muscular tension to the appropriate amount in the countless activities of daily living.[19]

TWO TYPES OF MOTOR NERVES INNERVATE MUSCLES

▨ **Alpha motor neurons:** Originating in the motor cortex of the brain, alpha motor neurons innervate the contractile muscle fibers (extrafusal fibers). A single alpha nerve excites a group of muscles fibers called the *motor unit*. As few as three fibers form the motor unit for the lumbricals of the hand, and up to 1600 muscle fibers form the motor unit of the gastrocnemius. The alpha motor neurons convey nerve impulses to the muscles for all movements, including voluntary muscle contraction and unconscious muscle activity involved in posture, balance, and habitual movement.

▨ **Gamma motor neurons:** Originating in the brainstem, gamma motor neurons innervate the muscle spindle (intrafusal fibers). These nerves carry unconscious information from the central nervous system to the muscle that sets the tone of muscle and are responsible through voluntary muscle contraction for fine muscular control. The alpha and gamma nerves fire at the same time (coactivation) to agonists, antagonists, and synergists for smooth and coordinated muscle action.

▨ **Dysfunction and injury:** Musculoskeletal injuries generate pain through tissue damage, chemical irritation from inflammation, and ischemia due to swelling. Pain and swelling lead to alteration in the function of the mechanoreceptors, causing changes in muscle and joint function. The outcome is decreased proprioception (position sense), balance disturbances, abnormalities in posture, decreased coordination, loss of fine motor control, slower reaction times, altered movement patterns, altered muscle firing patterns, and muscle weakness.[49] Chronic muscle dysfunction from adhesions (prior injury), immobilization, aging, or deconditioning can lead to sensory receptor atrophy.[49] If the dysfunction in sensory nerve function is not rehabilitated, it can lead to joint instability and problems with balance and coordination, leading to recurrent injuries, and can contribute to degeneration of the joint.[16] States of anxiety or emotional or psychological tension can cause an increase in the firing rate of the spindle cells. This increase causes the muscle tone to be "set" too high, creating hypertonicity and stiffness.[52]

▨ **Treatment implications:**
☐ Alterations in muscle activity after a painful injury do not necessarily return to normal even after the pain eventually resolves. Therefore, in the treatment of injuries and dysfunction of the sensory-motor system, it is essential for the therapist to focus on factors that improve proprioception, joint movement, muscle firing patterns, strength and stability, and sensory awareness. This neuromuscular reeducation is also called *sensory-motor rehabilitation* and involves therapy to improve the functional communication between the nervous system and the muscles.[49] Active participation of the client during treatment is much more effective for rehabilitation of the nervous system than is being passive.[16] Directing the client to concentrate during MET and bring focused attention and sensory awareness produces a reeducation of the central nervous system as well as rehabilitation of the motor and sensory nerves. Precise muscular contraction, which improves neuromuscular control, is an essential component of functional improvement.[48] It is important during MET for the therapist to provide feedback and guidance to the client to enhance proprioceptive reeducation.
☐ The therapist's touch, pressure, and movement stimulate the somatic sensory nerves. Each touch and movement sends a message to the spinal cord and brain, which, in turn, communicate with every other part of the client's body, including the centers of the person's emotions and psychology. Working within the client's comfort zone and using a gentle touch and a calm voice are critical because this induces relaxation and trust and helps to heal the whole person, not just the local tissue.
☐ Sustained muscle tension from injury or dysfunction indicates that the muscle spindles are set too high, like a thermostat set too high. There are two easy ways to decrease the firing rate of a spindle cell and therefore cause the muscle to relax. The first is to decrease the muscle length by bringing the origin and insertion toward each other. This method is emphasized in strain–counterstrain and positional-release techniques, which are incorporated into the STM described in this text. The second is to contract a muscle isometrically, as is done in MET. This technique causes the spindle activity to stop temporarily, allowing the muscle to be set to a new, more relaxed length.[61]

SENSITIZATION OF THE NERVOUS SYSTEM

▨ **Definition:** The term *sensitization* is used to describe the phenomenon in the nervous system in which there is an exaggerated response to normal stimuli. There are two principal causes:
☐ The limbic areas of the brain can cause an emotional exaggeration of pain, which can trigger the central nervous system to cause the muscles to become either too tight or too loose. This emotional exaggeration is caused by many factors, including culture, family history, pain history, and individual psychology.
☐ The other cause of sensitization happens at the level of the spinal cord. The area in the spinal cord that receives information about pain is next to the receptive field for movement (mechanoreceptors). Chronic inflammation can cause sensitization of the mechanoreceptors such that normal mechanical stimuli (e.g., movement of a joint within a normal range) cause the mechanoreceptor to be a pain producer.[62]

▨ **Treatment implications:** Massage and manual therapy, including MET and joint mobilization, can help to reeducate the mechanoreceptors. In addition to therapy, however, the client needs to gradually increase the amount of movement and learn that pain does not necessarily mean that the body is being injured.[55] Refer to the treatment implications above under "Somatic Nervous System" and to "Chronic Pain" below.

Part Four: Injury and Repair

MECHANICS OF SOFT TISSUE INJURY

ROLE OF COLLAGEN IN SOFT TISSUE INJURY

Soft tissues experience injury by excessive pulling (tension), compression, torsion (twisting), or shearing. There are two types of injury. One is described as *macrotrauma*, which implies a specific event. The injury is a rapidly applied load, such as a car accident, fall, or sport injury. The second type of injury is described as *microtrauma*, which is the result of repetitive or cumulative stress. Examples include tennis elbow, Achilles tendinitis, and carpal tunnel syndrome. Inflammation can result from either type of injury.

These two types of injuries can be illustrated by a stress–strain curve (Fig. 1-21). **Stress** is defined as the force per area applied to the tissue, and **strain** is described as the percent change in length. The degree of damage to the soft tissues is affected not only by the amount of stress, but also by the rate or acceleration of the stress. The higher the acceleration, the greater is the damage. This explains the whiplash phenomenon, in which low speed (7 mph) injury can damage the soft tissue. The injurious force is not the speed, but the high acceleration (300 milliseconds). Rapidly applied loads increase the stiffness and can damage the soft tissues.

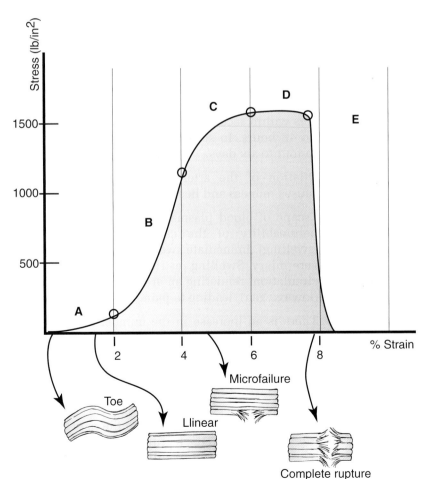

Figure 1-21. Stress–strain curve for a ruptured Achilles tendon. The five distinct regions are the **(A)** toe region, **(B)** linear region, **(C)** progressive failure region, **(D)** major failure region, and **(E)** complete rupture.

FIVE DEGREES OF SOFT TISSUE FAILURE

▨ **Toe region:** If the stress is small, the tissue returns to its normal length. The stress takes the slack out of the tissue by straightening the crimp. This is represented by the toe region of the curve. Tissue may be loaded with a 1.5% to 2.5% strain and return to normal. This elastic quality decreases with age, because the amount of crimp decreases with age.

▨ **Linear region:** If the strain is between 2.5% and 4%, all of the fibers have straightened out, the collagen tears at its outermost fibers first, which is called *microfailure*.[63] This degree of injury is represented by the linear area of the curve. The tearing of collagen is like a rope that frays from its outer fibers to the center. The client complains of stiffness with this amount of tearing.[46] Microfailure can occur within the normal physiologic range if there is repetitive stress on weakened tissue from a previously damaged structure.[64] Even with microfailure, the cells, fibers, and ground substance matrix are damaged, and an inflammatory response is initiated.

▨ **Progressive failure region:** A strain between 4% and 6% is called the *yield point*, at which point major tearing occurs.

▨ **Major failure region:** A strain of more than 6% involves many points of rupture.

▨ **Complete rupture:** An 8% strain causes the collagen fibers to tear completely apart.

▨ Following the tear of the collagen fibers, repair and regeneration of the tissue are carried out through the process of inflammation and repair.

INFLAMMATION AND REPAIR

FOUR CARDINAL SIGNS OF INFLAMMATION

▨ Redness

▨ Heat

▨ Swelling

▨ Pain

INFLAMMATION: THE BODY'S RESPONSE TO TWO TYPES OF IRRITANTS, LIVING AND NONLIVING

▨ **Living irritants:** Microorganisms, such as bacteria, are an example of a living irritant.

▨ **Nonliving irritants:** Trauma and repetitive stress are the primary causes of inflammation. Joint dysfunction, such as knock-knees, can irritate the cartilage and periarticular soft tissues, creating a microinflammatory environment, with the same cellular responses described in this chapter.

FUNCTIONS OF INFLAMMATION

▨ Protects the body from infection, removes debris, and kills foreign invaders such as bacteria.

▨ Repairs damaged tissue by stimulating new cell growth, which then synthesizes new fibers for repair.

TWO TYPES OF TRAUMA

▨ **Direct:** Occurs from blunt trauma, such as from contact sports, car accidents.

▨ **Indirect:**
   ☐ **Acute:** Occurs with sudden overloading.
   ☐ **Chronic:** Occurs as a result of repetitive or cumulative stress.
   ☐ **Acute on chronic:** Occurs as a result of a sudden tear of a chronically weakened area.

PHASES OF INFLAMMATION AND REPAIR

Vascular (Acute)

Begins within seconds of an injury and typically lasts 24 to 48 hours. In some cases, however, it may last from four to six days.

▨ Dilation of the arteries, veins, and capillaries causes redness and heat.

▨ Escape of blood plasma because of the increased permeability of the capillaries causes edema (swelling). Immediate swelling suggests a more severe injury. Swelling restricts lymph drainage and circulation, rendering an area acidic and ischemic (low oxygen), leading to pain.

▨ There is an increase in the number of fibroblasts. The fibroblasts increase in size and synthesize ground substance and collagen. This process begins within four hours of injury and can last four to six days. Collagen initially forms a weak, random mesh of fibers.

▨ Pain is produced by stimulation the pain receptors (nociceptors) from the tearing of the collagen fibers, by pressure from the swelling, and by chemical irritation.

- Pain causes muscle spasms, which decrease circulation, reducing the ability of an area to repair.

- Inflammation leads to stimulation of pain receptors that cause compensatory adaptations that either facilitate muscles, causing hypertonicity, or inhibit muscles, causing weakness.[65]

- Typically, with joint inflammation, the flexors of the joint become hypertonic, and the extensors become inhibited.[50]

Regeneration and Repair (Subacute)

The process of regeneration and repair begins two days after injury and lasts up to six weeks.

- Scar tissue is highly cellular, and new capillaries are formed. The capillaries are laid down in a random orientation unless the area is mobilized.

- Fibroblastic activity and collagen formation increases.

- Immature connective tissue is less dense, making it more fragile and therefore more easily injured. Pain does not indicate the level of repair, so care must be taken with the amount of pressure that is applied in a massage.

- In these early stages, collagen is laid down in a random, disorganized pattern, usually in a plane perpendicular to the long axis, and therefore has little strength (Fig. 1-22).[3] The collagen develops abnormal crosslinks, leaving the tissue with less flexibility.

Remodeling (Chronic)

The remodeling process can take three weeks to twelve months.

- The term *chronic* can mean different things depending on how it is used. It can indicate the final stage of healing, although regaining pre-injury strength may take up to two years. It may apply to an injury that lasts longer than three to six months and does not appear to be improving.[66] This latter condition is discussed below under "Chronic Pain."

- In the early stages of remodeling, collagen matures into a lattice that is completely disorganized. It can be palpated as thickened or fibrous tissue. A relative decrease in cellularity and vascularity occurs as collagen density increases.

- After approximately two months, fibroblastic activity decreases, and there is less collagen synthesis.

- Random orientation of collagen provides little support for tensile loads.

- Two months to one year later, collagen may develop a functional linear alignment in response to movement and may become reoriented to the line of stress. Tensile strength slowly increases as collagen remodels itself back to its normal parallel alignment from the introduction of movement, stretching, and exercise.

- Immobilization leads to significant adhesion formations; osteoporosis or loss of bone density; and the atrophy of muscles, capsules, and ligaments.

- During the remodeling phase, the tissue is vulnerable to reinjury. Challenging the tissue too much can overload it, creating chronic irritation or inflammation, or can lead to degeneration of the tissue.

- Chronic pain can cause sensitization of the mechanoreceptors, such that normal mechanical

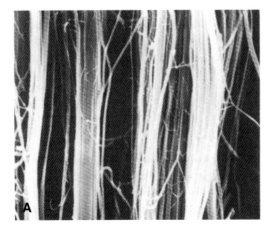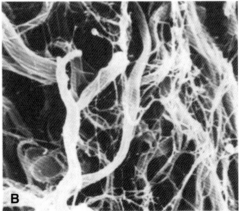

Figure 1-22. A. The normal longitudinal arrangement of a ligament. **B.** The random cross-weave of the collagen fibers in the early stages of repair after an injury to the ligament. (Reprinted with permission from Woo S, Buckwalter J. Injury and Repair of the Musculoskeletal Soft Tissues. Park Ridge, IL: American Academy of Orthopedic Surgeons, 1988.)

stimuli (e.g., movement of a joint within a normal range) cause the mechanoreceptor to be a pain producer.[62]

PAIN AND SOFT TISSUE

SOFT TISSUE IS A COMMON SOURCE OF PAIN

Nociception means the perception of harmful stimuli.[67] *Nociceptors* are specialized nerves embedded in soft tissue that monitor the body for evidence of injury. They are normally silent but are stimulated by excessive mechanical, thermal, or chemical stimuli. A common source of musculoskeletal pain is from the deep soft tissue. These tissues include the periosteum, joint capsule, ligaments, tendons, muscles, and fascia. The most pain-sensitive tissue is the periosteum and the joint capsule. Tendons and ligaments are moderately sensitive, and muscle is less sensitive.[46]

CAUSES OF SOFT TISSUE PAIN

Pain is elicited by harmful stimuli from three different classes of receptors: **mechanical, chemical,** and **thermal** receptors. **Acute** pain from trauma or cumulative stress is caused by damage to the tissue from excessive mechanical stress, such as compression, twisting, or pulling; inflammatory chemicals released after tissue damage; or excessive heat or cold. In **chronic** conditions, such as arthritis, pain is generated from ongoing tissue irritation or damage, emotional or psychological stress, or changes in the central nervous system that continue to send pain signals even when there is no harmful stimuli (Fig. 1-23). See below for further discussion. These basic categories can be expanded into the following six fundamental causes:[68]

- **Injury** creates inflammation and ischemia (low oxygen) due to swelling. Inflammation releases chemicals that irritate the pain fibers in the periosteum, joint capsules, bone, perivascular tissue, ligaments, synovial tissue, muscle and its fascia, and other soft tissues around the joint.

- **Mechanical irritation** is due to repetitive or cumulative stress to the periosteum, joint capsules, bone, tissue around the blood vessels (perivascular tissue), ligaments, muscle and its fascia, and other soft tissues around the joint. Mechanical irritation develops from abnormal tension, compression, or torsion (twisting) of the soft tissue. Abnormal alignment of the joint creates mechanical irritation of the soft tissue surrounding the joint.

- **Neurogenic pain** is caused by the irritation or inflammation of the sensory nerves themselves. This

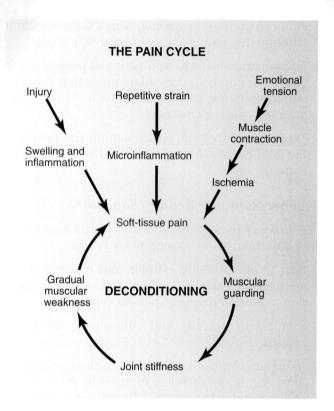

Figure 1-23. Soft tissue pain cycle. Chronic pain leads to gradual weakness and deconditioning.

inflammation then releases chemicals (neuropeptides) from the nerve endings. These chemicals irritate the pain fibers in the periosteum, joint capsules, bone, perivascular tissue, ligaments, synovial tissue, muscle and its fascia, and other soft tissues around the joint (see "The Nervous System").

- **Reflex hypertonicity** of muscles, induced by injury, stress, or arthrokinetic reflexes, creates stagnation in the tissue and decreased oxygen (ischemia), which causes pain.

- **Nerve entrapment** is caused by soft tissue swelling, adhesions in the connective tissue, or sustained muscle contraction. Entrapment of the nerve creates congestion and fluid stagnation. This reduces the flow within the nerve, leading to altered sensation (paresthesia). Entrapment also reduces oxygen to the nerve because of reduced blood flow, which leads to pain.

- **Psychological or emotional stress** stimulates the sympathetic nervous system and creates muscular hypertonicity, which leads to pain from decreased oxygen (ischemia) and increased acids in the tissue.

CHRONIC PAIN

- Chronic pain may be due to stress, degeneration in the joint, or a chronic inflammatory condition, such as rheumatoid arthritis. But in many clients with chronic pain, there are no objective findings, and the term *chronic* does not accurately reflect the physical condition of the body. Nerves can "backfire" in some clients and send pain impulses even when there are no harmful stimuli.

▨ Chronic pain often leads to depression and anxiety and pain avoidance behavior, which result in deconditioning.

▨ Clients who are in chronic pain need to focus on improving function and behavioral changes. They need to take several steps to reeducate their nervous system: become informed about pain and learn that "hurt does not necessarily mean harm," stay active, explore new ways to move, extend the "edges of pain" by moving a little more each week, and keep a positive attitude.[55]

▨ Treatment implications were discussed above in "Somatic Nervous System."

REFERRED PAIN

▨ Pain that originates in deep somatic tissue is usually referred into specific patterns called **sclerotomes** (Fig. 1-24). Sclerotomes are "those deep somatic tissues (fascia, ligaments, capsules, and connective tissue) that are innervated by the same spinal nerve."[46] The extent of the radiation depends on the intensity of the irritation to the tissue. When a tissue of a particular sclerotome is irritated, the pain can be perceived as originating from any and all of the tissue that is innervated by the same nerve.

▨ Referral of diffuse sclerotomal pain is distinguished from well-localized pain that is referred from irritation of the nerve roots. **Dermatomal pain** occurs if the sensory (dorsal) nerve root is irritated. The client will feel *sharp pain, numbing, or tingling that is well localized* in patches of skin called *dermatomes* that correspond to a specific nerve. Irritation of the motor (ventral) nerve root will elicit **myotomal pain**. Symptoms include deep, boring pain, well localized to specific muscles (myotomes), as well as potential weakness in the muscles supplied by that nerve root.[46] For further discussion of dermatomes, see Chapter 3, "Lumbosacral Spine," and Chapter 5, "Cervical Spine."

QUALITY OF PAIN FROM DEEP SOMATIC TISSUES

▨ Deep somatic pain is also called **sclerotomal pain** and is described as diffuse aching, numbing, and tingling.

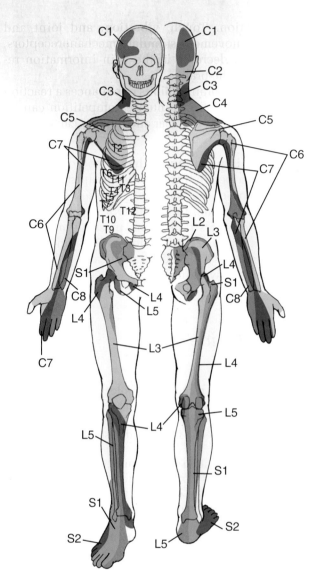

Figure 1-24. Irritation or injury of fascia, ligaments, tendons, joint capsules, or other connective tissues refers pain into regions innervated by the same spinal nerve. The pathways are called *sclerotomes*.

▨ Sclerotomal pain is often associated with autonomic disturbances, such as sweating, pallor, and feelings of nausea and being faint.

▨ Pain of sclerotomal origin and from the viscera sends impulses to the limbic and hypothalamus areas of the brain (the emotional centers) and may be responsible for emotional reactions of anxiety, fear, anger, and depression.

PAIN-GATE THEORY OF MELZAK AND WALL AND ITS RELATION TO MASSAGE

▨ The pain-gate theory proposes that there are two main factors that determine how pain is perceived:
  ☐ First, it depends on the balance between mechanoreceptor information and pain fiber

information. Touch, vibration, and joint and muscle movement stimulate mechanoreceptors, causing a decrease in the pain information received by the brain.

☐ Second, the brain inhibits or enhances a reaction to pain. Athletes in intense competition can ignore an injury, and fear and anxiety can exaggerate pain.

▌ **Treatment implication:** In the method of treatment that is described in this text, the therapist moves the entire region of the body being worked on, as well as the local tissue, to stimulate a large number of mechanoreceptors rather than pressing only at the site of the injury or dysfunction and keeping the rest of the body passive. This dramatically reduces the discomfort of working on these deep somatic tissues.

▌ *Study Guide*

Level I

1. Describe the new paradigm in biology and medicine.
2. Describe the characteristics of soft tissue injury.
3. Describe the arrangement of collagen fibers and how collagen is affected in injury, and describe the treatment implications.
4. Describe the function and dysfunction of ground substance and define thixotropy and its relevance to massage therapy.
5. Describe why movement in the early stages of repair is indicated.
6. Define tensegrity and piezoelectricity and describe their relevance to massage therapy.
7. List the causes of pain from soft tissue injury and dysfunction.
8. Describe a sclerotome and the quality of pain from those tissues.
9. Describe Janda's concept of soft tissue dysfunction and its relevance to massage therapy.
10. Describe Lauren Berry's concept of soft tissue dysfunction and its relevance to massage therapy.

Level II

1. Describe the pain-gate theory of Melzak and Wall and its relevance to massage therapy.
2. Describe the structural and neurological goals of treatment.
3. Describe joint play and joint dysfunction, and list the causes of joint dysfunction and its treatment.
4. Describe the functions of the following structures: muscle spindle, GTO, and alpha and gamma nerves.
5. List the eight causes of muscle dysfunction.
6. Describe how cartilage maintains its circulation and health.
7. Define the arthrokinetic reflex.
8. Describe the signs of impaired muscle function.
9. Describe the differences between the sympathetic and the parasympathetic nervous systems and the implication for massage therapy.
10. Describe the goals of joint mobilization.

▌ *References*

1. Covey A, Nunley R, Mehta S. Musculoskeletal education in medical schools: Are we making the cut? http://www.aaos.org/news/bulletin/marap07/reimbursement2.asp 2007.
2. Magee DJ, Zachazewshi JE, Quillen WS. Preface. In Magee DJ, Zachazewshi JE, Quillen WS, (eds): Scientific Foundations and Principles of Practice in Musculoskeletal Rehabilitation. St. Louis: Saunders, 2007.
3. Woo S, Buckwalter J. Injury and Repair of the Musculoskeletal Soft Tissues. Park Ridge, IL: American Academy of Orthopedic Surgeons, 1988.
4. Sutton GS, Bartel MR. Soft-tissue mobilization techniques for the hand therapist. J Hand Ther 1994; July–Sept:185–192.
5. Banes A, Lee G, Graff R, et al. Mechanical forces and signaling in connective tissue cells: Cellular mechanisms of detection, transduction, and responses to mechanical stimuli. Curr Opin Orthoped 2001;12:389–396.
6. Lieber RL. Skeletal Muscle Structure, Function, and Plasticity, 2nd ed. Philadelphia: Lippincott Williams & Wilkins; 2002.
7. Buckwalter JA. Musculoskeletal tissues and the musculoskeletal system. In Weinstein SL, Buckwalter JA (eds): Turek's Orthopedics, 6th ed. Philadelphia: Lippincott Williams & Wilkins, 2005, pp 3–56.
8. Liboff AR. Toward an electromagnetic paradigm in biology and medicine. J Altern Complement Med 2004;10:41–47.
9. Oschman J. Energy Medicine. Edinburgh: Churchill Livingstone, 2000.
10. Buckminster Fuller R. Synergetics: Explorations in the Geometry of Thinking. New York: Collier Macmillan, 1975.
11. Ingber DE. Tensegrity: The architectural basis of cellular transduction. Ann Rev Physiol 1997;59:575–599.
12. Oschman J. Energy Medicine in Therapeutics and Human Performance. Edinburgh: Butterworth Heinemann, 2003
13. Alenghat FJ, Ingber DE. Mechanotransduction: All signals point to cytoskeleton, matrix, and integrins. Sci STKE 2002;119:pe6.
14. Kibler WB, Herring SA. Functional Rehabilitation of Sports and Musculoskeletal Injuries. Gaithersburg, MD: Aspen Publishers, 1998.
15. Gulino M, Bellia P, et al. Role of water in dielectric properties and delayed luminescence of bovine Achilles tendon. FEBS Lett 2005;579:6101–6104.
16. Lederman E. The Science and Practice of Manual Therapy, 2nd ed. Edinburgh: Churchill Livingstone, 2005.
17. Porterfield J, DeRosa C. Mechanical Shoulder Disorders. St. Louis: Saunders, 2004.

18. Hertling D, Kessler RM. Management of Common Musculoskeletal Disorders. Philadelphia: Lippincott Williams & Wilkins, 2006.

19. Juhan D. Job's Body. Barrytown, NY: Station Hill Press, 1987.

20. Lundon K, Walker JM. Cartilage of human joints and related structures. In Magee DJ, Zachazewski JE, Quillen WS (eds): Scientific Foundations and Principles of Practice in Musculoskeletal Rehabilitation. St. Louis: Saunders, 2007.

21. Reid DC. Sports Injury and Assessment. New York: Churchill Livingstone, 1992.

22. Neumann DA. Kinesiology of the Musculoskeletal System. St. Louis: Mosby, 2002.

23. Woo S, An K-N. Anatomy, biology, and biomechanics of tendon, ligament, and meniscus. In Simon S (ed): Orthopedic Basic Science. Park Ridge, IL: American Academy of Orthopedic Surgeons, 1994, pp 45–88.

24. Zachazewski JE. Range of motion and flexibility. In Magee DJ, Zachazewshi JE, Quillen WS (eds): Scientific Foundations and Principles of Practice in Musculoskeletal Rehabilitation. St. Louis: Saunders; 2007, pp 527–556.

25. Engles M. Tissue response. In Donatelli R, Wooden M (eds): Orthopedic Physical Therapy. New York: Churchill Livingstone, 1989, pp 1–31.

26. Brukner P, Khan K. Clinical Sports Medicine, 3rd ed. Sydney: McGraw-Hill, 2006.

27. Kraushaar B, Nirschl R. Current concepts review: Tendinosis of the elbow (tennis elbow): Clinical features and findings of histological, immunohistochemical, and electron microscopy studies. J Bone Joint Surg 1999: 259–278.

28. Hitchcock T, Light T, Bunch W, et al. The effect of immediate constrained digital motion of the strength of flexor tendon repairs in chickens. J Hand Surg [Am] 1987;12: 590–595.

29. Hildebrand KA, Hart DA, Rattner JB, Marchuk LL, Frank CB. Ligament injuries: Pathophysiology, healing, and treatment considerations. In Magee DJ, Zachazewshi JE, Quillen WS (eds): Scientific Foundations and Principles of Practice in Musculoskeletal Rehabilitation. St. Louis: Saunders, 2007.

30. Wyke BD. Articular Neurology and Manipulative Therapy: Aspects of Manipulative Therapy. Edinburgh: Churchill Livingstone, 1985, pp 72–80.

31. Freeman MAR, Wyke B. Articular reflexes at the ankle joint: An electromyographic study of normal and abnormal influences of ankle-joint mechanoreceptors upon reflex activity in the leg muscles. Br J Surg 1967;54: 990–1001.

32. Hogervorst T, Brand R. Mechanoreceptors in joint function. J Bone Joint Surg 1998;80-A:1365–1378.

33. Cyriax J. Textbook of Orthopedic Medicine: Diagnosis of Soft Tissue Lesions, vol 1, 8th ed. London: Bailliere Tindall, 1982.

34. Moore K, Dalley A. Clinically Oriented Anatomy, 5th ed. Philadelphia: Lippincott Williams & Wilkins, 2006.

35. Becker R. The Body Electric. New York: William Morrow, 1985.

36. Turchaninov R. Research and massage therapy: Part 2. Massage Bodywork 2001;Dec/Jan:48–56.

37. Garrett WE, Best T. Anatomy, physiology, and mechanics of skeletal muscle. In Simon S (ed): Orthopedic Basic Science. Park Ridge, IL: American Academy of Orthopedic Surgeons, 1994, pp 89–125.

38. Matzkin E, Zachazewski J, Garrett W, Malone T. Skeletal muscle: Deformation, injury, repair, and treatment considerations. In Magee DJ, Zachazewshi JE, Quillen WS (eds): Scientific Foundations and Principles of Practice in Musculoskeletal Rehabilitation. St. Louis: Saunders, 2007, pp 97–121.

39. Levangie P, Norkin C. Joint Structure and Function, 3rd ed. Philadelphia: FA Davis Company, 2001.

40. Janda V, Frank C, Liebenson C. Evaluation of muscular imbalance. In Liebenson C (ed): Rehabilitation of the Spine, 2nd ed. Baltimore: Lippincott Williams & Wilkins, 2007, pp 203–225.

41. Wyke B. Articular neurology: A review. Physiotherapy 1972;58:94–99.

42. Lewit K, Simons D. Myofascial pain: Relief by postisometric relaxation. Arch Phys Med Rehabil 1984;65: 452–456.

43. Lewit K. Manipulative Therapy in Rehabilitation on the Locomotor System, 3rd ed. Oxford, UK: Butterworth Heinemann, 1999.

44. Janda V. Function of muscles in musculoskeletal pain syndromes. Seminar notes. Seattle, April 18–19, 1999.

45. Bullock-Saxton J, Murphy D, Norris C, Richardson C, Tunnell P. The muscle designation debate: The experts respond. J Bodywork Mov Ther 2000;4:225–241.

46. Lynch M, Kessler R, Hertling D. Pain. In Hertling D, Kessler RM (eds): Management of Common Musculoskeletal Disorders: Physical Therapy Principles and Methods, 3rd ed. Baltimore: Lippincott, 1996, pp 50–68.

47. Mankin H, Mow VC, Buckwalter JA, Iannotti J, Ratcliffe A. Form and function of articular cartilage. In Simon S (ed): Orthopedic Basic Science. Park Ridge, IL: American Academy of Orthopedic Surgeons, 1994, pp 1–44.

48. Woo SL-Y, An K-N, Arnoczky SP, Wayne JS, Fithian DC, Myers B. Anatomy, biology, and biomechanics of tendon, ligament, and meniscus. In Simon SR (ed): Orthopedic Basic Science. Park Ridge, IL: American Academy of Orthopedic Surgeons, 1994, pp 45–87.

49. Williams GN, Krishnan C. Articular neurophysiology and sensorimotor control. In Magee DJ, Zachazewski JE, Quillen WS (eds): Scientific Foundations and Principles of Practice in Musculoskeletal Rehabilitation. St. Louis: Saunders, 2007, pp 190–215.

50. Young A. Effects of joint pathology on muscle. Clin Orthop 1987;219:21–27.

51. Mennell J. Joint Pain. Boston: Little, Brown and Company, 1964.

52. Korr I. Proprioceptors and somatic dysfunction. J Am Osteopath Assoc 1975;74:638–650

53. Kisner C, Colby LA. Therapeutic Exercise, 5th ed. Philadelphia: FA Davis, 2002.

54. Wooden M. Mobilization of the upper extremity. In Donatelli R, Wooden M (eds): Orthopedic Physical Therapy. New York: Churchill Livingstone, 1994, pp 297–332.

55. Butler D, Moseley L. Explain Pain. Adelaide, Australia: Noigroup Publications, 2003.

56. Hanna T. Somatics. Menlo Park, CA: Addison-Wesley, 1988.

57. Guyton A, Hall J. Textbook of Medical Physiology, 10th ed. Philadelphia: WB Saunders, 2000.

58. Laskowski ER, Newcomer-Aney K. Refining rehabilitation with proprioception training: Expediting return to play. Phys Sportsmed 1997;25(10):89–102. http://www.postgradmed.com/issues/1997/oct/laskow.html.

59. Lewis MM. Muscle spindles and their functions: A review. In Glasgow EF (ed): Aspects of Manipulative Therapy, 2nd ed. Edinburgh: Churchill Livingstone, 1985, pp 55–58.

60. Wadsworth C. The wrist and hand. In Malone T, McPoil T, Nitz A (eds): Orthopedic and Sports Physical Therapy, 3rd ed. St. Louis: Mosby, 1997, pp 327–378.

61. Pearson K, Gordon J. Spinal reflexes. In Kandal E, Schwartz J, Jessell T (eds): Principles of Neural Science. New York: McGraw-Hill, 2000, pp 713–736.

62. Mense S. Nociception from skeletal muscle in relation to clinical muscle pain. Pain 1993;54:241–289.

63. Kellett J. Acute soft tissue injuries: A review of the literature. Med Sci Sports Exerc 1986;18:489–500.

64. Nordin M, Lorenz T, Campello M. Biomechanics of tendons and ligaments. In Nordin M, Frankel V (eds): Basic Biomechanics of the Musculoskeletal System, 3rd ed. Philadelphia: Lippincott Williams & Wilkins, 2001, pp 102–125.

65. Janda V. Pain in the locomotor system: A broad approach. In Glasgow EF (ed): Aspects of Manipulative Therapy, 2nd ed. Edinburgh: Churchill Livingstone, 1985, pp 148–151.

66. Lee AC, Quillen WS, Magee D, Zachazewski J. Injury, inflammation, and repair: Tissue mechanics, the healing process, and their impact on the musculoskeletal system. In Magee DJ, Zachazewski JE, Quillen WS (eds): Scientific Foundations and Principles of Practice in Musculoskeletal Rehabilitation. St. Louis: Saunders, 2007, pp 1–22.

67. Charman RA. Pain and nociception: Mechanisms and modulation in sensory context. In Boyling J, Palastanga N (eds): Grieve's Modern Manual Therapy, 2nd ed. Edinburgh: Churchill Livingstone, 1994, pp 253–270.

68. Zimmerman M. Pain mechanisms and mediators in osteoarthritis. Semin Arthritis Rheum 1989;18:22–29.

Suggested Readings

Corrigan B, Maitland GD. Practical Orthopaedic Medicine. London: Butterworths, 1983.

Greenman PE. Principles of Manual Medicine, 2nd ed. Baltimore: Williams & Wilkins, 1996.

Hertling D, Kessler RM. Management of Common Musculoskeletal Disorders, 4th ed. Philadelphia: Lippincott Williams & Wilkins, 2006.

Janda V, Frank C, Liebenson C. Evaluation of muscular imbalance. In Liebenson C (ed): Rehabilitation of the Spine, 2nd ed. Baltimore: Lippincott Williams & Wilkins, 2007, pp 203–225.

Levangie P, Norkin C. Joint Structure and Function, 3rd ed. Philadelphia: FA Davis, 2001.

Lederman E. The Science and Practice of Manual Therapy, 2nd ed. Edinburgh: Churchill Livingstone, 2005.

Magee DJ, Zachazewshi JE, Quillen WS (eds): Scientific Foundations and Principles of Practice in Musculoskeletal Rehabilitation. St. Louis: Saunders, 2007.

Oatis CA. Kinesiology: The Mechanics and Pathomechanics of Human Movement. Philadelphia: Lippincott Williams & Wilkins, 2004.

Oschman J. Energy Medicine. Edinburgh: Churchill Livingstone, 2000.

Oschman J. Energy Medicine in Therapeutics and Human Performance. Edinburgh: Butterworth Heinemann, 2003.

Reid DC. Sports Injury and Assessment. New York: Churchill Livingstone, 1992.

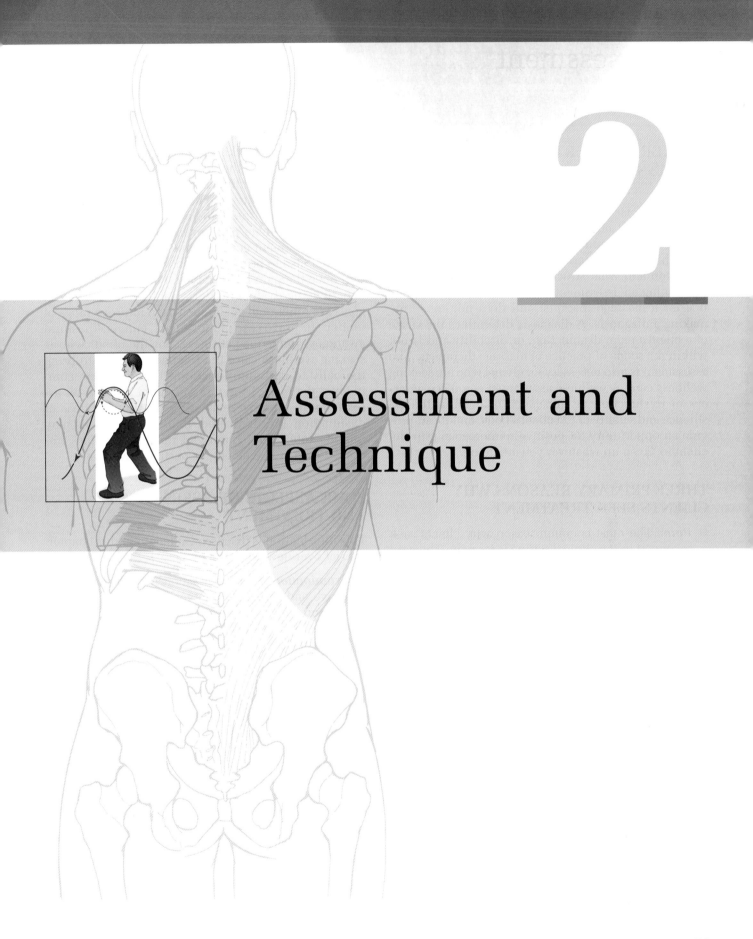

Assessment and Technique

Assessment

GENERAL OVERVIEW OF ASSESSMENT

Assessment is the process of gathering information from the client about his or her pain or dysfunction (taking a history) and performing an objective examination. This process determines the severity of the client's condition and what structures need to be worked on. Performing an assessment is within the scope of practice for a massage therapist and does not constitute making a diagnosis. A diagnosis determines the cause of a client's pain, dysfunction, or disability and is not within the scope of practice of massage therapists. The assessment is also necessary for clients who are seeking wellness care. A wellness assessment can discover areas of dysfunction or imbalance or confirm the resilience and vitality of the client's body, and it can provide an opportunity for positive reinforcement for the client to "keep up whatever you are doing."

THREE PRIMARY REASONS WHY CLIENTS SEEK TREATMENT

▨ *Pain:* The most common reason why clients seek treatment in the clinical setting is for pain. The pain may be due to an injury from a specific trauma, from repetitive or cumulative stress, from an acute exacerbation of an old condition, or from stress.

▨ *Dysfunction/disability:* The term *dysfunction* implies that the body is not functioning normally, and *disability* means a restriction or lack of ability to perform normal functions. The client might not be in pain but describes patterns such as an inability to elevate the arm overhead, stiff low back, or poor posture.

▨ *Wellness:* A significant contribution of massage and manual therapy is to promote optimum health. Whether the client is an athlete wishing to achieve maximum performance, someone seeking to achieve or enhance vitality, or a person wanting to reduce stress, massage and manual therapy are effective treatments to achieve those goals.

ESTABLISHING TREATMENT GOALS

The massage therapist who is working with pain and dysfunction has an expanded role compared with the therapist who is working in a spa environment. The primary goal for the therapist who is working in a spa is relaxation. In the clinical setting, the therapist's first task is to establish treatment goals with the client. For clients who are in pain, their primary goal will be to reduce or eliminate pain, even though for the therapist, the treatment goals are not only to eliminate the pain, but also to bring the structure to optimum function once the pain has resolved. For the client who is experiencing dysfunction or disability, the treatment goals are functional goals, such as to improve range of motion, improve ease of movement, enhance postural awareness, or reduce stiffness. For the client who is seeking wellness care, the treatment goal is to bring the body to optimum function. If there are no complaints, the task of the therapist is to perform an assessment to identify areas of dysfunction. If areas of dysfunction are discovered, the treatment goals may include relaxation, improved range of motion, improved ease of movement, or postural awareness.

FOUR ASPECTS OF ASSESSMENT AND TREATMENT

This information is discussed at length in this chapter. A brief overview is presented here.

▨ *Examination:* The examination has two parts: subjective and objective. The goal is to identify which structures are involved in the pain or dysfunction and, for the client who is seeking wellness care, to assess the general function of the musculoskeletal system.

▨ *Hypothesis and treatment plan:* Once the therapist has gathered the subjective and objective information, he or she establishes a hypothesis as to what structures need to be treated to reduce pain, improve function, and optimize wellness.[1] This hypothesis is preliminary and continues to evolve as the treatment progresses and more information is gathered from palpation, strength testing, and joint mobility. A treatment plan is suggested that is based on the severity and complexity of the condition.

▨ *Treatment and reevaluation:* The therapist must understand the patterns of pain and dysfunction and the effects of each treatment modality in order to apply the appropriate treatment to each client's condition. This information is presented below and in Chapter 1. The client's response to your treatment during the session forms part of your evaluation. Tenderness to your pressure, weakness or pain to muscle energy technique, and restricted movement are important aspects of your evaluation. A reevaluation is performed at the beginning of each session to reassess the function of the structures that are being treated in order to determine how the client is responding to care.

■ ***Discharge and future care:*** Once the functional goals have been achieved or there is no further objective improvement from treatment (maximum medical improvement), discharge and future care are discussed with the client. It is assumed that a self-care program has been established for anyone with pain or disability.

TWO PARTS OF THE ASSESSMENT

When working in the clinical setting, the therapist needs to take time at the beginning of the session to gather information from the client about the reasons the client is seeking care and to perform an objective examination. The client who is seeking wellness care might not have any specific complaints. In this case, the therapist will gather information on the client's history of previous injuries or complaints to help focus the objective examination. For clients who are seeking treatment for pain or decreased function, the process of gathering information is called *taking a history*. The subjective history and objective examination form the two elements of the assessment. The assessment helps to identify the stage of healing, that is, whether the condition is acute or chronic; identifies what structures need to be worked on; creates a clear intention about the treatment goals; provides a baseline of objective information to measure the effectiveness of treatment; helps to prevent treating conditions that are contraindicated; and indicates to the massage and manual therapist when to refer to a doctor or other health-care provider.

Subjective Examination: Taking a History

The first part of the examination is gathering information from the client about the chief complaint (i.e., the pain, dysfunction, or disability that led the client to seek treatment). This process is called *taking the history of the chief complaint* and is detailed below.

Objective Examination

The objective part of the examination includes the information that the therapist can observe or feel. It includes two aspects:

■ Observation

■ Examination

RECORDING INFORMATION

Providing massage therapy to clients who have pain, dysfunction, or disability requires that the therapist keep good records. Good record keeping provides the therapist with the information necessary to communicate with other health-care providers and forms an accurate record about what you were treating, the modalities of treatment you used, and the effectiveness of your treatment.

This text describes the essentials of performing an assessment for the massage therapist. The extent of your assessment depends on whether you are working under the direction of a doctor or another health-care provider or are working independently. In the former situation, it is the responsibility of the primary provider to take a thorough history, perform a complete examination, and inform the massage therapist regarding the client's condition. If you are working independently, it is your responsibility to take a history and perform an examination.

SUBJECTIVE, OBJECTIVE, ACTION (ASSESSMENT), AND PLAN (SOAP) NOTES

The health-care community has developed a standard format to record information in the client's chart. These notes form a medical and legal record. If you are working independently, create a chart for each patient. If you are working under the direction of another provider, you will still need to take notes about your session. Some clinics want you to write your notes in the client's chart; other clinics want you to communicate verbally to the primary therapist or doctor or to write your notes in a separate file that you keep with you.

There are four different categories of information that you need to record in your notes. These categories can be remembered with the acronym *SOAP*, which stands for "subjective, objective, assessment/action, and plan."

■ ***Subjective:*** The subjective information is the client's present complaint, that is, the client's symptoms. If the client does not have any symptoms, write down, "Wellness treatment." To find out the details of the symptoms, use the format described below called *history of the chief complaint*. Abbreviate "subjective" with the letter "s" with a circle around it.

■ ***Objective:*** This information is a summary of the examination findings. These findings are called ***signs,*** that is, what the therapist can objectively observe. Examination includes: observation, active range of motion (ROM), passive ROM, isometric testing, special tests, and palpation. Abbreviate "objective" with the letter "o" with a circle around it.

■ *Assessment/action:* In the medical community, "A" stands for assessment. Assessment is the working hypothesis about what structures or condition could be responsible for the client complaint. In the realm of manual therapy, the letter "A" also stands for the action taken, that is, what treatment was given to address those structures. As a massage therapist, briefly describe what techniques you performed and on what major areas you worked. Often, a client says, "Whatever you did last time worked like a miracle," and unless the treatment approach was written down, the therapist might not remember what created such a positive response. Abbreviate "action" with the letter "a" with a circle around it.

■ *Plan:* The plan is an outline of your treatment goals. How many treatments do you recommend? How often? What structures do you want to work on next session, and what tests do you want to perform? If you are working under the direction of a primary provider, you will not be making the decision about how many treatments or how often, but recommendations from the massage therapist are important in the decision. Abbreviate "plan" with the letter "p" with a circle around it.

PROGRESS NOTES

■ The notes in the client's chart are called *progress notes*. The first visit requires taking a history of the chief complaint unless a primary provider has performed the examination. If you are working independently, keep a chart on the client to record the notes about your examination findings and the treatments performed. You need to record only the significant examination findings. If the only positive examination finding is a loss of approximately 50% of right cervical rotation in active ROM and that motion elicited a pain in the right scapular region, it is necessary to write only that finding.

■ The first visit in which an established client presents with a new problem requires taking a history, however brief. Do not make the mistake of assuming that a client's chronic low back pain is the same as always unless you specifically ask whether there have been any new incidents, injuries, or symptoms. Since last seen, your client could have had an acute low-back strain and, unless asked, might not tell you about it.

■ The next four to six visits typically require only a brief notation regarding present symptoms, positive objective findings, the treatment you performed, and the plan for what you want to work on next time. If you are treating someone who is in acute distress, reassess the positive objective findings in each follow-up visit.

■ The primary provider typically performs a reevaluation approximately every six treatments. If you are practicing independently, you will need to perform this examination yourself. This allows you to measure the effectiveness of your treatment by determining whether there are gains in the client's functional status. Do not rely solely on a change in symptoms to measure progress. Improvement of function is the measure of effective treatment.

■ This information will form your progress notes. That is, you should note if the condition is getting better, worse, or staying the same.

SUBJECTIVE EXAMINATION: TAKING A HISTORY

When you ask clients about the condition for which they seek treatment, this is called *taking a history*. With experience, this part of your session becomes the foundation for the rest of your treatment. Gathering accurate information from the client on the nature of his or her complaint helps you to determine what structures you will be treating, the severity of the condition, whether the condition is acute or chronic, whether your treatment needs to be extremely gentle or more vigorous work is indicated, whether massage is contraindicated, and whether a referral to another provider is indicated. The history becomes a critical aspect to your session. What follows are the essential points to cover in your questions. We will assume that the client is seeking treatment for pain, but the condition may be loss of motion, loss of strength, numbness or tingling, or various other symptoms.

LOCATION

Ask the client to point to the area of complaint. A shoulder pain does not indicate where the pain is. Shoulder pain could mean the upper trapezius, the lateral humerus, or many other areas.

ONSET

Did the condition (pain, loss of motion, etc.) arise suddenly or gradually? Was there an incident of injury? A gradual onset suggests an overuse syndrome, postural stresses, or somatic manifestations of emotional or psychological stresses. When you ask about the onset, you are gathering information about the recent episode of pain or dysfunction. A separate question addresses when the client first noticed this condition (see "History of Area of Chief Complaint") and thus helps to determine any previous incident or injury prior to the current episode that involved this same region.

FREQUENCY

How often does it hurt, or how often does the client notice the dysfunction or disability? Is it once a day, once a week, ten times a day, constant? The simplest types of sprains and strains to the muscles, tendons, and ligaments hurt when these are being used and are relieved with rest. Constant pain is a red flag, that is, a symptom that is usually associated with a severe injury or pathology. Severe inflammation may hurt constantly, but so do tumors and fractures. A client with constant pain needs a referral to a doctor. Many people use the phrase "It hurts all the time" to mean that it hurts frequently rather than that it hurts at every moment.

DURATION

How long does it last when it hurts? The more serious the condition, the longer it will last.

QUALITY

Typical words that are used to describe the chief complaint are as follows:

- **Stiff, achy, tight:** These words are associated with muscles, tendons, ligaments, and joint capsules and their associated connective tissue and usually describe a simple tension or a mild overuse of the soft tissue. If an ache is more than mild, is frequent, and lasts a long time, it is more serious and represents inflammation. A thorough examination is required to rule out a more serious condition.

- **Sharp:** This describes a more severe soft tissue injury, joint problem, or a nerve root condition. A muscle or ligament tear can be sharp when the muscle or ligament is used, but it is usually relieved at rest. A nerve root inflammation can elicit a sharp pain, but the pain is often independent of movement. The protocols for how to distinguish between these two conditions are described in the section entitled "Objective Examination."

- **Burning:** Burning pain is associated with nerve inflammation. It is safe to perform massage on a client with burning pain, but the client typically needs a referral to a chiropractor or osteopath to assess the need for spinal manipulation.

- **Tingling, numbing:** These words describe a nerve compression, either near the spine or in the extremities. If a series of four treatments does not resolve mild tingling and numbing, refer the client to a chiropractor or osteopath.

- **Throbbing:** This is associated with acute inflammation and swelling, such as an acute bursitis. Gentle muscle energy technique (MET), passive joint movement, and soft tissue mobilization (STM) are indicated with mild throbbing pain to help reduce the swelling and resolve the inflammation. Severe throbbing is a contraindication to massage.

- **Gripping:** This word is typically used to describe a serious condition, often a nerve root injury (see Chapter 3, "Lumbosacral Spine," and Chapter 5, "Cervical Spine"). If the client describes a mild gripping pain, gentle treatment may be performed. Severe gripping pain is a contraindication to massage and requires a referral to a doctor.

RADIATION

Is there pain, numbing, or tingling in the arms or legs? As was mentioned in Chapter 1, there are three basic types of referred pain: sclerotomal, myotomal, and dermatomal. Sclerotomes are deep somatic tissues (fascia, ligaments, capsules, and connective tissue) that are innervated by the same spinal nerve. When a tissue of a particular sclerotome is irritated, the pain may refer into specific patterns called **sclerotomes,** which are all the tissue innervated by the same nerve (see Fig. 1-14 in Chapter 1). Usually, sclerotomal pain is described as *deep, aching, and diffuse.* The extent of the radiation depends on the intensity of the irritation to the tissue.

A **myotome** consists of the muscles that are supplied by the motor root(s) of the spinal nerve(s). If there is irritation or compression of the motor (ventral) nerve root, in addition to deep, boring pain, there may be a weakness in the muscles that are supplied by that nerve root (myotome) and a decrease in the response in the corresponding reflex. A **dermatome** is an area of skin that is supplied by the sensory (dorsal) root of a spinal nerve. Irritation of the sensory nerve root elicits a *sharp pain, numbing, or tingling* that is well-localized in dermatomes corresponding to the root, called **dermatomal pain.** The most common cause of nerve root irritation is disc herniation. Nerve root pain is much more serious and requires an assessment by a chiropractor or osteopath.

SEVERITY

Ask your clients to rate their pain on a 0 to 10 scale, with 10 being the worst pain ever experienced and 0 being no pain. The number 10 should be used for incapacitating pain (i.e., the client cannot work or perform household duties with pain that severe). Moderate pain (5 to 9) interferes with a person's ability to perform work or household duties. Mild pain (1 to 4) does not interfere with a person's activities of daily living.

AGGRAVATING FACTORS

What activities make the condition worse? Does sitting, standing, walking, twisting, bending, or resting aggravate the pain? The simplest strains and sprains of the musculoskeletal system are irritated with too much movement and relieved by rest. When a condition hurts more with rest, either an inflammation or a pathology is indicated.

RELIEVING FACTORS

What activities make the condition better? Does resting, moving, or applying ice or heat relieve the pain? As the soft tissue heals, it feels good to move the injured area. Stretching tight muscles, shortened ligaments, and joint capsules feels good, despite some mild discomfort. Acute injuries involving the soft tissue are painful with large movements and are relieved with rest.

NIGHT PAIN

Inflammation and tumors are worse at night. Constant, gripping pain that is worse at night is a red flag and needs a referral to a doctor. An area that hurts at night but is relieved with movement indicates inflammation.

PRIOR TREATMENTS AND THEIR EFFECTS

Are you the first therapist to treat this condition? If so, you need to perform a careful history and examination to determine whether massage is contraindicated and when to refer. It is also important to know whether the client has had massage and manual therapy before and whether it was helpful.

PROGRESS

Is the client getting better, getting worse, or staying the same? If a client is getting worse, then use extra care in your history and examination to determine whether a referral is indicated.

HISTORY OF AREA OF CHIEF COMPLAINT

Have there been any accidents, injuries, or surgeries to the area of complaint in the client's past? The longer the history, the more challenging is the condition.

MEDICATIONS

If a person has taken pain medication within four hours of your assessment and treatment, you need to be cautious, because the pain medication could be giving the client a false sense of comfort with the examination and depth of the therapist's work.

DIAGNOSTIC STUDIES PERFORMED

Have X-rays, magnetic resonance imaging (MRI), or other diagnostic tests been performed? If, so, get a copy of the report for your file. Does the report indicate a severe condition?

OBJECTIVE EXAMINATION

The objective examination includes observation and examination. There are five elements to the examination: active movements, passive movements, isometric testing, special tests, and palpation. Accurate examination requires that the therapist follow a specific sequence of procedures and apply those steps to the area of the body under examination. This ensures that all the relevant information is being gathered. Each chapter in this book describes the specific examination procedures for a particular region of the body. However, it is important first to understand the basic principles of the examination and why each aspect of the examination is performed.

OBSERVATION

Observation begins as soon as the therapist greets the client. Notice body posture; ease of movement; whether the client has a dysfunctional gait, such as a limp; getting up and down from the chair; and removing outer garments. Facial expression and tone of voice are clues to the level of discomfort.

- *Posture:* Notice the client's posture in both standing and seated positions and the posture or position of the area of complaint. For example, notice if the shoulder is held in an elevated or forward posture on one side.

- *Redness, swelling:* Redness or swelling indicates inflammation, and special precautions are necessary for red, hot, swollen tissue. The therapist needs to be extremely gentle in the application of treatment. The first goal is to reduce the swelling by performing gentle MET and passive ROM.

- *Scars:* Scars indicate either prior surgery or prior injury and reveal that the area is compromised. Ask the client to describe how he or she received the scar.

- *Atrophy:* Atrophy is a loss of muscle tone. Either the area has been deconditioned from lack of use or there is neurological involvement. Simple atrophy can be a result of immobilization caused by prior fracture, lack of use due to pain, or sedentary lifestyle, common in the elderly. Complex atrophy is a long-standing condition that involves the damage or dysfunction of the nerve(s) innervating the afflicted muscles. Do not work vigorously on an atrophied muscle. The area needs MET to reestablish the neurological communication and exercise.

MOTION ASSESSMENT

The next part of the examination is divided into two sections. In active motion assessment, the therapist asks the client to perform movements in specific directions. In passive motion assessment, the therapist moves the client. Injuries and dysfunctions of the musculoskeletal system hurt when the injured area is moved; and more complex conditions such as inflammation of the nervous system, systemic conditions such as heart disease, or pathologies such as tumors are not significantly aggravated by movement. If an area does not hurt at rest but does hurt with movement, then the simplest of conditions—the sprains and strains of soft tissue—are indicated.

Active Movements

The therapist notes the following categories:

▓ **Range of motion (ROM):** Is the range of motion normal, decreased, or increased? Determining normal ROM is more complex than it might seem. You need to consider the client's age and sex. There is less ROM as we age, and women typically have greater ROM than men. If the complaint is in the extremities, then begin with the noninvolved side, and always compare both sides.
   □ **Decreased ROM** is caused by either pain or changes in the joint or soft tissue. If the loss of motion is not a result of pain, then the therapist needs to gather more information to determine whether the lack of motion is caused by adhesions in the joint capsule, ligaments, myofascia, spastic muscles, degeneration in the joints, or other causes.
   □ **Increased ROM** that is significantly different from the other side indicates a moderate to severe injury to the ligaments, joint capsule, or both. Increased ROM on both sides compared with normal ROM suggests a generalized *hypermobility syndrome* and potential instability in the joints.

▓ **Pain:** If movement is painful, ask the client to describe its location, quality, and severity. The three stages of healing elicit pain at different ranges of the movement, as follows:
   □ **Acute** conditions yield pain before the normal ROM.
   □ **Subacute** conditions give pain at the end of that normal range.
   □ **Chronic** conditions may elicit pain with overpressure at the end of active or passive motion.

Passive Movements

Passive motion testing includes two categories: (1) testing for the ROM, pain, and quality of the soft tissue as it is being stretched at its end range, called the *end feel*, and (2) moving the joint passively to determine the range and quality of accessory motion (*joint play*). The first category originated with James Cyriax, MD, who developed a system of soft tissue assessment called *selective tension testing*.[2] He made the simple but profound observation that muscles and tendons and their associated connective tissues can be accurately examined by means of isometric testing, since muscles are contractile tissues, and that noncontractile soft tissues, such as the joint capsule, ligaments, fascia, bursae, dura mater, and dural sheath, can be accurately examined with passive motion testing. This principle helps to differentiate muscle-tendon strains from ligamentous sprains and therefore helps to determine where and how to apply the treatment. These principles are utilized in the examination of each region of the body.

TESTING FOR PASSIVE RANGE OF MOTION, PAIN, AND END FEEL

When performing passive motion on the client, note the following three categories:

▓ **ROM:** Passive ROM is typically greater than active ROM.

▓ **Pain:** Note the location, quality, and severity of the pain. To help determine the stage of healing, note when pain is felt during the range of passive motion.
   □ **Acute** conditions yield pain before the normal ROM.
   □ **Subacute** conditions give pain at the end of the normal range.
   □ **Chronic** conditions may elicit pain with overpressure at the end range.

▓ **End feel:** This term, which was developed by James Cyriax, is defined as the feeling that is transmitted to the therapist's hands as a slight overpressure is applied at the end of the joint's passive ROM.[2] The end feel gives important information about the type of injury or dysfunction and its severity. For example, elbow flexion normally has a soft tissue approximation end feel as the biceps and other soft tissues are being compressed. A bony end feel in elbow flexion would be abnormal and would indicate degeneration of the elbow joint. Seven categories of end feel are differentiated:
   □ **Soft tissue approximation:** A soft end feel, as is felt in flexing the elbow, as the biceps and forearm muscles are pressed together.

- ☐ **Muscular:** A more rubbery feeling than a soft tissue approximation, as is felt in stretching the hamstrings.
- ☐ **Bony:** An abrupt, hard end feel, as is felt in extending the elbow.
- ☐ **Capsular:** A thick, tight feeling, similar to that of stretching leather, as is felt in external rotation of the shoulder.
- ☐ **Muscle spasm:** A tight, bound feeling, ending before the normal ROM, as is felt in a muscle spasm. Palpation confirms the assessment.
- ☐ **Springy block:** A feeling of the joint rebounding or springing, associated with a decreased ROM. A classic finding with a torn meniscus of the knee as the joint is brought to passive extension.
- ☐ **Empty:** The client stops further passive motion because of pain, even though the therapist cannot detect any tissue tension or other resistance to the motion. Typical with acute bursitis, emotional guarding, or a pathology.

TESTING FOR PASSIVE ACCESSORY MOTION (JOINT PLAY)

The second type of passive motion testing is to determine the range and quality of movement between the joint surfaces, called *accessory motion* or *joint play*. These tests are performed during the examination described in each chapter and as part of specific soft tissue and joint mobilizations during the treatment. Joint dysfunction is a loss of joint play movements, as each joint needs slight passive movement to function normally. See "Joint Movement" in Chapter 1 (p. 36) for further discussion.

ISOMETRIC TESTING

Isometric contraction is an assessment of the contractile structures (e.g., muscles, tendons, and their associated connective tissues) and the nervous system. These tests are performed as part of contract-relax (CR) MET (see "Muscle Energy Technique," p. 76). During the contraction, the therapist notes two things: the **strength** of the resistance and whether the client experiences **pain.** Isometric testing yields three possible findings:

- **Strong and painless** contraction indicates a normal structure.

- **Painful** contraction indicates an injury or dysfunction in the tested muscle-tendon-periosteal unit.

- **Weak and painless** contraction may indicate one of nine possibilities:
  - ☐ The muscle is inhibited because of hypertonic antagonist.

- ☐ The muscle is inhibited because of dysfunction or injury in a local joint that the muscle crosses.
- ☐ Fixation or subluxation of a vertebra of the spine, causing irritation to the motor nerve and weakness in the muscles that are innervated by that nerve.
- ☐ Nerve injury (e.g., rupture of a disc), which can create pressure on the nerve root, causing the muscle that the root innervates to weaken.
- ☐ The muscle is deconditioned from lack of use.
- ☐ An atrophied muscle from previous injury or disease.
- ☐ Reflexive weakness caused by visceral imbalance, which is called the *viscerosomatic reflex* and may be assessed by means of applied kinesiology.
- ☐ Stretch weakness describes a condition in which a muscle is kept in a habitually stretched position that causes it to weaken.
- ☐ Tightness-weakness, a condition in which a muscle is habitually short and tests weak, even if tested at its resting length.[3]

PALPATION

This text assumes that the therapist has been trained in the fundamentals of palpation. See Hoppenfeld[4] and Chaitow[5] for textbooks on palpation.

As was mentioned in Chapter 1, touching another human being is an act of giving and receiving information. It conveys not only our skill, but also our sensitivity and compassion. The therapist wants to convey through touch that the client is completely safe physically and emotionally. The client should be able to relax completely under the therapist's touch.

Our touch is also a powerful assessment tool. Our hands receive information about the condition of the tissue under our fingers as well as the client's general health and emotional and psychological state. As a general rule, the palpation that is described in this text is done while performing the strokes.

Five Characteristics of Soft Tissue the Therapist Can Palpate

Five characteristics of soft tissue can be palpated to inform the therapist about the state of health of the tissue and the stage of healing. Acute injuries, which create inflammation, will manifest as hot and swollen tissue. In subacute and chronic conditions, it is necessary to compare both sides of the body to determine abnormalities.

Temperature
- Heat is an indication of inflammation, and coldness in an area of the body compared to the other side indicates compromised circulation.

Texture

Texture is determined by two qualities: water content and fiber content. Healthy tissue has a distinct feel that is hard to describe but has a balance between fiber and water.

- **Water content:** Healthy tissue is well hydrated and feels like a water balloon filled with water. Inflamed tissue has a tight, resistant feel due to the swollen tissue, like a water balloon filled with too much water. Deconditioned or atrophied tissue feels mushy because there is too little water. Healthy tissue is pliable (has "give") and resilient (springs back).

- **Fiber content:** The feeling of healthy soft tissue is also due to the fiber. Too little fiber from deconditioning or atrophy makes the tissue feel mushy. Too much fiber from adhesions or scarring feels thick and dense.

Tenderness

The therapist can gain information about the severity of the condition by palpation. Pressing into tissue and taking out all the slack puts the tissue in tension. Normally, there is no pain with pressing into the soft tissue, only a sense of pressure.

- **Acute:** The client feels pain before tissue is in tension. This is due to inflammation in acute conditions and due to ischemia (low oxygen) in chronic conditions. Inflammation is localized pain; ischemia is more diffuse.

- **Subacute:** The client feels pain at tissue tension.

- **Chronic:** The client might feel pain with overpressure (i.e., pressing further into the tissue after the tissue is in tension).

Tone

Four categories of tone are used to differentiate healthy tissue and between acute and chronic conditions.

- **Normal:** The soft tissue feels resilient, homogeneous, relaxed, and fluid without being watery.

- **Acute:** The soft tissue feels watery owing to the swelling (edema) and warm or hot, depending on the extent of the inflammation.

- **Chronic (adhesions):** The soft tissue feels fibrous, gristly, dry (decreased water), thickened, stiff, and tight.

- **Chronic (atrophy):** The soft tissue feels mushy and flaccid, owing to a loss of tone (i.e., decreased fiber content).

Mobility

- **Normal:** Soft tissue is normally pliable (has "give"), resilient (springs back), and extensible (ability to stretch).

- **Hypomobile:** Decreased movement is called *hypomobility*. The soft tissue may be tight from excessive muscle tension or muscular guarding due to injury or from emotional or psychological stress, or it may be thick because of adhesions from joint injury or dysfunction.

- **Hypermobile:** Increased movement in the soft tissue is called *hypermobility*. It may be caused by prior injury, inhibition of normal neurological tone, atrophy, immobilization, or heredity, which would manifest as increased mobility throughout the body (hypermobility syndrome).

SPECIAL TESTS

Each region of the body requires special orthopedic tests to help isolate the structures that are the source of the client's pain or dysfunction. For example, in Chapter 3, "Lumbosacral Spine," a special test is the straight-leg-raising test, which is used to determine whether the client has nerve root pressure. Each chapter lists special tests for each region.

PATTERNS OF SOFT TISSUE AND JOINT DYSFUNCTION, INJURY, AND DEGENERATION

After performing the history and objective examination, gather all the pieces of information to form an assessment of the client's condition. Patterns will emerge within the countless types of injuries and dysfunctions in the body. Knowing these patterns helps to guide the therapist in determining the type of injury or dysfunction and therefore helps to create an appropriate treatment. It can be frustrating for the client and the therapist to assume that the client merely has tight muscles when examination findings suggest degeneration in the joint. These categories overlap, and most clients present with several categories at the same time. Understanding what structures to treat dramatically increases the effectiveness of the treatment.

We apply each of these patterns to each region of the body in the subsequent chapters of this book.

ARTHRITIS, OSTEOARTHRITIS, AND DEGENERATIVE JOINT DISEASE

The word **arthritis** means inflammation of a joint. In common language, the word *arthritis* or **osteoarthritis** usually refers to chronic pain or stiffness in a joint. The more accurate term for chronic degeneration of the joint is **arthrosis** or **degenerative joint disease.** Following common usage, this text uses *osteoarthritis* and *degenerative joint disease* interchangeably, and these terms imply a chronic condition unless specified otherwise. The term *joint degeneration* refers to degeneration of the cartilage.

■ Active and passive ROM are decreased. If the joint is inflamed or contractures have developed, then movements are limited and painful. Chronic degeneration often has crepitation (grinding sounds) with active and passive movement.

■ Resisted (isometric) movements are usually painless but may be weak. The patterns of muscle weakness are described in each chapter.

■ Passive motion elicits a capsular end feel with mild to moderate degeneration and a bony end feel in more advanced conditions.

CAPSULITIS

Capsulitis is an inflammation of the joint capsule. As with arthritis, the term is often used for chronic conditions, as in adhesive capsulitis of the shoulder. Technically, chronic adhesions in the capsule are a **capsulosis.**

■ Active and passive ROMs are decreased and painful during the inflammatory stage. In chronic conditions, such as adhesive capsulitis, the person has limited ROM that might not be painful until the tissue is stretched through the tension barrier.

■ Resisted (isometric) contraction is usually painless.

■ Passive motion reveals an empty end feel if there is inflammation and a thickened, leathery (capsular) end feel if the condition is chronic.

TENDINITIS/TENDINOPATHY

Tendinitis is a tear to the collagen fibers of a tendon, caused by an acute injury or cumulative overuse syndrome. This leads to inflammation of the tendon. Chronic dysfunction and pain of a tendon are called *tendinopathy* and describe a degeneration of the tendon rather than inflammation. To palpation, an inflamed tendon will be tender before tissue tension, whereas chronic tendinopathy will be tender with overpressure.

■ Active motion can be limited and painful, depending on the extent of the injury.

■ Passive stretching can be painful when the tendon is fully stretched.

■ Isometric testing with mild tendinitis is typically strong unless the tissue is fatigued with repeated testing. With moderate to severe conditions, testing is weak and painful. The severity of the condition

is proportional to the limitation and pain during active motion and the degree of pain and weakness during isometric challenge.

MUSCLE STRAIN

A **muscle strain** is a tear to the muscle and its associated connective tissue as a result of an acute episode or a cumulative overuse syndrome.

■ Active motion can be painful and limited, depending on the extent of the injury.

■ Passive movement is usually not painful except by fully stretching a muscle and putting overpressure at the end of normal range.

■ Isometric testing is typically strong with mild injuries and elicits pain or discomfort at the site of injury. Moderate to severe strains test weak and painful. Mild strains are not painful to isometric testing unless the muscle is challenged repeatedly to a state of fatigue. As with tendinitis, moderate to severe conditions test weak and painful. The severity of the condition is proportional to the limitation and pain during active motion and the degree of pain and weakness during isometric challenge.

LIGAMENT SPRAIN

A **ligament sprain** is a tear to the ligament and its associated connective tissue due to an acute episode or a cumulative overuse syndrome.

■ Active ROM is decreased and painful.

■ Passive motion is typically decreased in one plane of motion and elicits pain at the site of the injury.

■ Isometric testing is not painful.

■ Moderate to severe ligament sprains create hypermobility in the associated joint.

BURSITIS

A **bursitis** is an inflammation of the fluid-filled bursal sac, typically a result of repetitive overuse of the muscle that overlies the bursa. This friction irritates the bursa, stimulating excessive fluid buildup and pain caused by the pressure within the bursa.

■ Active ROM is decreased and painful.

■ Passive motion that compresses the bursa elicits pain, limited motion, and an empty end feel.

■ Isometric contraction of the muscle overlying the bursa can be painful, depending on how acute the bursitis is. In an acute bursitis, isometric contraction of the muscle is painful.

DISC LESION (HERNIATION, BULGE, PROTRUSION)

A disc injury is a tear of the fibrocartilage between the vertebrae of the spine. The tear may be contained, called an *internal derangement,* or there may be a displacement of the nucleus, causing the outer rim of the disc to bulge or protrude, called a *herniation.* This bulge often presses against the nerve roots, leading to pain, numbing, or tingling in the extremities.

▨ Observation often shows an **antalgic posture** (i.e., sustained lateral flexion), caused by the pain in either the trunk or the cervical spine.

▨ Active ROM and passive ROM are limited and painful, especially in extension.

▨ With cervical discs, isometric testing may reveal weakness in the muscles of the arm, hand, or both; with lumbar discs, a weakness in the muscles of the leg and foot can result.

IMPAIRED MUSCLE FUNCTION

As was mentioned in Chapter 1 in the section "Muscle Dysfunction," muscles may become weak (inhibited) or hypertonic (facilitated) because of reflex activity from joint dysfunction (arthrokinetic reflex), prior muscle injury, poor posture, and emotional stress. Muscle imbalances cause uneven distribution of forces through the joint, and though typically painless, they can lead to impaired movement and degeneration in the associated joint.

▨ Active ROM and passive ROM of the associated joint are often normal.

▨ Isometric testing is the best way to identify muscle weakness. Sustained muscle contraction is best identified by palpation.

MYOFASCIAL PAIN SYNDROME (TRIGGER POINTS)

Myofascial pain syndrome is defined as a chronic, regional pain syndrome characterized by myofascial trigger points.[6] The trigger point is a hyperirritable area in a tight band of muscle, eliciting dull, aching pain. Some potential causes include acute and chronic overload of the muscle and postural stresses. The author's clinical experience supports studies that show that trigger points are effectively and painlessly treated with postisometric relaxation (PIR) MET.[7]

▨ The trigger point is a hypersensitive palpable nodule in a taut band, which is painful on compression.

▨ There is often decreased ROM and decreased strength in the muscle and increased pain with stretching.

SOFT TISSUE POSITIONAL DYSFUNCTION

Lauren Berry, RPT, contributed the concept of positional dysfunction of the soft tissue. The fascicles or bundles of fibers of the muscles, tendons, ligaments, and nerves can roll out of their normal position relative to the other fascicles. As a result, the entire muscle, tendon, ligament, and nerve can become misaligned in relation to the joint and neighboring soft tissues. The author has theorized that this misalignment creates an abnormal torsion or twist (interfascicular torsion) in the fibers and fascicles and decreased function. Positional dysfunction is caused by poor posture, joint injury or dysfunction, and emotional or psychological stress.

▨ Active ROM and passive ROM of the associated joint are typically not painful.

▨ Isometric testing does not reveal positional dysfunction, although positional dysfunction of the muscle can create muscle weakness.

▨ Palpation reveals an increased tension in the soft tissue, chronic positional dysfunction leads to adhesions, and the tissue will feel thick and fibrous.

JOINT DYSFUNCTION (JOINT FIXATION OR SUBLUXATION)

Joint dysfunction is the loss of passive glide (joint play) of the joint surfaces. It is often asymptomatic. If the joint "locks," it is typically described as a painful catch. The pain is usually of sudden onset and is often sharp and well localized. Joint dysfunction is typically accompanied by hypertonic muscles in the area of dysfunction. If massage does not reduce muscle tension, then the underlying cause may be reflex activity from the joint dysfunction.

▨ Active and passive movements in one direction are decreased.

▨ Passive mobilization of the joint identifies loss of normal play in the joint.

▨ Isometric testing typically is not used to detect joint fixation, but muscles that are innervated with the nerves that emerge from the level of spinal fixation are often weak.

NERVE ENTRAPMENT OR COMPRESSION SYNDROMES

Nerves are susceptible to compression within the spinal canal due to stenosis (narrowing), from protrusions of the intervertebral disc or bony spurs; as they exit the spine through the intervertebral foramen; and as they travel through muscles (e.g., through the scalenes) and fibro-osseous tunnels, such as the carpal tunnel. Typical symptoms include numbing and tingling (paresthesias) unless the nerve root is affected, in which case pain is the predominant symptom. Compression of the motor nerve root causes muscle weakness in the associated myotome.

■ Increased compression of an already compressed nerve elicits or increases the symptoms. For example, Phalen's test compresses the median nerve and increases the symptoms of carpal tunnel syndrome

(see Chapter 7, "The Elbow, Forearm, Wrist, and Hand").

■ Stretching an entrapped or compressed nerve increases the symptoms. For example, the straight-leg-raising test increases pain, numbing, or tingling in the leg if the lumbosacral nerve roots are irritated (see Chapter 3).

■ Manually stroking across an entrapped nerve can temporarily increase a numbing and tingling sensation.

Technique

The technique section is divided into three parts. The first part provides a brief overview of the three techniques that are used in this text and introduces concepts that help the therapist to stay energized and relaxed while performing the treatment. The second part describes each of the three techniques in detail. The third part provides guidelines for how to apply these three techniques in acute, subacute, and chronic conditions.

OVERVIEW OF TREATMENT TECHNIQUES

As was mentioned in Chapter 1, this text introduces a unique combination of three techniques, performed in a specific protocol or "recipe" that has been found in over 30 years of clinical practice to achieve the most efficient and effective success in the treatment of musculoskeletal conditions. One of the unique contributions of this method of therapy is that it combines profound relaxation with effective soft tissue therapy. Relaxation optimizes the healing potential of the body and the most successful outcome. Each of the subsequent chapters describes how to apply these three techniques to each region of the body.

The three techniques are as follows:

■ *Soft tissue mobilization (STM):* This text introduces a new style of STM (massage) called ***wave mobilization***, which rhythmically mobilizes the soft tissue transverse to the fiber in a rounded, scooping motion.

■ *Muscle energy technique (MET):* This is a method of manual therapy in which the client provides ac-

tive resistance to the therapist's pressure. Osteopaths, chiropractors, and physical therapists have successfully used MET for decades. The active participation of the client with the therapist can change neurological patterns that improve proprioception, improve soft tissue and joint function, and dramatically change chronic pain patterns.

■ ***Joint mobilization:*** To induce passive movement to the joints helps to reduce swelling and pain, decreases muscle spasms, provides lubrication and nutrition to the joint, and can be profoundly relaxing. Because the joints are a primary source of pain and disability, joint mobilization is essential for optimum care for musculoskeletal pain and dysfunction.

GUIDELINES FOR STAYING ENERGIZED AND RELAXED WHILE PERFORMING TREATMENT

A key to optimizing the healing potential of the treatment and to maintaining a healthy career in massage and manual therapy is to learn to stay energized and relaxed during treatment. The first step is for the therapist to focus attention not only on *what* he or she is doing, but also on *how* he or she is doing it. It requires a balance in the therapist's attention between what is felt *in the client's body* and what the therapist feels *in his or her own body,* with a continuous focus on relaxation for the client *and* the therapist. The client's relaxation response creates the neurological and emotional environment for healing; and for the therapist to work in a calm and relaxed manner not only prevents injuries, but also creates an internal environment for self-healing. In other words, giving a treatment can promote healing in both the client and the therapist. We will first discuss the guidelines for the therapist.

First Goal for the Therapist: Creating Inner Calmness

The effects of treatment begin even before you touch your client. As was described in Chapter 1, research has found that humans radiate a biomagnetic field and that this field can, in theory, be focused for healing. To maximize the benefits of treatment, the therapist would benefit from taking time at the beginning of each day to engage in some practice that establishes inner calmness. This might be focused breathing, prayer, meditation, yoga, tai chi, or any other centering practice. Most of us have many thoughts and feelings moving through us at any given moment, potentially making us feel "scattered." Centering practices create inner stillness by bringing our attention to the present moment. The easiest way to achieve that is to focus on your breathing. Feel the breath coming into the nostrils, and feel it moving out of the nostrils, or feel the rising and falling of the abdomen as you inhale and exhale. Focusing on the sensations of your breath helps you to be grounded, that is, to stay in the present moment, in your present experience. This creates inner **coherence**, a state in which our thoughts and feelings are focused. It is similar to taking light that has many different wavelengths that are out of phase and bringing them all to one wavelength and all in phase. This coherence of light is called a *laser*, a very penetrating beam, analogous to the focused, penetrating touch that develops from the inner coherence of the therapist.

Second Goal for the Therapist: Heartfelt Intention

Each of us is transmitting a message to the world by our thoughts, feelings, and actions. We are like radio stations, broadcasting our programs. We can sense that in each other. We have met people who have "negative energy" or the opposite, "beautiful energy." We have a great deal of control over what we are communicating to the world with our thoughts and feelings. The heart is the primary source of the electricity streaming through the body and is therefore the primary source of our electromagnetic field. It is a hundred times stronger than the electrical signal from our brains. A profound way to increase the effectiveness of your treatment is to breathe into your heart for a few minutes before your workday and create an intention to be of help to the people you will treat that day.

Third Goal for the Therapist: Being Present

Being present is a state in which thoughts, emotions, and body movements are all focused on what we are doing in the present moment. This focused awareness in not easily achieved and represents a lifelong practice. Many traditions call this *being awake*. To be fully present creates the internal environment for optimum healing. To be fully attentive to what you are doing from moment to moment brings focus, depth, and precision to your work. When we are not fully present, we are not only thinking about the past or future, or daydreaming, we may have thoughts of insecurity or judgment, and we don't notice if our bodies are uncomfortable or straining. A simple method to bring attention back to the present moment is for the therapist to focus on his or her breath and on the sensations of his or her body. It is natural for the attention to drift. Without any judgment or criticism, gently bring your attention back to present moment.

Fourth Goal for the Therapist: Effortless Work

Massage and manual therapy are work. Effortless work is akin to taking a walk; it is relaxing and energizing even though it requires work. As in walking, learn to use your legs to perform most of the work. Balance the work required from the legs with the effortless quality of moving from the center of your body. Performing effortless work is based on three principles:

- Proper ergonomics
- Relaxation
- Whole body movement

First Principle: Ergonomics

Rule No. 1: Keep Your Joints in the Open (Resting) Position

The resting position of a joint is the position in its ROM at which the joint is under the least amount of stress.[3] As was mentioned in Chapter 1, the human body is a tensegrity structure; that is, the muscles, tendons, and connective tissue (the myofascial system) are the tension members of the body. These tension members keep the body upright and provide the force that moves our body. The bones and joints are the compression members. The myofascial system is designed to perform the work of giving a massage, because it absorbs the pressure (reaction force) as you push into the client and prevents overloading the cartilage of the joints, preventing degeneration. Giving a massage with the myofascial system providing the work requires the joints to be in the resting position and not in the closed-packed (tight) position.

In the closed-packed position, the fingers, wrists, elbows, and knees are all extended. In this position, the joints are under maximum compression, and the ligaments and joint capsules are maximally tight. The repetitive stresses of giving a massage load the cartilage of the joint and accelerate the degeneration of the joint.

To achieve the open-packed (loose) position of the joints, the following posture is assumed (Fig. 2-1):

- **Spine:** The spine is upright, midway between flexion and extension. Excessive lordosis (swayback) is avoided by tucking your pelvis, keeping a slight curve in the lumbar spine.

- **Temporomandibular joint (TMJ):** The teeth are slightly apart. The top of the tongue is lightly touching the upper palate.

- **Elbow:** The elbow is in approximately 70° of flexion. Always keep some flexion in the elbows, because this allows the muscles to absorb the pressure of pushing into the client.

- **Wrist:** The wrist is in neutral position, midway between flexion and extension, or extended as much as 20°.

- **Metacarpophalangeal (MCP) joints (the knuckles):** The open position is slight flexion.

- **Interphalangeal (IP):** The open position is slight flexion.

- **Knee:** The knees are in slight flexion.

Rule No. 2: Keep Your Wrist and Hand in the Position of Function as Much as Possible

In the *position of function* of the wrist and hand, the intrinsic musculature and the extrinsic musculature are in balance and under equal tension. It is the position in which finger and thumb flexion can occur with the least effort.[3]

- **Wrist:** In a neutral position, midway between flexion and extension, or extended as much as 20° with slight ulnar flexion.

- **Fingers:** The knuckle joints (MCP joints) and the joints of the fingers are all in slight flexion.

An easy way to determine the position of function of the hands is to stand in a relaxed posture, with the arms hanging at the sides. The wrist and hands automatically assume the resting position (Fig. 2-2**A**). If the elbows are flexed approximately 70°, they are now relaxed and open, the best position for performing the massage (Fig. 2-2**B**).

Second Principle: Relaxation

To induce profound relaxation in the client requires that the therapist be relaxed. In all exceptional

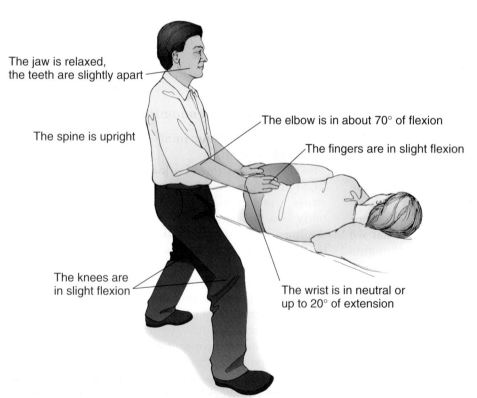

The jaw is relaxed, the teeth are slightly apart

The spine is upright

The elbow is in about 70° of flexion

The fingers are in slight flexion

The knees are in slight flexion

The wrist is in neutral or up to 20° of extension

Figure 2-1. Open position of the joints in the standing posture. The knees are slightly bent; the elbows are flexed about 70°; the wrist is in neutral, midway between flexion and extension, or up to 20° of extension; the fingers are flexed slightly; the spine is upright; and the jaw and teeth are held slightly apart.

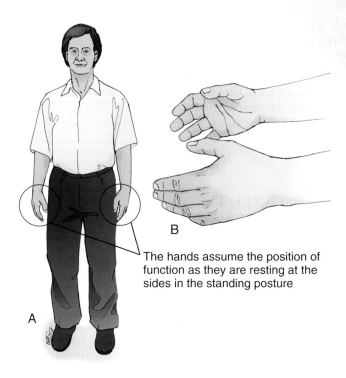

The hands assume the position of function as they are resting at the sides in the standing posture

A

B

Figure 2-2. **A.** An easy way to determine the position of function of the hands is to stand in a relaxed posture, with the hands hanging at the sides. **B.** The hands automatically assume a resting position, also called the *position of function*. If the hands are kept in this position and the elbows are flexed, the hands remain in the best position for performing a massage: open and relaxed. Try to keep your hands and wrists in this position as much as possible while performing the massage.

performances, whether dance, music, sports, or massage and manual therapy, a person's greatest potential is expressed by being relaxed and letting movement happen through oneself. This is called *being in the zone* and indicates a sense of getting out of the way and letting some greater force move through you. Relaxation also helps to conserve vital energy, whereas excess tension drains the body's energy. The basic guidelines are as follows:

▨ Relax your entire body—the hands, wrists, arms, shoulders, back, belly, and jaw.

▨ Minimize muscular effort. Effort is often felt as invasive by clients, and they resist your effort by tensing somewhere else in their body.

▨ Breathe from your belly. Make sure that your breathing is relaxed and that the sensations in your body are comfortable.

▨ Keep your hands soft and relaxed. Imagine a stream of energy moving through your hands.

Third Principle: Whole Body Movement

This is the fundamental principle of martial arts and sports. In martial arts, it is called *moving from the center.*

To achieve a powerful tennis serve, baseball throw, or golf swing requires that the force be generated from the center of the body (the pelvis) and move into the arms and hands as centrifugal force. In manual therapy, we are pushing on the body during soft tissue work, and the easiest and deepest work comes when the therapist is generating the force from the pelvis and legs.

Move your hands by moving your whole body. Even if your stroke is 1 inch long, rock your whole body into that stroke. This moves the mass of your body into the area where you are working.

The pelvis should face the area you are working. The legs are the "engines" that drive the strokes, and the pelvis is the "steering wheel." Point the pelvis straight into the strokes.

USING HEALING ENERGY (CHI) IN YOUR MASSAGE

Chi is a Chinese word that means life force (literally, "breath"). It is a fundamental concept of Taoism, a religion that was founded in China by Lao Tzu, who is said to have been born in 604 B.C. Literally, *Tao* means "the way," and it means the way things are, the way to live one's life, and the essence or source of the universe.

The Taoists observed nature and especially water as embodying the essence of the Tao. Water is so yielding that it takes the shape of whatever container you put it in, yet it is so powerful that it dissolves rocks and forms canyons.

Taoists believe that you can actually draw chi from the universe, and they developed exercises such as tai chi ch'uan and chi gung to build a person's chi. The expression of this energy in daily life was to practice the path of *wu wei*, which can be translated as "effortless effort." The goal is to combine two seemingly incompatible conditions: activity and relaxation. This effortless effort is supple, never forced or strained.

From tai chi, we learn that "the motion should be rooted in the feet, released through the legs, controlled by the waist, and manifested through the fingers."[8] The therapist bends the knees and imagines the legs extending into the earth as roots, drawing water up through the center of the foot. It rises up the legs into the belly and the heart and then moves out from the heart, into the arms and hands as waves of healing energy (chi).

All parts of the body should move together so that there is not only an economy of motion, but also a concentration of power and increased effectiveness. When performing wave mobilization, first move the body weight backward onto the back leg, gathering chi, like water ebbing back to the ocean. Release the chi by moving the whole body forward, similar to an ocean wave flowing forward. Use the entire mass of the body to rock the client and perform the stroke. Rock the client forward as you perform the massage stroke, and let the client rock back as you release the stroke, or gently pull the client back slightly as you move your body back. The therapist's body and the client's body move as one. Imagine a cloud of energy streaming through your hands and through your client rather than pressing on the client.

The therapist's muscles should remain relaxed, and the joints should remain open (i.e., in some flexion), because this allows the energy to flow. Tightening your muscles constricts your chi. Remain supple and relaxed, maintaining a slow and even breath from the belly.

THE SCIENCE OF HEALING ENERGY (CHI)

A new paradigm in biology and medicine has been hypothesized that was discussed in Chapter 1. Current research is discovering that electromagetic energy controls cellular function, including repair and rejuvenation. And it has been found that each person emits an electromagnetic field, which can, in theory, be focused for healing.[9] The energy that the word *chi* describes is infinitely bigger than a person's own electromagnetic field. In the author's opinion, it describes two different fields of energy. One is the earth's magnetic field. One portion of this field is called *Schumann resonances*, which are electromagnetic waves in the extremely low frequency spectrum, generated by 40 million lightning discharges that occur daily, which pump energy in the cavity formed by the earth's surface and the ionosphere. The lowest resonant frequency is 7.83 hertz, which is the speed of light divided by the earth's circumference. Research shows that this is the same frequency as is found in a deep meditative state and the frequency of brain wave activity that is common to all healers while they are working.[9] It is therefore plausible that therapists can learn to quiet their minds and resonate with the micropulsations of the earth's field and be able to utilize this energy for healing. It is possible that one of the reasons why the Taoists looked to nature as a source of inspiration was that they were able to enter deeper meditative states in nature because they were coupling their field with Schumann resonances.

The word *chi* also implies universal energy. In the author's opinion, this is the same as what quantum physicists call "zero point field (ZPF)."[10] ZPF describes the waves of energy that can still be detected at absolute zero freezing point, at which all molecular motion stops. They are waves of energy on the subatomic level conceptualized like waves in the ocean and represented in Figures 2.6, 2.7, and

2.8 below. Physicists describe 95% of the energy in the universe as invisible, so-called dark energy and dark matter, and many people believe that ZPF and this invisible energy are the same. This vast ocean of energy runs through each of us, and wave mobilization is theoretically one method that allows ZPF and Schumann resonances to be focused for healing.

THE THREE TECHNIQUES: WAVE MOBILIZATION, MUSCLE ENERGY TECHNIQUE, AND JOINT MOBILIZATION

SOFT TISSUE MOBILIZATION: THE WAVE MOBILIZATION STROKE

The wave mobilization stroke was developed by the author during the course of 30 years of clinical practice and daily practice of tai chi. The stroke was developed by using the insights of the Taoists on the nature of water, the principles of tai chi, and the insights of the author's mentor, Lauren Berry, RPT. Wave mobilization is a practical means to theoretically focus the biomagnetic field for healing. The development of wave mobilization was motivated by three objectives: (1) to translate the extraordinary clinical results of the quick, soft tissue manipulation techniques used by Lauren Berry into gentle massage strokes; (2) to create a massage style that is relaxing and nurturing while maintaining superb clinical results; and (3) to develop a massage technique that is also relaxing and energizing for the therapist. These goals were realized with **wave mobilization.**

Nature of Water

- Water is so supple that it will take the shape of whatever container it occupies.

- Water is so powerful that it will dissolve rocks to form canyons.

- Water makes up two-thirds of the body, surrounding every cell. Evidence suggests that unlike ordinary water, water inside the body is largely structured, having a density much higher than that of ice, allowing molecules to pack tightly together.[11] As was discussed in Chapter 1, water and protein (collagen) are charged molecules (dipole), forming tight structural bonds with each other. This water–protein complex forms tightly packed, highly ordered arrays that act like a liquid crystal, being extremely sensitive to weak electromagnetic fields such as those emitted by the hands of the therapist.

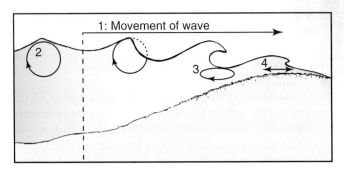

Figure 2-3. Ocean wave characteristics. *1.* The waves move perpendicular to the shoreline and perpendicular to the ground. *2.* A water molecule moves in a circular pattern by the passage of a wave. *3.* As the water becomes more shallow, the waves become flatter and more elliptical. *4.* Just above the sea floor, the wave moves not in a circular pattern but forward and backward.

▨ The highly organized structured water in the body results in a coherent system; that is, the water and protein complexes throughout the body tend to vibrate together.

▨ Water acts as a conductor of electricity.[12] When we compress and stretch the body, we are generating electricity due to the piezoelectric property of soft tissue. These waves of electrical charge (streaming potentials) are carried instantaneously to every cell in the body.

Characteristics of Ocean Waves

▨ Ocean waves move perpendicular to the shoreline (Fig. 2-3).

▨ The energy that moves through the ocean moves the water in a circular motion.

▨ As the ocean wave approaches shallower water, the interaction with the bottom slows the wave, making it more elliptical and flatter.[13]

▨ Waves just above the sea floor move back and forth instead of in a circular motion.

▨ Ocean waves ebb and flow in rhythmic cycles.

▨ Strong waves, such as storm waves, create a rounded, digging motion that erodes the beach (Fig. 2-4).

Wave Mobilization Strokes Mimic Ocean Waves

▨ The author has taken this natural pattern of how energy moves through ocean water and applied it to soft tissue therapy.

▨ The strokes are transverse (perpendicular) to the line of the fiber of the soft tissue.

▨ Just as water molecules are displaced in a circular pattern by the ocean wave, we want to mobilize the

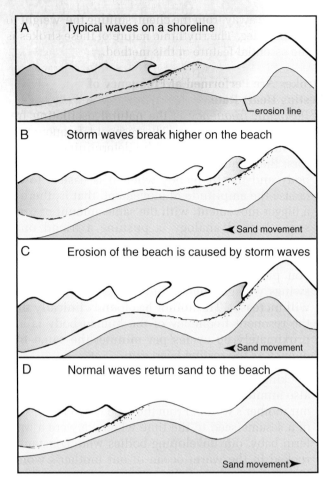

Figure 2-4. Strong waves, such as storm waves, create a digging motion that erodes the beach.

tissue in a circular pattern. The stroke is a circular scooping motion, in which you apply one-half of a circular motion as you scoop down into the soft tissue.

▨ The stroke becomes flatter, more elliptical, if you encounter greater resistance in the tissue or if the tissue is near the bone.

▨ For tissue that is next to the bone, we apply back-and-forth flatter strokes or transverse friction strokes. This is akin to the movement of water against the sea floor.

Characteristics of Wave Mobilization Strokes

Strokes Are Performed Rhythmically

▨ An essential feature of the wave mobilization strokes is that they are repetitive movements that are performed rhythmically, in what may be described as *rhythmic oscillations*. The therapist moves his or her body toward the client, compressing the tissue in a rounded, scooping motion, and then moves his or her body away from the client, shifting the weight to the back leg. The rhythmic nature of these strokes is the essential feature of this method.

Strokes Are Performed at Frequency of Resting Heart Rate

▨ *Resonant frequency* is the natural oscillating frequency of a structure. The resonant frequency of the human body is found by determining two factors: the frequency when it is easiest to move the body and the frequency when it is easiest to increase the amplitude of movement, that is, there is a bigger movement, with the same amount of pressure. A good analogy is pushing a friend on a swing. If you push the swing randomly, you will not be able to get your friend moving very well. If you push at a specific time in each swing, the swings will get higher and higher (the amplitude will increase). The author has found clinically that the resonant frequency of the human body is approximately 60 cycles per minute, the same frequency as the resting heart rate.

▨ Rocking the body at the frequency of the heartbeat also mimics the rhythmic waves we felt as babies in our mother's womb. From the time we were the size of a sesame seed to the time when we were a full-term baby, our developing bodies were constantly rocked in the warm ocean of our mother's womb by our mother's heartbeat. Every cell in our body formed while being rocked in the gentle rhythm of the heartbeat. Rocking a client to the rhythm of the heartbeat may be described as *heart-wave resonance*.

Rhythmic Strokes Conserve Energy

▨ Performing strokes rhythmically means that work is interspersed with rest. Because the therapist is working during only one-half of the cycle, energy is conserved.

▨ Performing the strokes rhythmically utilizes two mechanisms to conserve energy.[14] The first is the pendulum action of shifting the body back and forth with the strokes; the second is the use of the elastic energy. As the therapist moves his or her body onto the back leg in the first part of the stroke, he or she generates potential energy, called *elastic strain energy*, by loading the muscles and fascia of the calf and quadriceps. This potential energy is converted to kinetic energy that is used to move the body forward and perform the stroke.

▨ We also utilize the elastic quality of the client's muscles, tendons, ligaments, capsules, and fascia. As the therapist presses into the client, some of the kinetic (movement) energy from the therapist is stored in the client's tissues and is returned to the therapist as elastic energy.

Transverse Strokes Induce Order into the Body and Increase Energy

▨ As we learned in Chapter 1, a consequence of injury and dysfunction is that the normally highly ordered, parallel fibers are repaired in random orientation. Wave mobilization strokes are performed transverse to the fiber in a highly ordered, rhythmic sequence. From the second law of thermodynamics, we learn that order in a system contains energy and disorder loses energy. The author's hypothesis is that imparting a highly ordered, rhythmic mobilization to the body that realigns the fibers and fascicles adds coherence (order) and energy to the body.

The Stroke Is Typically One Inch Long

The wave mobilization strokes are short, rhythmic scooping strokes that are about 1 inch long. When these strokes are repeated over an area for a period of time, the tension decreases. Instead of needing to press harder into the tissue in order to go deeper, as the strokes are repeated in an oscillating rhythm during the initial session or subsequent treatments, the superficial tissue is transformed from a thick gel to its healthier liquid state, and deeper tissues are easily worked on without needing extra force.

Rhythmic Strokes Entrain the Client into the Heart Rhythm

The term *entrainment* describes the situation when two rhythms that have nearly the same frequency become coupled with each other so that they have the same rhythm. After the therapist establishes internal coherence (order) by quieting the mind and focusing on the present moment through the breath, he or she can entrain the client to this calm healing state by rocking the client's body rhythmically at the frequency of the heartbeat. Therapist and client are moving together, entrained to the rhythm of the heart.

Three Intentions of Each Stroke

First Intention: Mobilize (Rock) the Body

The wave mobilization strokes are applied in an oscillating rhythm like the ebb and flow of the ocean. The typical frequency is between 50 and 70 cycles per minute. Studies have found that babies are rocked to sleep most effectively when this frequency of rocking is used.[15] Rocking the body rhythmically induces relaxation in both the muscles and the nervous system (central nervous system sedation). It is noteworthy that many spiritual traditions involve whole body rocking to enter deep trance states.

Second Intention: Mobilize the Joint

Mobilize the whole segment where you are working. If you are working on the thenar pad of the thumb, mobilize the thumb joint. To release the deltoid, mobilize the glenohumeral joint; to release the erector spinae, mobilize the spinal joints. Each of these procedures is described in the subsequent chapters.

Third Intention: Mobilize the Soft Tissue

The soft tissue is mobilized transverse to the fiber in a rounded, scooping motion. One of the primary differences between this technique and classic massage is that soft tissue is always mobilized along with the joint and body mobilization. By mobilizing the joint, mechanoreceptors are stimulated that have a relaxation effect on the surrounding muscles. By mobilizing the whole body, the central nervous system is brought into a parasympathetic state, reducing blood pressure, heart rate, and respiration.

Therapist–Client Relationship

- The client should be able to completely relax when receiving this work. There may be some discomfort when tight or injured areas are worked on, but the treatment should not be painful.

- To achieve client relaxation, especially in the case of a first-time client, it is helpful to say something like "I may touch some sore or painful areas as I work. If you cannot completely relax into my pressure, please tell me and I will lighten up the pressure. I have found that the greatest therapeutic results come when you are comfortable and completely relaxed."

- Clients need to allow their body to rock when stroked. The wave mobilization strokes cannot achieve its profound results in the "chair massage" style of client positioning or if the client is prone. With these positionings, the therapist is pressing through the client into a rigid surface, losing the rocking motion, which is an essential component of the treatment benefit.

- Instruct clients to avoid bracing or tensing their body in any way. If clients tense, pull away, or hold their breath, then you are working too hard.

- If an area is tender, then lighten your pressure, soften your hands, and slow down.

- If an area still remains too painful for manual work, use reciprocal inhibition or CR MET (see "Muscle Energy Technique") to reduce the pain and hypertonicity, or work in another area.

- This work should relax the whole person, not just the muscle on which you are working.

- To increase the effectiveness of the therapy, ask clients to participate in the session with their conscious attention. During manual techniques, ask clients to place their attention on the muscle you are trying to relax. Guide them mentally by saying, "Feel this muscle relaxing." During MET, ask the client to become consciously aware of when a muscle is contracting and when it is relaxing. Bringing conscious attention to the therapy engages the client's higher brain functions and dramatically increases the effectiveness of the therapy through the changes effected in the central nervous system.

Psychological Environment for Healing

- Create a mental image of healing for the client. It can be dramatically helpful to say, "I think that you are going to feel a lot better," if you believe that it is a reasonable possibility. It is important not to create false hope, but it is equally important to help create a mental image of healing.

- It is very valuable to explain the treatment to the client. When you describe your exam findings, the tretment plan, and the effects of the treatment, it builds trust and confidence in the client, which allows the client to relax and gain the maximum benefit.

- When you feel the muscle relaxing, giving positive feedback induces greater relaxation and improves a sense of well-being.

Create Emotional Environment for Healing

- Pain is an emotional experience. Clients might be depressed, anxious, or fearful about their pain or dysfunction. Or clients might seek wellness care and have extra stress that puts them "on edge." Touch and movement affect emotions through your words and your touch.

- Create a relaxing, caring environment to achieve the most effective treatment.

Table Height, Client and Therapist Positioning

Client Position

- To minimize your reach, bring the client as close to the edge of the table as is comfortable. In the side-lying position, the legs are tucked into a fetal position, and the arms are flexed in a similar "prayer position."

- It is essential that the client remain in a neutral position in the side-lying position. That is, the client's shoulder and hips should be aligned vertically over each other and not rotated forward or backward. If the client is not in the neutral position, then he or she cannot be rocked easily.

Therapist Positions

▨ Four basic positions are described in this text. The four positions refer to the direction of the therapist's pelvic region. They are described relative to the massage table. The head of the massage table is where the client's head is positioned. The three standing positions are given for teaching purposes, because it is assumed that the therapist is facing his or her work, whatever the exact angle.

▨ 45° headward.

▨ 45° footward.

▨ 90° to the table. In this position, the therapist is facing the table.

▨ Sitting.

Table Height

Because wave mobilization is performed by keeping the knees slightly bent, the table height is lower than usual. The proper table height is determined by first having the therapist stand with his or her side next to the table. When the arms are in a relaxed position hanging at the sides and the fingers are hanging down, the top of the table should be at the tip of the fingers.

Practice of the Wave Mobilization Stroke

The following description takes the therapist step by step through the wave mobilization stroke. This stroke may be performed as an energy exercise (*chi gung*) by repeating it for several minutes with one leg forward and switching sides, then repeating it with the opposite leg forward. The description is followed by an exercise in working with a fellow therapist to practice the stroke.

Beginning Posture to Perform the Wave Mobilization Stroke

▨ Take a "bow stance" by placing your heels together, with the feet 45° from the midline (Fig. 2-5**A**).

▨ Bend your knees slightly. Place all of your weight on your right foot, then move your left foot shoulder width apart and approximately 12 inches in front of you. Turn the left foot to face the same direction as your pelvis and not 45° from the midline, as is the right foot (Fig. 2-5**B**).

▨ Your hips continue to face forward. Move 70% of your weight forward onto the left foot. Your left knee should be over the left toes.

▨ Hold a "golden sphere of energy" in front of your belly. The hands are relaxed, approximately 1 foot apart. The wrists are straight, and the elbows are

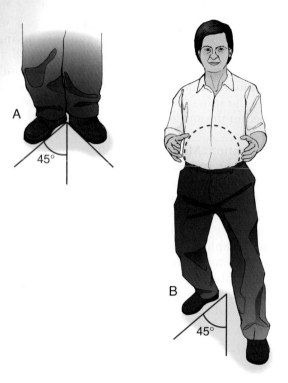

Figure 2-5. **A.** Basic standing posture to perform the wave mobilization stroke involves being in a "bow" stance. To begin, place the heels together with the feet spread apart 45° from the midline. **B.** The bow stance, with the hands holding a golden sphere of energy. The back leg continues to face 45° from the midline. The front foot faces in the same direction as the pelvis. The knees are over the toes.

flexed approximately 70°. The fingers and thumb are in slight flexion, the position of function.

▨ Your whole body—hands, arms, shoulders, back, belly, jaw, face—is relaxed but not limp. You are alert and awake. Tuck your chin slightly to lengthen the neck and to keep your head upright.

▨ The wave mobilization stroke has three phases: drawing back (ebbing), scooping in (flowing), and rolling through.

First Movement: Draw Back or Gathering Chi

▨ Inhale, and move 70% of your weight onto your back leg, gathering your chi (Fig. 2-6). Keep your trunk on one level as you move back. Your trunk neither rises up nor sinks down, and it does not tip from side to side. The only exception to this is if you are working on a large client or a client whose muscles are particularly thick. In these cases, let your body sink down approximately 1 inch by bending the knees a little more as you move your weight onto your back leg.

▨ As you move your weight back, your hands rise up slightly in a rounded motion, as if you are moving over a ball.

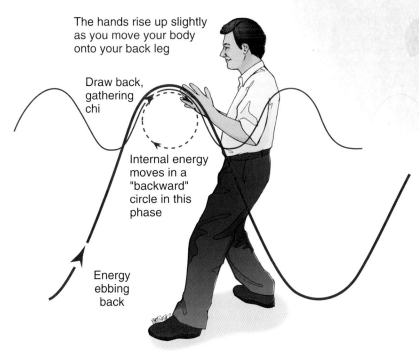

The hands rise up slightly as you move your body onto your back leg

Draw back, gathering chi

Internal energy moves in a "backward" circle in this phase

Energy ebbing back

Figure 2-6. The first movement of the wave mobilization stroke, which is called "drawing back, gathering chi." The first part of all the massage strokes that are performed in the standing posture is to move approximately 70% of the body weight onto the back leg. This movement is essential because it allows the therapist to move the whole body into the massage stroke. If you are working on a particularly tense client or on a large body, allow your body to sink down approximately 1 inch by bending your knees a little more as you move your weight onto your back leg.

Second Movement: Move Forward or Scoop in or Sinking Chi

▨ As you begin to exhale, begin to move your whole body forward, and allow the hands to sink in another rounded motion (Fig. 2-7). The hands remain in the position of function.

▨ As your body moves forward, imagine your hands sinking into the tissue the way a wave of energy moves through water.

Third Movement: Roll Through or Dispersing Chi

▨ During the finishing portion of the stroke, lighten the pressure, allowing your hands to rise up. Imagine rolling your hands through the tissue, as if your thumbs are rolling over the lip of a bowl (Fig. 2-8). This movement is akin to the curling action of the ocean wave as it breaks.

▨ At the end of the stroke, your left knee should be over your left toes. The end of the body movement

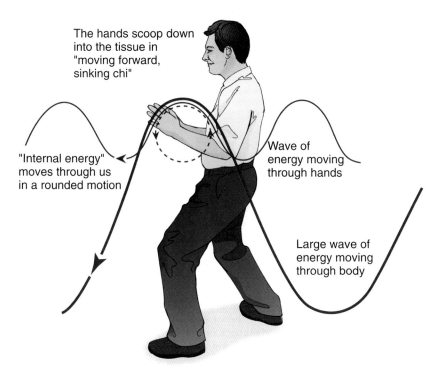

The hands scoop down into the tissue in "moving forward, sinking chi"

"Internal energy" moves through us in a rounded motion

Wave of energy moving through hands

Large wave of energy moving through body

Figure 2-7. The second movement of the wave mobilization stroke, which is called "moving forward, sinking chi." The whole body moves as one piece. The legs, pelvis, and arms all move together. The hands remain in a position of function. As the body moves forward, the hands press into the tissue. The greater the resistance in the tissue, the more elliptical (flatter) the stroke. As was mentioned in Figure 2-6, when working on tight areas, you have allowed your body to sink down approximately 1 inch in the first movement. If you are in this lower position, the second movement involves elevating the body approximately 1 inch as you move forward. In working on most clients, the therapist's body remains on a level plane as it moves forward and backward.

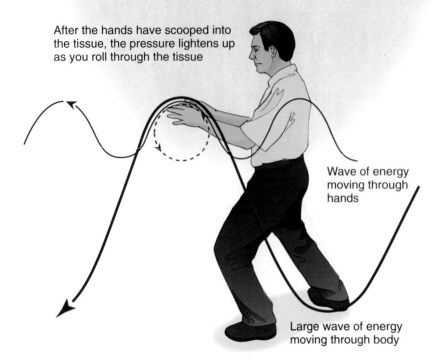

After the hands have scooped into the tissue, the pressure lightens up as you roll through the tissue

Wave of energy moving through hands

Large wave of energy moving through body

Figure 2-8. The third movement of the wave mobilization stroke, which is called "roll through, dispersing chi." After the hands have pressed into the tissue during the second movement, the finishing portion of the stroke involves rolling through the tissue. The pressure lightens, and you feather out the tissue as if you are rolling over the lip of a bowl. This is akin to the breaking of the wave.

should be coordinated with the end of the stroke. Therapists commonly make the mistake of stopping their body movement while continuing the stroke with their hands. This, however, creates excessive work for the muscles of the hands and arms.

Practicing with a Fellow Therapist

▨ **Intention:** The following description of how to perform the basic wave mobilization stroke can be applied to any area of the body. For demonstration purposes, this practice stroke is applied to the muscles of the thenar pad at the base of the thumb. It is described in the context of a classroom situation with a fellow therapist, who will assume the role of the client for practice purposes.

▨ **Client position:** The client sits on the massage table with a pillow on the lap and the right hand resting on the pillow with the palm up. The therapist assumes the bow stance (see "Beginning Posture to Perform the Wave Mobilization Stroke") with the pelvis facing perpendicular to the thenar pad. The therapist then places both thumbs on the thenar pad and holds the dorsal surface of the shaft of the thumb.

First Movement: Draw Back or Gathering Chi
▨ Inhale, and move 70% of your weight onto your back leg, gathering your chi (Fig. 2-9**A**). Keep your trunk on one level as you move back.

▨ As you move your weight back, draw the skin back approximately 1 inch, and rotate the shaft of the thumb slightly toward you (Fig. 2-9**B**).

Second Movement: Move Forward or Scoop in or Sinking Chi
▨ As you begin to exhale, begin to move your whole body forward (Fig. 2-10**A**). Let the body movement move the thumbs into the muscles of the thenar pad in a rounded, scooping motion (Fig. 2-10**B**). Gently squeeze your fingers to stabilize the back of the client's thumb, which allows your thumbs to sink into the muscles.

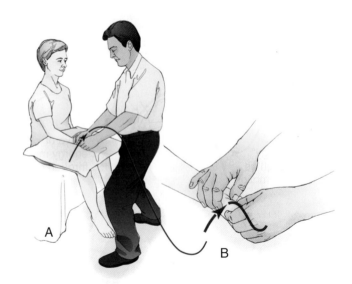

A   B

Figure 2-9. A. Standing position to practice the wave mobilization stroke on the thenar eminence. During the first movement, move your weight back onto your back leg. **B.** During the first movement, draw the skin back, and rotate the shaft of the thumb slightly toward the palm.

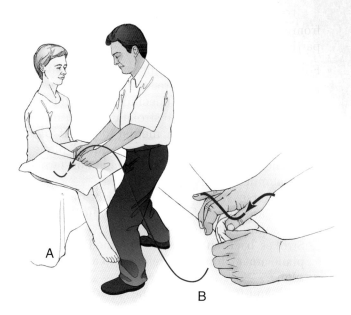

Figure 2-10. A. During the second movement, the whole body moves forward. As the body moves forward, the mass of the body moves the therapist's thumbs into the soft tissue of the client's thenar pad. The pelvis faces the direction of your stroke. Keep the entire body relaxed. **B.** Both thumbs sink into the soft tissue of the thenar eminence in a rounded, scooping motion, perpendicular to the shaft of the thumb. Work only within the client's comfortable limit. The fingers stabilize the shaft of the client's thumb in the sinking portion of the stroke rather than mobilizing it.

Third Movement: Roll Through or Dispersing Chi

The finishing portion of the stroke involves moving the body, thumbs, wrists, and arms together. As the body continues to move forward, the thumbs perform a rounded, scooping motion approximately 1 inch long, rolling a wave of pressure through the tissue as if rolling over the lip of a bowl (Fig. 2-11**A**). The stroke does not slide over the skin. At the same time that you are performing the stroke, gently mobilize the client's thumb by rotating it away from the palm (laterally) (Fig. 2-11**B**). Your body continues to move forward until the stroke is finished.

Release the pressure on the skin, place your thumbs on a slightly different spot, and move your body as you pull the skin back approximately 1 inch to perform the stroke again. Practice for several minutes, and then perform the same strokes on the other hand.

Massage Strokes Overview

Four Types of Transverse Strokes

All of the wave mobilization strokes are applied transverse to the line of the fiber. Transverse strokes dissolve adhesions, broaden the tissue, stimulate cellular synthesis, and realign the fibers to their normal parallel array without imposing longitudinal stress that can

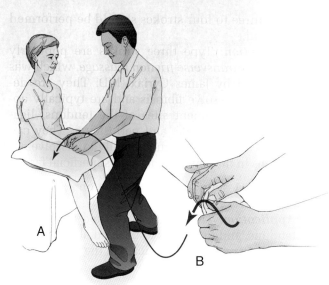

Figure 2-11. A. During the finishing portion of the stroke, the therapist's body continues to move forward. If the body stops moving, the hands should stop also. **B.** The finishing portion of the stroke involves decreasing the pressure of the stroke and feathering out the client's soft tissue, as if rolling over the lip of a bowl. You might feel the soft tissue fibers rolling under your thumbs.

disrupt healing fibers. The two exceptions to this transverse protocol are described below in the section entitled "Two Basic Longitudinal Strokes."

Type one: The fundamental wave mobilization stroke is a short, rounded, scooping stroke, approximately 1 inch in length. As has been mentioned, the stroke becomes flatter and more elliptical as resistance is encountered in the tissue (see "Wave Mobilization Mimic Ocean Waves"). This stroke does not slide over the surface of the skin but moves through the skin.
☐ *Application:* This stroke is typically applied to the fibers and fascicles of the tendons, ligaments, joint capsules, muscle bellies, and associated fascia throughout the entire body. It can be applied to all the soft tissue, including the nerves.

Type two: Short, back-and-forth strokes. These strokes may be applied slowly or with medium speed. They are slower than a type three stroke.
☐ *Application:* These strokes are applied to myotendinous junctions, tenoperiosteal junctions, areas of thickening within the muscle belly, tendons and tendon sheaths, and ligaments. It is a deeper stroke than a type one stroke but not as deep as a type three stroke.

Type three: Short, brisk, transverse friction strokes. These strokes are flat and not rounded or elliptical. The speed of the stroke is also an essential feature; three to four strokes should be performed per second.

- [ ] *Application:* Type three strokes are popularly known as *transverse friction massage,* which was pioneered by James Cyriax, MD. They are designed to dissolve fibrosis and are typically applied to attachment sites of the tendons, ligaments, joint capsule, and periosteum. They can also be applied more superficially to dissolve adhesions in the skin, dermis, and superficial fascia.

- **Type four:** A short, brisk, unidirectional, rounded scooping stroke.
  - [ ] *Application:* This stroke is applied to muscles, tendons, and ligaments to unwind abnormal torsion or to realign the fascicles in the muscle, tendon, or ligament.

Two Basic Longitudinal Strokes

These strokes are classic deep tissue strokes in the tradition of Ida Rolf. They are designed to lengthen fascia that has shortened and thickened. Although postisometric relaxation (PIR) technique (see "Muscle Energy Technique" below) is effective in lengthening the muscle and its deep fascia, it occasionally is necessary to apply longitudinal strokes to stretch the fascia that forms the superficial sleeve around a structure or that forms the deep fascial compartments. For example, the crural fascia of the anterior compartment of the leg is a thick structure and often requires deep longitudinal strokes to lengthen the fascia. These strokes are applied only as needed, because they can be uncomfortable to receive and stressful for the therapist to perform.

- A long, continuous, stroke that slides over the skin.
  - [ ] *Application:* These strokes are applied at various depths. Superficially, they are designed to lengthen the superficial fascia and to dissolve adhesions between the fascia and the surrounding structures. These strokes may be applied to the deep fascia to lengthen the coverings of the muscles (epimysium), separate muscles that have adhered to each other, or dissolve adhesions between the muscle and the muscle's fascial compartment.

- A slow, deep stroke that does not slide over the skin.
  - [ ] *Application:* These strokes are applied to localized adhesions ("knots") within the muscle that do not respond to either the transverse strokes or the MET. Because these strokes are typically uncomfortable, they are applied only after the other techniques have been tried.

Stroke Direction

- The direction of the strokes is described in two ways: (1) in one specific direction, for example, from medial to lateral, and (2) back and forth in a particular plane.

- For clarification, when the instructions are given to perform types two and three transverse strokes that move back and forth in a specific plane of the body, it is easier to describe the stroke direction in common terms, such as the medial-to-lateral plane, rather than to use the exact anatomical plane or axis. The correspondence of the common terms to the anatomical terms is as follows:
  - [ ] Transverse strokes in the anterior-to-posterior plane are also referred to anatomically as the *horizontal or transverse plane.*
  - [ ] Strokes back and forth in the medial-to-lateral plane are anatomically referred to as the *coronal plane.*
  - [ ] Back-and-forth strokes in the superior-to-inferior plane are anatomically referred to as the *sagittal plane.*

Guidelines for Stroke Application

- The client must be able to relax completely into the strokes for them to have the greatest clinical benefit. The intention is to engage the parasympathetic nervous system, which regulates healing and regeneration within the body. To engage this part of the nervous system, the client needs to be able to relax completely.

- The strokes are performed rhythmically, without sudden changes in speed.

- The more acute the condition, the lighter the strokes and the more gentle the rocking. In chronic conditions, deeper strokes and greater rocking may be applied.

- The more watery the tissue, the lighter the stroke. The more fibrous the tissue, the deeper the stroke.

- The closer we are to the attachment point, the shorter the stroke. The more the stroke is in the muscle belly, the larger is the amplitude and the broader the stroke.

- Mobilize the entire segment where you are working, not just the tissue under your hands.

- Keep your hands as relaxed as possible, even though you may be working deeply.

MUSCLE ENERGY TECHNIQUE

- *Definition:* MET is a procedure that involves a voluntary contraction of a patient's muscle in a precisely controlled direction, at varying levels of intensity, against a distinctly executed counterforce applied by the therapist.[16]

History: The origins of MET date to the 1940s, when Kabat developed techniques of active patient participation to strengthen muscles that were neurologically impaired.[17] He called these types of muscular reeducation techniques *proprioceptive neuromuscular facilitation*. During the 1950s, Fred Mitchell, Sr, DO, and other osteopaths applied these techniques to mobilize joints and called it *muscle energy technique*. MET has been refined by many practitioners, including Philip Greenman,[16] Karel Lewit,[18] Vladimir Janda and colleagues,[19] and Leon Chaitow.[20] It is important to realize that although MET has been used by osteopaths to move a vertebra through a specific restriction barrier,[21] these techniques can also be applied to the soft tissue.

Application for massage therapists: It is not the goal of the massage therapist to move a vertebra in a specific direction. For the massage therapist, MET is used to treat the soft tissue and nervous system. Because MET uses voluntary effort, we are using the highest part of the central nervous system to reprogram involuntary patterns in the muscles. A secondary effect is that active muscle contraction helps to mobilize the joints. MET has many clinical uses, which are described below.

Clinical Uses

- To decrease sustained contraction in hypertonic muscles and to lengthen shortened fascia within the muscles.

- To increase the extensibility and reduce the sensitivity of the periarticular tissue (the soft tissue surrounding the joint).[7] As the ligaments, joint capsule, and periosteum interweave with the fascial expansion of the muscles at the tenoperiosteal attachments, muscle contraction places a stretch on the connective tissues around the joint.

- To strengthen a weakened muscle or group of muscles. Isometric contraction provides increased tonus and performance because of increased muscle fiber participation.

- To reestablish normal firing patterns in the muscle. If a muscle is weak, then other muscles substitute for its action. MET can reeducate the muscle to perform its normal action.

- To reduce localized edema in acute injuries, as muscle contraction acts to pump the lymphatic and venous systems.

- To reestablish normal movement patterns, mobilize restricted joints, normalize joint play, and increase their ROM. These techniques are helpful prior to chiropractic adjustments or osteopathic manipulations.

- To provide pain management through reciprocal inhibition and mechanoreceptor stimulation.

- To facilitate sensory-motor integration, which brings the client's awareness to areas of habitual contraction and corrects what Thomas Hanna[22] calls "sensory motor amnesia."

- To reduce trigger points in a fast and painless way.[19,7,23]

- One form of CR MET involves isometric contraction. Voluntary isometric contraction is used not only to reduce muscle hypertonicity, but also for assessment purposes.[24] We note whether the muscle is weak, painful, or strong and painless (see "Isometric Testing").

- MET is an excellent treatment for hospitalized, bed-ridden, and frail clients because effective results can be achieved with very light pressure.

Using MET to Induce Neurological and Mechanical Relaxation in a Muscle

Neurological Basis of MET

Although the practice of MET has a large following among osteopaths, chiropractors, and physical therapists, there is still debate in the literature about how MET works. Some authors focus on the Golgi tendon organs,[20] whereas others focus on the muscle spindle.[21] The essential neurological role of muscle spindles can be summarized as follows:

- MET employs the conscious, voluntary contraction of isolated muscles. Isolated voluntary contraction of a muscle is different from the muscle contraction that is used in most daily activities. Because higher brain centers are used to isolate muscle contraction, unique neurological effects are achieved compared with those that are accomplished in functional activities.

- As has been mentioned, there are two types of muscle fibers: extrafusal and intrafusal. The extrafusal fibers provide the force of muscle contraction and are innervated by alpha motor nerves. The intrafusal fibers, also called *muscle spindles*, are innervated by gamma nerves and act as sensory receptors to help regulate the length and tone of a muscle.

- During sustained muscle contraction in which muscles are unconsciously or involuntarily tightened, gamma motor neuron activity is thought to be abnormally set to a higher gain or firing rate. This keeps the muscle's tone too high (hypertonic) and its resting length abnormally short.

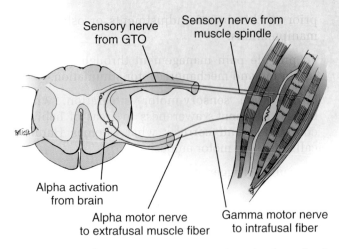

Figure 2-12. Voluntary isometric contraction stimulates the alpha motor neurons, causing contraction of the extrafusal muscle fibers. This causes a relaxation of the intrafusal fibers, temporarily silencing the muscle spindles. This pause in spindle activity causes a relaxation of muscle tone.

- Voluntary isometric contraction shortens the muscle belly, slackening the intrafusal fibers and unloading the muscle spindle, turning it off temporarily (Fig. 2-12).[25] Because isolated voluntary isometric contraction requires only alpha motor nerve activity, the gamma motor nerve is not firing to the muscle spindle.

- As the muscle relaxes after voluntary isometric contraction, the alpha motor nerve turns off, and the muscle belly lengthens. During this relaxation phase, the gamma motor nerves begin to fire to reset the muscle's resting tone. Theoretically, because the gamma motor nerves have just been turned off, the new rate at which they are firing has been reduced, decreasing the resting tone of the muscle.

- Sherrington's law of reciprocal inhibition states that when a muscle (agonist) contracts, it has an inhibiting effect on the opposing muscle, the antagonist.

Mechanical Basis of Muscle Relaxation Using MET

- Muscles that are in an adaptive, shortened position or held in a sustained contraction have an increased stiffness. Relaxation after isometric contraction increases muscle temperature and reduces this stiffness because of the thixotropic property of muscle.[26]

Using Muscle Energy Technique to Lengthen Muscles and Reduce Trigger Points

- Muscle contraction increases muscle temperature because the stored energy from the contraction is released as heat as the muscle relaxes. The increase in temperature increases the elasticity and extensibility of the connective tissue (fascia of the muscle-

tendon unit) and decreases the viscosity of the ground substance.

- When a muscle contracts isometrically, the muscle fibers shorten, and the connective tissue lengthens to keep the muscle at the same length. This lengthening dissolves abnormal crosslinks in the collagen, allowing more normal gliding of the fibers and permitting the muscle to be stretched to a new length.

- The pain and dysfunction associated with trigger points are relieved when the muscle is restored to its full length.[7]

Therapeutic Principles of Muscle Energy Technique

There are many styles of MET. The style listed below has proved most effective clinically.

- The most important principle is that MET should never be painful. It may be mildly uncomfortable but never painful. If it is even mildly painful, stop. The therapist should then attempt to use less pressure until a level of pressure is found into which the client can completely relax.

- If it is still painful, use RI (see "Reciprocal Inhibition"). If a contraction still elicits pain, work with any muscle related to the associated joint that is not painful. For example, if resisted internal rotation and external rotation of the shoulder are painful, try resisted adduction, flexion, or extension.

- Perform MET on the hypertonic or shortened muscles first, because those tissues inhibit their antagonists. After you have released the hypertonic muscles, use MET to strengthen the weakened muscles.

- The muscle is typically positioned in its mid-range position, halfway between its fully stretched position and its fully relaxed position. This position is the most accurate measure of its strength and is usually the most comfortable position. If a muscle cannot be placed at its mid-range position, it is placed at its pain or resistance barrier.

- The therapist instructs the client to resist the pressure that the therapist exerts. This is important, because the therapist wants to be in complete control of the effort that the client is exerting. Otherwise, some clients believe that their strongest effort is what is required, and they might strain or overwhelm the therapist. The therapist could say, "I am going to try to move you in a certain direction. Your job is to resist me and not let me move you. Tell me if there is anything more than a slight discomfort. It should not be painful." Then the therapist applies pressure gradually.

- The therapist typically applies only modest pressure that requires only 10% to 20% of the client's available strength to resist the therapist's force. In acute conditions, only a few grams of pressure is required to make a neurological change. In chronic conditions, as much as 50% effort may be applied to create more heat and a greater stretch on the connective tissues.

- The client resists the therapist's effort for 5 to 10 seconds in acute conditions, and the therapist may have the client hold longer for chronic conditions. Gently tap on the muscle that is being contracted to bring sensory awareness to an area of unconscious hypertonicity. The therapist might say, "Feel this muscle working," as it contracts, and then, "Feel this muscle relaxing," as it relaxes.

- This contract (resist)-relaxation cycle typically is repeated three to five times, but it may be repeated as many as 20 times in chronic conditions.

- It is often helpful to add a contraction to the opposite muscle (antagonist) after the contraction of the agonist. This is especially helpful after PIR MET, as it not only adds a deeper level of relaxation, but also "sets" the involved muscle in a relaxed state in its lengthened position. This is accomplished through reciprocal inhibition.

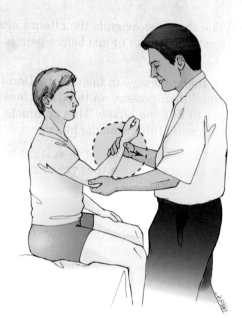

Figure 2-13. CR MET and RI MET can be demonstrated with the biceps and triceps muscles. During CR MET, the therapist holds the distal forearm and instructs the client to "not let me move you" as the therapist attempts to pull the forearm slowly and gently toward himself or herself (extend the elbow). To perform RI MET on the biceps, the therapist instructs the client to "not let me move you" as the therapist attempts to push the forearm away from himself or herself (flexing the elbow). In resisting, the client contracts the triceps, the antagonist of the biceps.

Types of Muscle Energy Procedures

MET can be applied to almost any muscle in the body. This text describes the most commonly used techniques in each region of the body. MET is specific, and the direction of the resistance must be precise to be effective.

Contract Relax (CR)

- *Intention:* The purposes in applying CR are to achieve relaxation in hypertonic muscles, to bring sensory awareness to a muscle, and to assess weakness or pain in the muscles.

- *Position:* The therapist places the client's elbow into a resting position, halfway between full flexion and full extension, or until a resistance barrier is felt (Fig. 2-13).

- *Action:* The therapist holds the forearm and stabilizes the elbow and gives the client the following instructions: "Don't let me move you," while attempting to pull the elbow into extension. Once the therapist has educated the client, the therapist can simply say, "Resist" or "Hold," but in the beginning, it is often confusing for the client if the therapist says only, "Hold." If the therapist says, "Don't let me move you," the client does not have

to think about the exact direction or what muscle is working.

- The client resists the therapist's pressure for 5 to 10 seconds. Make sure the client is not holding his or her breath.

- Tell the client, "Relax." Wait a few seconds until the client is completely relaxed.

- Repeat the CR cycle three to five times or until you feel the muscle relax.

Reciprocal Inhibition (RI)

- *Intention:* RI is used in acute conditions. If contraction of a muscle is painful even with minimal effort from the client, RI on the muscle that has the opposite action, that is, the antagonist of the painful muscle, sends a neurological message to the agonist to inhibit its contraction. RI is also useful to alternate with CR MET or at the end of a series of PIR procedures. This reinforces the relaxation after the CR MET and sends a message to the agonist to relax in its more lengthened state after a PIR technique. In the following example, we assume that the biceps is hypertonic and painful with any isometric contraction.

- *Position:* The therapist extends the client's elbow until the resistance barrier or just before pain is felt (see Fig. 2-13).

- *Action:* The therapist says to the client, "Don't let me move you," then presses on the distal forearm and attempts to flex the elbow. This contracts the triceps, reciprocally inhibiting the biceps.

- The therapist instructs the client to relax, waits a few seconds, and then repeats the cycle three to five times.

Postisometric Relaxation (PIR)

- *Intention:* The purpose in applying PIR is to lengthen shortened muscles and the associated fascia and to relieve trigger points. The finger flexors are used as an example, because they are typically short and tight.

- *Position:* The client is supine with the elbow extended and the forearm supinated, with the wrist over the edge of the table. The therapist places his or her fingers on the palmar surface of the client's fingers and a stabilizing hand on the client's distal forearm.

- *Action:* The therapist slowly and gently presses the client's fingers into extension until just before the stretch elicits pain or until the therapist feels a resistance to stretch in the muscle and fascia (Fig. 2-14A). The therapist then instructs the client, "Don't let me

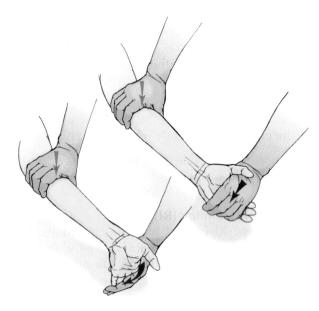

Figure 2-14. PIR MET is easily demonstrated with the finger flexors. The client is supine with the elbow extended. The therapist places one hand on the fingers and slowly presses the fingers into their comfortable limit of extension. Next, the therapist instructs the client to "not let me move you" while slowly and gently pressing on the fingers. After approximately 5 seconds, the therapist relaxes for a few seconds and then presses the fingers into further extension to their comfortable limit. This contract-relax-lengthen cycle is repeated several times.

move you," and has the client resist as the therapist slowly presses on the fingers for approximately 5 to 10 seconds, attempting to press the fingers toward greater extension (Fig. 2-14**B**).

- The therapist tells the client, "Relax," and waits a few seconds until the client is completely relaxed.

- After the client relaxes, the therapist slowly and gently presses the fingers until just before the stretch elicits pain or until a resistance to stretch is felt in the muscle and fascia.

- Starting from this new barrier, the therapist repeats the contract (resist), relax, lengthen, contract cycle three to five times.

- If the therapist cannot increase the stretch, the client should be told to resist for 20 to 30 seconds at the comfortable resistance barrier for several cycles, and then the stretch should be attempted again. Sometimes an increase in the ROM can be achieved only 1 inch at a time.

Contract-Relax-Antagonist Contract

- *Intention:* The intent in using contract-relax-antagonist-contract (CRAC) cycle is to stretch adhesions, lengthen the connective tissue, and reduce hypertonicity in muscles. The CRAC technique adds an RI to the PIR technique by having the client actively contract the antagonist. This contraction has an inhibitory effect on the stretched muscle, and it is effective for stretching chronically shortened muscles. This technique is for chronic conditions only. The gastrocnemius serves as an example.

- *Position:* The client is supine. The therapist places one hand on the client's knee. The other hand holds the heel, and the forearm rests on the ball of the foot (Fig. 2-15).

- *Action:* The client actively pulls the foot into dorsiflexion, and the therapist keeps contact with the forearm against the ball of the foot. The therapist instructs the client to relax in this position. The therapist then instructs the client, "Don't let me move you," and has the client resist as the therapist slowly leans his or her body weight toward the head of the table, pressing the forearm against the ball of the client's foot, attempting to pull the foot further into dorsiflexion. The therapist holds for 5 seconds, then instructs the client to relax. Next, the therapist tells the client to actively pull the foot into dorsiflexion (headward) until a new resistance barrier is encountered.

- The therapist repeats the CRAC sequence three to five times per session or as needed. The sequence is then repeated on the client's other side.

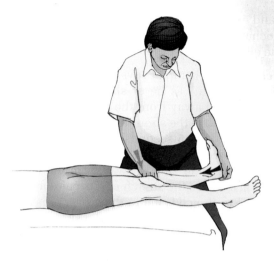

Figure 2-15. CRAC MET can be demonstrated with the gastrocnemius muscle. The client is supine with the knee extended. The therapist places one hand on the client's heel and rests the forearm on the ball of the client's foot. Next, the therapist instructs the client "Do not let me move you" while slowly and gently pressing his or her forearm into the ball of the client's foot for approximately 5 seconds. The therapist relaxes for a few seconds and then instructs the client to actively pull the foot toward the head, dorsiflexing the ankle and lengthening the gastrocnemius. The CRAC cycle is repeated several times.

Eccentric Contraction

- *Intention:* The intent in using eccentric contraction is to dissolve adhesions and lengthen the connective tissue. This procedure must be done with care, because excessive force can irritate the soft tissue. It is contraindicated for deconditioned or frail clients or clients who have had joint replacements. This technique is for chronic conditions only. The biceps is used as an example.

- *Position:* The therapist extends the elbow until just before the stretch elicits pain or until a resistance to the stretch in the muscle and fascia is felt (see Fig. 2-13).

- *Action:* The therapist says to the client, "Don't let me move you," while attempting to pull the elbow into extension. The therapist may use a moderate force, having the client resist with approximately 50% of his or her maximum effort for 5 to 10 seconds. Next, the therapist instructs the client to "Keep resisting, but now let me move you very slowly." The therapist overcomes the client's resistance by pulling the elbow into further extension while the client is attempting to pull the elbow into flexion.

- The therapist instructs the client to relax and repeats the procedure three to five times, beginning at the new resistance barrier and moving the elbow to its greatest extension in the pain-free range.

- Eccentric MET should be incorporated into practice with only light resistance at first.

Concentric Muscle Energy Technique

- *Intention:* If muscles are weak, concentric MET can help to restore proper neurological firing patterns and increase muscle tone. This technique must be done as a precise and controlled movement, with emphasis on precision in isolating the muscle contraction rather than on strength. For this example, we will assume that the deep neck flexors and hyoid muscles are weak but not painful. This technique should not be performed if the client is experiencing acute neck pain.

- *Position:* The client is supine. The client bends the knees and brings his or her feet flat on the table (Fig. 2-16).

- *Action:* The client is asked to slowly raise the head off the table a few inches to look toward his or her feet by first tucking the chin. The therapist watches to see whether the head is extending on the neck (i.e., if the chin is jutting away from the throat) or the head is being flexed with the neck as the chin moves closer to the throat. If the deep neck flexors are of normal strength, then the chin moves toward the throat and not up to the ceiling. If the deep cervical flexors are weak, the sternocleidomastoid and scalenes substitute for the deep cervical flexors, extending the head and jutting the chin toward the ceiling.

- This action is repeated several more times. The client should perform this movement as an exercise until the muscles are strong and the client is using the muscles in a precise and controlled way.

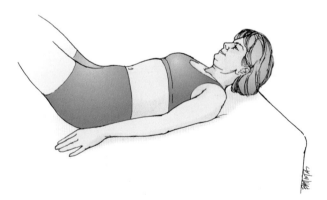

Figure 2-16. A demonstration of concentric MET may be performed on the deep cervical flexors and hyoid muscles. These muscles are often weak, and substitution for their action is performed by the sternocleidomastoid and scalenes. With the client lying on his or her back on the table, with knees bent and feet on the table, the therapist instructs the client to lift his or her head slowly off the table a few inches by tucking the chin and rotating it toward the throat.

Muscle Energy Technique to Increase the ROM in Joints

■ **Intention:** One application of MET is to increase the ROM of a joint. As the ligaments, joint capsule, and periosteum interweave with the fascial expansion of the muscles at the tenoperiosteal attachments, muscle contraction places a stretch on the connective tissues around the joint. Isometric contraction can increase the extensibility of the soft tissue surrounding the joint.[7] Neurologically, it is not well understood why voluntary muscle contraction affects the joint capsule, but Freeman and Wyke[27] and others have documented that reflexes exist between muscles and ligaments. All of the styles that are described above can be used to increase the ROM of a joint rather than to focus on affecting the muscle and its associated fascia. It can be confusing, however, for the therapist to attempt to determine which muscles are involved if there is a decrease in the ROM of a joint. Therefore, do not think of muscles; simply determine the direction of decreased motion, and have the client resist your attempts to move the joint into the restricted direction. This approach has proved valuable for capsular adhesions. Decreased internal rotation of the shoulder is used as an example.

■ **Position:** The client is sitting and places one hand on the lower back (Fig. 2-17). If this is difficult, the

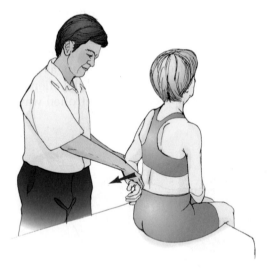

Figure 2-17. To increase the range of medial rotation of the shoulder joint, have the client sit on the table and place the back of one hand on his or her back. The therapist places a hand between the client's hand and the back. The therapist instructs the client to "not let me move you" while slowly and gently attempting to pull the client's arm away from the back for approximately 5 seconds. The therapist relaxes for a few seconds and then slowly and gently pulls the hand further away from the back until it is uncomfortable or a resistance barrier is felt. Again, the therapist instructs the client to "not let me move you" while slowly and gently attempting to pull the arm further away from the back, increasing the medial rotation of the glenohumeral joint.

hand is placed on the sacroiliac joint or greater trochanter area. The therapist holds one hand on the elbow and the other hand on the distal forearm.

■ **Action:** The therapist says to the client, "Don't let me move you," as he or she attempts to pull the client's hand away from the lower back, that is, attempts to move the shoulder into greater medial rotation. Hold for 5 seconds. The client then relaxes for a few seconds during which the therapist pulls the client's hand slowly away from the lower back until just before the stretch elicits pain or until a resistance to stretch is felt in the fascia. This is usually only approximately 1 inch. If the stretch is painful, the therapist releases the pull until it is comfortable again. This action is repeated three to five times.

■ Remember that in working with joints, even a slight change in the ROM can translate into a significant change of function.

JOINT MOBILIZATION

■ **Definition:** Joint mobilization can be defined as a form of passive joint movement.[28] The movement may be described as being between the two bones, called *osteokinematics*, or being between the joint surfaces, called *arthrokinematics*. Flexion and extension of the knee, for example, describe the movement between bones in one plane. During knee flexion, the ends of the tibia and femur are also rolling and sliding on each other, which is arthrokinematic movement. Each joint has a slight passive movement that is referred to as *accessory motion* or *joint play*, which is necessary for full ROM. The three specific accessory motions are roll, slide, and spin.

■ **Indications:**
  ☐ Acute, swollen tissue, because active motion would be painful.
  ☐ Pain, muscle spasm
  ☐ Stiff (hypomobile) joint, whether from degeneration, decreased joint play, or capsular thickening
  ☐ Decreased ROM
  ☐ To promote optimum function of the joint and surrounding muscles

■ **Clinical effects of joint mobilization:**[28,29]
  ☐ Pain relief through mechanoreceptor stimulation, closing the pain gate (see Chapter 1).
  ☐ Decreases muscle guarding by stimulating Type I and II mechanoreceptors[30]
  ☐ Relaxation is also achieved by reflexes, which influence muscle tone[30]
  ☐ Decreases adhesions and minimizes formation of contractures
  ☐ Maintains accessory motion (joint play) and ROM (osteokinematics)

□ Promotes circulation to increase nutrition and oxygen in the tissue and the removal of waste products. For example, this reduces congestion at the nerve root, a major source of pain.[31]

□ Stimulates the synovial membrane to increase nutrients and lubrication (synovia) within the joint to enhance the health of articular cartilage, as well as intra-articular fibrocartilage of the menisci and the intervertebral discs.

□ Increases water content in tissue that has dehydrated because of adhesions from injury or immobilization.

□ Improves proprioception by stimulating mechanoreceptors surrounding the joint

Types of Joint Mobilization

Flexion and Extension

▦ *Intention:* Gentle, pain-free, passive joint motion in flexion and extension reduces swelling and pain.

▦ *Position:* One example of this type is flexion and extension of the knee. The client is supine. The therapist brings the involved knee to a comfortable degree of flexion (Fig. 2-18).

▦ *Action:* Gently flex the knee to its comfortable limit. Slowly pump the knee in small arcs of pain-free flexion and extension to pump the excess fluid out of the knee. This is typically performed after CR MET, which also helps to disperse swelling.

Unidirectional Mobilization

▦ *Intention:* Most joints have a typical pattern of fixation or loss of normal joint play. Some examples include the anterior fixation of the femur in the acetabulum and the anterior fixation of the humerus in the glenoid fossa. The intention in this example is to restore the anterior to posterior glide of the femur in the acetabulum.

▦ *Position:* For mobilization of the femur, the client is supine. Place both hands next to each other below the inguinal ligament, midway between the anterior superior iliac spine and the pubic symphysis (midline of the body) (Fig. 2-19).

▦ *Action:* Gently push the proximal femur posteriorly in brisk, oscillating pulses. Repeat several times.

Rhythmic Oscillations Combined with Soft Tissue Mobilization

▦ *Intention:* The intention is to unwind the muscles and joint capsule and to passively mobilize the joint. This improves accessory motion, mobilizes periarticular tissue, reduces muscle spasms, improves lubrication of the joint, provides pain management, and reduces abnormal torsion in the soft tissue. This type of joint mobilization forms the basis of the wave mobilization strokes in which soft tissue and joint mobilizations are combined. One example is the glenohumeral joint.

▦ *Position:* The client is supine. Hold the client's arm with your inferior hand at 90° abduction, then lift it off the table slightly to bring the superficial tissue into slack (Fig. 2-20).

▦ *Action:* Hold the deltoid muscle with your superior hand such that the shaft of your thumb is in line with the shaft of the humerus. Perform a series

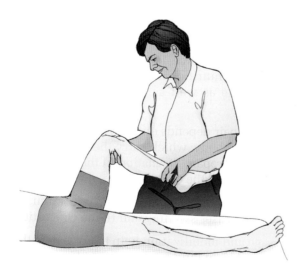

Figure 2-18. Gently flex the client's knee to its comfortable limit. Slowly pump the knee in small arcs of pain-free flexion and extension to pump the excess fluid out of the knee. This is typically performed after CR MET for knee flexion and extension, which also helps to disperse swelling.

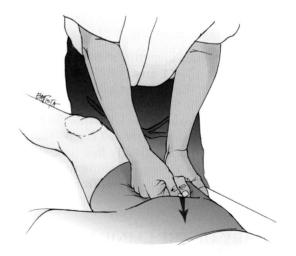

Figure 2-19. To help restore anterior-to-posterior glide of the femur in the acetabulum, place both hands next to each other below the inguinal ligament, midway between the anterior superior iliac spine and the pubic symphysis (midline of the body), and gently push the proximal femur posteriorly, in brisk, oscillating pulses. Repeat several times.

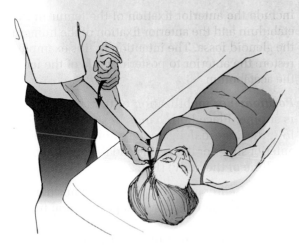

Figure 2-20. Hold the deltoid muscle with your superior hand such that the shaft of your thumb is in line with the shaft of the humerus. Perform a series of short, scooping strokes in a superior direction with your thumb as you rock the client's arm in small arcs of external rotation.

of short, scooping strokes in a superior direction with your thumb as you rock the client's arm in small arcs of external rotation.

Multidirectional Motion to Improve Joint Function

- *Intention:* Passive joint motion improves accessory motion, mobilizes periarticular tissue, reduces muscle spasms, improves lubrication of the joint, and provides pain management. One example of this type is figure-eight mobilization of the cervical spine.

- *Position:* The client is supine. Find the vertebral facets by first locating the spinous processes in the midline. Move slightly laterally to touch the medial extensor muscles. Move your fingertips over that muscle bundle, and you will feel a bony indentation, which is the facet (Fig. 2-21).

- *Action:* With your fingertips at the vertebral facets starting at the C7–T1 area, gently induce a slight movement with the hands in a figure-eight pattern. For example, the client's head is rotated to the right, then side flexed to the left while the fingertips of your left hand push on the left facets. Then rotate the client's head left, laterally flex it right, and so on. This is a slow, extremely gentle procedure, and there should be no pain. Repeat from the C7–T1 to the C1–C2 area.

SUMMARY OF THE CLINICAL EFFECTS OF SOFT TISSUE MOBILIZATION, JOINT MOBILIZATION, AND MUSCLE ENERGY TECHNIQUE

- Increases the synthesis of new cells to promote repair and healing of injured or compromised tissue.

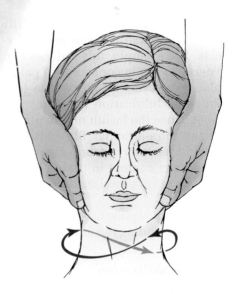

Figure 2-21. Find the vertebral facets by first locating the spinous processes in the midline. Move slightly laterally to touch the medial extensor muscles. Move your fingertips over that muscle bundle, and you will feel a bony indentation, which is the facet. With your fingertips placed at the vertebral facets starting at the C7–T1 area, gently induce a slight movement with the hands in a figure-eight pattern.

- Crossing transverse to the fiber in the soft tissue creates a tensile (stretching) force on the collagen, which increases the activity of the fibroblasts and leads to the synthesis of collagen and ground substance.

- All cells in the body are stimulated to increase their activity with mechanical stimulation. The longitudinal pulling force of active muscle contraction of MET increases muscle regeneration through synthesis of satellite cells.

- The normal functioning of the cells depends on movement.

- Promotes fluid exchange of blood, lymph, synovial fluid, and interstitial fluids (ground substance) to increase the nutritional exchange and oxygenation of the tissue as well as the elimination of waste products.

- Healthy repair depends on the free movement of the fluids of the body, which carry the cells, fibers, and nutrition for repair. Stagnation in the tissue leads to poor repair and the accumulation of waste products.

- Massage and mobilization facilitate circulation, which decreases swelling and tissue congestion.

- Massage and mobilization help to normalize the articular synovial fluid by one of two effects: stimulation of the synovial membrane through joint mobilization or stimulation of excess fluid release by mobilization of the joint in a flexion and extension pumping action.

- Winding and unwinding of the joint capsule through joint mobilization rehydrates the articular cartilage.

- Rhythmic oscillations (rocking movements) promote circulation and decrease joint swelling.

- Compression and decompression of the STM strokes act like a pump to increase and decrease the pressure within the tissue, promoting the exchange of fluids.

- Compression from the massage strokes creates heat, which creates a thixotropic effect on the ground substance, increasing its water uptake.

- MET through muscle contraction can stimulate the circulation deep within the body (down to the bone) and within the joint, reducing swelling.

- STM and MET help to realign and strengthen connective tissue fibers, especially collagen.

- Crossing transverse to the fiber imparts tension (stretch) to the elastic component (collagen), like pulling on a spring or crossing the string of a musical instrument. When the stretch is released, the energy imparted into the stretched fiber is released as heat. Heat promotes lubrication and nutritional exchange at the microscopic level.

- Crossing transverse to the fibers spreads the fibers, dissolving abnormal crosslinks and adhesions, resulting in a greater ability of the tissue to lengthen and an increase in the ROM of the joints.

- CR MET creates tensile forces (pulling or stretching) that increase collagen synthesis, resulting in greater tissue strength. It also provides a pulling force through muscle contraction that elongates the connective tissue and helps to realign the collagen fibers into their normal parallel alignment.

- PIR or CRAC MET provides stretching to the connective tissue that dissolves abnormal crosslinks in the fascia within the muscle, allowing for greater length and elasticity in the tissue.

- Normalizes the function of the muscles.

- STM and MET reduce muscle hypertonicity.

- MET helps to restore normal firing patterns in the muscle.

- MET increases the length of the fascia within the muscle and the myotendon.

- Isotonic and CR MET strengthen a weakened muscle or group of muscles.

- PIR MET can eliminate trigger points.

- Normalizes positional dysfunction.

- STM and MET realign tissue that has developed an abnormal torsion or twist.

- STM and MET correct interfascicular torsion by unwinding the abnormal torsion.

- STM and MET help to realign the collagen fibers into their normal parallel alignment.

- Establishes normal neurological function in the soft tissue through manual techniques and MET.

- STM and MET decrease adhesions that entrap nerve fibers and decrease neurological flow.

- MET helps to normalize the arthrokinetic reflex, reducing reflex facilitation or inhibition.

- Facilitates sensory-motor integration by bringing the client's conscious awareness to areas of habitual contraction or weakness, correcting what Thomas Hanna[22] calls "sensory motor amnesia."

- Mobilizes restricted joints and helps to promote healthy cartilage.

- Mobilization and STM promote the exchange of synovial fluid into and out of the joint by winding and unwinding the joint capsule.

- Mechanical stimulation through massage, mobilization, and muscle contraction (MET) stimulates the synthesis of chondrocytes and cartilage repair.

- Massage, mobilization, and MET decrease adhesions, allowing for increased ROM in the joints.

- Provides pain management.

- Mobilization increases mechanoreceptor stimulation, which reduces pain sensations because of the pain gate and reoxygenation of the tissue.

- Massage, mobilization, and MET decrease swelling in the tissues and joints by promoting fluid exchange.

- Massage, mobilization, and MET increase circulation, which increases the oxygenation in the tissues and the elimination of lactic acid and other waste products, which are pain producers.

- Creates a piezoelectric effect.

- Stretching the fibers by longitudinal or transverse strokes creates a piezoelectric current that increases synthesis of new cells and the creation of electrical potentials that realign the fibers.

- Massage, mobilization, and MET create an electromagnetic field effect.[32]

- The cells, fibers, and fluids in the body are a "liquid crystal" that emits a biomagnetic field. Collagen is a semiconductor that, when stimulated (piezoelectric effect) through movement, massage, or manipulation, generates an electric field. Electric currents emit a magnetic field.

■ Living systems respond to external energy fields, and biomagnetic fields are emitted from the hands of the therapist.

■ Energetic pulses precede action, so a healing intention from the therapist is critical.

TREATMENT GUIDELINES FOR SOFT TISSUE DYSFUNCTION AND INJURY

ACUTE PHASE (BEGINS WITHIN MINUTES AND LASTS UP TO SIX DAYS)

Treatment Rationale

■ Inflammation stimulates the body's defense and repair mechanisms. However, in soft tissue injuries, excessive or prolonged inflammation can delay healing and lead to negative tissue changes.[33] The body has an extraordinary innate ability to heal injuries, and all treatment is aimed at maximizing the body's regenerative capacity. Injury, whether of rapid or gradual onset, creates inflammation. This creates swelling (edema), which then prevents normal circulation, leading to ischemia (low oxygen) and increased concentration of pain-producing chemicals, such as histamine and lactic acid. The swelling creates pain through stimulation of pressure receptors, and the acids create pain through irritation of chemoreceptors. Pain leads to muscle spasms. Muscle spasms decrease blood flow, creating greater ischemia and pain, leading to more muscle spasms. A pain-spasm-pain cycle is established. Prolonged edema not only prolongs pain, but also causes the deposition of excessive crosslinks in the collagen, creating adhesions and thick stagnant tissue. Joint swelling creates a reflex inhibition of the surrounding muscles and muscle atrophy.

In the acute stage of rehabilitation, preserving as much mobility and strength as possible in the injured area through **STM** and **joint mobilization** is now recommended.[34] *Joint mobilization* is defined as simply passive joint movement.[28,31] Pain-free passive joint movement, especially in flexion-extension planes, provides a pumping action to promote circulation and reduce swelling. Joint mobilization also stimulates the joint mechanoreceptors, which reduces pain and promotes a relaxation response, both to the local muscles and to the whole nervous system.[30] Passive mobiliza-

tion maintains mobility in the joints, ligaments, tendons, and muscles; increases nutrition to the joint to maintain health in the cartilage; stimulates cellular synthesis; and helps to realign healing fibers. STM supplies healthy stimulation to the tissue, which reduces swelling and promotes circulation, improving oxygen and nutrition and reducing the concentration acids; reduces muscle spasms; promotes the synthesis of new cells to repair the area; prevents adhesions; and maintains mobility. When an area is mobilized, loose connective tissue develops, allowing for strong and mobile new tissue at the site of injury and ensuring painless restoration of normal function in the soft tissue and joint. Immobilization leads to the formation of dense, irregular connective tissue and the area becomes dense and hard.[35] Even micromovements (i.e., millimeters of movement) and grams of pressure promote nutritional exchange and cellular regeneration and help to realign the healing fibers. Gentle **CR MET** with light resistance also reduces swelling and muscle spasms and stimulates cellular synthesis. MET creates a pumping action deep into the tissue, which increases lymphatic movement to remove wastes, promotes circulation of oxygen and nutrition to the cells, and promotes the normal parallel alignment of the healing fibers. MET may also minimize muscle atrophy.

Factors Indicating Acute Phase

■ Pain at rest, especially pain at night.

■ Swelling, redness, heat.

■ Muscle spasms, which guard against movement.

■ Painful, limited joint movement.

■ Tender to palpation before tissue tension.

Treatment Goals for Acute Phase

■ Decrease pain.

■ Control inflammation by reducing swelling.

■ Restore normal fluid movement, improving oxygen and nutrition to the injured site and excretion of waste products.

■ Reduce hypertonicity in muscles.

■ Reestablish full, pain-free joint movement as quickly and comfortably as possible.

■ Stimulate cellular synthesis.

■ Help to align healing fibrils and fibers.

■ Induce a relaxation response.

■ Minimize muscular inhibition.

Treatment Guidelines

▧ Palpate the area to determine the amount of heat and swelling. A hot, swollen area indicates acute inflammation, and massage is **contraindicated** on the site of inflamed tissue, because pressure can disturb the healing fibers. However, passive movement and pain-free MET are recommended. Massage may be performed near the site of inflammation or on an area that is warm, as the inflammation is mild or resolving. The intensity or dose of treatment is the art of clinical practice. Treatment intensity is based on several factors: degree of pain, age of patient, degree of conditioning, extent of loss of ROM, and degree of muscle spasms. Pressure should be light so as not to disturb the healing fibrils. Always work within the comfortable limits of your client. The client should be able to completely relax, even if the treatment is uncomfortable. Some clients can tolerate only a few grams of manual pressure, a few degrees of passive motion, or a few ounces of resistance with MET. Any movement is beneficial if it does not increase the pain or inflammation.

▧ **Joint mobilization.** Passive joint movement in the pain-free range should begin as quickly and comfortably as possible to prevent adhesions and loss of motion and to promote circulation.[36] Slow, small-amplitude oscillations are performed in the beginning of the range of joint movement (grade I) or within the free range of the joint motion (grade II). Frequency varies from one per second for painful conditions to two or three per second if there is less pain.

▧ **Muscle energy technique.** Gentle pain-free isometrics of very low intensity should be performed immediately to prevent or minimize muscular inhibition and to decrease swelling. With muscle injury, MET should be performed with the muscle in the resting position so as to not stretch or stress the healing filaments. Perform CR MET and RI MET with very light pressure. MET should always be pain free.

▧ **Soft tissue mobilization.** STM is performed cautiously and gently, with very light, slow wave mobilization strokes transverse to the line of the fiber on tendons, ligaments, joint capsules, and other soft tissues. Keep your hands relaxed, your touch gentle, and your pace slow when working with tender tissue. STM is akin to small, gentle waves in a protected bay on a calm day.

▧ **Stretching is contraindicated.** PIR MET, CRAC MET, and eccentric MET all attempt to stretch the connective tissue. These techniques are contraindicated in the inflammatory phase, because they disturb the newly formed tissue.

SUBACUTE PHASE (REPAIR/REGENERATION PHASE) (TWO DAYS TO SIX WEEKS)

Treatment Rationale

▧ In the second phase of repair, there is a dramatic increase in collagen fiber production, but the fibers are organized in a random weave. As a result, an abnormal number of crosslinks develop between the collagen fibers, inhibiting the normal glide of connective tissue structures relative to one another. The tissue shortens, leading to increased stiffness and pain in both the local tissues and the associated joint. Muscles lose length because of soft tissue shortening and strength because of disruption of muscle fibers and articular nerves. Joint capsules thicken, leading to abnormal movement patterns, joint stiffness, and eventual joint degeneration. Abnormal joint movement also leads to strength/weakness imbalances in the muscles through the arthrokinetic reflex. The intention of STM is to promote the movement of connective tissue structures to glide in relation to each other. This promotes the health of the tissues by increasing lubrication and nutrition. Joint mobilization (passive joint movement) is used to help orient the healing fibers; promote the synthesis of collagen, chondrocytes (cartilage cells), and synoviocytes (cells of the synovial lining), which increase strength, lubrication, and nutrition to the joint and cartilage matrix; and stretch the myofascia and capsular tissues that can cause decreased joint motion. MET is used to maintain or increase muscular strength, promote proper neuromuscular function, promote cellular synthesis, help to restore the normal function of nerves, promote nutritional exchange, promote alignment of the healing fibers, reduce hypertonicity, and increase joint motion. Your client's response to your treatment is the best guide as to how quickly or vigorously to proceed.

Factors Indicating Subcute Phase

▧ Signs of inflammation have decreased.

▧ Swelling and heat have reduced or resolved.

▧ Pain or discomfort after activity, during activity, or with a particular movement.

▧ Muscles are not spastic but will be either tight and short, or weak.

▧ Joints will still have some discomfort/pain at the end ranges and often decreased ROM.

▧ Tender to palpation at tissue tension at site of injury.

Treatment Goals for Subacute Phase

- Continue to decrease swelling and hypertonicity.

- Promote collagen synthesis.

- Restore the ability of soft tissue to glide relative to other tissues.

- Realign the developing fibrils to normal parallel alignment.

- Unwind torsion within the tissue, and reposition the soft tissue to restore functional alignment.

- Dissolve abnormal crosslinks and adhesions.

- Improve extensibility (length).

- Help to restore normal neurological function.

- Restore normal ROM in the involved joint.

- Correct the posture.

Treatment Guidelines

- Patient response is the best guide as to how quickly or vigorously to progress.

- **Joint mobilization (passive joint movement).** Passive joint mobilization can be performed to mobilize the tissue at the tension barrier (grades III and IV).

- **Muscle energy technique.** MET, including CR and RI, is performed within pain-free limits with greater pressure to engage more muscle fibers and connective tissue. Place the muscle in a relaxed position rather than a stretched position to prevent disrupting healing fibers. PIR MET to gently stretch the tissue may be used as the client progresses. Always work within the client's comfort zone.

- **Soft tissue mobilization.** It is important that the STM should remain fairly light; otherwise, you run the risk of breaking down the immature collagen fibers. The depth of the STM may be increased slightly during the subacute phase but always within the client's comfort level.

CHRONIC PHASE (REMODELING PHASE) (THREE WEEKS TO TWELVE MONTHS)

Treatment Rationale

- From three weeks to about two months, there is an abundance of collagen that becomes thicker and reorients in response to stresses place on it.[29] Unless the area is mobilized, adhesions in the soft tissue and stiffness in the joints develop. Movement from exercise and stretching is something that clients can do on their own, but there often remain impairments in the injured area. Collagen molecules are held together by weak bonds for up to ten weeks after an injury and can be easily remodeled during that period. As the collagen matures, it changes to stronger bonds and is more resistant to remodeling. If the tissue is not properly mobilized and stretched during the first few months after an injury, it becomes less responsive, and greater effort is required to change it. To prevent chronic pain, adhesions must be dissolved, the length in the connective tissue must be restored, the joint play (accessory movement) and ROM in the joint must be normalized, and strength must be returned to weakened muscles. Chronic pain is the result of two very different healing processes. The area is either (1) unstable owing to weakness in the musculature and overstretched or atrophied ligaments (including the joint capsule) or (2) restricted owing to thick, shortened soft tissue around the joints, loss of joint play, or degeneration of the joint surfaces, leading to stiff joints with decreased ROM and tightness-weakness imbalances in the muscles that cross the joint. A combination of these two conditions can also be present in the same joint. For example, the knee can have an overstretched medial collateral ligament; a weak vastus medialis; a short, thick iliotibial band; and a tight biceps femoris.

Factors Indicating Chronic Phase

- No signs of inflammation.

- May have painful or painless limitation of full active motion. Much of the pain may be due to stress placed on adhesions and joint impingement.

- Pain or feeling of tightness or discomfort at end of passive stretch.

- Palpation of adhesions.

- Sustained muscular weakness or tightness.

- Poor balance (neuromuscular control).

Treatment Goals for Stiff Soft Tissue and Joints in the Remodeling Phase

- Restore pain-free, full ROM to the joint.

- Eliminate pain in deep connective tissues.

- Dissolve adhesions and restore flexibility and alignment to the soft tissue, including ligaments, joint capsules, and periosteum.

- Restore strength, sensory awareness, and normal firing patterns in the weakened muscles.

- Eliminate hypertonicity in short, tight muscles.

- Help to restore normal proprioception.

Treatment Guidelines

- **Joint mobilization (passive joint movement).** Mobilizations through tissue barrier (grade IV) may be used in the chronic condition. Performed to restore accessory motions (joint play), promote full ROM, rehydrate the joint, improve nutrition to the area, promote cellular synthesis, increase joint mobility, and improve muscle performance.[37]

- **Muscle energy technique.** PIR, CRAC, and eccentric MET can be used to lengthen the connective tissue, dissolve adhesions, increase ROM in the joint, and help to restore normal neurological function. CR MET is used to promote the normal firing pattern and strength in a muscle. Eccentric MET is used with chronic conditions; with thick, fibrotic tissue; and in the well-conditioned client.

- **Soft tissue mobilization.** STM can be performed at an increased depth to muscles, tendons, ligaments, and the joint capsule to dissolve adhesions. Transverse friction massage can be used to release the tissue attachments to the periosteum at the bone. Chronic restrictions may involve deep "scars" or adhesions. Deep friction creates mild hyperemia, which accelerates the repair and stimulates mechanoreceptors, which inhibit pain.[38] The art of manual therapy is to match the force of the strokes to the stage of the healing. To restore the functional properties of thickened soft tissue in the remodeling phase, greater depth needs to be applied to overcome the restrictive barriers.

Treatment Goals for Unstable Joints and Weak Soft Tissue in the Remodeling Phase

- Identify hypertonic muscles. Use CR MET or PIR MET if the muscles are tight, because hypertonic muscles have an inhibiting effect on their antagonists, owing to the law of reciprocal inhibition.

- Identify weak muscles. Perform CR MET on weak muscles to help strengthen them, promote normal neurological communication, and promote lymphatic circulation and nutritional exchange.

- Identify areas of the joint that may be restricted, even though unstable, and mobilize the restricted area.

- Suggest strengthening and stabilization exercises, or refer the client for rehabilitation therapy.

- For help in maintaining benefits of the treatment, a daily exercise program is encouraged. This exercise program should include exercises to stretch tight areas and to strengthen weak areas as well as exercises of balance and coordination to help restore neurological function.

Chronic Pain or Dysfunction Requires a Comprehensive Program of Rehabilitation

- It is important to remember that continuing problems for the nervous system from soft tissue injury can manifest as problems in coordination, balance, movement, posture, weakness, hypertonicity, and stiffness. Your recommendations for treatment should include balance and coordination exercises as well as posture, strength, and flexibility training.

Contraindications to Massage and Manual Therapy: Red Flags

Red flags are signs and symptoms that are rarely encountered in benign (nonpathological) forms of pain. Your goal is to quickly identify clients who might have a pathological condition in which massage and manual therapy might be contraindicated and to distinguish them from the vast majority of clients who would benefit from massage and manual therapy.

HISTORY QUESTIONS FOR THE CLIENT TO RULE OUT SERIOUS PATHOLOGY

- Do you have constant pain that is worse at night and not relieved by any position? (Tumors and infections, as well as significant inflammation, are often worse at night.)

- Do you have constant writhing or cramping pain? (Rule out tumor and infection.)

- Do you have intense local pain that developed after a recent significant trauma? (Rule out fracture.)

- Do you have any fevers? (Rule out infection.)

- Do you have a history of cancer or other serious medical problems?

- Have you had any unintended weight loss? (Weight loss is often associated with cancer.)

- Do you have bowel or bladder control problems? (These may indicate pressure on spinal cord)

- Do you have significant, unexplained lower limb weakness? (This can indicate pressure on the spinal cord or significant nerve root compression)

If a client answers yes to any of the above questions, it is important that a doctor evaluate the client. If the client has severe pain, has a red flag, and has not been seen by a doctor before his or her office visit to you, refer that client for evaluation prior to your session.

If the client is in moderate pain, that is, the pain is interfering with work or activities of daily living, and the client has red flags, you may treat the client if he or she can comfortably lie on your table in the fetal position without pain.

If the client is in pain in the fetal position, refer the client to a doctor before you provide treatment. If the client can lie on your table in the fetal position comfortably, use the MET and the massage strokes slowly and gently. Work only within pain-free limits. At the end of the session, inform the client that you recommend that a doctor evaluate him or her. You could say, "I need to have more information to treat you effectively." Or you might say, "There are many causes of pain, and I recommend that you see a doctor to make sure you don't have a more serious condition." If your client has mild pain and a red flag, you can safely provide treatment, but the client needs to be referred to a doctor also.

CONDITIONS IN WHICH DEEP PRESSURE IS CONTRAINDICATED

STM uses a wide range of pressures that the therapist can apply to the client and includes the practice of the "laying of hands," which uses the electromagnetic field from the therapist's hands as the therapeutic modality. With this in mind, there are no contraindications to the laying of hands. It takes years of practice in the art of massage to know the proper amount of pressure to apply to a particular condition. However, deep pressure is contraindicated in certain conditions:

- Osteoporosis

- Disc herniation

- Pregnancy

- Inflammation

Guidelines for Referring Clients

In addition to knowing the red flags that indicate when massage is contraindicated, it is important to know that certain conditions are best treated in conjunction with other practitioners. A good clinician knows when to refer to other health-care providers for further evaluation or treatment. Throughout this text, it is indicated when a referral is recommended. The three providers who are most often referred to include:

- A medical doctor (MD) to diagnose a client who has a red flag and to rule out a pathological condition.

- A doctor of chiropractic (DC) or doctor of osteopathy (DO) to evaluate and provide adjustment or manipulation for the spine and the extremities.

- A registered physical therapist (RPT) or specialist in exercise rehabilitation (e.g., personal trainer, Pilates trainer, yoga instructor).

Listed below are symptoms that typically indicate the need for a referral. Because the vast majority of pain and dysfunction in the body is a problem of function and not pathology, most of the referrals are to specialists in problems of functional disturbance (chiropractors and osteopaths) and not to specialists in disease and pathology (medical doctors).

- Clients with radiating pain and/or numbing or tingling in the arms or legs should be evaluated.

- Any chronic pain (not soreness) should be evaluated.

- If muscles do not relax after several treatments, the client might need treatment to normalize joint function.

- Sharp localized pain, as distinguished from an ache, that does not improve in three days should be assessed.

Overview of Treatment

GENERAL TREATMENT GUIDELINES

- Massage typically lasts one hour, although the length of the session can vary greatly. Chiropractic doctors have effectively used the techniques described in this text in 15-minute sessions prior to the adjustment. Massage and manual therapy can be effective in 30-minute sessions.

- Treatments are typically given weekly for four to six weeks to treat most conditions. A client who is in acute distress can be treated more frequently. Clients who are in chronic pain might have weekly treatments for several months and then graduate to two times per month for several months, then once a month, and so forth until the point of maximum medical improvement has been reached. This is the point at which there are no further gains in the subjective or objective findings. Treatment frequency is then determined by how well the client can maintain his or her functional gains. In chronic conditions, STM, joint mobilization, and MET can help to support functional gains.

- The client should be evaluated after approximately every six treatments to determine the need for continuation of care. The goal in reevaluating is to identify subjective and objective improvement, gather objective examination findings for future treatments, and assess the need for a referral if there is little or no improvement.

- Massage and manual therapy are also designed for health enhancement (wellness care) and improvement in sports, dance, and recreation. Many clients elect to be treated on an ongoing basis.

TREATMENT PROTOCOL FOR THE CLIENT WITH AN ACUTE CONDITION

- It is important to determine the severity of the client's condition to determine your treatment protocol. Once you have ruled out red flags through your history questions and determined that the client is a candidate for massage therapy, perform the assessment.

- Begin your work on the noninvolved side in injuries or dysfunctions of the spine, not only because it is easier for the client, but also because a relaxation response is transferred from one side of the body to the other.

- As has been mentioned, tell your client that she or he should be able to completely relax into the massage and MET.

- In work on the spine, begin the session with gentle rocking movements of the whole body, as described in the first series of strokes in Chapter 3. This helps you to make contact with your client in a noninvasive way and determine the level of guarding. If the client's body is resistant to the rocking, slow down until you feel a relaxation response. You might say in a gentle voice, "Allow me to move your body. This rocking is like putting a baby to sleep. Just relax."

- Once the client is more relaxed, you may elect to perform CR MET or RI MET if the muscles are extremely tender and hypertonic. Typically, spend only a few minutes at a time with MET, and then perform more strokes. Alternate the MET with the strokes throughout the session.

- The greater the client's distress, the lighter the strokes should be. Rock the client slowly and with a small amplitude. Small, gentle movements can be soothing and help to disperse swelling. Large, brisk movements can be irritating.

■ Remember that pain relief does not mean the restoration of normal function. Once the pain is resolved, assess the area again to ensure that the ROM is normal and that the length and strength of the muscles in the region are balanced.

TREATMENT PROTOCOL FOR THE CLIENT WITH CHRONIC PAIN

■ A general treatment for most clients with chronic pain typically involves a "spinal session," that is, performing Level I strokes on the lumbosacral, thoracic, and cervical areas of the spine. Then focused work is performed on the specific area of complaint.

■ The strokes are usually applied more deeply, as it is necessary to dissolve adhesions in the soft tissue. We often perform manual work in areas that are uncomfortable, and we need to remind the client that he or she should be able to completely relax into the massage strokes, even if they are uncomfortable. Otherwise, ask the client to always let you know if he or she cannot relax into what you are doing.

■ Perform MET throughout the session, interspersing it with the strokes.

■ Mobilize the client with bigger movements in areas of fibrosis, and perform only small-amplitude mobilizations in areas of instability.

■ Instruct your client in the correct posture. The cumulative stresses from poor posture can create chronic tension patterns that can be the source of a client's pain.

■ It is essential that clients with chronic pain have proper exercise instruction that includes strength and stabilization training in addition to instruction in coordination and balance.

■ Rehabilitation has two categories: passive care and active care. **Passive care** is care that is done to the client, including massage therapy. **Active care** is care that the client does on his or her own. It is now well recognized that activity decreases the disability associated with chronic pain.[39]

CLIENTS WHO ARE REACTIVE TO TREATMENT: SIDE EFFECTS

■ If a client develops **side effects** of increased pain after your session, assume that you worked too hard

for too long in an area. Massage therapists are often enthusiastic, which can lead to working too hard, especially when learning a new technique. If your client is mildly sore for a day or two, as if she or he went to a new exercise class, that is considered normal. This soreness is often associated with the first sessions. Moderate to severe discomfort after a session or the next day could mean that your treatment was much too vigorous.

■ All interventions have potential side effects. This is well known and easily accepted in allopathic medicine when a patient develops side effects from a drug. It is not as easily accepted when a client has side effects from massage or physical therapy or from chiropractic or any other manual intervention. The goal of the therapist is to minimize side effects, because it is unreasonable to assume that your treatments will never have side effects. The more experienced the practitioner, the fewer the side effects.

■ You might be missing an underlying joint problem. For example, if the joint is inflamed and you work too hard, your client might have increased pain the day after the treatment.

■ You might be missing underlying emotional distress. Massage can change habits of muscle function and posture, and even a positive change can be unconsciously sensed as a distress to that person's homeostasis. Inquire whether your client is experiencing a period of high stress.

■ You might be missing an underlying pathology. Even if your client's symptoms do not fall into the category of the red flags, there could be a subclinical pathology.

CLIENTS WHO ARE UNRESPONSIVE TO THERAPY

If your client does not show some improvement in response to your treatments after a trial of four sessions, there are several possible causes:

■ Your client might be deconditioned or atrophied and lack enough muscle tone to hold the changes that you introduce. The client might lack proper exercise habits to support the changes you make in these sessions.

■ Poor posture places stress on the system that can undermine your therapy. You can perform brilliant work to help reestablish normal function in the neck and shoulders that is undone between your sessions as the client sits in front of the computer all week with poor posture.

▧ You might not have enough experience and might need to refer your client to a more advanced practitioner.

▧ An underlying joint problem, pathology, or emotional problem might exist.

▧ The personality match between the client and the therapist might be poor. If the client is not improving under your care and you do not suspect the need for further assessment, refer your client to another practitioner.

▧ The client might need a different kind of treatment, such as myofascial release, Active Release Technique, Feldenkrais, or Rolfing, to name a few.

▧ *Study Guide*

Level I

1. Describe the five characteristics of soft tissue that the therapist can palpate.
2. Describe the three treatment modalities that are used in the method described in this text.
3. Describe the treatment goals for each stage of inflammation and repair.
4. Describe the open position of the joints and its implication for a massage therapist.
5. Describe the position of function of the wrist and hand and why it is important for the massage therapist.
6. Describe the three intentions of wave mobilization strokes.
7. Name three characteristics of wave mobilization strokes that are similar to ocean waves.
8. Describe why pain-free movement is typically recommended in the early stages of rehabilitation.
9. List six clinical uses of MET.
10. Define RI MET, CRAC MET, and PIR MET, and describe how to increase the ROM of a joint with MET.

Level II

1. Describe the four aspects of assessment and treatment.
2. Define the acronym *SOAP*.
3. List four questions that will help to determine whether massage is contraindicated (the red flags).
4. List six categories of information that you want to gather in taking a history.
5. Describe the categories of information from an active motion assessment, and explain what information helps to determine the stage of healing from active ROM.
6. List five different reasons why a muscle tests weak to isometric challenge.
7. Describe three clinical effects of joint mobilization.
8. Describe the hypothesis about how muscle energy technique relaxes a hypertonic muscle.
9. Describe the eight categories of end feel.
10. Describe four symptoms that indicate the need for a referral.

▧ *References*

1. Andrade C-K, Clifford P. Outcome-Based Massage, 2nd ed. Philadelphia: Lippincott Williams & Wilkins, 2008.
2. Cyriax J. Textbook of Orthopedic Medicine: Diagnosis of Soft Tissue Lesions, vol 1, 8th ed. London: Bailliere Tindall, 1982.
3. Levangie P, Norkin C. Joint Structure and Function, 3rd ed. Philadelphia: FA Davis, 2001.
4. Hoppenfeld S. Physical Examination of the Spine and Extremities. New York: Appleton-Century-Crofts, 1976.
5. Chaitow L. Palpation Skills. New York: Churchill Livingstone, 1998.
6. Travel J, Simons D. Myofascial Pain and Dysfunction. Baltimore: Lippincott Williams & Wilkins, 1999.
7. Lewit K, Simons D. Myofascial pain: Relief by post-isometric relaxation. Arch Phys Med Rehabil 1984;65:452–456.
8. Lo B, Inn M, Amaker R, Foe S. The Essence of T'ai Chi Ch'uan. Berkeley, CA: North Atlantic Books, 1985.
9. Oschman J. Energy Medicine. Edinburgh: Churchill Livingstone, 2000.
10. McTaggart L. The Field. New York: Harper, 2002.
11. Pollack GH. Cells, Gels, and the Engines of Life. Seattle: Ebner & Sons, 2001.
12. Rosenberg B. Electrical conductivity in proteins. J Chem Phys 1962;36:816–823.
13. Garrison T. Oceanography, 3rd ed. Pacific Grove, CA: Brooks/Cole/Wadsworth, 1999.
14. Lederman E. Harmonic Technique. Edinburgh: Churchill Livingstone, 2000.
15. Lederman E. The Science and Practice of Manual Therapy, 2nd ed. Edinburgh: Churchill Livingstone, 2005.
16. Greenman PE. Principles of Manual Medicine, 2nd ed. Baltimore: Williams & Wilkins, 1996.
17. Voss D, Ionta M, Myers B. Proprioceptive Neuromuscular Facilitation, 3rd ed. Philadelphia: Harper and Row, 1985.
18. Lewit K. Manipulative Therapy in Rehabilitation on the Locomotor System, 3rd ed. Oxford: Butterworth Heinemann, 1999.
19. Janda V, Frank C, Liebenson C. Evaluation of muscular imbalance. In Liebenson C (ed): Rehabilitation of the Spine, 2nd ed. Baltimore: Lippincott Williams & Wilkins, 2007, pp 203–225.
20. Chaitow L. Muscle Energy Techniques. New York: Churchill Livingstone, 1996.
21. Mitchell F. Elements of muscle energy technique. In Basmajian J, Nyberg R (eds): Rational Manual Therapies. Baltimore: Williams & Wilkins, 1993, pp 285–321.
22. Hanna T. Somatics. Reading, MA: Addison-Wesley, 1988.
23. Liebenson C, Tunnell P, Murphy DR, Gluck-Bergman N. Manual Resistive techniques. In Liebenson C (ed): Rehabilitation of the Spine, 2nd ed. Philadelphia: Lippincott Williams & Wilkins, 2007, pp 407–463.
24. Kendall F, McCreary E, Provance P, Rodgers M, Romani W. Muscles: Testing and Function, 5th ed. Baltimore: Lippincott Williams & Wilkins, 2005.
25. Kandel E, Schwartz J, Jessell T. Principles of Neural Science, 4th ed. New York: McGraw-Hill, 2000.
26. Lorenz T, Campello M. Biomechanics of skeletal muscle. In Norkin M, Frankel V (eds): Basic Biomechanics

of the Musculoskeletal System, 3rd ed. Philadelphia: Lippincott Williams & Wilkins, 2001, pp 148–174.

27. Freeman MAR, Wyke B. Articular reflexes at the ankle joint: An electromyographic study of normal and abnormal influences of ankle-joint mechanoreceptors upon reflex activity in the leg muscles. Br J Surg 1967; 54:990–1001.

28. Hertling D, Kessler RM. Management of Common Musculoskeletal Disorders. Philadelphia: Lippincott Williams & Wilkin, 2006.

29. Kisner C, Colby LA. Therapeutic Exercise, 5th ed. Philadelphia: FA Davis, 2002.

30. Wyke BD. Articular neurology and manipulative therapy. In Glasgow EF (ed): Aspects of Manipulative Therapy, 2nd ed. Edinburgh: Churchill Livingstone, 1985, pp 72–80.

31. Brukner P, Khan K. Clinical Sports Medicine, 3rd ed. Sydney: McGraw-Hill, 2006.

32. Oschman J. Energy Medicine. Edinburgh: Churchill Livingstone, 2000.

33. Woo S, Buckwalter J. Injury and Repair of the Musculoskeletal Soft Tissues. Park Ridge, IL: American Academy of Orthopedic Surgeons, 1988.

34. Kibler WB, Herring SA, Press J, Lee P. Functional Rehabilitation of Sports and Musculoskeletal Injuries. Gaithersburg, MD: Aspen, 1998.

35. Reid DC. Sports Injury and Assessment. New York: Churchill Livingstone, 1992.

36. Kellett J. Acute soft tissue injuries: A review of the literature. Med Sci Sports Exerc 1986;18:489–500.

37. Edmond SL. Joint Mobilization/Manipulation, 2nd ed. St. Louis: Mosby, 2006.

38. Palastanga N. Soft-Tissue Manipulation Techniques. In Boyling JD, Palastanga N (eds): Grieve's Modern Manual Therapy, 2nd ed. Edinburgh: Churchill Livingstone, 1998, pp 809–822.

39. Liebenson C. Active Self-Care: Functional Reactivation for Spine Pain Patients. In Liebenson C (ed): Rehabilitation of the Spine, 2nd ed. Philadelphia: Lippincott Williams & Wilkins, 2007, pp 295–329.

▨ Suggested Readings

Basmajian J, Nyberg R, eds. Rational Manual Therapies. Baltimore: Williams & Wilkins, 1993.

Chaitow L. Palpation Skills. New York: Churchill Livingstone, 1998.

Greenman PE. Principles of Manual Medicine, 2nd ed. Baltimore: Williams & Wilkins, 1996.

Hoppenfeld S. Physical Examination of the Spine and Extremities. New York: Appleton-Century-Crofts, 1976.

Kendall F, McCreary E, Provance P, Rodgers M, Romani W. Muscles: Testing and Function, 5th ed. Baltimore: Lippincott Williams & Wilkins, 2005.

Lederman E. The Science and Practice of Manual Therapy, 2nd ed. Edinburgh: Churchill Livingstone, 2005.

Magee D. Orthopedic Physical Assessment, 3rd ed. Philadelphia: WB Saunders, 1997.

3

Lumbosacral Spine

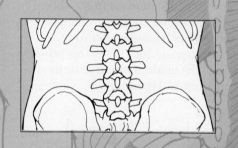

Problems with the **lumbosacral spine,** or low back, are some of the most common complaints that clients present to the massage therapist. **Low back pain (LBP)** is the second leading symptom for which adult patients consult their primary care physicians.[1] Disorders of the low back are the leading cause of disability in people younger than 45 years of age.[2] Every year 50% of the adult population in the United States experiences at least one day of back pain, yet 80% of LBP is nonspecific, meaning that the cause is unknown.[3] It has been estimated that at least 98% of LBP results from mechanical disorders of the spine, that is, problems of function rather than a structural pathology.[4] Sustained muscle contraction is a primary cause of dysfunction and pain,[5] and a recent analysis of treatments for low back pain showed that massage therapy was effective for persistent back pain.[6]

Anatomy, Function, and Dysfunction of the Lumbosacral Spine

GENERAL OVERVIEW

■ The spine consists of 33 bones divided into five regions: **cervical, thoracic, lumbar, sacral,** and **coccygeal** (Fig. 3-1).

■ There are 24 distinct vertebrae: seven cervical, twelve thoracic, and five lumbar.

■ Five vertebrae are fused to form the **sacrum,** and four are fused to form the **coccyx.**

■ The lumbopelvic region consists of five lumbar vertebrae, the right and left innominate **bones,** which function as lower-extremity bones, and the sacrum, which functions as part of the spine. The pelvis has three joints: a **symphysis pubis** and two **sacroiliac joints.**

PRIMARY AND SECONDARY CURVES

When the body is viewed from the side, there are three visible curves: the lumbar, the thoracic, and the cervi-cal. The sacrum and the coccyx, which are not visible, form a fourth curve. The thoracic and coccygeal curves are called **primary curves** because the vertebral column at birth has one curve that is convex posteriorly. The cervical and lumbar curves are convex anteriorly and are called **secondary curves** because they develop after birth in response to the infant's lifting his or her head and standing upright, respectively.

The degree of curve in the healthy spine represents the balance between stability and mobility. The curves enhance the load-bearing capacity of the spine by allowing it to "flex." With too little curve, the spine is stiff. With too much curve, the spine is often hypermobile and unstable. However, an increase in the thoracic curve, which is often caused by bony changes such as osteoporosis, represents bone degeneration.

Pelvic rotation, or anterior/posterior tilt, is the primary factor that determines the amount of curve in the spine (Fig. 3-2). Pelvic rotation is determined by many

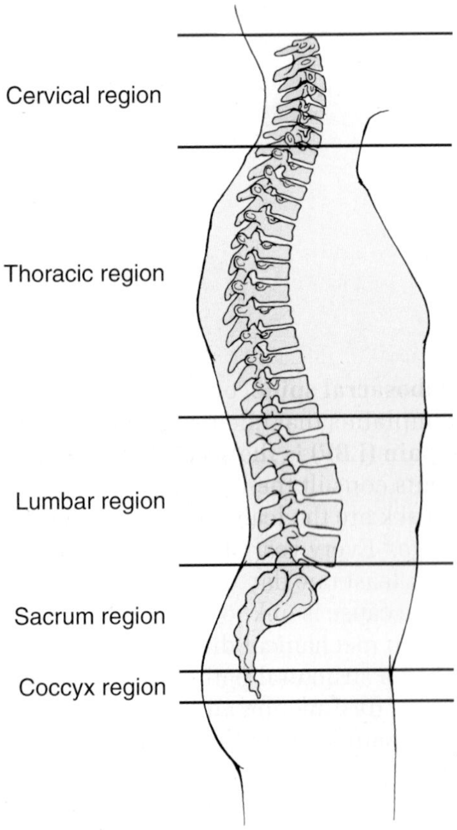

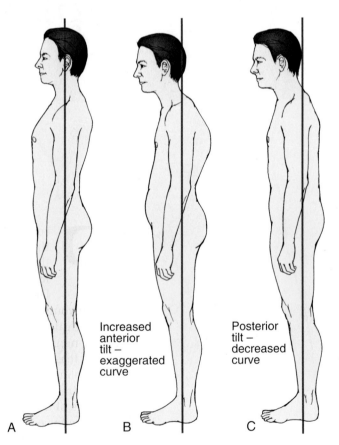

Cervical region

Thoracic region

Lumbar region

Sacrum region

Coccyx region

Figure 3-1. Lateral view of the spine showing the five regions and the four curves.

Increased anterior tilt – exaggerated curve

Posterior tilt – decreased curve

A   B   C

Figure 3-2. A, Normal spinal curves. **B,** Increased anterior pelvic tilt and exaggerated curve. **C,** Decreased curve due to a posterior pelvic tilt.

factors, including genetics, muscle balance, pronation, and posture. Anterior rotation of the pelvis creates an increase in the lumbar curve, and all other curves are increased to keep the body in gravitational balance. Posterior rotation of the pelvis creates a flattening of the lumbar curve and a decrease of the thoracic and cervical curves. As is discussed in this chapter, many muscular factors contribute to the amount of pelvic rotation.

POSTURE

Posture is determined by many factors, including genetics, structural abnormalities caused by disease, habits of work and play, mimicking parents and peers, compensations resulting from injury, emotional and psychological factors, and gravity.[7]

GENERAL ANATOMY OF THE VERTEBRAE

There are five vertebrae in the lumbar spine. Each vertebra consists of an anterior and a posterior portion (Fig. 3-3).

■ The anterior portion is composed of the **vertebral body** and **intervertebral disc,** which form a **fibrocartilaginous** or **amphiarthrodial joint.**

■ The posterior portion is composed of two vertebral arches formed by a pedicle and lamina; two transverse processes; a central spinous process; and paired articulations, the **inferior** and **superior facets,** which form **synovial joints.** Each vertebra forms three joints with the vertebra above and three joints with the vertebra below (or the sacrum). This three-joint complex includes an intervertebral disc and two facet joints.

■ There are three openings through which the spinal cord and spinal nerves travel. The central canal is called the vertebral foramen, and is located behind each vertebral body. The spinal cord travels through this canal from C1 to L5. The paired intervertebral foramen are openings between two adjacent vertebrae through which the nerve roots travel. They are discussed in more detail below.

INTERVERTEBRAL DISC

■ **Definition:** The **intervertebral disc (IVD)** is a fibrocartilage structure that binds two vertebral bodies together.

■ **Structure:** The IVD is composed of a nucleus and an annulus.
  □ **Nucleus:** The nucleus is a colloidal gel contained within a fibrous wall that is 80% to 90% water, which changes its shape and releases and absorbs water. The nucleus obtains nutrition by movement, and this water-binding capacity decreases with age.
  □ **Annulus:** Concentric layers of interwoven fibrocartilaginous fibers form the annulus. The fibroelastic tissue is primarily elastic but becomes more fibrous with age and therefore loses some shock-absorbing ability. The outer third of the annulus is innervated by mechanoreceptors and free nerve endings (pain receptors) that have automatic, unconscious (i.e., reflexive) communication with the surrounding muscles.[1]

■ **Function:** The IVD provides a shock-absorbing hydraulic system that permits a rocker-like movement of one vertebra upon the other because of a fluid

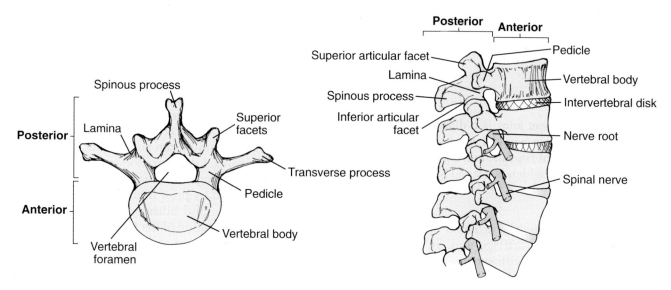

Figure 3-3. Vertebral anatomy. The anterior portion of the vertebrae consists of the vertebral body and the intervertebral disc. The posterior portion consists of a pedicle and lamina, two transverse processes, a central spinous process, and the inferior and superior facets.

shift in the nucleus and an elasticity of the annulus. The disc also provides proprioceptive and nociceptive functions. Disc nutrition into the annulus occurs by movement of the spine, which pumps fluids into the disc through cycles of compression and decompression.

■ **Dysfunction and injury:** The IVD is prone to both acute injury and chronic degeneration and is a major source of LBP. Chronic degeneration involves loss of fluid in the nucleus and loss of elasticity of the annulus.

 □ Repetitive torsion forces (that is, repetitive bending and twisting) can cause an **internal disruption** due to small tears of the annulus. The annulus may become lax owing to these tears creating bulges around the circumference of the disc. This is called a **disc bulge.** The bulge may develop into a **herniated disc,** which is a displacement of disc material. Herniation has two types: either a small, localized displacement or a broad-based herniation. The term *protrusion* or *extrusion* can be used for herniation. Finally, a **sequestered disc,** also called a prolapse, is a leaking of disc material into the spinal canal.

 □ When injured, the disc leaks inflammatory material that can be a source of LBP and referred pain caused by irritation of the nerve root.

■ **Treatment implications:** The Hendrickson Method of soft tissue mobilization introduces a new style of soft tissue and joint mobilization called *wave mobilization* that theoretically helps to promote fluid exchange to the disc. Through rhythmic cycles of posterior to anterior (P–A) mobilization, the author postulates that this cycle of compression and decompression pumps the disc to help rehydrate a degenerated disc and helps to disperse excess fluids of an inflamed disc, helping to resolve venous stasis, which is the vascular congestion at the nerve root, a significant source of pain.

FACET JOINT

■ **Definition:** The **facet joint** is a diarthrodial or synovial joint, containing a synovial space surrounded by a connective tissue joint capsule, adipose tissue fat pads, and a fibromeniscus, which is a small meniscoid structure located near the edge of the joint (see Fig. 3-3).

■ **Structure**
 □ **Articular surface:** The articular surface is covered by hyaline cartilage and, in the healthy state, is lubricated with synovial fluid.
 □ **Joint capsule:** The joint capsule is composed of an inner synovial layer and an outer fibrous layer. It is reinforced anteriorly with the ligamentum flavum and posteriorly with the multifidus muscle. The joint capsule is one of the most richly innervated structures of the spine. It contains proprioceptive and nociceptive nerve fibers.

■ **Function:** The facets determine the range and direction of movement and have some weight-bearing capacity. In the healthy state, they are designed to slide on each other. Extension closes the facets, and flexion opens them. Compression squeezes fluid out of the hyaline cartilage, and the cartilage is rehydrated as the fluid is reabsorbed with the release of the compression. Activities of daily life, such as walking, move the spine through these cycles of compression and decompression, thus promoting normal lubrication in the facets. Sitting, on the other hand, is only compressive and dehydrates the facets.

■ **Dysfunction and injury:** Dysfunction of the facets is common, even in childhood, owing to poor posture and injury, such as a fall. This dysfunction implies that the facets are not moving normally relative to each other. This loss of normal motion alters the mechanics, creating irritation and inflammation and eventual fibrosis and thickening of the soft tissue surrounding the joint. This fibrosis or thickening creates joint stiffness and eventual degeneration if it is not corrected. Nearly everyone over 30 years old has some degeneration of the spine, especially in the cervical spine and the lumbar spine. Degeneration of the spine is usually asymptomatic, and there is no correlation between X-rays and symptoms. Pain from the facet joints can vary from sharp pain to a deep ache and can refer achy pain into the buttock and thigh. There are four broad categories of dysfunction and injury of the facets.

 □ **Hypomobility:** Restricted motion at the lumbosacral facets implies a loss of the normal gliding motion on the cartilage surfaces. This is called a **joint fixation.** Restricted motion of the facet results in a reflex that typically creates hypertonicity of the muscles at the same vertebral level. Hypomobility can lead to degeneration.

 □ **Degeneration:** Degeneration is the loss or thinning of the normal cartilage on the surface of the facet. This thinning can be mild, moderate, or severe. Advanced degeneration is called "arthritis" or degenerative joint disease (DJD). Degeneration can be caused by prior injury, repetitive stresses, hypomobility, and muscle or movement imbalances. Degeneration of the facet also involves loss of the synovial fluid and causes the joint to "dry out." Sustained contraction of the paraspinal muscles (muscles on either side of the spine) increases the compression to the facets and accelerates their degeneration.

☐ **Acute facet syndrome:** The cause of "locked back" is not well understood. One chiropractic theory proposes a fixation or microadhesion of the facet surfaces, and manipulation introduces normal movement by releasing the fixation. Other current theories suggest that the cause is an entrapment of the fibromenisci between the facets.

☐ **Joint capsule injury:** Injuries to the joint capsule are called **sprains,** as the outer capsule is ligamentous. Because the capsule is highly innervated, sprains are painful, potentially giving local and referred pain into the leg. Injury also affects the mechanoreceptors, resulting in altered movement patterns, dysfunctions of coordination and balance, and altered reflexes to the muscles, creating either weakness or hypertonicity.

▨ **Treatment implications:** One of the intentions of the wave mobilization style of soft tissue therapy is to induce P–A mobilization into the facets in rhythmic oscillations of compression and decompression. This helps to restore the normal gliding characteristics of the facets, helps to reduce hypertonicity in the surrounding muscles and stimulates the synovial lining of the capsule to increase lubrication to rehydrate the cartilage. If the facets are swollen, the author theorizes that this same mobilization helps to disperse excess fluids. Patients who have chronic LBP need balance and coordination exercises as part of their rehabilitation to reeducate the proprioceptors. Wave mobilization is especially effective with hypomobility and degeneration, whereas an acute facet syndrome often requires manipulation to correct the fixation. With a joint capsule injury, mobilization of the soft tissue and joints help to promote a healthy repair by reducing adhesions in the joint capsule.

INTERVERTEBRAL FORAMEN

▨ **Definition:** The **intervertebral foramen (IVF)** is an opening (foramen) formed by:
1. Two pedicles from the superior and the inferior vertebrae that form the roof and floor;
2. The disc, posterior longitudinal ligament, and vertebral body anteriorly;
3. The facets, anterior capsule and ligamentum flavum posteriorly.

▨ **Function:** The IVF provides an opening for the motor and sensory nerve roots that originate at the spinal cord.

▨ **Dysfunction and injury:** Narrowing of the IVF can cause compression of the nerve roots, creating pain, numbing, tingling, and weakness in the legs. The diameter of the IVF is narrowed by many factors: disc degeneration, disc protrusion, thickening and fibrosis of the ligamentum flavum and joint capsule, facet position, facet degeneration and calcification, and increased lordosis of the lumbar spine. If the narrowing is significant, it is called **foraminal stenosis.**

NERVES OF THE LUMBOSACRAL SPINE

Ventral (motor) and **dorsal (sensory)** nerve roots originate from the spinal cord and merge at the IVF. The union of these two roots is called a **spinal nerve.**

Dorsal Root Ganglion
The **dorsal root ganglion** (DRG) is a cluster of cell bodies of the sensory root and typically lies in the IVF near the disc. The DRG has been postulated to be a major site of pain, called radicular (which means *root*) pain.[7] It is also mechanically sensitive, so altered movement patterns may initiate reflex activity that results in sustained muscle contraction.

A **dermatome** is an area of skin supplied by the sensory (dorsal) root of a spinal nerve. Irritation of the DRG elicits a sharp pain in the dermatome corresponding to the root, called **dermatomal pain** (Figs. 3-4 and 3-5).

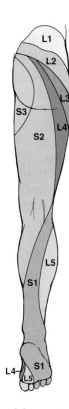

Figure 3-4. Dermatomes of the posterior lower limb.

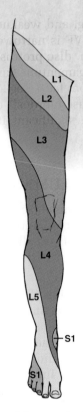

Figure 3-5. Dermatomes of the anterior lower limb.

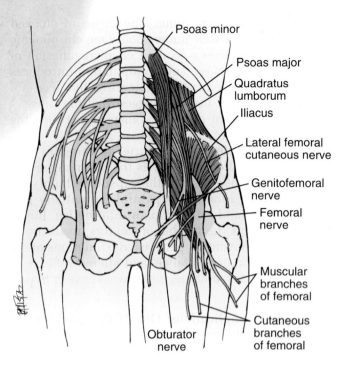

Figure 3-6. Muscles and nerves of the anterior pelvis. The lumbar plexus consists of nerves from L1 to L4 and travels through the psoas muscles. It divides into many branches, including the femoral, lateral femoral cutaneous, obturator, and genitofemoral nerves.

VENTRAL ROOTS

▪ A **myotome** consists of the muscles that are supplied by the motor root(s) of the spinal nerve(s). Irritation of the motor (ventral) root elicits muscle weakness and potential atrophy.

▪ The corresponding myotomes of the lumbar nerve roots are L2—hip flexion (iliopsoas), L3—knee extension (quadriceps), L4—ankle dorsiflexion (anterior tibialis), L5—great toe extension (extensor hallucis longus), S1—foot eversion (peroneals), and S2—knee flexion (hamstrings). If weakness is detected in these muscles, one source of the weakness might be nerve root irritation. However, it takes a great deal of clinical experience to determine that the nerve root is the source of the weakness. In the author's experience, the most common cause of weakness is fixation of the vertebral facet of the vertebra corresponding to the involved myotome.

▪ Assessment of a nerve root involvement involves the straight-leg-raising (SLR) test to determine abnormal root tension (see p. 126, "Assessment"). The most common cause of increased root tension is a swollen or bulging disc.

LUMBAR PLEXUS

Branches of nerves that communicate with other branches of nerves form a nerve plexus.

The **lumbar plexus** consists of nerves from L1 to L4 and travels through the psoas muscle (Fig. 3-6). It innervates the anterior, medial, and lateral thigh, leg, and foot. It includes the femoral, lateral femoral cutaneous, obturator, and genitofemoral nerves.

SACRAL PLEXUS

The **sacral plexus** consists of nerves from L4–L5 and S1–S3. It forms the sciatic nerve, which is actually two nerves within the same sheath, the common peroneal and tibial nerves. These nerves supply the posterior thigh, leg, and foot, as well as the anterior and lateral leg and the dorsum of the foot.

SACROILIAC JOINT

▪ **Definition:** The **sacroiliac joint (SIJ)** is a synovial joint consisting of the articulation of the sacrum with the right and left ilia.

▪ **Structure:** As in all synovial joints, its joint capsule is a pain-sensitive structure. The articular surfaces are different from those of any other joint in the body in that the hyaline articular cartilage of the sacrum faces the fibrocartilage surface of the ilium. The joint has a corrugated design, with ridges and depressions; that is, it is a self-locking mechanism, like a keystone of an arch.

▥ **Function:** The main movements of the SIJ are a forward tilting of the sacrum called *nutation* and a backward tilting called *counternutation*. The main movement of the iliac bones is also anterior and posterior rotation. The symphysis pubis has a superior and an inferior translatory movement. Stability comes from the close-fitting joint surfaces, the muscles, the ligaments, and the fascia that cross the joint.

▥ **Dysfunction and injury:** The SIJ is a common source of LBP as a result of trauma such as a fall on the buttock, repetitive stresses such as weight-bearing imbalances due to a leg-length difference, and mechanical irritation due to loss of normal movement.

  ☐ Subluxation or fixation of the SIJ, in which the undulating ridges and depressions are no longer complementary (subluxation) and/or the normal movement of the SIJ is decreased (fixation), is a common dysfunction. This loss of normal motion may be due to ligamentous shortening, muscular hypertonicity, and roughened articular surfaces leading to articular adhesions.

  ☐ Pain from SIJ dysfunction or injury can be sharp, dull, or aching and typically refers to the buttock, groin, posterior thigh, and occasionally below the knee.

▥ **Treatment implications:** Because the SIJ is stabilized with the muscles that attach to the pelvis and sacrum, assessment should consider the length, strength, and movement patterns of the major muscles of the SIJ. Since the SIJ is a synovial joint with lubricated surfaces with some movement, part of our intention is to mobilize the SIJ in posterior-anterior (P–A) glide to help restore motion and rehydrate the cartilage surfaces. Increased deposition of fiber along the SI joint line often requires transverse friction massage.

LUMBOSACRAL SPINE LIGAMENTS

▥ **Description:** In addition to the dynamic stability provided by the musculature, a "continuous ligamentous stocking" wraps around the bones and interweaves with the superficial and deep fascia, as well as the muscles, providing essential passive stability to the lumbopelvic region.[8]

▥ **Structure:**
  ☐ **Anterior longitudinal ligament:** The anterior longitudinal ligament (ALL) is a dense band that runs along the anterior and lateral surfaces of the vertebral bodies and discs from the second cervical vertebra to the sacrum. The ALL serves as an attachment for the crura of the diaphragm and resists extension.

  ☐ **Posterior longitudinal ligament:** The posterior longitudinal ligament (PLL) runs within the vertebral canal along the posterior surfaces of the vertebral bodies from the second cervical vertebra to the sacrum. The PLL resists flexion.

  ☐ **Neural arch ligaments:** The ligamentum flavum, interspinous ligament, supraspinous ligament, and intertransverse ligament compose the neural arch ligaments. The ligamentum flavum attaches to the lamina of each vertebra and reinforces the wall of the vertebral canal posterior to the intervertebral foramen (IVF). The interspinous ligament is continuous with the ligamentum flavum, which is a continuation of the joint capsule, which is continuous with the supraspinous ligament, which is attached to the thoracolumbar fascia.

  ☐ **Sacrotuberous ligament:** The sacrotuberous ligament is a triangular structure that extends from the posterior iliac spine, the SIJ capsule, and the coccygeal vertebrae to the ischial tuberosity. The biceps femoris, multifidus, and thoracolumbar fascia all interweave with this ligament.

  ☐ **Sacrospinous ligament:** The sacrospinous ligament arises from the lateral margin of the sacral and coccygeal vertebrae and the inferior aspect of the SIJ capsule and attaches to the ischial spine.

  ☐ **Short and long dorsal (posterior) sacroiliac ligaments:** These sacroiliac ligaments are a complex array of multilevel, multidirectional ligaments. The long dorsal SIJ ligament travels under the sacrotuberous ligament, from the posterior superior iliac spine (PSIS) to the lateral sacral crest. This ligament resists counternutation.

  ☐ **Iliolumbar ligament:** The iliolumbar ligament arises from the transverse processes of L4–L5 and attaches to the iliac crest and adjacent region of the iliac tuberosity.

  ☐ **Inguinal ligament:** The inguinal ligament is formed by the inferior margin of the aponeurosis of the external abdominal oblique. It arises at the anterior superior iliac spine (ASIS) and inserts into the pubic tubercle.

▥ **Function:**
  ☐ The ligaments of the lumbosacral region provide passive stability to the spine and pelvis. These ligaments and fascia serve as attachment sites to the major muscles of the spine.

  ☐ The ligaments and joint capsules have a neurosensory role. They have nociceptors and proprioceptors that play an important role in initiating reflex activity in the musculature, providing instantaneous information to the muscles regarding position and movement of the joint.[2]

■ **Dysfunction and injury:**
  ☐ Ligament injury decreases mechanoreceptor and proprioceptive functions, leading to reflexive muscle hypertonicity and weakness, altered movement patterns, altered coordination and balance, and instability.[9]
  ☐ Ligament injury can also lead either to laxity and consequent joint instability or to shortening and thickening of the ligaments that lead to stiffness in the joint. Both outcomes alter joint mechanics and neurologic function.

■ **Treatment implications:** Treatment of injured ligaments consists of four primary intentions:
  1. Rehydrate the tissue through cycles of compression and decompression while performing the wave mobilization strokes.
  2. Reestablish normal neurologic communication between the muscle and the ligament with muscle energy technique (MET).
  3. Release adhesions with transverse massage and MET. As the fascia of the myotendon unit is attached to the ligaments, muscle contraction mobilizes the ligaments, helping to reduce adhesions.
  4. Exercise the ligament. If the ligaments have become weakened or have a diminished capacity to signal the muscle regarding movement information, exercise rehabilitation is the most effective therapy. In addition to strength training, balance and coordination exercises are essential.

THORACOLUMBAR FASCIA

■ **Definition:** The **thoracolumbar fascia (TLF)** is a sheet of dense connective tissue that covers the muscles of the back of the trunk.

■ **Structure:** The TLF is divided into posterior, middle, and anterior layers.
  ☐ The posterior layer is located under the skin and subcutaneous fat and begins as a continuation of the aponeurosis of the latissimus dorsi. It is thick and fibrous and is attached to the lumbar spinous processes and the supraspinous ligament and surrounds the erector spinae and multifidus. The TLF continues to the sacrum and ilium and blends with the fascia of the gluteus maximus (G. max.).
  ☐ The middle layer attaches to the transverse processes and intertransverse ligaments of the lumbar vertebrae and blends with the anterior layer.

■ The anterior layer surrounds the quadratus lumborum and attaches laterally to the transverse abdominus and the internal oblique.

■ **Function:** The TLF plays an important role in lumbosacral function because it can be dynamically engaged through the muscles that attach to it. The latissimus dorsi, G. max., transverse abdominus, and internal oblique tighten the TLF and stabilize the lumbosacral spine when they contract.

■ **Dysfunction:** In the client who has chronic LBP, the fascia typically palpates as thickened and lacks resilience. Theoretically, this thickening and lack of resilience are caused by the laying down of excessive collagen resulting from sustained hypertonicity in the latissimus dorsi and the pushing force on the fascia resulting from broadening of the erector spinae muscles when they contract. The TLF forms a container or septa for the muscles within it, and these muscles are designed to slide relative to this container. Fibrosis constricts these normal gliding characteristics.

■ **Treatment implications:** Because the fascia is often thickened from sustained muscle contraction, MET and soft tissue mobilization (STM) are used to reduce the hypertonicity in the muscles contained within the fascia, to lengthen the fascia, and to dissolve the adhesions between the muscles and the fascia.

MUSCLES OF THE LUMBOSACRAL SPINE

■ **Structure:** The muscles of the trunk can be divided into posterior, anterior, and lateral muscles. The muscles of the back, or posterior region, can be divided into seven fascial layers (see Table 3-2) and two groups: the superficial (extrinsic) group, which affect the movement of the trunk, arm, and respiration, and the deep (intrinsic) group, which move the trunk, maintain posture, and stabilize the spine.

■ Superficial back muscles: trapezius, latissimus dorsi, levator scapula, rhomboids, serratus posterior superior and inferior, and splenius capitus and cervicus.

■ Deep back muscles can be further divided into three groups: erector spinae group (sacrospinalis), including the iliocostalis, longissimus and spinalis; the transversospinalis group, including the semispinalis, multifidus, and rotatores; the deepest layer, consisting of the interspinalis and intertransversarii. Bogduk and Twomey[10] have further divided the erector spinae into a superficial or costal portion and a deep or vertebral portion. The deep portion is not described in most texts but can be palpated by experienced therapists. It consists of lumbar fibers of the iliocostalis and longissimus (see Fig. 3-52 later in the chapter).

■ The anterior muscles include the flexors of the lumbosacral spine, which include the abdominals and the iliopsoas. The abdominals consist of four muscles: the rectus abdominus, internal oblique, external oblique, and transverse abdominus.

▓ The lateral muscle of the lumbosacral spine is the quadratus lumborum. It is a lateral flexor and significant stabilizer of the spine.

▓ **Function:** The muscles of the lumbar region provide dynamic stabilization to the spine. Stabilizing muscles may be divided into two groups: dynamic, phasic muscles and postural, tonic muscles. The first group includes large, movement-producing muscles. These include the rectus abdominus, the external oblique, and the thoracic portions of the longissimus and iliocostalis. The postural, tonic muscles connect directly to the lumbar vertebrae and provide segmental stability. They include the multifidus, the psoas, the quadratus lumborum, the lumbar portions of the longissimus and iliocostalis, the diaphragm, and the internal oblique and transverse abdominus.[11] The deep intrinsic muscles of the transversospinalis group have a very high concentration of muscle spindles. They function as proprioceptors, allowing the spine to make precise adjustments to movement and position. Co-contraction of the deep abdominals and multifidi is now the foundation of exercise rehabilitation of the low back. Muscles are not only the engines of voluntary and involuntary movement in the body, but they also act to elongate the spine.[12] It is important to remember that muscle strength, not our bones, holds us upright. Strong muscles decompress the spine and help us to stand tall. Muscles also unconsciously (reflexively) communicate with all of the other structures of the body, including the skin, nervous system, and connective tissue, including the ligaments and joint capsules. Muscles express our emotions and reflect our comfort or distress. It is important to remember that muscles of the hip region, including the gluteals, tensor fascia lata, rectus femoris, and hamstrings, all have a profound influence on lumbosacral function.

▓ **Dysfunction:** Muscle contraction is often a primary source of lumbosacral dysfunction and pain.[5] In LBP or dysfunction, it is typical for the erector spinae to be held in a sustained contraction. Hypertonicity limits movement in the joints, creating an inhibition of the normal gliding of the facets, known as a fixation. This stimulates the joint mechanoreceptors, which have neurologic reflexes to the surrounding muscles. Some muscles increase their tension, such as the erector spinae, and others become inhibited, such as the multifidi. The multifidi are especially important in LBP, as the fibers interweave with the joint capsule. Sustained contraction adds a compressive load to the joint, and weakness de-

creases the stability of the lower back. Both of these conditions accelerate the degeneration process.

Jull and Janda[13] have discovered predictable patterns of muscle imbalance. These imbalances alter movement patterns and therefore add a continuing stress to the joint system. Hypertonicity is also a major source of pain. It is critical to understand these muscle imbalances because they may be a dominant factor in the cause of musculoskeletal pain and a major factor in the continuance of the pain. In the lumbopelvic region, Jull and Janda[13] call this muscle imbalance **lower (pelvic) crossed syndrome,** because the tight iliopsoas and erector spinae and the weak abdominals and G. max. form a cross (Fig. 3-7).

LOWER (PELVIC) CROSSED SYNDROME: MUSCLE IMBALANCES OF THE LUMBOSACRAL REGION

▓ **Muscles that tend to be tight and short:** The iliopsoas, the lumbar portion of erector spinae, the piriformis, the rectus femoris, the tensor fascia lata (TFL), the quadratus lumborum (QL), the adductors, and the hamstrings are examples of tight, short muscles. (Although the lumbar erectors are usually tight and short, they often test weak. A muscle is weak in its shortened position, and sustained contraction weakens a muscle.)

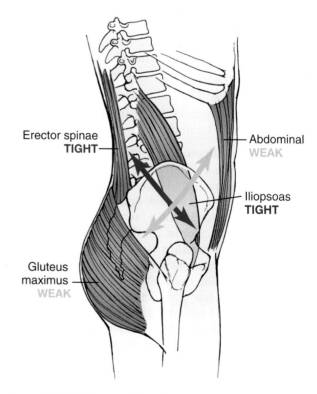

Figure 3-7. Pelvic crossed syndrome.

- **Muscles that tend to be inhibited and weak:** The G. max., medius, and minimus and the abdominals are examples of inhibited, weak muscles.

Postural Signs of the Lower Crossed Syndrome

- Lumbar hyperlordosis caused by short erector spinae.

- Anterior pelvic tilt and protruding abdomen caused by weak G. max. and abdominals and tight iliopsoas.

- Hypertonic muscles at thoracolumbar junction resulting from compensation for a hypermobile lumbosacral junction.

- Foot turned outward because of a tight piriformis.

Positional Dysfunction of the Lumbosacral Muscles

- The erector spinae roll into a medial torsion (toward the midline). Most people with LBP assume some flexion, that is, they bend forward slightly, to decompress the spine. Because the erector spinae muscles attach toward the midline, as the person tilts forward, the erectors are pulled into a medial torsion.

- The iliopsoas rolls into a medial torsion. One cause of this is the effect of gravity on the human body. In dysfunction or after an injury, we "collapse into gravity." The trunk tilts forward, the arms internally rotate, the arches collapse, and the iliopsoas rolls medially, creating an internal or medial torsion to the iliopsoas.

- Gluteals and external rotators of the hip tend to roll into an inferior torsion.

- **Treatment implications:** Clinically, it is essential to release the hypertonicity in a muscle and lengthen a shortened muscle and its connective tissue before trying to strengthen a weak or inhibited muscle. As described by Sherrington's law of reciprocal inhibition (RI), a tight agonist inhibits its antagonist. For example, a tight iliopsoas inhibits the G. max. Sometimes the muscle is weak because of this neurologic inhibition, and strength can be reestablished within a few contract-relax (CR) METs. If the muscle does not respond after a few sessions, then refer the client to a chiropractic or osteopathic doctor for assessment of joint fixation, which is the next most likely cause of muscle weakness. A muscle may also be atrophied, in which case the client would be referred to a physical therapist or personal trainer.

- Use MET to help your client reestablish normal movement patterns through precise, controlled muscle contractions. If a muscle is weak, then other muscles will substitute for that muscle's action. For example, in hip abduction, if the G. medius is weak, the TFL will substitute. This creates an internal rotation of the hip with abduction, which is a dysfunctional pattern.

- Manually reestablish the normal position and length of the muscles by releasing their abnormal torsion. For example, reposition the psoas medial to lateral, and reposition the G. max. and piriformis inferior to superior.

Relationship of Muscles to Lumbosacral Balance

See Table 3-1.

Table 3-1	Relationship of Muscles to Lumbopelvic Balance

Muscles that Increase the Lumbar Curve and Create an Anterior Pelvic Tilt

- Tight/short iliopsoas
- Tight/short sartorius, rectus femoris, and TFL
- Tight/short adductors: pectineus, adductor brevis, longus, magnus (anterior part), gracilis
- Tight/short thoracic fibers of longissimus (bowstring effect)
- Weak abdominals, weak or inhibited gluteals, especially gluteus maximus

Muscles that Decrease the Lumbar Curve

- Tight/short gluteus maximus and posterior portion of the adductor magnus
- Tight/short hamstrings
- Tight/short abdominals
- Weak erector spinae muscles

Muscles that Cause a Lateral Pelvic Tilt (Pelvic Obliquity)

- A lateral pelvic tilt typically is caused by tight adductors and weak/inhibited hip abductors, a tight quadratus lumborum (QL), tight tensor fascia lata (TFL) and tight iliotibial band (ITB)
- Adductor hypertonicity can cause a high ilium on the side of contracture, an apparent short leg, and an abduction of the opposite hip
- Abductor hypertonicity can cause a low ilium on the side of contracture, an apparent long leg, and adduction of the opposite hip
- A tight TFL and ITB tilt the pelvis down on that side
- Gluteus medius weakness causes the pelvis to be high on the corresponding side
- QL and lateral abdominal contracture elevates the ilium on the high side

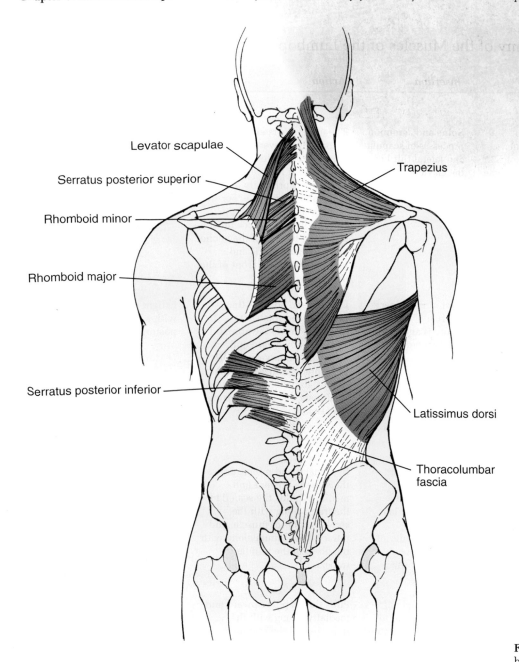

Levator scapulae

Serratus posterior superior

Rhomboid minor

Rhomboid major

Serratus posterior inferior

Trapezius

Latissimus dorsi

Thoracolumbar fascia

Figure 3-8. Superficial layer of back muscles.

ANATOMY OF THE MUSCLES OF THE LUMBOSACRAL REGION: THE SEVEN LAYERS OF THE BACK

The back muscles can be divided into seven layers (Fig. 3-8). See Table 3-2.

MUSCULAR ACTIONS OF THE TRUNK

The trunk is capable of seven different movements: flexion, extension, lateral flexion to the right and left, rotation to the right and left, and circumduction. Flexion opens the lumbar facets, and extension

closes the facets, taking the spine into its close-packed position.

The extent of motion in the nonacute spine is determined by many factors, including the tightness of the muscles, the extensibility of the ligaments, the elasticity of the articular capsule, and the fluidity and elasticity of the disc. If a client is experiencing pain, muscular guarding and swelling will also limit movement.

▨ Flexion
  ☐ Rectus abdominus: compresses the abdomen.
  ☐ External abdominal oblique: causes lateral flexion to the same side and rotation to the opposite side.

Table 3-2	Anatomy of the Muscles of the Lumbopelvic Region			
Muscle	*Origin*	*Insertion*	*Action*	*Dysfunction*
First Layer				
Trapezius	Medial one-third of superior nuchal line, spinous processes of C7 and all thoracic vertebrae	Spine and acromion processes of scapula and lateral third of the clavicle	The upper fibers elevate the scapula, the lower fibers depress it, and the middle fibers retract the scapula. The trapezius is primarily a muscle of the shoulder girdle. For the scapula to be elevated, the anterior head and neck must be stabilized by way of the anchor of the longus capitis and longus colli on the front of the neck	The upper fibers are tight and short, whereas the lower fibers are weak and long, allowing the scapula to migrate headward, decreasing its stability for movement of the arm.
Latissimus dorsi	Spinous processes of lower six thoracic vertebrae, spinous processes of all lumbar and sacral vertebrae, crest of ilium, and lower three ribs	Crest of the lesser tubercle of the humerus and floor of intertubercular groove	Extends and adducts the humerus and rotates it medially, draws the arm and shoulder downward and backward, interweaves with the thoracolumbar fascia, and has a stabilizing effect on the lumbosacral spine by tensing the fascia.	Is tight and short, especially with a rounded-shoulders posture.
Second Layer				
Rhomboid minor	Spinous processes of C7 and T1	Vertebral border of the scapula, superior to the spine of scapula	Both major and minor: draws the scapula upward and medially, holds the scapula to the trunk along with the serratus anterior muscle, and retracts the scapula along with the fibers of the middle trapezius.	Rhomboids are weak, which contributes to a rounded-shoulder posture.
Rhomboid minor	Spinous processes of T2–T5	Vertebral border of the scapula below the spine of the scapula		
Levator scapula	Posterior tubercles of the transverse processes of C1–C4. Significant attachment site as four major muscles blend into each other at this point: splenius cervicis, posterior scalene, longissimus capitis, and levator scapula	Superior angle of the scapula and to the base of the spine of the scapula	Pulls the scapula upward and medially (along with the trapezius); if the scapula is fixed, pulls the neck laterally; acts similar to the deep fibers of the erector spinae (see below) to prevent forward shear caused by cervical lordosis.	Levator eccentrically contracts in the head-forward posture.
Third Layer (see Fig. 3-9)				
Serratus posterior superior	Spinous processes of C7, T1, and T2	Second to fifth ribs	Elevates the second to fifth ribs	Serratus tends to be weak, demonstrated by winging of the scapula.
Serratus posterior inferior	Spinous processes of T11 and T12 and L1 and L2	Lower four ribs: T9–T12	Draws the lower four ribs downward and backward	

Table 3-2	Anatomy of the Muscles of the Lumbopelvic Region (*Continued*)			
Muscle	**Origin**	**Insertion**	**Action**	**Dysfunction**

Fourth Layer (*see Fig. 3-9*)

Muscle	Origin	Insertion	Action	Dysfunction
Splenius capitis	A large, flat muscle from the spinous processes of C3–C7 and T1–T3	Lateral third of the superior nuchal line and the mastoid process of the temporal bone	Muscles of both sides acting together extend the head and neck; one side acting alone rotates the head to the same side. Accentuates the cervical lordosis.	Both muscles tend to be short and tight, which hyperextends the cervical spine, compressing the joints.
Splenius cervicis	A large, flat muscle from the spinous processes of T4–T6	Posterior tubercles of transverse processes of the upper three cervical vertebrae (C1–C3)	Muscles of both sides acting together extend the head and neck; muscle of one side rotates the neck and the head to the same side. Accentuates the cervical lordosis.	

Fifth Layer: Erector Spinae (*see Fig. 3-9*)

Bogduk and Twomey[10] describes a deep and superficial layer to the iliocostalis and longissimus muscles.

Iliocostalis (Lateral Column): Ilium to Ribs

Muscle	Origin	Insertion	Action	Dysfunction
Lumbar fibers of iliocostalis (deep layer of iliocostalis)	Lumbar component consists of four to five overlying fascicles; attaches on iliac crest just lateral to the PSIS	Lateral aspect of the lumbar transverse processes L1–L4	Contracting unilaterally, acts as lateral flexors of the lumbar vertebrae. Acting bilaterally, extends the spine. The deep fibers help to stabilize the lumbar vertebrae to the pelvis and, along with the psoas act as guy wires in the A–P plane. These fibers also decrease the lumbar curve, which is the opposite action as the psoas.	The erector spinae tend to be tight and weak. The position of dysfunction is for the fibers to roll into a medial torsion. This is due to the tendency of the spine to seek flexion when it is injured or with forward-head posture. As the attachments of the erectors merge toward the sacral base, dysfunction and injury will cause the fascicles to roll toward the midline.
Thoracic fibers of iliocostalis (superficial layer of iliocostalis)	By a tendinous sheet of fascia referred to as the erector spinae aponeurosis to the PSIS, the dorsal surface of sacrum, the posterior sacroiliac ligament, and the sacrospinous ligament	Angle of ribs T12–T4	As it does not attach to lumbar vertebrae, acting bilaterally can have a bowstring effect, causing increased lumbar lordosis. Unilaterally, they can laterally flex thoracic cage. They contract eccentrically when the trunk flexes forward. Through concentric contraction, they extend the spine; isometrically, they control the position of the rib cage relative to the pelvis.[2]	
Iliocostalis cervicis	Angles of ribs 3–6	Posterior tubercles of the transverse processes of C4–C6	Acting bilaterally, extends the spine; unilaterally, causes lateral flexion	

(continued)

Table 3-2   Anatomy of the Muscles of the Lumbopelvic Region (*Continued*)

Muscle	Origin	Insertion	Action	Dysfunction
Fifth Layer: Erector Spinae (*continued*)				
Longissimus (Intermediate Column): Sacrum to Transverse Process				
Lumbar fibers of longissimus (deep layer)	Composed of five fascicles, each attaching to the anterior-to-medial aspect of the PSIS, L5 fascicle is most medial	Transverse processes of all lumbar vertebrae	Same as lumbar fibers of iliocostalis described above.	
Thoracic component of longissimus (superficial layer)	Attaches to a broad tendinous sheet called the erector spinae aponeurosis, which attaches to the entire length of the medial sacral crest and the lateral sacral crest, where it blends with the sacrotuberus and dorsal sacroiliac ligaments	Divided into two parts: the medial insertions reach the tips of the transverse processes of all thoracic vertebrae T1–T12, and the lateral insertions reach the ribs at the inferior margin, between the tubercle and the inferior angle	Same as thoracic fibers of iliocostalis described above.	
Longissimus cervicis	Lies under the splenius capitis, lateral to the semispinalis group and attaches to the t.p.s of upper four to six thoracic vertebrae (T1–T6)	Posterior tubercle of the transverse processes of C2–C6		
Longissimus capitis	Transverse and articular processes of lower four cervical vertebrae	Posterior margin of mastoid process deep to the sternocleidomastoid (SCM) and splenius capitis	Acts as a significant stabilizer of the cervical spine along with the SCM and the posterior scalene. These muscles act as guy wires in three planes.[2] The longissimus capitis and cervicis also laterally flex and rotate the spine and head to the same side.	
Spinalis (Central Column): Spinous Process to Spinous Process				
Spinalis thoracis	Spinous processes of T11 and T12 and of L1 and L2	Spinous processes of T1–T10		
Spinalis cervicis (not always present)	Spinous process of C7	Spinous process of C2		
Spinalis capitis (usually fused with semispinalis capitis)	C7 through T3 transverse processes	Attaches with the semispinalis capitis between the superior and inferior nuchal lines of the occipital bone	Erector spinae muscles of both sides acting together extend the vertebral column and assist in maintaining erect posture; muscles on one side acting alone bend the vertebral column to the same side.	

Table 3-2	Anatomy of the Muscles of the Lumbopelvic Region (*Continued*)

Muscle	Origin	Insertion	Action	Dysfunction
Sixth Layer: Transversospinalis Muscles (see Fig. 3-10)				
The transversospinalis muscles consist of two groups that run from the transverse process to the spinous process.				
Rotatores	Vertebral transverse processes	Base of the spinous process of the first or second vertebra above	Rotatores are highly innervated with muscle spindles and act to sense movement between the vertebrae.	Weakness (inhibition) of the rotatores leads to balance disturbances and instability.
Multifidus	Largest and most medial of the lumbar back muscles; from the posterior sacrum, the aponeurosis of the erector spinae, the medial surface of the PSIS, and the posterior sacroiliac ligaments; and the sacrotuberous ligament	To the spinous process of L1 to L5; fibers also attach to joint capsule of lumbar facets and protect the capsule	Stabilizes the lumbar spine; helps to control flexion and the shear force in the lower lumbar spine in forward flexion. Counters the action of the psoas.[2] Rotatores and multifidi, when acting bilaterally, extend the vertebral column; when acting unilaterally, they bend the vertebral column to the same side and rotate the vertebrae to the opposite side. Multifidi protect the joint capsule from being caught between the joint surfaces.[10]	Mutlifidus is typically in a sustained contraction with an acute injury. This compresses the facets, adding to continuing pain. In the chronic state, the multifidi typically become weak, leading to instability.
Semispinalis group: Muscles run from transverse process to spinous process of the fourth to sixth vertebrae above.				
Semispinalis capitis (largest muscle in the back of the neck)	C7 through T6 transverse processes and C4 through C7 articular processes	Covered by the trapezius and splenius capitis in the cervical region, it inserts between the superior and the inferior nuchal lines of the occipital bone	Extension of the cervical spine and head; increases cervical lordosis. Helps to maintain the upright posture of the head.	Semispinalis capitus can entrap the greater occipital nerve, which travels though it, leading to pain and burning sensation on the occiput.
Semispinalis cervicis	Transverse processes of T1–T6	Spinous processes of C2–C5	Has a significant attachment to the spinous process of C2 and an important stabilizing effect on C2. Palpation: The semispinalis cervicis and capitis palpate as a rounded muscle bundle lateral to the cervical spinous processes. The trapezius and splenius muscles are flat by comparison.	
Semispinalis thoracis	Transverse processes of T6–T12	Spinous processes of T1–T6	Semispinalis group, when acting bilaterally, extends the vertebral column, especially the cervical vertebrae and head, and rotates the head backward; when acting unilaterally, draws the head to the opposite side.	

(continued)

Table 3-2 Anatomy of the Muscles of the Lumbopelvic Region (*Continued*)

Muscle	Origin	Insertion	Action	Dysfunction
Seventh Layer				
Interspinales	Spinous processes of each vertebra	Adjacent spinous processes		
Intertransve-rsarii	Vertebral transverse processes	Adjacent transverse processes	It has been suggested that these muscles may contribute to proprioceptive input.[2]	
Gluteal Region (*see Fig. 3-11*)				
Gluteus maximus	Arises from posterior line of ilium, posterior aspect of the sacrum, coccyx, and sacrotuberous ligament	Ends in a thick tendinous lamina, passes lateral to the greater trochanter, and attaches to the iliotibial tract of the fascia lata; deeper fibers of the lower part attach to the gluteal tuberosity of the femur between the vastus lateralis and the adductor magnus	Extensor and powerful lateral rotator of thigh. Inferior fibers assist in adduction; upper fibers are abductors. Balances trunk on femur, balances knee joint by means of the ITB, and is associated with bringing the trunk upright.	Gluteus maximus is typically weak, inhibited by sustained contraction on the hip flexors, especially the iliopsoas, causing overuse of the hamstrings. Because of this weakness, hip extension may be initiated by the hamstrings, causing a dysfunctional gait pattern.
Gluteus medius	Broad, thick muscle arises from the outer surface of the ilium, between the anterior and the posterior gluteal lines, and the external aspect of ilium	Converges to a strong, flat tendon that is attached to the superior aspect of the lateral surface of the greater trochanter	Principal muscle of abduction. Anterior fibers medially rotate and may assist in flexion; posterior fibers laterally rotate and may assist in extension of hip.	If weak, leads to lateral pelvic tilt; pelvis is high on the side of weakness; if contracted, the pelvis is low on side of contracture.
Gluteus minimus	Deep to the gluteus medius, smallest of three gluteals. Fan-shaped origin arises from outer surface of ilium between ASIS and greater sciatic notch	Attached to a ridge in the lateral surface of the anterior-superior portion of the greater trochanter and the hip joint capsule	Acting with the gluteus medius, abducts the hip; the anterior fibers of the minimus rotate the hip medially. Both may also act as flexors of hip.	Tightness causes abduction and medial rotation of the thigh. In standing, there will be a lateral pelvic tilt, low on the side of shortness, accompanied by medial rotation of the femur.
Deep Lateral Rotators of the Hip				
Piriformis	Anterior surface of the sacrum among and lateral to sacral foramina one to four; margin of greater sciatic foramen and pelvic surface of sacrotuberous ligament	Passes out of the pelvis through the greater sciatic foramen and attaches by a rounded tendon to the superior-posterior border of greater trochanter; often blended with common tendon of obturator internus and gemelli	Laterally rotates the extended thigh; abducts the hip when hip is flexed.	Sustained contraction in the piriformis may compress the sciatic nerve as it emerges through the sciatic notch, eliciting an ache, numbing, or tingling down the posterior thigh.

Table 3-2	Anatomy of the Muscles of the Lumbopelvic Region (*Continued*)			
Muscle	**Origin**	**Insertion**	**Action**	**Dysfunction**
Deep Lateral Rotators of the Hip (continued)				
Quadratus femoris	Proximal part of the lateral border of the tuberosity of ischium	Attaches to the posterior femur, extending down the intertrochanteric crest	Laterally rotates and adducts the hip.	
Obturator internus	Internal or pelvic surface of the obturator membrane and margin of the obturator foramen, the inferior ramus of the pubis and ischium	Travels from its origin toward the lesser sciatic foramen, making a right-angled bend over the surface of the ischium between the spine and the tuberosity; blends with the two gemelli, forming the "triceps coxae," inserting on the medial superior surface of the posterior greater trochanter	The strongest lateral rotator of the hip with the gluteus maximus and the quadratus femoris. It acts as an abductor in the flexed position.	Lauren Berry, RPT, theorized that the obturator internus rolls into an inferior torsion with low back dysfunction, and this torsion could create a pulling force on the loose irregular connective tissue suspending the sciatic nerve, creating sciatica.
Gemellus superior	External surface of the spine of the ischium	Attaches with obturator internus on the medial surface of the greater trochanter	The two gemelli assist the obturator internus	
Gemellus inferior	Upper part of the tuberosity of the ischium, below the groove for obturator internus	Attaches with the obturator internus (as above)	.	
Obturator externus	Flat, triangular muscle covering the external surface of the anterior pelvic wall, arising from bone around the obturator foramen	Trochanteric fossa of the femur	Lateral rotation of the hip and assists in adduction	
Lateral Pelvic Region (see Fig. 3-6)				
Quadratus lumborum (QL)	Internal lip of the iliac crest and the iliolumbar ligament; QL has fibers oriented in three directions	Anterior surfaces of L1–L4 transverse processes and twelfth rib	Concentric contraction causes lateral flexion of the trunk to the same side; eccentric contraction controls the rate of lateral bending to the opposite side; isometrically, act as guy wires to help stabilize the lumbar spine.[2]	A short QL will elevate the ilium. A weak QL will lead to lumbar instability.

(continued)

Table 3-2	Anatomy of the Muscles of the Lumbopelvic Region (*Continued*)			
Muscle	**Origin**	**Insertion**	**Action**	**Dysfunction**
Anterior Pelvic Region				
Psoas major and minor	Divided into a superficial and a deep part: the deep part arises from the transverse processes, L1–L5 and the superficial part from the intervertebral discs of T12–L5 and the vertebral bodies T12–L5; lumbar plexus of nerves travels between the two parts and is susceptible to entrapment; psoas minor is an inconstant muscle from T12–L1 and inserts on the iliopubic eminence	Travels with the iliacus over the lateral pubic ramus to insert onto the lesser trochanter of the femur	Because the psoas and the iliacus have the same insertion point and the same action, they are often described as one muscle, the iliopsoas; however, they are two distinct muscles. They are the main flexors of the hip; they also laterally rotate the hip; with the extremity fixed, the psoas flexes the trunk; unilateral contraction causes rotation of trunk to the opposite side. Acts to stabilize the lumbar spine on the pelvis and as an anterior guy wire to balance the effect of the deep erectors.	Shortens, often owing to extensive sitting. This causes an increased lordosis, an anteriorly rotated pelvis, and an increased compressive load to the lumbar facets.
Iliacus	Upper margin of iliac fossa and the inner lip of the iliac crest	Lesser trochanter	Has the same action as the psoas; they are the main flexors of the hip; also laterally rotates the hip; with the extremity fixed, the iliacus flexes the trunk; unilateral contraction causes rotation of the trunk to the opposite side. A sustained contraction causes an anterior torsion of the ilium, bringing the ASIS forward and down, and an extension of the lumbar facets, causing increased compression.[2]	
Abdominal Muscles				
Rectus abdominus	Pubic crest and symphysis of pubic bone	Fifth to seventh cartilage of rib cage and xiphoid process	Flexes the vertebral column; pulls the sternum toward the pubis (antagonist of erector spinae); tenses the abdominal wall; all the abdominal muscles act to stabilize the trunk. They also eccentrically and isometrically contract to prevent excessive rotation and lateral flexion in the trunk.[2]	The rectus and external oblique act as postural stabilizers, and weakness decreases lumbar stability.
External oblique	Largest and most superficial of the abdominals, it attaches by fleshy digitations from the lower eight ribs, interdigitating with the serratus anterior	Attaches on the external lip of the iliac crest; on the inguinal ligament and the outer layer of the rectus sheath	Both sides acting together flex the vertebral column, rotate the trunk to the opposite side, and resist anterior torsion of the ilium.	

Table 3-2	Anatomy of the Muscles of the Lumbopelvic Region (*Continued*)			
Muscle	*Origin*	*Insertion*	*Action*	*Dysfunction*
Abdominal Muscles (continued)				
Internal oblique	Intermediate lip of iliac crest; thoracolumbar fascia; lateral two-thirds of the inguinal ligament	Attaches on fleshy digitations to the lower three ribs (9–12); the linea alba and aponeurosis help in formation of rectus sheath; also attaches with the transverse abdominus to the thoracolumbar fascia	Same as for external oblique, except rotates toward same side, and bends the body laterally; also stabilizes the spine through the thoracolumbar fascia.	Weakness of the internal oblique and transverse abdominus decreases lumbar stability. The abdominal muscles are weak in a client with LBP, which causes an anterior pelvic tilt, increased lumbar lordosis, and a rounded-shoulder posture. Weak abdominals decrease the stability of the lumbopelvic region. They are often inhibited by tight extensors. Strengthening the abdominals decreases tension in the erector spinae, decreases the lumbar curve, and increases the stability of the lumbopelvic region. Shortness in the abdominals depresses the chest and contributes to thoracic kyphosis.
Transverse abdominus	Costal—deep surfaces of costal cartilages of lower six ribs Vertebral—the thoracolumbar fascia from the t.p.s of the lumbar vertebrae Pelvic—internal lip of iliac crest, lateral third of inguinal ligament	Aponeurosis helps form the rectus sheath; attaches to the xiphoid process and pubic crest	Flattens the abdominal wall. Fibers run horizontally around the abdomen.	

- ☐ Internal abdominal oblique: causes lateral flexion and rotation to the same side.
- ☐ Psoas major: flexes and rotates the hip laterally.

■ Extension

Extension occurs mostly in the lumbar region of the spine.
- ☐ Erector spinae (sacrospinalis), including the iliocostalis, longissimus, and spinalis: extend, rotate, and laterally flex the trunk on the side of the trunk to which they are attached.
- ☐ Semispinalis thoracis: acts bilaterally to extend the trunk or acts unilaterally, laterally flexing the trunk and rotating it to the opposite side.
- ☐ Multifidus: acts bilaterally to extend the trunk and neck or acts unilaterally, laterally flexing and rotating the trunk and the neck to the opposite side.
- ☐ Quadratus lumborum: causes lateral flexion.

■ Lateral Flexion

Practically all trunk flexor and extensor muscles contribute to lateral flexion.
- ☐ External and internal abdominal oblique
- ☐ Quadratus lumborum

■ Rotation
- ☐ External and internal abdominal oblique
- ☐ Erector spinae
- ☐ Semispinalis thoracis
- ☐ Multifidus
- ☐ Rotatores

■ Circumduction

Circumduction results from a sequential combination of flexion, lateral flexion, hyperextension, and lateral flexion to the opposite side.

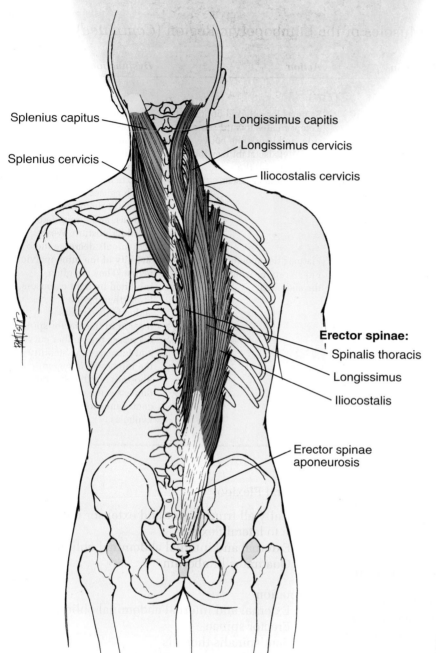

Splenius capitus

Splenius cervicis

Longissimus capitis

Longissimus cervicis

Iliocostalis cervicis

Erector spinae:

Spinalis thoracis

Longissimus

Iliocostalis

Erector spinae
aponeurosis

Figure 3-9. Third, fourth, and fifth layers of back muscles.

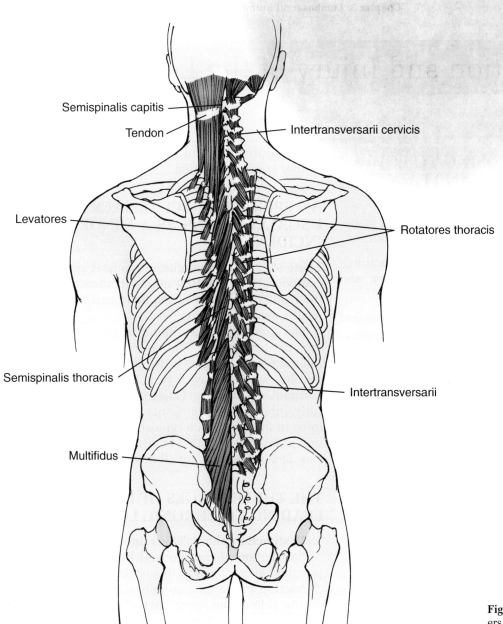

Semispinalis capitis

Tendon

Intertransversarii cervicis

Levatores

Rotatores thoracis

Semispinalis thoracis

Intertransversarii

Multifidus

Figure 3-10. Sixth and seventh layers of back muscles include the transversospinalis group.

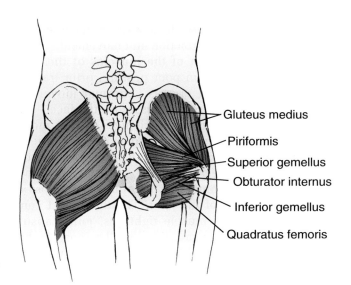

Gluteus medius

Piriformis

Superior gemellus

Obturator internus

Inferior gemellus

Quadratus femoris

Figure 3-11. Gluteal muscles and deep rotators of the hip.

Dysfunction and Injury of the Lower Back

FACTORS PREDISPOSING TO LOW BACK DYSFUNCTION AND PAIN

- **Lifestyle factors:** Sitting at a desk excessively, manual labor, excessive driving, obesity, lack of exercise.
- **Functional factors:** Posture, joint dysfunction, muscle imbalances, deconditioning, fatigue, altered movement patterns, emotional tension.
- **Structural factors:** Rheumatologic, endocrine or metabolic, neoplastic (tumors), vascular diseases, infection, congenital anomalies, pelvic and abdominal disorders.

PATHOGENESIS OF LOW BACK PAIN

The cause of LBP is controversial. A rational hypothesis, described by Kirkaldy-Willis and Bernard,[5] is outlined below.

THREE MOST COMMON FACTORS PREDISPOSING A PERSON TO AN EPISODE OF LOW BACK PAIN

1. **Emotional upset,** such as tension, stress, anxiety, fear, resentment, uncertainty, and depression. Emotional upset causes local areas of vasoconstriction and sustained muscle contraction that lead to muscle fatigue. These changes result in altered patterns of muscle contraction and movement.
2. **Abnormal function of the muscles** of the lumbopelvic girdle from poor posture, prior trauma, or deconditioning creates abnormal movement patterns and excessive stresses on the facets and disc. The result of these changes is that movement becomes restricted and painful. These restrictions of movement lead to fibrosis around the joint.
3. **Facet joint hypomobility (fixation)** is the loss of normal gliding of the joint. The three most common causes are muscle tightness, joint capsule adhesions, and intra-articular adhesions. As has been mentioned, this hypomobility has reflexive changes in the surrounding muscles, setting up a continuing cycle of muscle dysfunction and further joint dysfunction.

AN EPISODE OF ACUTE BACK PAIN USUALLY BEGINS AS A MINOR INCIDENT

These stresses on the musculoskeletal system can be compensated for until a minor incident overwhelms the resilient capacity of the body and tissue damage results, leading to acute pain.

The client reports a minor incident, such as gardening or reaching for a light object, and experiences an intense pain in the low back. The symptoms may also develop within a day or two. There are two different mechanisms of injury: (1) a rotational strain that typically injures the facet joints and (2) a compression force in flexion, which typically injures the disc. It is important to realize that in any given injury, the muscles, facets, and disc are all involved to some degree.

THE THREE STAGES OF DEGENERATION LEADING TO CHRONIC LOW BACK PAIN

1. **Dysfunction phase:** This minor trauma leads to inflammation of the synovial lining of the capsule, called synovitis, and to sustained hypertonic contraction in the erector spinae muscles, usually on one side of the lower back. The inflammation releases enzymes that cause minimal degeneration of the articular cartilage. Changes in the disc begin in the dysfunction phase with small circumferential tears in the annulus that become larger and form a radial tear that passes from the annulus to the nucleus. These tears increase until there is internal disc disruption, which can lead to a disc herniation in which the nucleus shifts position.
2. **Instability phase:** The dysfunction phase is often followed by a phase of instability, which is demonstrated by abnormal, increased movement of the facets. There is laxity in the joint capsule and the annulus of the disc and subluxation (partial dislocation) of the facets.
3. **Stable phase:** The last phase of pathogenesis is the stable phase, in which the body responds to the continuing degeneration by laying down connective tissue and bone. Continuing degeneration leads to bony spurs under the periosteum, enlargements of the inferior and superior facets, periarticular

fibrosis, and loss of motion. With further degeneration, the normal disc height is reduced, owing to the loss of proteoglycans and water.

DIFFERENTIATION OF LOW BACK PAIN

LBP can be caused by primary problems due to dysfunction, injury, or degeneration of the musculoskeletal system in the low back or from secondary problems. These secondary problems are diverse but may be categorized as follows:

- Visceral diseases such as kidney stones or endometriosis

- Vascular diseases such as aneurysms

- Tumors, especially cancer that has metastasized from another site

- Stress-related disorders, such as adrenal exhaustion

TYPICAL PATTERNS OF SYMPTOMS

The vast majority of LBP is caused by a mechanical disorder, that is, a problem of function and not pathology. The precise cause of mechanical LBP can be difficult to determine. Sometimes it is a case of a frank injury, but more often, there is an underlying hypomobility of the facets of the lumbar spine or SIJ, chronic muscle imbalance, poor posture, or emotional stress. Assuming that the client's pain is caused by a mechanical disorder, there are three broad categories of symptoms in the low back:

- Tight, stiff: an acute presentation of these symptoms implicates a muscle strain; chronic stiffness is typically a degenerated disc and joint.

- Ache: an acute, mild to moderate ache can be muscle, ligament, or joint strain/sprain complex; a severe ache implicates the disc.

- Sharp: a sharp pain in the low back indicates a joint involvement. It can be a mild irritation, moderate inflammation, or severe damage to the cartilage and associated soft tissue.

THERE ARE TWO TYPES OF PAIN THAT REFER INTO THE LEGS FROM THE LOW BACK

There are two fundamental types of pain that refer into the leg(s): sclerotomal and radicular. The two types are differentiated by the quality of pain. These two types of referral are important to distinguish, because it helps you to differentiate a simple mechanical disorder from a serious condition, such as a herniated disc.

- **Sclerotomal pain,** the first type of referred pain, is caused by an injury to the paraspinal muscle, ligament, facet joint capsule, disc, or dura mater and can manifest locally and be referred to an extremity. For example, pain from a muscle strain in the lumbar region may be felt as a pain in the thigh in addition to the lower back. Usually, the sclerotomal referred pain is described as *deep, aching, and diffuse.*

- **Radicular pain,** the second type of referred pain, is caused by an irritation of the spinal nerve root. If the sensory (dorsal) root is irritated, *sharp pain, numbing, or tingling that is well localized* in dermatomes occurs. If there is compression of the motor (ventral) nerve root, in addition to deep, boring pain, there may be a weakness in the muscles supplied by that nerve root (myotome) and a decrease in the response in the corresponding reflex. The most common cause of nerve root irritation is disc herniation. Nerve root pain is much more serious and requires an assessment by a chiropractor, osteopath, or orthopedist.

With these three types of low back symptoms and two categories of referral in mind, we can enumerate nine common types of LBP. Note that these are artificial categories and that an injury or dysfunction usually has several of these causes of pain at the same time. For example, with a simple overuse injury of the lower back, muscles, ligaments (including joint capsule), and joint dysfunction would all typically be involved. These categories should be used as a guide to help differentiate simple from more complex problems.

COMMON TYPES OF DYSFUNCTION AND INJURY TO THE LOWER BACK

MUSCLE STRAIN

- **Cause:** Strains may be categorized as an acute episode, such as a sport injury; a cumulative stress, such as standing at work all day; or an acute episode overlaying a chronic problem.

- **Symptoms:** Pain is usually described as diffuse and achy, either across the low back or on one side. Client reports being stiff and tight, especially with certain movements. Rest is relieving. An acute injury may present as a gripping spasm in the lower back that can be worse with active motion.

- **Signs:** Active motion localizes the area or line of pain. On palpation, muscles are tight and tender.

Passive motion is not painful, except with full muscle stretch.

- **Treatment:** The primary intention in treating **acute** injuries is to reduce pain, swelling, and muscle spasms. Perform the Level I series of strokes, beginning on the non-involved side. Gentle, rhythmic rocking of the body in the side-lying position is deeply relaxing. Perform RI or CR MET on the tight and tender muscles, interspersed with your massage strokes. For **chronic** conditions, the intention is to identify short, tight muscles; fibrous tissue; weak muscles; and hypomobile joints. Perform both Level I and Level II strokes. Perform CR MET for the lumbar erectors (MET #3), and postisometric relaxation (PIR) MET to the piriformis, quadratus lumborum, and iliopsoas as needed. Identify weak muscles, and perform CR MET to help recruit them. The wave mobilization strokes are now performed more deeply to dissolve adhesions, and the P–A mobilization of the spine is performed more deeply to increase the motion to the joints. Depending on the severity of the injury, an acute strain resolves in 1 to 4 weeks.

LIGAMENT SPRAIN (INCLUDING JOINT CAPSULE)

- **Cause:** The ligaments may be disrupted owing to an acute injury, such a lifting a heavy object, a cumulative stress such a repetitive twisting while gardening, or an acute episode overlaying a chronic problem.

- **Symptoms:** Pain is well localized and can be sharp in certain movements.

- **Signs:** Active and passive motion can be painful. Passive overstretch is typically painful. Resisted motion usually is not painful. We assess the ligaments by movement characteristics in response to wave mobilization strokes. Ligamentous thickening in the lumbosacral region is either localized or diffuse. Localized thickening feels like a dense, leathery resistance to movement as P–A mobilization is introduced in that specific area. Diffuse thickening, such as that present in degenerative arthritis, reveals this same dense, leathery resistance to motion but in a more diffuse area. We can palpate ligaments over the SIJ, and they feel thick and fibrous if they have shortened.

- **Treatment:** The first goal in treating an **acute** ligament injury is to reduce pain, inflammation, and muscle guarding as quickly as possible. Gentle rocking in the side-lying position induces relaxation in the muscles and central nervous system. Begin on the non-involved side. Perform CR and RI MET for the lumbar spine to reduce hypertonicity,

and then perform the Level I strokes. The P–A glide of the wave mobilization strokes will provide a gentle movement to the ligaments, promoting repair and preventing adhesions. The goal for **chronic** injuries is to reduce the adhesions in the ligaments, reduce protective muscle spasms, and promote normal joint motion. Perform Level I strokes to scan for areas of restriction and hypertonicity. Use CR MET to reduce excess tightness and PIR MET to lengthen shortened muscles. Perform Level II strokes, especially the third and fourth series for the multifidi and joint capsule. Identify areas of fibrosis, and perform back-and-forth and friction strokes on areas of fibrosis. Encourage the client to perform balance exercises to restore normal function to the mechanoreceptors in the ligaments. Ligaments often take 6 weeks to 1 year to heal.

FIXATION OR SUBLUXATION OF THE VERTEBRAL FACETS (FACET SYNDROME)

- **Cause:** A sudden onset of acute back pain is typically caused by a mechanical blocking of the facet joint. There are many theories to explain this phenomenon: subluxation (a partial dislocation), fixation (an adhesion of the articular surfaces of the joint), or an entrapped meniscoid, to name a few. Injury, poor posture, muscle imbalances, emotional or psychological tension leading to muscle hypertonicity, fatigue, and deconditioning all predispose to altered joint movement and potential fixation of the facets.

- **Symptoms:** Fixation or subluxation may be completely painless. Acute back pain may present as either a sudden or an insidious onset of well-localized unilateral or bilateral paravertebral pain. Pain may radiate to the groin, buttock, or thigh.

- **Signs:** Active extension may cause a "catch" or abrupt restriction in the area of the fixation. A decrease in lateral bending may occur, and flexion is cautious and limited. Hypertonicity and tenderness may be present in the paravertebral muscles. Motion palpation of the joint reveals loss of normal passive motion at the end range. SLR is normal.

- **Treatment:** Clients with **acute** LBP are most comfortable in the side-lying fetal position with a pillow between the knees. Begin the Level I series of strokes on the non-involved side, with gentle rocking to induce relaxation. Perform a scanning palpation of the gluteal and lumbar regions to assess areas of tenderness and spasticity. Perform CR and RI MET for the lumbar erectors and piriformis. Perform wave mobilization strokes with a slow rhythm and light pressure until a comfortable depth has been established. The P–A mobilization to the facets will help to reduce swelling, reduce hypertonicity, and induce normal mobility to the facets. Perform CR MET for subacute back pain (MET #3), if it is within client's comfort zone, to reduce hypertonicity at a deeper level. If your client does not show significant improvement after four treatments, refer the client to a chiropractor or osteopath to assess the need for spinal manipulation. **Chronic** fixations are hypomobile joints and the primary intention of the treatment is to mobilize the restricted segment. Identify hypomobility with motion palpation. Begin with Level I series of strokes, scanning the body for areas of hypertonicity, and use MET on those hypertonic muscles. Perform Level II strokes, especially the third and fourth series to release the multifidi and to mobilize capsular adhesions, which will allow for greater movement at the facets. When performing the wave mobilization strokes, sink deeply into the tissue within the patient's tolerance to induce deep P–A mobilization on the restricted segments.

SACROILIAC JOINT DYSFUNCTION AND INJURY

▨ **Cause:** SIJ dysfunction refers to either hypomobility or hypermobility of the joint. As with the facet joints, hypomobility may also be described as a fixation or subluxation, meaning that the joint is in a sustained misalignment. The SIJ may be injured by trauma, such as a fall on the buttock, or by repetitive twisting motion, such as in golf, gardening, or ballet. SIJ pain is also common after pregnancy. Predisposing factors for dysfunction are leg-length discrepancy, muscle imbalances, and sustained muscle tightness. Refer to the causes of joint fixation described above.

▨ **Symptoms:** Pain in the buttock, groin, and posterior thigh can be sharp, dull, or aching; occasionally, pain below the knee occurs.

▨ **Signs:** Unleveling of the pelvis measured at the PSISs or the ASISs, tenderness to palpation at the PSIS on one or both sides, positive Kemps test eliciting pain to the SIJ, and diminished passive mobilization in P–A glide at the SIJ.

▨ **Treatment:** The primary intention of treating **acute** SIJ pain is to reduce the pain and inflammation. Perform Level I strokes with emphasis on the piriformis, quadratus lumborum, erector spinae, and iliopsoas. Perform CR and RI MET for the lumbar erectors (METs #1 and #2). Refer to the treatment protocol for acute facet fixations described above for general guidelines in treating acute joint pain of

the spine. If your client does not show significant improvement after four treatments, refer the client to a chiropractor or osteopath to assess the need for spinal manipulation. **Chronic** SIJ dysfunction typically involves the entire pelvic girdle. Scan the region by performing Level I strokes to identify areas of hypertonicity and fibrosis. The short, tight muscles will typically include the piriformis, lumbar erectors, QL, iliopsoas, lumbar erectors, hamstrings, rectus femoris, and TFL. See Chapter 8: The Hip, p. 382, for METs for those muscles (METs #3, #5, and #10). Use MET for the erector spinae (MET #3) to release the fascia that inserts on the SIJ. Perform Level II strokes with emphasis on the sacrotuberous, iliolumbar, and posterior sacroiliac ligaments to dissolve fibrosis. Emphasize the P–A mobilization with the third and fifth series of Level II strokes to help rehydrate the joint.

PIRIFORMIS SYNDROME

▨ **Cause:** Piriformis syndrome is caused by a hypertonic piriformis muscle, often caused by excessive sitting, such as during a car trip or desk work; by SIJ dysfunction; or by overuse resulting from pelvic obliquity that leads to weakness of the G. medius of the ipsilateral side (the piriformis will overwork, trying to substitute as an abductor[1]). In approximately 10% of the population, the sciatic nerve travels through the piriformis muscle, which causes a predisposition to sciatica when the muscle is in a sustained contraction. In the other 90%, the sciatic nerve travels under the muscle and is vulnerable to a sciatic irritation if the muscle is short and tight.

▨ **Symptoms:** Pain occurs in the middle of the buttock, and an achy pain can radiate down the posterior thigh but rarely past the knee.

▨ **Signs:** Palpation reveals a tight and tender piriformis muscle; stretching the piriformis muscle by adducting the flexed hip over the supine client's extended leg increases buttock pain; straight leg raise (SLR) test with internal rotation can increase the pain, which is relieved when the hip is externally rotated.

▨ **Treatment:** For **acute** piriformis syndrome, perform CR and RI MET for the piriformis (MET #4) with light pressure to assess the degree of irritability. Repeat MET with increasing pressure to engage more of the muscle if technique remains within the client's comfort level. Perform Level I series with emphasis on the gluteal region. As you perform the strokes, palpate the tissues to assess for hypertonicity, and perform MET and wave mobilization as indicated. For **chronic** conditions, first reduce the hypertonicity with MET #4. Then perform PIR MET (MET #5) to lengthen the muscle. Also use MET to lengthen all the external rotators of the hip (see MET #4 in Chapter 8: The Hip, p. 384). Next perform deep STM on the piriformis, Level I third series, to reduce any adhesions and help to unwind the muscle. If you have identified that the G. medius is weak, perform MET to facilitate this muscle (MET #8 in Chapter 8).

COCCYDYNIA

▓ **Cause:** Many patients report falling on the buttocks or giving birth as the initial event. The ligaments of the coccyx are easily sprained, and increased muscle tension keeps the coccyx from returning to proper alignment. Often, articular and soft tissue changes such as coccygeal ligamentous fibrosis, spasm in the muscles of the pelvic floor, and subluxation of the sacrococcygeal joint occur. Pain may be referred from the lumbar spine, SIJ, or pelvic viscera.

▓ **Symptoms:** Clients may experience coccyx pain, especially when sitting. It rarely refers to another location.

▓ **Signs:** Indicators of coccydynia are pain at the coccyx when sitting and the presence of thick, fibrotic ligaments about the coccyx.

▓ **Treatment:** Coccydynia treatment necessitates the release of the ligaments of the sacrococcygeal joint and the balancing of the musculature of the pelvic region. Perform all of the Level I strokes, with emphasis on the second series, focusing on the ligaments attaching to the coccyx and sacrum. If your client does not respond to the soft tissue therapy, refer the client to a chiropractic or osteopathic doctor to assess the need for manipulation.

ARTHROSIS (ARTHRITIS): DEGENERATION OF VERTEBRAL FACETS

▓ **Cause:** Degeneration is by definition a chronic condition. Fibrosis of the joint capsule and loss of cartilage cause a loss of lubricant in the joint, leading to hypomobility and stiffness. Clients are often told that they have "arthritis," but the term typically describes a degeneration of the vertebral facets, correctly termed *arthrosis*. Degeneration is caused by previous injury to the facets, chronic fixation of the facets, sustained muscle tension, muscle imbalances that create altered movement patterns through the joint, poor posture, deconditioning, and obesity.

▓ **Symptoms:** Clients experience a dull, achy pain that is worse in the morning, better after moving around for several minutes, and worse again at the end of the day. Clients typically feel diffuse stiffness in the entire lower back.

▓ **Signs:** Chronic loss of lumbar extension with localized damage or a more complete loss of lumbar motion with diffuse changes in the affected joints is a sign of degeneration. Examination reveals a loss of passive motion ("joint play") at the involved facets.

▓ **Treatment:** The primary goal of treatment is to rehydrate the joints, lengthen capsular tissues, and reduce excessive tension in the multifidi muscles, which interweave with the joint capsules. Perform MET #3 to reduce lumbar hypertonicity and increase extensibility of the capsular tissues, and perform MET #9 in Chapter 4: Thoracic Spine for the transversospinalis group. Perform Level I strokes, concentrating on the sixth series, and the fourth series in Level II for the multifidi. Perform strong P–A mobilization with the strokes, mobilizing the facets to rehydrate the joints. As you perform the Level I strokes, identify areas of tightness, and perform MET as indicated. Clients who have degeneration need to move, such as brisk walking, and they need to stretch. Some discomfort accompanies increased movement, but it is a necessary discomfort to recover function in the joint. The general rule is that the client should be able to relax completely into the discomfort of moving the involved area.

SPONDYLOSIS (DISC DEGENERATION)

▓ **Cause:** Spondylosis has the same factors described above for arthrosis.

▓ **Symptoms:** Clients report stiffness and a diffuse, dull ache across the lower back and gluteal region, relieved by short periods of rest. Long periods of rest increase stiffness. Stiffness and pain are worse in the morning.

▓ **Signs:** Decreased range of motion (ROM), especially extension, is an indicator of spondylosis. Disc degeneration is clear on X-rays.

▓ **Treatment:** Disc degeneration and degeneration of the facets are intimately related, and the treatments for the two conditions are identical. Follow the protocol for arthrosis, described above. Disc and facet degeneration will often lead to lower (pelvic) crossed syndrome, described earlier in the chapter. As you perform the Level I and Level II strokes, identify areas of tightness by palpation and areas of weakness with MET. Release the tight muscles first, then use CR MET to help strengthen the weak muscles. A stretching program, such as yoga, is helpful. In addition, clients should walk briskly for 20 minutes or more per day. Traction on a slant board may be performed to promote fluid uptake in the disc.

DISC HERNIATION (DISC BULGE, PROTRUSION)

■ **Cause:** Disc herniation is most common in young adults, between 30 and 40 years old. It is probably a result of repetitive stresses and eventual tearing of the annulus fibrosis, especially in rotation and forward flexion. However, some authors such as Kirkaldy-Willis and Bernard[5] suggest that the condition may start as a dysfunction caused by muscle imbalance. A sedentary lifestyle and obesity are risk factors.

■ **Symptoms:** Disc protrusion causes a sharp, nagging, or gripping pain in the gluteal region and the middle of the lower back. With disc herniation, pain, numbing, or tingling refers into the legs with irritation of the nerve root. Even at rest, pain is still present. Sitting usually worsens the symptoms.

■ **Signs:** Often, the client presents to your office in slight forward flexion or in sustained lateral flexion (**antalgia**). All active motion is painfully limited.

Coughing, sneezing, and moving the bowels may increase pain. The client usually has a positive SLR and well-leg-raising test, sensory changes in specific dermatomes, or weakness in the legs.

■ **Treatment:** The goal of treatment is to reduce the pain and inflammation as quickly as possible. Place the client in side-lying fetal position, which is the position of greatest comfort for acute back pain. Perform RI and CR MET (METs #1 and #2) to reduce swelling and muscle spasms. Although reflex muscle guarding typically accompanies an acute disc problem, it is important to realize that the goal of treatment is to reduce *excessive* tension in the muscles. Deep release of the muscles is **contraindicated,** as it may destabilize the spine. Perform Level I strokes with a gentle, light pressure, and slow, small rocking motions. Palpate the muscles as you perform the strokes, and perform CR MET on the tight muscles, typically the QL, piriformis, and iliopsoas. As the client improves, deeper P–A mobilization may be applied with the wave mobilization strokes to restore normal passive motion to the facets. Work under the supervision of a doctor (chiropractic, osteopathic, or medical). Treatment should include strengthening, stabilizing, and proprioceptive reeducation.

Assessment

BACKGROUND

One of the primary intentions of lumbosacral assessment for the massage therapist is to differentiate an acute disc injury from injuries and dysfunctions to the muscles, ligaments, and joints. The details from your client's history regarding symptoms and onset will guide your examination. The physical exam will rule in or rule out an acute disc injury from other dysfunctions and injuries. This objective is accomplished primarily through active ROM and the SLR test. A herniated disc will severely limit lumbar ROM, have a positive SLR test, and manifest as leg pain greater than back pain. The second goal is to assess the passive motion of the intervertebral joints. The third goal is to assess the soft tissue through isometric testing and palpation. One clinical use of MET is to assess the muscles for pain and strength. Assessment through palpation is accomplished primarily through performing the strokes.

HISTORY QUESTIONS FOR CLIENTS WHO HAVE LOW BACK PAIN

Once you have ruled out the "red flags" (see Chapter 2, "Assessment and Technique") that may indicate a serious pathology and the need for an immediate referral to a doctor, you need to determine the level of distress in your client, that is, you need to know how bad the pain is. Questions such as "Did you sleep comfortably last night?" "Is the pain sharp or diffuse?" and "Do you have pain, numbing, or tingling in your legs?" will help you to determine (1) the appropriate depth of your massage strokes, (2) the appropriate amount of joint mobilization, (3) the strength of the pressure used in MET, (4) the necessity of referring your client to a doctor for further evaluation, and (5) the recommendations for follow-up treatments. Refer to the section "Subjective Examination: Taking a History" in Chapter 2: Assessment and Technique for more information.

DID YOU SLEEP COMFORTABLY LAST NIGHT?

Pain that occurs when a client rolls over in bed is usually benign and caused by a mechanical problem. Pain that has decreased after a night's sleep usually indicates a mechanical problem, that is, muscle, ligament, or joint injury or dysfunction. Pain that is constant, even at rest, is indicative of inflammation, such as a disc herniation, or a more serious pathology, such as a tumor, and needs referral to a doctor.

IS THE PAIN SHARP OR DIFFUSE?

A sharp pain in the lower back or SIJ area usually indicates a joint problem. A referral of sharp and gripping pain into the legs indicates a nerve root problem. Diffuse LBP can be muscle, ligament, or joint dysfunction or injury. Your active ROM assessment helps to differentiate these various conditions (see "Summary of Possible Findings of Active Range of Motion," p. 124).

DO YOU HAVE PAIN, NUMBING, OR TINGLING IN YOUR LEGS?

If the client answers yes, you need to perform the SLR test before you begin your massage (see p. 126). If the SLR test creates intense, sharp pain in the legs, it typically indicates a nerve root problem, and you need to refer your client to a doctor. If your client can lie on the table comfortably in the fetal position, you may perform gentle massage. The intention is to relax the client and not attempt to perform deep release of the muscles as that could be destabilizing. If the SLR creates a diffuse pain, numbing, or tingling in the legs, it is usually a sclerotomal pain (see "Differentiation of Low Back Pain" above), and STM is indicated. As has been mentioned, a constant, gripping pain in the legs needs an immediate referral, and massage on the lower back is contraindicated.

OBSERVATION: CLIENT STANDING

Note any redness or swelling of the skin that may indicate inflammation and the need for much lighter pressure in your strokes. Also, notice any scars that might indicate a previous serious injury or surgery.

Observe any asymmetry in your client's posture from the posterior and side views. A detailed postural assessment is for clients with chronic pain. If the client is experiencing acute pain, perform a postural assessment to determine if the sustained position, usually lateral bending (antalgia) or forward flexion, is a result of

muscle spasms. If these postures are associated with acute pain, it usually indicates a facet syndrome or a disc protrusion. Postural assessment for acute pain is brief.

POSTERIOR VIEW

▓ **Is the client listing to the side?** It might be a result of chronic muscle and joint imbalance. If the client cannot straighten because of the pain, it usually indicates a disc protrusion or muscle strain in the QL or the iliopsoas.

▓ **Is the spine vertical?**
  ☐ **Position:** Have your client stand in front of you.
  ☐ **Action:** Place your index and middle finger on either side of the C7 spinous process, and slowly move your fingers down the spine to L5.
  ☐ **Observation:** Does your client have a lateral curvature, called scoliosis, in the thoracic or lumbar spine? Lumbar scoliosis may be caused by sciatic neuritis, joint dysfunction, muscle spasm, irritation of the disc, or degenerative joint disease. (See Chapter 4 for further assessment of scoliosis.)

▓ **Are the iliac crests level?** (Fig. 3-12)
  ☐ **Action:** Place your fingertips on the iliac crests.
  ☐ **Observation:** If they are uneven, then make a note of the high side in your chart. Compare this

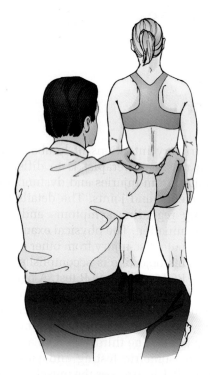

Figure 3-12. Assessment of iliac crests. To assess whether the iliac crests are level, place your fingertips on the top of the iliac crests.

finding with a seated assessment. If the iliac crests are uneven in standing and level sitting, there might be a leg-length difference or pronation in the ankle on the short side. If they remain uneven in standing and sitting, it indicates a muscle and joint dysfunction in the lumbopelvic region.

▨ **Is the head tilted to one side or balanced in the midline?**

▨ **Are the shoulder heights equal?** Place your index fingers horizontally under the inferior angles of the scapulae.

SIDE VIEW

▨ The earlobe should be in line with the upright acromion process. The most common dysfunction is forward-head posture.

▨ **Observe the lumbar curve from the side to see whether it is increased or decreased.**
  ☐ **Observation:** A neutral spine has a mild curve in the low back, midway between flat and lordotic.

▨ **Correct the client's standing posture.**

▨ **Action:** Adjust the lumbar spine so that the client has a mild curve in the low back. Next, bring the head back if necessary so that the opening of the ear is over an upright acromion.

MOTION ASSESSMENT

Start by asking your client whether any particular motion brings up the pain. Have your client perform that motion last. While the client performs the movements, note the ROM and whether the movement is painful. If it is painful, ask the client about the quality of the pain and its location.

FORWARD FLEXION

▨ **Position:** Have your client stand in front of you, feet placed shoulder width apart.

▨ **Action:** Ask the client to bend forward as far as is comfortable, with knees straight (Fig. 3-13).

▨ **Observation:** Flexion is a combination of hip, lumbar, and thoracic motion. The trunk should flex at least to 90°, that is, parallel to the floor. You can measure the distance from the fingertips to the floor. Observe the spine from the side. The lumbar curve should flatten in bending forward. If

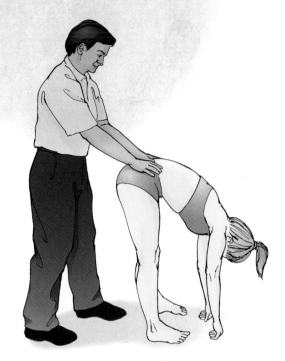

Figure 3-13. Assessment of active flexion. To assess active flexion in the lumbopelvic region, ask the client to bend forward as if she is going to touch her toes. Tell her to stop if it becomes painful. Have her bend her knees when coming back to standing.

the lumbar lordosis is maintained, it indicates erector spinae muscle spasms or hypomobility of the joints. Painless limitation is usually due to tight hamstrings. Diffuse soreness or pain in the lower back indicates an injury to the muscle, ligament, or joint. A sharp pain in the lower back indicates joint involvement. A dramatic limitation of motion indicates inflammation and swelling and a more serious injury, usually disc involvement.

EXTENSION

▨ **Position:** The therapist stands at the client's side and asks the client to stand with feet shoulder width apart and palms on the lower back (Fig. 3-14).

▨ **Action:** Have the client bend backward to a comfortable limit, keeping the knees straight.

▨ **Observation:** The ROM of lumbar extension is approximately 30°. Does the lumbar spine curve? Or is the client bending only at the hips? Active extension is the best test for joint dysfunction and injury, since extension compresses the facets. A sharp local pain in extension indicates a facet syndrome. With a facet syndrome, diffuse pain, numbing, or

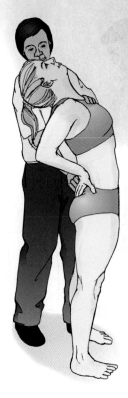

Figure 3-14. Assessment of extension. To assess extension, have the client place her hands on her lower back and bend backward to her comfortable limit.

tingling may refer into the gluteal region, thigh, and leg. A sharp, dermatomal pain in extension often indicates a nerve root problem, as extension also closes down the IVF slightly.

For clients who have chronic pain or dysfunction, a more accurate assessment of pure lumbar extension may be done with the client lying prone on the massage table, resting on his or her elbows, with the pelvis remaining on the table. Is there a round curve in the lumbar spine? If there is limitation of this motion, it indicates a chronic degenerative condition or hypomobility of the joints. A loss of motion and stiffness indicates muscle and connective tissue shortening, including ligaments.

SIDE FLEXION

▓ **Position:** The client stands with feet shoulder width apart and arms at the sides. The therapist stands behind the client and places both hands on the client's hips to stabilize the pelvis so that it does not sway or rotate (Fig. 3-15).

▓ **Action:** Ask the client to slide one hand down the side of his or her leg without rotating the trunk.

▓ **Observation:** The client should be able to slide his or her hand down equally on both sides, almost to knee

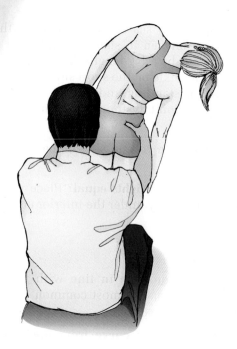

Figure 3-15. Assessment of lateral flexion. To assess lateral (side) flexion, stand behind your client and hold her pelvis to prevent any rotation or swaying. Ask her to slide her hand down the side of her leg to her comfortable limit.

level (approximately 30°). The lumbar spine should form a smooth curve in side bending. A sharp angle indicates hypomobility at the facet joints. Pain on the bending side indicates a joint problem because the facet is being compressed. Pain, stiffness, or tightness on the opposite side often indicates stiffness of the erectors and QL on the opposite side.

KEMPS TEST (QUADRANT TEST)

▓ **Intention:** To help differentiate narrowing of the IVF caused by degeneration or SIJ problems.

▓ **Position:** The client and therapist assume the same positions as in the side-bending test.

▓ **Action:** Have the client slide his or her hand down the back of the leg, one leg at a time, to a comfortable limit.

▓ **Observation:** Kemps test compresses the IVF and SIJ slightly and elicits referral of sharp pain into the leg with disc problems, diffuse referred pain with SIJ problems, or LBP with sacroiliac or lumbar joint dysfunctions and injuries (Fig. 3-16).

SUMMARY OF POSSIBLE FINDINGS OF ACTIVE RANGE OF MOTION

A dramatic limitation of the ROM is indicative of a facet syndrome, disc injury, severe DJD, or moderate

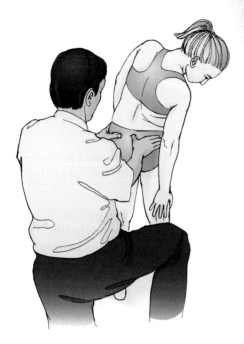

Figure 3-16. Kemps test. Kemps test is used to help differentiate sacroiliac problems and compression of a nerve caused by narrowing of the IVF. Have your client slide her hand down the back of her leg. This combines rotation and extension of the spine and compresses the IVF on the side of turning.

to severe strain or sprain of the musculoligamentous tissues. If the ROM is normal and the movement elicits diffuse LBP, then it is usually a muscle problem. If active motion is slightly decreased and the motion elicits a sharp back pain, then it often indicates a joint or ligament problem. If there is a generalized loss of all motions without pain, just stiffness, there is often a diffuse arthrosis or spondylosis in the lumbosacral spine. Diffuse loss of motion, joint stiffness, and referral of pain into the legs with extension and Kemps test may indicate foraminal encroachment, a degenerative condition in which the IVF is narrowed and the nerve root is compressed. This requires a referral to a chiropractic or osteopathic doctor.

BALANCE ASSESSMENT

- **Intention:** To assess the client with chronic LBP, which often leads to balance problems from instability and dysfunction of the proprioceptors.

- **Position:** Have your client stand next to the wall so that he or she can place a hand on the wall for support while performing this test if needed. The therapist stands facing the client.

- **Action:** Ask your client to lift one foot off the ground a few inches and attempt to balance on the other leg for 20 seconds. Repeat on the other side.

- **Observation:** Chronic LBP patients and geriatric patients often have problems with balance. If your client cannot balance comfortably on each leg, then have him or her do this as an exercise at home for 30 seconds to 1 minute on each leg, once a day.

SEATED ASSESSMENT

- **Place your thumbs under the PSISs to see whether they are level.** An unlevelling is called a pelvic obliquity. This may be a result of muscle spasms, DJD, sciatic neuritis, disc herniation, or joint fixation in the SIJs or lumbar spine.

- **Assess sitting posture.** Is the client's posture slumped? Correct a slumped posture by introducing a slight lumbar curve and placing the client's head so that the opening of the ear is over the upright acromion (see Fig. 5-12).

PALPATION

SCANNING EXAMINATION

- Most of the soft tissue palpation is done while performing the strokes. As you perform each stroke, feel for temperature, texture, tenderness, and tone.

- A scanning palpation is done in a few areas to rule out a serious lower back problem. Severe pain with medium pressure to the bone is a red flag for serious pathology. With the client seated, press with a medium amount of pressure on the following structures: the sacrum, the SIJs medial to both PSISs, each spinous process in the lumbar spine, and the paraspinal muscles.

MOTION PALPATION OF THE JOINTS AND PARASPINAL SOFT TISSUE

- **Intention:** Perform motion palpation to assess the condition of the soft tissue and joints of the lumbosacral region. The goal is to detect loss of joint play (hypomobility) in the intervertebral and SIJs and hypertonicity in the muscles. An experienced

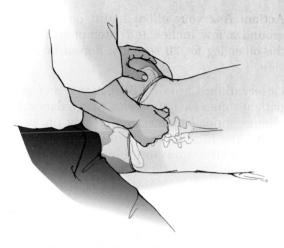

Figure 3-17. Palpation in the side-lying position. Assess the soft tissue and the motion of the spine.

practitioner can differentiate stiffness in the joints from tightness in the muscle.

- **Position:** Ask the client to lie in the fetal position, with a pillow between the knees. This is the most relaxed position for the soft tissue of the spine.

- **Action:** Begin by rocking the client gently. This rocking movement introduces a wave into the body and, like sonar, returns information to the therapist regarding the client's level of relaxation. A guarded, tense person feels rigid in response to this motion, and a relaxed, open person is pliable and resilient. Next, use the supported-thumb or soft fist position to perform a series of P–A wave mobilization strokes along the SIJ and the facets of the lumbar spine, which lie under the erector spinae (Fig. 3-17).

- **Palpation findings:**
  - ☐ A healthy lumbosacral spine is resilient and bends with your pressure. The movements are relaxing and completely pain-free.
  - ☐ Inflamed tissue is painful. The degree of pain indicates the level of inflammation.
  - ☐ Hypertonic muscles have a tight, springy resistance to movement.
  - ☐ Thickened soft tissue in the ligaments and capsule has a thick resistance to your movement.
  - ☐ A localized degeneration has a hard resistance to movement, whereas more diffuse degeneration has a similar hard resistance in a broader area.
  - ☐ A hypermobile spine has excessive, abnormal movement between the vertebrae. This is due to loose ligaments and deconditioned muscles. There are many causes, such as a prior injury that didn't heal properly owing to immobilization.

NERVE TENSION TEST

STRAIGHT-LEG-RAISING TEST

- **Intention:** Perform the SLR test if the client has pain radiating to the leg (Fig. 3-18). The test helps to differentiate a nerve root lesion from sclerotomal pain.

- **Position:** The client is supine. The therapist stands at the side of the table by the leg with the referred pain.

- **Action:** The therapist grasps the client's leg just proximal to the ankle and slowly lifts it up, keeping the knee straight, until there is pain or until an elevation of 70° is attained.

- **Observation:** The test is positive if lifting the leg increases or initiates leg pain, numbing, or tingling below the knee before 70° of elevation. Note the quality and location of the pain. Intense, sharp pain usually indicates nerve root tension, probably an injury to the disc. Pain that is only in the back indicates a ligament sprain or facet syndrome. A pulling discomfort behind the knee at about 70° is from a tight hamstring and is considered normal. If the client has a positive SLR test, perform the SLR test on the "good" leg. If this test elicits pain below the knee on the involved leg, it indicates a much more severe disc problem. If the SLR test is negative, that is, there was no aggravation of leg pain with elevation of the leg, and the client reports that he or she often has referral of diffuse pain into the leg, the client has sclerotomal pain coming from a joint, muscle, tendon, or ligament (see "Differentiation of Low Back Pain").

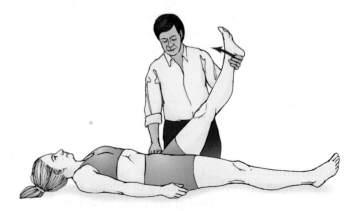

Figure 3-18. SLR test. The SLR test is performed if there is pain, numbing, or tingling into the leg. The therapist slowly lifts the client's leg off the table until there is pain in the leg or until there is tissue tension; this usually occurs at approximately 70°.

Techniques

GUIDELINES TO APPLYING TECHNIQUES

A thorough discussion of treatment guidelines can be found on p. 86 in Chapter 2: Assessment and Technique. In the method of treatment described in this text, we make two underlying assumptions: (1) that pain or dysfunction in one localized area affects the entire region, so we assess and treat an entire region rather than localized pain, and (2) that pain that localizes in one tissue affects all of the structures in the region. LBP, for example, typically involves muscles, tendons, ligaments, joints capsules, facet joints, and intervertebral discs. This is called, *somatic dysfunction*, a term developed by osteopaths that is defined as "impaired or altered function of related components of the somatic (body framework) system; skeletal, arthrodial (joint), and myofascial structures; and related vascular, lymphatic, and neural elements."[14] A simple muscle strain, for example, is not an isolated condition but affects the associated joints, nerves, and muscles that are compensating for the strain, as well as the vascular and lymphatic systems. The treatment described in this text addresses all the components of somatic dysfunction through three techniques: muscle energy technique (MET), soft tissue mobilization (STM), and joint mobilization (JM). These techniques can be applied to every type of back pain, but the "dose" of the technique varies greatly from slow movements and light pressures for acute conditions to stronger pressures and deeper-amplitude mobilizations for chronic problems. Each aspect of the treatment is also an assessment to determine pain, tenderness, hypertonicity, weakness, and hypomobility or hypermobility. We use the philosophy of treating what we find when we find it. Remember that the goal of treatment is to heal the body, mind, and emotions. Keep your hands soft, keep your touch nurturing, and only work within the comfortable limits of your client so that he or she can completely relax into the treatment.

THE INTENTIONS OF TREATMENT FOR ACUTE CONDITIONS ARE AS FOLLOWS

▓ To stimulate the movement of fluids to reduce edema, increase oxygenation and nutrition, and eliminate waste products.

▓ To maintain as much pain-free joint motion as possible to prevent adhesions and maintain the health of the cartilage, which is dependent on movement for its nutrition.

▓ To provide mechanical stimulation to help align healing fibers and stimulate cellular synthesis.

▓ To provide neurological input to minimize muscular inhibition and help to maintain proprioceptive function.

 CAUTION: *Stretching is* **contraindicated** *in acute conditions.*

THE INTENTIONS OF TREATMENT FOR CHRONIC CONDITIONS ARE AS FOLLOWS

▓ To dissolve adhesions and restore flexibility, length, and alignment to the myofascia.

▓ To dissolve fibrosis in the ligaments and capsular tissues surrounding the joints.

▓ To rehydrate the cartilage and restore mobility and range of motion to the joints.

▓ To eliminate hypertonicity in short, tight muscles; strengthen weakened muscles; and reestablish the normal firing pattern in dysfunctioning muscles.

▓ To restore neurological function by increasing sensory awareness and proprioception.

Clinical examples are described below under "Soft Tissue Mobilization."

MUSCLE ENERGY TECHNIQUE

THERAPEUTIC GOALS OF MUSCLE ENERGY TECHNIQUE

A thorough discussion of the clinical application of MET can be found on p. 76. The MET techniques described below are organized into one section for teaching purposes. In the clinical setting, the METs and STM techniques are interspersed throughout the session. METs are used for assessment and treatment. A healthy muscle or group of muscles is strong and pain-free when isometrically challenged. MET will be painful if there is ischemia or inflammation in the muscles or their associated joints. The muscle will be weak and painless if the muscle is inhibited or the nerve is compromised. During treatment, MET is used as needed. For example, when you find a tight and tender piriformis, use contract-relax (CR) MET to reduce the hypertonicity and tenderness. If the piriformis is painful while contracting, perform a reciprocal inhibition (RI) MET for the piriformis, which contracts the adductors, inducing a neurological relaxation to the piriformis. If the G. max. is weak and inhibited, first release the tight hip flexors, especially METs #6 and #8 for the iliopsoas and rectus femoris, and then use isotonic MET to recruit/strengthen the G. max.

MET is very effective for an acute, painful back, but the pressure that is applied must be very light, so as not to induce pain. Gentle, pain-free contraction and relaxation of the lumbar flexors and extensors and related muscles provide a pumping action to reduce swelling, promoting the flow of oxygen and nutrition and eliminating waste products.

THE BASIC THERAPEUTIC INTENTIONS OF MET FOR ACUTE CONDITIONS ARE AS FOLLOWS

- Provide a gentle pumping action to reduce pain and swelling, promote oxygenation of the tissue, and remove waste products.

- Reduce muscle spasms.

- Provide neurological input to mimimize muscular inhibition.

- Help to maintain as much pain-free joint motion as possible.

THE BASIC THERAPEUTIC INTENTIONS OF MET FOR CHRONIC CONDITIONS ARE

- Decrease excessive muscle tension

- Strengthen muscles.

- Lengthen connective tissue.

- Increase joint movement and increase lubrication to the joints.

- Restore neurological function.

The MET section below shows techniques that are used for most clients: two techniques (MET #1 and #2) for acute, painful conditions and one technique (MET #8) for chronic conditions only.

Remember that MET should not be painful. Mild discomfort as the client resists the pressure is normal if the area is irritated or inflamed. Refer to Chapter 8 for METs for the hip abductors, adductors, rectus femoris, hamstrings, TFL, and iliotibial band (ITB).

MUSCLE ENERGY TECHNIQUE FOR ACUTE LOW BACK PAIN

1. *Contract-Relax for the Lumbar Erector Spinae*

- **Intention:** We begin with the client in a side-lying position. This places the lumbar spine in flexion, which opens the facet joints, reducing lumbar pain. It is also the most relaxed position for the spinal muscles. An acute low back can be irritated if the facet joints are moved too much. A safe and effective way to decrease pain and edema and reduce muscle hypertonicity in the lumbosacral region is isometric contraction of the lumbar extensors. If this motion is painful, then begin with an RI MET, illustrated below.

- **Position:** The client is side-lying in the fetal position, with a pillow between the knees and hips flexed to 90°. To prevent trunk rotation, make sure the client lines up the top shoulder over the lower shoulder and the top hip over the lower hip. The therapist places one hand on the sacrum and one hand on the midthoracic region.

- **Action:** Instruct the client to resist as you press P–A on the spine for approximately 5 seconds. Cue the client by saying, "Don't let me move you." Press for 5 seconds, and then have the client relax. Remember, the client's body should not move as he or she resists your pressure. These are isometric contractions. I often alternate the CR and RI techniques several times, which reduces the hypertonicity in the lumbar erectors and decreases the pain in the lower back.

2. *Reciprocal Inhibition for the Lumbar Erector Spinae for Acute Back Pain*

- **Intention:** An acute low back may be irritated if the extensor muscles are contracted. A safe and effective way to reduce muscle hypertonicity in the lumbosacral region is isometric contraction of the flexors of the trunk, the iliopsoas. When the iliopsoas contracts, the lumbar extensors relax by means of reciprocal inhibition (Fig. 3-19).

- **Position:** The client is side-lying in the fetal position, with a pillow between the knees and hips flexed to 90°. The therapist places one hand on the anterior thigh just above the knee and the other hand on the lower back.

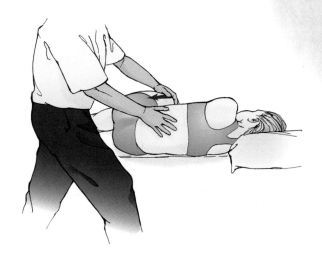

Figure 3-19. RI MET for the lumbar erector spinae. To perform RI on the extensors of the spine, have your client resist as you gently try to pull her thigh into extension.

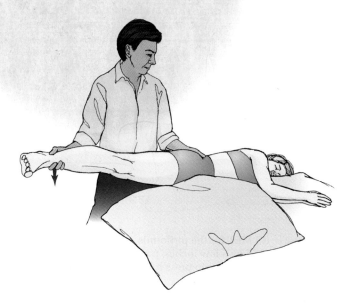

Figure 3-20. CR MET for the lumbar erector muscles in the subacute or chronic phases. To release hypertonicity in the extensors in the client who is not in acute pain, have her straighten her leg and gently lift it off the pillow. Have her resist as you lean your body into her leg, attempting to push it forward.

▨ **Action:** Have the client resist your attempt to lightly pull the thigh into extension, that is, toward the foot of the table. Cue the client by saying, "Don't let me move you." Hold for 5 seconds. Alternate the CR and RI techniques several times, which reduces the hypertonicity in the lumbar erectors and decreases the pain in the lower back.

▨ **Observation:** The lumbar spine should not arch during the RI. Place your hand on the client's back and have him or her keep the spine against your hand as the client resists.

MUSCLE ENERGY TECHNIQUE TO RELEASE HYPERTONIC MUSCLES OF THE LUMBOPELVIC REGION

3. *Contract-Relax Muscle Energy Technique for the Lumbar Erector Muscles in the Subacute or Chronic Phase*

▨ **Intention:** To reduce muscle hypertonicity by performing CR MET. Hip extension engages the lumbar erectors. If the erectors palpate as hypertonic, then CR MET is a safe and effective way to reduce their hypertonicity (Fig. 3-20).

▨ **Position:** The client is side-lying in the fetal position. Have the client straighten the top leg, making sure the knee is fully extended, and lift the leg off the pillow and into a few degrees of extension.

▨ **Action:** Instruct the client to resist as you attempt to press the client's extended leg forward for approximately 5 seconds. It is often helpful to tap lightly on the lumbar extensors to give a sensory cue to the muscles. You might say, "Feel these muscles working," as they contract. Have the client put the leg

back on the pillow and lie in the fetal position. Next, place your hand on the top of the client's thigh just above the knee, and have the client resist as you very lightly attempt to pull the thigh into extension, as was described in the section "Reciprocal Inhibition for the Lumbar Erector Spinae for Acute Back Pain." Repeat this cycle three to five times.

4. *Contract-Relax and Reciprocal Inhibition Muscle Energy Techniques for the Piriformis*

▨ **Intention:** To perform CR MET to release the hypertonicity of the piriformis. This technique is also used for problems with the hip.

▨ **Position:** The client is side-lying in the fetal position with a pillow between the knees.

▨ **Action:** Have the client lift his or her leg off the pillow and resist as you gently attempt to press the leg back down to the pillow for approximately 5 seconds (Fig. 3-21). To perform RI MET on the piriformis, have your client squeeze his or her knees together. This contracts the adductors and reciprocally inhibits the piriformis. You can give a sensory cue by lightly attempting to pull the client's knees apart.

5. *Postisometric Relaxation of the Piriformis*

▨ **Intention:** The intention is to lengthen the piriformis. The piriformis is typically short and tight,

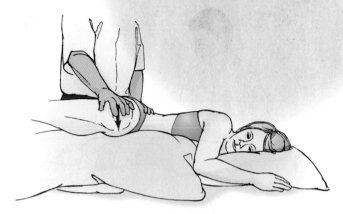

Figure 3-21. CR MET for the piriformis. Have your client lift her leg off the pillow a few inches, parallel to the floor, and resist as you gently attempt to press it back down to the pillow for approximately 5 seconds.

so it compresses not only the SIJ but also the sciatic nerve. PIR of the piriformis should be performed for chronic conditions only.

- **Position:** The client is supine. To lengthen the right piriformis, have the client cross the right leg over the left, placing the right foot on the table on the outside of the left knee (Fig. 3-22). You may stand on either side, facing the table (although I prefer to stand on the client's left side). Use your superior hand to hold the client's right ASIS to stabilize the pelvis, and place your left hand on the lateral aspect of the client's right distal thigh.

- **Action:** Have the client resist as you attempt to pull the leg across the body and push the knee toward the table for approximately 5 seconds. Relax, and as the client relaxes, pull the leg further across the body and press the knee further toward the table, until there is pain or you feel the resistance barrier. Repeat this CR–lengthen cycle several times.

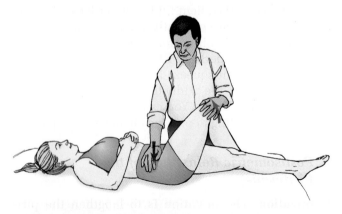

Figure 3-22. PIR of the piriformis.

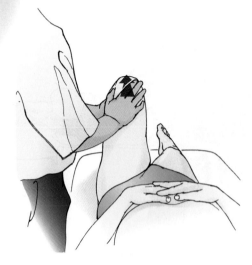

Figure 3-23. CR MET of the iliopsoas. The therapist stands in the 45° footward position and places both hands on the client's distal thigh. Have the client resist as you press gently in an inferior direction on the top of her thigh for approximately 5 seconds.

6. Contract-Relax Muscle Energy Technique for the Iliopsoas

- **Intention:** Use CR MET to reduce the hypertonicity of the iliopsoas.

- **Position:** Stand in the 45° footward position, and place both your hands on the client's distal thigh.

- **Action:** Have the client resist as you press gently in an inferior direction on the top of the thigh for approximately 5 seconds (Fig. 3-23).

7. Reciprocal Inhibition Muscle Energy Technique for the Iliopsoas

- **Intention:** To perform RI MET to reduce the pain and hypertonicity of the iliopsoas by contracting the hip extensors, antagonists of the iliopsoas.

- **Position:** Stand in a 45° headward direction, and place both your hands on the client's shin or posterior thigh.

- **Action:** Have your client resist as you press gently in a headward direction for approximately 5 seconds. This engages the hip extensors and reciprocally inhibits the iliopsoas, the main hip flexor (Fig. 3-24).

8. Length Assessment and Postisometric Relaxation for the Iliopsoas and the Rectus Femoris (Chronic only)

- **Intention:** To assess the length and to perform PIR for the iliopsoas and the rectus femoris (Fig. 3-25). The iliopsoas is a significant contributor to acute place the other hand on the flexed leg. Ask your client to tuck his or her chin, and then rock the client back onto the table, resting the head on a pillow. The right leg will hang over the edge of the table. The knee should be pulled to the chest just enough to keep the lower back flat on the table.

- **Observation:** If the length of the iliopsoas is normal, then the right thigh will be parallel to the floor or lower. If the length of the rectus is normal, the lower leg will be perpendicular to the floor. If the TFL is short, the leg will be abducted slightly.

- **Action:**
  - ☐ To lengthen the iliopsoas, perform PIR. Have the client resist as you press down on his or her right thigh. Press for 5 seconds, and after the client has relaxed for a few seconds, press down on the distal thigh to a new resistance barrier, stretching the iliopsoas and anterior hip joint capsule.
  - ☐ To lengthen the rectus femoris, have the client resist as you use your leg to press into the client's leg, attempting to press the leg into further flexion. Press for 5 seconds, have the client relax, then press again into a new resistance barrier.
  - ☐ Repeat the CR–lengthen cycle several times.

9. Contract-Relax and Postisometric Relaxation of the Quadratus Lumborum (QL)

- **Intention:** To lengthen the QL (Fig. 3-26). The QL is typically tight in chronic LBP, and performance of PIR is a safe and effective way to lengthen it.

- **Position:** The client is side-lying with the knees flexed into the fetal position for the first technique. In the PIR technique, maintain the side-lying position but with the top leg straightened and the bottom leg flexed. You might need to cue the client by asking him or her to hike the hip toward the shoulder to resist you as you pull the leg away from the pelvis. Explain that you want the client to use the muscles on the top of the hip (crest of the ilium) to lift the hip toward the shoulder, resisting your pull.

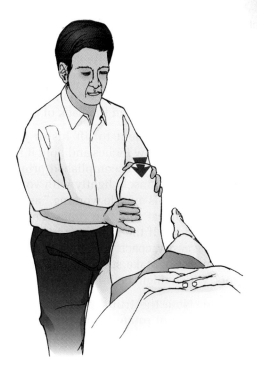

Figure 3-24. RI MET of the iliopsoas. Have your client resist as you press in a superior direction on her shin or posterior thigh.

and chronic LBP. A short iliopsoas increases the lumbar curve, compressing the facets and inhibits the normal function of the lumbar extensors through reciprocal inhibition (RI).

- **Position:** Instruct your client to sit on the end of the table, then to grasp the left leg and pull it to the chest. Support the client's head with one hand, and

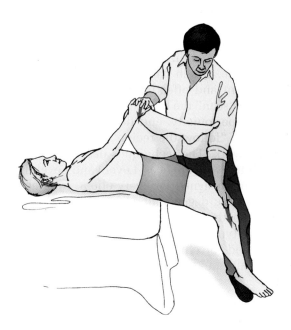

Figure 3-25. Length assessment and postisometric release of the iliopsoas lund rectus femoris.

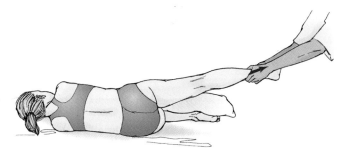

Figure 3-26. PIR of the QL.

■ **Action:**

☐ If the QL is painful or if you want to cue your client on how to how to fire the QL, perform a simple CR MET. First, flex the client's hips in the fetal position. Face footward, place your hands on the iliac crest, and ask client to resist as you gently push the ilium inferiorly (toward the foot of the table). Touch the QL and say, "Feel this muscle working." This technique is also a good way to train your client on how to "find" the QL and what action you are looking for in the next technique.

☐ Hold the client's leg above the ankle, and abduct the leg approximately 20° from the midline. Instruct the client to resist, saying, "Don't let me move you," as you pull the leg for approximately 5 seconds. Make sure the client's body is neutral and not rotated forward or backward. If the leg is too heavy or creates discomfort in this position, then place pillows under the top leg to support it, or tuck the leg under your armpit. After the client holds for 5 seconds, have him or her relax, and as the client relaxes, pull the leg and stretch the quadratus. Repeat the CR–lengthen cycle a few times. At the end of the PIR cycle, use RI to help "set" the QL in its new lengthened position. Place your fist on the heel of the client's straightened leg, and have the client resist as you push headward for approximately 5 seconds.

10. *Isotonic Muscle Energy Technique for the Gluteus Maximus*

■ **Intention:** Hip extension is accomplished primarily by the G. max. and hamstrings and secondarily by the erector spinae (Fig. 3-27). Weakness in the G. max. is common and may cause the hamstrings and lumbar

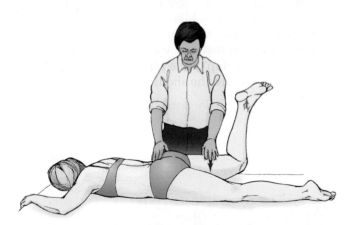

Figure 3-27. Isotonic MET for the gluteus maximus. With her knee flexed, have the client slowly lift her thigh off the table. It is important to perform the movement slowly to isolate the gluteus maximus.

erectors to initiate hip extension, which hyperextends the lumbar spine and compresses the facets. This MET helps to facilitate (strengthen) the G. max.

■ **Position:** Have the client lie face down on the table and bend one knee to 90°. Place one hand on the G. max. and the other hand on the back of the thigh.

■ **Action:** Instruct the client to lift his or her thigh slowly off the table a few inches and hold it for 5 seconds. This movement is accomplished primarily by the G. max. Tap the muscle lightly with your fingertips and say, "Feel this muscle working," as the client is contracting. Repeat this five times. Perform this MET on both sides. If the muscle is weak and does not strengthen easily, coach your patient in this MET as a home exercise. Make sure you have release the hip flexors, which might be inhibiting the G. max.

■ **Observation:** Note the trunk position. Make sure your client does not rotate his or her trunk to perform this motion.

SOFT TISSUE MOBILIZATION

BACKGROUND

A thorough discussion of the clinical application of STM can be found on p. 68. In the Hendrickson Method of therapy described in this text, the STM movements are called wave mobilization and are a combination of joint mobilization and STM performed in rhythmic oscillations with a frequency of 50–70 cycles per minute, except when performing brisk transverse friction massage strokes, which can be 2–4 cycles per second, or if a person is in extreme distress, when the rhythm might be slower than 50 cycles per minute. These mobilizations are presented in a specific sequence, which has been found to achieve the most efficient and effective results. This allows the therapist to "scan" the body to determine areas of tenderness, hypertonicity, and decreased mobility. It is important to "follow the recipe" until you have mastered this work. The techniques described below are divided into two sequences: Level I and Level II. Level I strokes are designed for every client, from acute injury to chronic degeneration, to enhance health and bring the body to optimum performance. Level II strokes are typically applied after Level I strokes and are designed for chronic conditions. Guidelines for treating acute and chronic conditions are listed below.

GUIDELINES FOR THE THERAPIST

■ **Acute:** The primary intention of treatment is to decrease pain and swelling as quickly as possible, maintain as much pain-free joint motion as possible, and induce relaxation. In this method of treatment, the soft tissue is compressed and decompressed in rhythmic cycles. This provides a pumping action, which helps to promote fluid exchange, reducing swelling. We perform the strokes for the lumbar spine in the side-lying position, which keeps the joints in their open position. This is the resting position for the spine and the most pain-free position. The strokes that are applied to the client who is in acute pain need to be performed with a very gentle touch, a very slow rhythm, and small amplitude. There is no uniform "dose" or depth of treatment. The depth of treatment is based on the client's level of pain. If the soft tissue does not begin to relax, return to gently rocking the body, and then use more METs to help reduce muscle guarding. As was mentioned previously, intersperse your STM work with MET. Remember that **stretching is contraindicated** in acute conditions.

▪ **Chronic:** The typical exam findings in clients with chronic back problems are short and tight erector spinae and iliopsoas and weakness in the gluteus maximus and abdominals (the lower crossed syndrome). The joints are typically hypomobile, with thick, fibrotic ligaments and capsular tissues. Some patients demonstrate the opposite: hypermobility in the joints, weak, deconditioned muscles, and atrophy in the ligaments and capsular tissues. This latter condition is described as *instability*. The primary goals of treatment depend on the patient. For patients who are hypomobile, the treatment goals are to reduce the hypertonicity of the muscles; promote mobility and extensibility in the connective tissue by dissolving the adhesions in the muscles, tendons, ligaments, and capsular tissues surrounding the joints; rehydrate the cartilage of the facet joints and discs; establish normal joint play and range of motion in the joints; and restore normal neurological function by stimulating the proprioceptors and reestablishing the normal firing patterns in the muscles. Patients who are unstable need exercise rehabilitation. Our treatments can support their stability by reducing tension in the tight muscles and performing MET to the weak muscles to help reestablish normal firing patterns and rehabilitate the proprioceptors. With chronic lumbar conditions, it is also important to treat tightness in the TFL and ITB, hamstrings, external rotators of the hip, rectus femoris, and gastrocnemius. With chronic conditions, we use stronger pressure on the soft tissue and more vigorous mobilizations on the joints. In the Level II sequence, we add deeper soft tissue work and work on attachment points, using transverse friction strokes if we find fibrosis (thickening). As was mentioned in the "Acute" section above, intersperse your soft tissue work with METs.

Clinical Example: Acute

Subjective: RA is a 42-year-old minister who presented with acute back pain on her right side, which occurred two days previously after she lifted one of her children. She described the pain as a deep ache with occasional sharp pain. She denied any referral of pain into the legs.

Objective: Examination revealed that lumbar flexion was limited to 50% of normal with an achy pain in the low back. Extension was 25% of normal and elicited a pain in the right L5–S1 region. SLR test was negative. Palpation revealed spastic and tender gluteal and lumbar muscles and a loss of passive glide at the L5 vertebra.

Assessment: Muscle strain with a loss of normal accessory glide (fixation) of the facet.

Treatment (Action): The treatment began with the patient in the side-lying position, painful side down, and a pillow between the knees. I began with slow, gentle rocking of the whole body to determine the level of guarding and pain and to induce a relaxation response. I began Level I wave mobilization strokes in the gluteal region slowly and gently, using very little pressure. The intention was to provide gentle movement to the soft tissue and joints, to reduce swelling, to promote cellular synthesis, and to realign the healing fibers. Palpation revealed that she was quite tight and tender in the piriformis. Very gentle CR and RI MET (#4) for the piriformis were performed several times. This reduced hypertonicity and provided a pumping action for the lymph and blood, reducing intramuscular edema and promoting reoxygenation of the tissue. The muscles were much less tender after three to four MET cycles. The treatment continued with the Level I series of strokes. The erector spinae were also hypertonic and tender. I used MET #3 to reduce the tension and pain. I performed the wave mobilization strokes over the lumbar and thoracic spine for several minutes. These movements create a P–A glide to the facet joints, which stimulates the normal fluid exchange to the cartilage and induces a general relaxation response. The muscles began to relax, and the movement of the spine became much more comfortable and resilient. The same treatment was applied to her other side. Next, with the patient supine, palpation revealed a very tender and tight iliopsoas (IP). A series of very gentle METs (#6 and #7) were used for the IP, followed by slow and gentle STM, including passive movement to the hip. The session ended with gentle work on her cervical spine. She reported feeling much better after the session. She was able to stand and move about the treatment room with much less discomfort.

Plan: I recommended weekly visits for four weeks. The same treatment described above was repeated. At the time of her last visit, she reported being pain free and was able to lift her children and perform her other daily activities without pain. Examination demonstrated full and pain free range of motion and normal motion in the soft tissue and joints. She was discharged from active care but elected to return in one month for wellness care.

Clinical Example: Chronic

Subjective: BM is a 74-year-old gardener who presented to my office complaining of chronic stiffness in the low back. He denied a prior injury but reported that his back has been stiff upon awakening for years and "goes out" a couple times a year, requiring him to stop work for a few days.

Objective: Examination revealed a significant loss of lumbar extension and significant loss of passive motion of the intervertebral joints. The soft tissue of the spine was thick and dense with very little resilience.

Assessment: Hypomobility of the lumbar spine with adhesions in the soft tissues.

Treatment: I attempted gentle rocking of his whole body in the side-lying position to induce a relaxation response and to determine the level of resilience in the spine. As I pressed him forward to induce the wave mobilization into his body, his body felt rigid and resistant to movement. I performed MET #1 several times. His body began to relax and allow the wave mobilization. I began the first series of Level I strokes and palpated thick, dense muscles in the gluteal region. I used MET #4 to induce relaxation into the region, had him lie supine, and performed a PIR MET for the piriformis to lengthen the tissue. I returned him to side-lying and began another series of strokes to the QL. The QL was thick and tight. I performed PIR MET for the quadratus (MET #9) to dissolve adhesions and lengthen the connective tissue.

The sixth series of strokes revealed hypertonic erector muscles along the lumbar and thoracic spine, with a thick, fibrotic feel, and a loss of P–A glide to the spine. The wave mobilization strokes were interspersed with MET #3 to help reduce the hypertonicity and rehydrate the tissue. I performed the strokes with deep pressure and a strong P–A component to help induce increased lubrication in the joints and greater joint play. Although there was mild discomfort to the mobilization, he said that the movements felt great. I ended the treatment with him supine and performed a series of METs and Level I cervical strokes. He was in a profound state of relaxation at the end of our session. Upon moving about the treatment room, he felt a sense of ease and fluidity that he had not felt in years.

Plan: I recommended a series of weekly visits for one month. I repeated the same basic treatment each visit. As I penetrated deeper into the tissue, I used shorter, more brisk transverse friction strokes on the multifidi, joint capsules, and iliolumbar ligaments (Level II, series 4 and 5). I also used MET #8 to lengthen the iliopsoas. The patient reported feeling less stiff in the mornings. Upon examination, there was a significant decrease in muscular tension, the tissue was more pliable and less fibrotic, there were better glide and greater range of motion to the facet joints, and active extension had improved and was pain free. I recommended another series of weekly visits for one month and a daily walking and stretching program.

Table 3-3	Essentials of Treatment

- Rock the client's body while performing the strokes
- Shift your weight while performing the strokes.
- Perform the strokes rhythmically, about 50 to 70 cycles per minute.
- Keep your hands and whole body relaxed.

Table 3-3 lists some essentials of treatment.

LEVEL I: LUMBOSACRAL

1. *Release of Gluteus Medius, Minimus, and Piriformis*

- **Anatomy:** Gluteal fascia; gluteus maximus, medius, and minimus; piriformis; and superior cluneal nerves (Fig. 3-28)

- **Dysfunction:** The G. medius is a strong abductor of the hip, and its dysfunction contributes to pelvic unleveling and LBP. Although the G. medius and minimus tend to be weak, they may also be hypertonic, known as *tightness weakness,* or weak because of reciprocal inhibition by hypertonic adductors. The piriformis is typically short and tight. Hypomobility and hypertonicity may cause the superior cluneal nerves to become entrapped in thickened, fibrous, gluteal fascia just below the crest of the ilium.

Position
- **Therapist Position (TP):** Standing, facing the line of the stroke
- **Client Position (CP):** Side-lying, in the fetal position, with a pillow under the head and between the knees, with the hands resting on each other in a "prayer position"

Strokes
This first series of strokes is how we begin all of the spinal sessions. In fact, in this method of therapy, most sessions begin with side-lying spinal work because it is profoundly relaxing and provides a foundation for all the extremity work. Begin your spinal sessions by placing both hands on the gluteal region and gently rocking the client's entire body with a rhythm of approximately one cycle per second. This rocking creates a wave in the client's body that is like sonar, reflecting the client's level of relaxation or guarding. It is also a way to make nurturing contact with the client and induce profound relaxation. Next, we scan the gluteal region to assess tenderness and hypertonicity. There are three basic lines, described below. Begin superficially with broad, scooping strokes, and proceed with deeper strokes as the area releases. Possible hand positions include double thumb, braced thumb using the pisiform of the opposite hand, and the fifth metacarpophalangeal area of a soft fist.

1. The first line of strokes begins midway between the greater trochanter and the iliac crest in the belly of

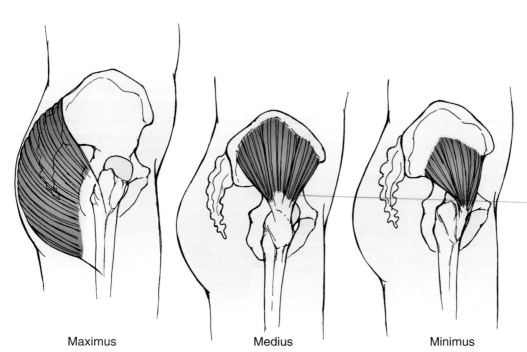

Maximus · Medius · Minimus

Figure 3-28. Gluteus maximus, medius, and minimus.

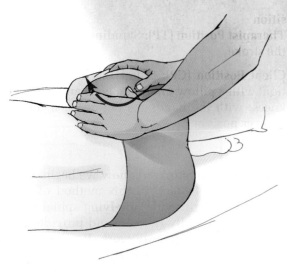

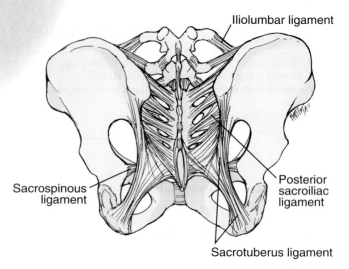

Figure 3-29. Double-thumb technique to release the gluteal fascia, cluneal nerves, and gluteus medius and minimus.

Figure 3-30. Sacrotuberous and sacrospinous ligaments.

the G. medius (Fig. 3-29). Perform a series of 1-inch scooping strokes, perpendicular to the line of the G. medius. Begin another series of strokes approximately 1 inch below your previous stroke, and continue this line of strokes to the piriformis, which travels between the PSIS and greater trochanter.

2. A second line of strokes begins approximately 1 to 3 inches from the greater trochanter at the myotendinous junctions of G. medius, G. minimus, and piriformis. Start at the superior aspect of this area, and work inferiorly in 1-inch scooping strokes around the greater trochanter.

3. The third line is along the superior portion of the iliac fossa to release the gluteal fascia, superior cluneal nerves, and superior portion of the G. medius and minimus. Begin at the most lateral-superior aspect of the ilium, using 1-inch scooping strokes, and move your hands more medially and inferiorly as you work down the iliac fossa.

2. *Release of Gluteus Maximus and Sacrotuberous Ligaments*

▧ **Anatomy:** G. max. and the sacrotuberous ligament. Work the G. max. superficially; work the sacrotuberous ligament and posterior aspect of the fascia lata deeply (Fig. 3-30).

▧ **Dysfunction:** In dysfunction, the G. max. is weak. In some cases, it may be hypertonic, especially with hypertonic hamstrings, and a loss of the lumbar curve might occur. The ligaments tend to develop fibrotic changes because of excessive tension caused by pelvic obliquity (unleveling), hyperlordosis, anterior pelvic tilt, or inflammation from trauma. Microscopically, the sacrotuberous ligament tends to develop an inferior torsion and needs

to be stroked superiorly. Fibrosis of the ligaments of the coccyx is a common cause of coccydynia (coccyx pain).

Position
▧ **TP:** Standing

▧ **CP:** Side-lying, fetal position, with the top part of the client's body angled diagonally forward on the table and the pelvic area at the back edge of the table, with the ischial tuberosity facing toward you

Strokes
1. Lift the G. max. muscle in short, scooping, 45° headward strokes from below the PSIS to the greater trochanter. Begin another series of strokes just below the first line, from the lateral portion of the sacrum and coccyx, and continue to the posterior surface of the femur to release the posterior gluteal fascia, which merges into the fascia lata.

2. Perform a series of deep, scooping strokes, in a 45° headward direction from the ischial tuberosity to the coccyx and lower portion of the sacrum to release the sacrotuberous ligament (Fig. 3-31).

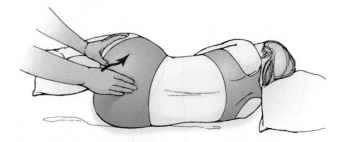

Figure 3-31. Release of the sacrotuberous ligament from the ischial tuberosity to the sacrum and coccyx.

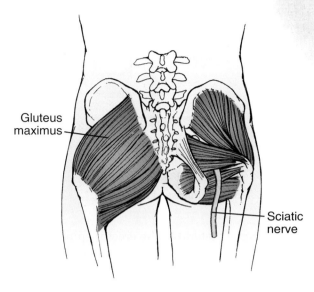

Figure 3-32. Deep rotators of the hip and the sciatic nerve.

3. Release of Deep External Rotators and Sciatic Nerve

▨ **Anatomy:** Piriformis, inferior gemellus, quadratus femoris, superior gemellus, obturator internus, sciatic nerve (Fig. 3-32).

▨ **Dysfunction:** These muscles roll into an inferior torsion, especially the obturator internus, which makes a right-angled bend under the sacrotuberous ligament at the ischial tuberosity. Lauren Berry, RPT, believed that this inferior torsion of the obturator internus and its fascia could have a tethering effect on the sciatic nerve, creating sciatica. The sciatic nerve can become entrapped under a hypertonic piriformis, which is a condition called *piriformis syndrome.* The sciatic nerve can also become entrapped in the space between the ischial tuberosity and the greater trochanter and at the inferior-lateral border of the ischial tuberosity, where it can become entrapped under the biceps femoris.

Position
▨ **TP:** Standing

▨ **CP:** Side-lying, fetal position

Strokes
1. Palpate the piriformis and perform a CR and RI MET for this muscle (MET #4).
2. Perform a series of lifting, scooping strokes perpendicular to the line of the fiber of the piriformis (Fig. 3-33). Begin in the belly of the muscle, midway between the PSIS and the greater trochanter. Perform a series of strokes first toward the greater trochanter, and then perform another series that moves from the mid-belly toward the PSIS.

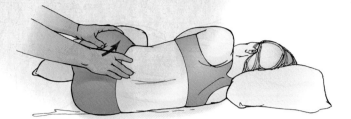

Figure 3-33. Double-thumb release of the piriformis. Begin your strokes just below the PSIS, and continue to the greater trochanter.

3. Perform a series of strokes in the inferior-to-superior (I–S) direction, covering the entire area between the ischial tuberosity and the greater trochanter and posterior femur.
4. Perform a series of strokes on the obturator internus along the superior and lateral border of the ischial tuberosity. Lift the soft tissue in a series of strokes in the I–S direction, and as you come to the superior portion of the ischial tuberosity, perform the strokes in a circular motion, scooping laterally to medially, following the contour of the bone (Fig. 3-34).
5. Perform a series of 1-inch scooping strokes with the thumbs, in the medial-to-lateral (M–L) plane, going from the lateral surface of the ischial tuberosity to the greater trochanter. If your client has some mild numbing and tingling down the leg and does not have a positive SLR test, these strokes will also release an entrapped sciatic nerve in this area (Fig. 3-35). An entrapped sciatic nerve normally manifests some mild numbing and tingling down the leg as it is being released. *Perform this stroke no more than six times if it increases the tingling.*

 CAUTION: *Do not repeat this stroke if pain radiates toward the spine, as that usually indicates a nerve root irritation, in which case crossing the nerve only aggravates the condition.*

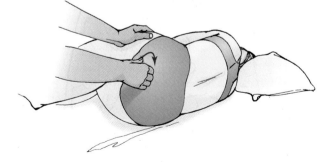

Figure 3-34. Supported-thumb technique to release the obturator internus. Lift the soft tissue in a circular motion, scooping laterally to medially along the superior and lateral border of the ischial tuberosity.

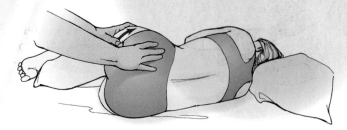

Figure 3-35. Release of a peripheral entrapment of the sciatic nerve from the trough formed between the ischial tuberosity and the greater trochanter.

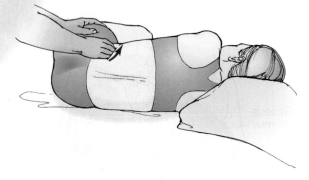

Figure 3-37. Fingertip release of the QL.

4. Transverse Release of the Quadratus Lumborum

▨ **Anatomy:** QL (Fig. 3-36)

▨ **Dysfunction:** The quadratus tends to shorten with both acute and chronic lower back dysfunction. If it is in a sustained contracture on one side only, due to trauma, or postural faults, for example, it will laterally flex the lumbar spine to that side, called *antalgia*. Antalgia may be caused by many factors, including a protruding disc.

Position

▨ **TP:** Standing, 45° headward or 45° caudally

▨ **CP:** Side-lying, fetal position, with back close to edge of table

Strokes

1. Facing 45° headward, use fingertips (Fig. 3-37) or a supported thumb, and place your hand just above

the iliac crest lateral to the erector spinae. Perform a series of 1-inch scooping strokes on the QL in an M–L direction. The series begins at the most lateral aspect of the QL, and each new stroke begins 1 inch more medially. The supporting hand compresses the ilium slightly headward with each stroke, bringing the origin and insertion of the QL together, helping to relax the QL by turning off the muscle spindles.

2. Begin another series of strokes superior to the previous series, working into the belly of the QL, releasing the entire muscle from the iliac crest to the twelfth rib.

3. An alternative position is to face 45° caudally and use a double-thumb technique to perform these same strokes (Fig. 3-38).

 CAUTION: *Do not use strong pressure under the last rib, as the kidneys lie in this region and could be irritated by too much pressure.*

5. Release of the Thoracolumbar Fascia and Erector Spinae Aponeurosis

▨ **Anatomy:** TLF (Fig. 3-39), erector spinae aponeurosis (tendinous sheet of attachment)

▨ **Dysfunction:** The most common form of chronic lumbosacral dysfunction is hypomobility or lack of move-

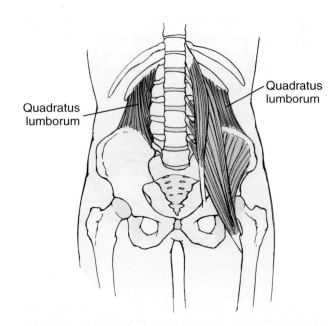

Quadratus lumborum

Quadratus lumborum

Figure 3-36. Quadratus lumborum.

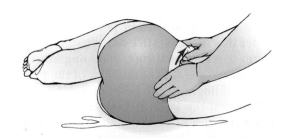

Figure 3-38. Double-thumb technique to release the QL.

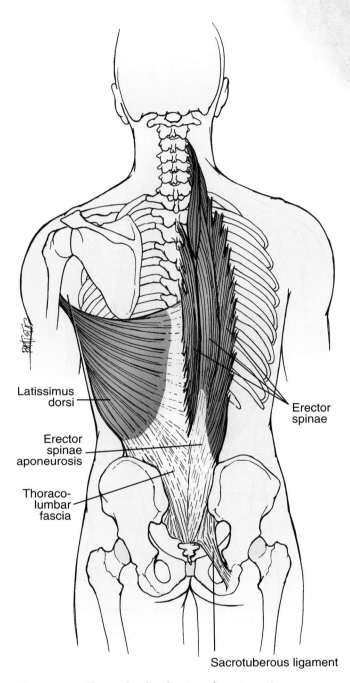

Latissimus dorsi

Erector spinae aponeurosis

Thoraco-lumbar fascia

Erector spinae

Sacrotuberous ligament

Figure 3-39. Thoracolumbar fascia and erector spinae aponeurosis.

ment. The erectors tend to be tight, compressing the facets and the intervertebral discs. This tightness dehydrates these tissues, leading to degeneration. The fascia and aponeurosis tend to shorten and dehydrate, leading to fibrosis. The positional dysfunction of the erector spinae is a medial torsion, pulling the erectors to the midline. This pulling is demonstrated by the finding that most patients who have LBP are in some sustained trunk flexion. Since the erectors attach toward the midline, a forward trunk increases this pulling to the midline.

Position
- **TP:** Standing, facing the table at a 45° angle inferiorly for longitudinal strokes and at a 90° angle for transverse strokes; emphasize a lengthening between the thoracic cage and the pelvis

- **CP:** Side-lying, fetal position

Strokes
There are two series of strokes, one directed caudally and the other laterally. These strokes also introduce a P–A glide into the spine. This mobilization technique promotes hydration of the facet joints, the intervertebral discs, the ligaments, and the muscles that have dehydrated due to fibrosis from previous inflammation or hypertonicity. This mobilization "resuscitates" the spine. Use gentle rocking if the client is in acute pain and deeper rocking if the client's pain is chronic.

1. Using a supported-thumb technique, perform a series of strokes approximately 1 inch long that are directed caudally (Fig. 3-40). Begin immediately next to the spinous processes near L4, that is, near the top of the ilium, and work down to the apex of the sacrum. Begin another series approximately 1 inch laterally, and include the entire area between the lumbar spinous processes and the ilium. The more superficial strokes release the fascia and the aponeurosis of the erector spinae muscles. The deeper strokes affect the multifidi, ligaments, joints, and discs.

2. Using a supported-thumb technique, perform a series of transverse strokes to release the TLF and erector spinae aponeurosis, working medially to laterally (Fig. 3-41). Begin at the lumbar spinous processes, scooping laterally. Release the entire

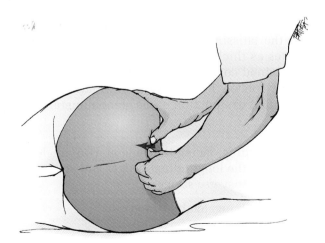

Figure 3-40. Supported-thumb technique to release the thoracolumbar fascia and erector spinae aponeurosis in a superior-to-inferior direction.

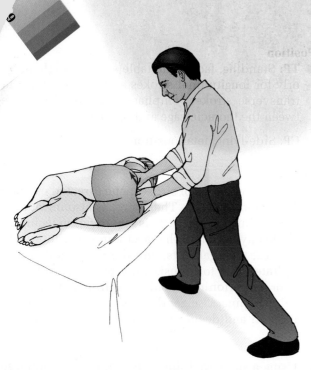

Figure 3-41. Supported-thumb technique to release the thoracolumbar fascia and erector spinae aponeurosis in an M–L direction.

soft tissue between the lumbosacral spine and the ilium, working from L4 down to the sacral apex.

6. *Transverse and Longitudinal Release of Soft Tissue of the Lumbar Spine from L4 to T12*

▧ **Anatomy:** Latissimus dorsi, TLF, erector spinae (Fig. 3-42)

▧ **Dysfunction:** The latissimus dorsi is eccentrically loaded in chronic LBP; that is, it is long and tight. With the trunk typically in some sustained flexion, the latissimus contracts to assist the extensors and the TLF to which it attaches. The aponeurosis of the latissimus blends with the fascia and palpates as thickened if there is a history of LBP. A sustained contraction in the latissimus also internally rotates the humerus, contributing to the position of dysfunction of the glenohumeral joint.

Position
▧ **TP:** Standing, facing the table at a 45° angle headward for the longitudinal strokes and at a 90° angle for the transverse strokes

▧ **CP:** Side-lying, fetal position

Strokes
There are two types of strokes in two lines. Release the TLF, latissimus, and trapezius (at T12) superficially; release the erector spinae and multifidi deeply.

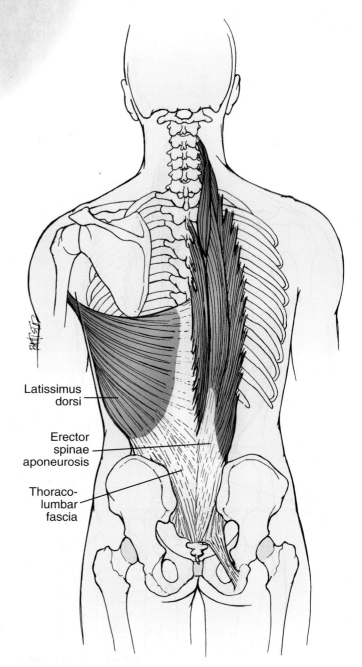

Latissimus
dorsi

Erector
spinae
aponeurosis

Thoraco-
lumbar
fascia

Figure 3-42. Latissimus dorsi, thoracolumbar fascia, and erector spinae.

These strokes are all scooping strokes approximately 1 inch long.

1. Using a supported-thumb technique, perform a series of I–S strokes beginning near L5. Remember that L4 is at the same level as the crest of the ilium. The first line of strokes is next to the spinous process of the vertebrae (Fig. 3-43). The second line is approximately 1 to 2 inches more laterally, posterior to the transverse processes. Use your support hand to rock the body.

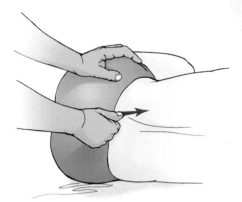

Figure 3-43. Supported-thumb technique to release the first line of the thoracolumbar fascia and erector spinae muscles in an I–S direction.

2. Perform a series of M–L strokes on the two lines described above (Fig. 3-44). The first line begins next to the spinous processes, scooping laterally in 1-inch strokes. The second line is approximately 1 to 2 inches more laterally.

> *Clinical Reminder: Remember: Pull the skin back 1 inch as you move onto your back leg; scoop into the tissue as you shift your body forward onto your front leg. Stay relaxed. Move your hands with each new stroke, and get into a gentle, calm rhythm as you work. These strokes are deeply relaxing when performed correctly.*

7. Transverse Release of the Psoas and Iliacus

■ **Anatomy:** Psoas major and iliacus (Fig. 3-45)

■ **Dysfunction:** The iliopsoas tends to roll into a medial torsion, which is often demonstrated as a genu valgum (knock-knees) and pronated ankles, a common weight distribution dysfunction. The iliopsoas tends to be tight, increasing the lordosis of the lumbar spine, which causes a compression of the lumbar facets. Sitting shortens the iliopsoas.

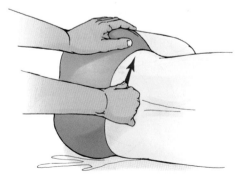

Figure 3-44. Supported-thumb technique to release the thoracolumbar fascia and erector spinae muscles in an M–L direction.

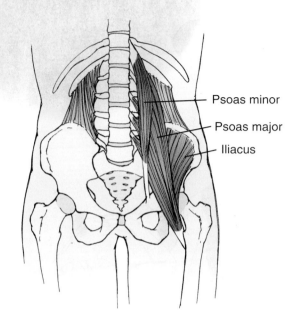

Psoas minor
Psoas major
Iliacus

Figure 3-45. Psoas minor, psoas major, and iliacus muscles.

 CAUTION: *Do not perform deep iliopsoas work on a pregnant woman.*

Position
■ **TP:** Standing, facing the direction of your stroke

■ **CP:** Supine

Strokes
1. Palpate the psoas (Fig. 3-46), and perform CR and RI MET on the iliopsoas with the hip at 90° flexion (MET #6 and #7).
2. To release the psoas, assume a 45° headward position, flex the client's hip and knee, and stabilize the client's lower leg against your body (Fig. 3-47). Place the fingertips of both hands on the iliopsoas; rock your body and your client's body rhythmically back and forth as you stroke back and forth on the iliopsoas, parallel to the inguinal ligament. You can also place your flexed knee on the table to stabilize the client's leg.
3. Using the same hand position described in the second stroke, palpate the iliacus by first placing your fingertips on the ASIS. Gently roll your fingertips over the bone and into the iliac fossa, feathering the abdominal cavity away with the back of your fingers/hand. Maintain contact with the iliacus covering the bone by flexing your fingertips so as not to compress the viscera. Release the iliacus with gentle, superficial-to-deep and lateral-to-medial, scooping strokes, following the contour of the bone as if you are cleaning the inside of a bowl. Begin at the ASIS, and then perform another series of strokes 1 inch superiorly and medially. Continue

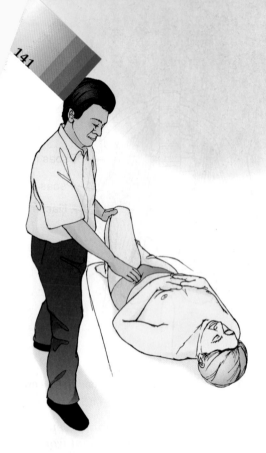

Figure 3-46. Palpation of the psoas. Find the psoas by first plac-ing your fingertips on the ASIS. Move medially approximately 2 to 3 inches, along the inguinal ligament. Gently roll your finger-tips slowly into the abdominal tissue just over the superior sur-face of the ligament. Have your client begin the motion of lifting his thigh toward his chest. You will feel the psoas contract un-der your fingertips. If the client is ticklish or sensitive to being touched in this area, have him place his hand on top of your hand. This reduces the sensitivity.

in 1-inch segments, covering the entire iliac fossa. Rock the client's leg in a lateral-to-medial direction with your strokes.

4. Bring the client's hip into approximately 90° flex-ion. Using your fingertips, scoop the iliopsoas laterally in 1-inch strokes as you move the client's hip in circles of abduction (Fig. 3-48). You sink into the tissue as the hip is being flexed and scoop later-ally as the hip is abducted. Then release your fingers as the thigh is being brought to the midline, and re-peat the scooping stroke in a slightly new area.

LEVEL II: LUMBOSACRAL

1. Transverse Release of Soft Tissue Attachments to the Crest of the Ilium

■ **Anatomy:** TLF, internal and external abdominal obliques, erector spinae aponeurosis, transverse ab-dominus, iliocostalis lumborum, QL (Fig. 3-49).

■ **Dysfunction:** The iliac crest is a significant attach-ment site for fascia and muscles, which act as stabi-lizers for the pelvis and the lumbar spine. The soft tissue here thickens with chronic irritation associ-

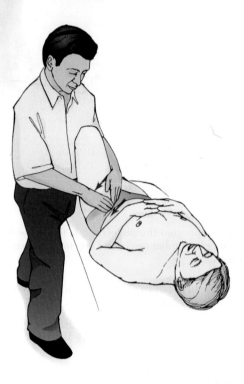

Figure 3-47. Release of the iliopsoas. Place the fingertips of both hands on the iliopsoas, and move the client's entire leg with your strokes.

ated with injuries and dysfunctions of the lum-bosacral spine. The abdominal muscles can be strained at their attachments to the lateral iliac crest, called a "**hip-pointer**" injury. This area also thickens owing to chronic muscle imbalance.

Position

■ **TP:** Standing, 90° to the crest of the ilium, or 45° caudally

■ **CP:** Supine; or side-lying, fetal position

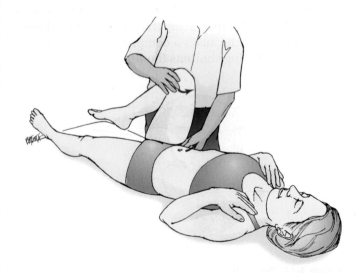

Figure 3-48. Fingertip release of the torsion of the iliopsoas. Move the hip in circles of abduction and external rotation as you roll the fibers of the iliopsoas laterally.

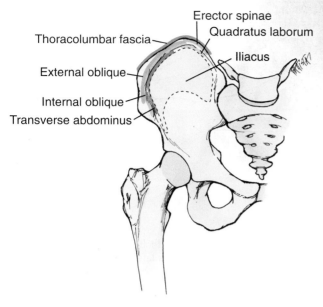

Figure 3-49. Soft-tissue attachments on the iliac crest. From superficial to deep: thoracolumbar fascia, erector spinae aponeurosis, iliocostalis lumborum, external and internal abdominal obliques, the transverse abdominus, and the QL.

Strokes

From superficial to deep, the attachments on the iliac crest are the TLF, which blends with the aponeurosis of the latissimus dorsi, iliocostalis lumborum, external abdominal oblique, internal abdominal oblique, transverse abdominus, quadratus lumborum, and iliolumbar ligament.

1. Facing 45° inferiorly and using a double- (Fig. 3-50) or supported-thumb technique, perform a series of 1-inch scooping strokes in an M–L direction along the crest of the ilium. Begin at the lateral aspect of the external lip of the iliac crest, and move in 1-inch segments more medially with each new stroke. The intention is to "clean the bone." Your strokes should move along the surface of the bone without digging into the bone. A healthy attachment site feels glistening and smooth. Tissue that has been under excessive load or that has been previously injured feels fibrotic.

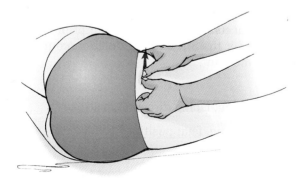

Figure 3-50. Double-thumb technique to release the crest of the ilium.

2. Repeat the same stroke in two more lines on the intermediate and internal lip of the iliac crest. You body faces more caudally with these strokes. As you perform these strokes, move the entire pelvis in the direction of your stroke.
3. To release the abdominal attachments from the ASIS to the most posterior portion of the iliac crest, ask your client to lie on his or her back, with legs extended. You may place a pillow under the client's knees. Using the fingertips-over-thumb technique, perform scooping strokes from anterior to posterior on the iliac crest (Fig. 3-51). Begin the strokes at the ASIS, and work more posteriorly with each stroke.

2. Transverse Release of the Soft Tissue Attachments to the Posterior Superior Iliac Spine

Anatomy: From superficial to deep, the attachments on the PSIS and the medial aspect of the iliac crest are the thoracic fibers of iliocostalis lumborum, lumbar fibers of the iliocostalis, and lumbar fibers of longissimus (Fig. 3-52).

Dysfunction: As was mentioned in the anatomy section, Bogduk and Twomey[10] have described a superficial and deep portion of the erector spinae. Now the deep attachments to the PSIS are addressed. The lumbar fibers of the iliocostalis and longissimus stabilize the lumbar spine and act to prevent anterior shear of the vertebrae relative to the sacrum and ilium.[2] Injury or dysfunction shortens and thickens soft tissue. Attachment points dry out, becoming ischemic and eventually fibrous. The intention is to dissolve the fibrosis, broadening and rehydrating the tissue.

Position

TP: Standing, facing the direction of your stroke

CP: Side-lying, fetal position

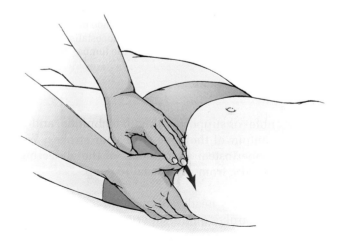

Figure 3-51. Release of the abdominal attachments to the lateral aspect of the ilium.

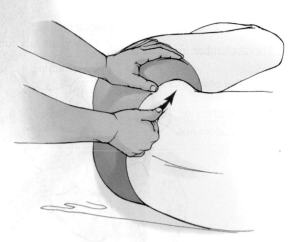

Figure 3-53. Supported-thumb technique to release the lateral portion of the iliac crest and the lateral portion of the PSIS.

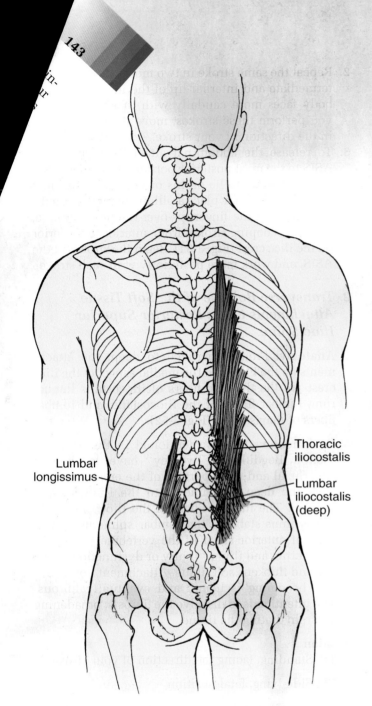

Lumbar longissimus

Thoracic iliocostalis

Lumbar iliocostalis (deep)

Figure 3-52. Deep portion of the erector spinae muscles. Shown here are the thoracic fibers of the iliocostalis lumborum, the lumbar fibers of the iliocostalis, and the lumbar fibers of the longissimus.

Strokes

Use a double- or supported-thumb technique, and follow the contour of the bone with your strokes. Work on the tenoperiosteal attachments of the above muscles to the PSIS, from superficial to deep.

1. Facing slightly headward, perform a series of M–L scooping strokes on the superior portion of the PSIS and the adjoining portion of the iliac crest (Fig. 3-53) to releases the thoracic fibers of the iliocostalis.

2. Continue this series of 1-inch scooping strokes in an I–S direction on the medial and inferior portion of the PSIS following the contour of the bone. This releases the lumbar fibers of the iliocostalis. As you sink more deeply with these strokes, you are on the lumbar fibers of the longissimus, which are the deepest muscle fibers attaching to the PSIS.

3. Release of the Soft Tissue Attachments to the Sacrum

■ **Anatomy:** From superficial to deep, the attachments on the sacral base are the TLF; the erector spinae aponeurosis, which is a continuation of the tendon of the thoracic fibers of longissimus; the multifidus; and the posterior sacroiliac ligaments which are next to the bone (Fig. 3-54).

As the thoracic fibers of longissimus run headward, they angle approximately 10° to 15° laterally. Deep to the fibers of the longissimus is the multifidus. The muscle mass that you palpate medial to the PSIS is the multifidus.

■ **Dysfunction:** Soft tissue tends to shorten and become fibrotic with overuse or as a consequence of a prior injury. The multifidus attaches to the joint capsules of the vertebral facets, and releasing the multifidus at the sacrum assists in the release of the lumbar facets. Fibrotic tissue from prior strain can extend over the SIJ, limiting nutation/counternutation in the joint.

Position

■ **TP:** Standing, facing direction of stroke

■ **CP:** Side-lying, fetal position

Strokes

1. To release the thoracic fibers of longissimus, use the supported-thumb technique. Face caudally,

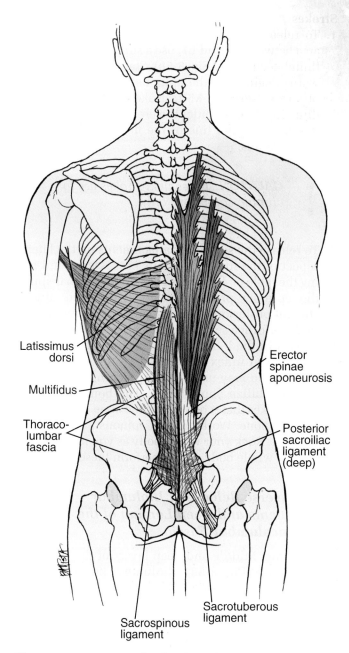

Figure 3-54. From superficial to deep, the attachments to the sacrum are the thoracolumbar fascia, erector spinae aponeurosis, a continuation of the thoracic fibers of longissimus, the multifidi, and the posterior sacroiliac ligaments.

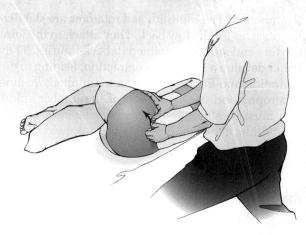

Figure 3-55. Release of the thoracic fibers of the longissimus. Use a supported-thumb technique, and perform a series of M–L strokes that are angled slightly inferior.

2. To release the multifidi attachments on the sacral base stand in the 45° headward position. Using the supported-thumb technique, perform a series of 1-inch, M–L scooping strokes in an approximately 45° headward direction (Fig. 3-56). Work at a deeper level than the previous stroke. Begin at the midline of the sacrum, and work to the PSIS. Cover one-half of the sacrum.

3. Use your palpation skills to feel for thickened, fibrous tissue in the the posterior sacroiliac ligaments. If you feel areas of fibrosis, use the same technique described in the previous stroke, and perform short, strokes transverse to the line of the fibrotic fiber. Place your supporting hand on the ilium, and rock the client's body in short oscillations with each stroke. These deep strokes on the ligaments are used **only as needed** to release fibrotic tissue.

4. Release of Multifidi and Rotatores from L5 to L1

Anatomy: multifidus, rotatores (Fig. 3-57)

and place your working hand just medial to the PSIS at the superior part of the sacrum (Fig. 3-55). Your supporting hand is on the ilium next to the working hand. Perform a series of 1-inch M–L strokes that are angled in a slightly inferior direction. Your first stroke is next to the PSIS, and each new stroke begins a little closer to the midline of the sacrum. The second line of strokes begins slightly below the first line. Work in 1-inch segments to the lowest part (apex) of the sacrum, covering one-half of the entire sacrum.

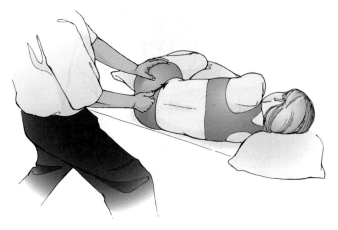

Figure 3-56. Release of the multifidi. Standing in a 45° headward stance, scoop in an M–L direction.

■ **Dysfunction:** The multifidi and rotatores are stabilizing muscles for the low back. They attach to the joint capsule and are often strained in back injuries. They either develop a sustained contraction, leading to dehydration and fibrosis, or become inhibited, leading to atrophy and destabilization of the lumbar spine. You must be able to palpate the difference, as it is contraindicated to work deeply on atrophied tissue.

Position

■ **TP:** Standing, facing headward

■ **CP:** Side-lying, fetal position

Strokes

1. To release the multifidus and rotatores from the area between L5 and L1, use a supported- or double-thumb technique (Fig. 3-58). Stand facing 45° headward. Begin near the spinous process of L5, and perform a series of M–L strokes in a 45° headward direction. Scoop under the erector spinae, working transverse to the line of the fiber of the multifidi and rotatores.

 CAUTION: These next strokes are for chronic conditions only.

2. To release the soft tissue attachments on the lateral aspect of the lumbar spinous processes, stand facing the table or 45° headwards. In the lumbar spine, the spinous processes (SP) are angled almost straight posteriorly. Using a supported-thumb position, perform a series of short, brisk, back-and-forth strokes in the I–S plane on the spinous processes. Your flexed index finger rests on the other side of the SP. You may use a slight pinching grasp of the SP to stabilize your thumb. The bone is cleaned with strokes that scoop across the bone. Do not press into the bone. Work on each spinous process, from L5 to L1. Rock your whole body as you mobilize the client's whole body as you perform these strokes.

5. Transverse Release of Iliolumbar Ligaments and Deep Lamina of the Thoracolumbar Fascia

■ **Anatomy:** Middle and deep layers of the TLF (alar ligaments) (Fig. 3-59), iliolumbar ligaments (Fig. 3-60).

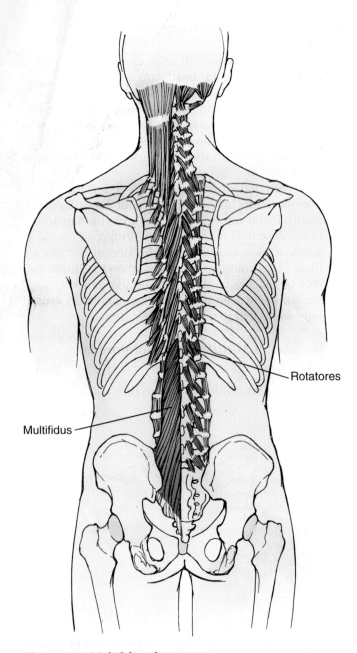

Figure 3-57. Multifidi and rotatores.

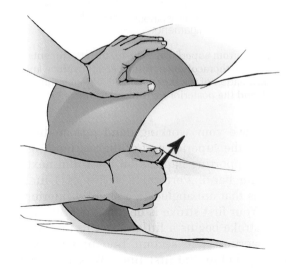

Figure 3-58. Supported-thumb release of the multifidi and rotatores.

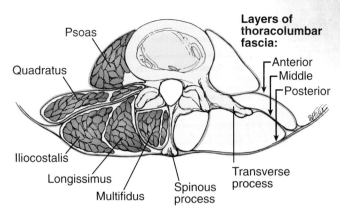

Figure 3-59. Anterior, middle, and deep layers of the thoracolumbar fascia. The three layers travel from the spinous and transverse processes of the lumbar vertebrae to the ilium.

▓ **Dysfunction:** L4 and L5 vertebrae experience the greatest stress in the lumbar spine because the lumbar lordosis tips these vertebrae down, creating a shear. The iliolumbar ligaments provide stability to the SIJ and the L5–S1 vertebrae. These ligaments shorten and thicken in chronic LBP. The deep lamina of the TLF travels from the lumbar transverse processes to the ilium.

Position
▓ **TP:** Standing, facing headward

▓ **CP:** Side-lying, fetal position; you might need to increase the lumbar curve slightly by bringing the knees away from the client's chest slightly to put the erector muscles in more slack.

Strokes
Now you are working the deepest layers of soft tissue between the medial aspect of the ilium and the spin-

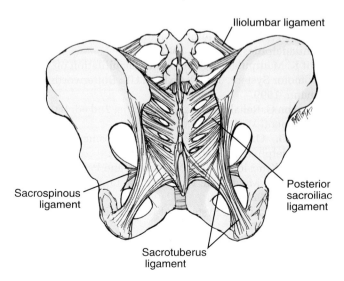

Figure 3-60. Iliolumbar ligaments.

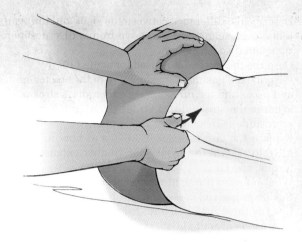

Figure 3-61. Supported-thumb release in three lines for the middle and deep layers of the thoracolumbar fascia and the iliolumbar ligaments.

ous and transverse processes on the lowest lumbar vertebrae. The intention is to scoop transverse to the line of the fiber, broadening these fibers to release any fibrosis. It takes a great deal of preparation to work this deeply. These strokes are for chronic conditions only.

1. Using the supported-thumb position (Fig. 3-61), place your working hand next to the spinous process of L4, which is at the level of the iliac crest. Your supporting hand rests on the ilium. Perform a series of 1-inch scooping strokes in a superior direction between the L4 vertebra and the ilium, transverse on the deep lamina of the TLF and iliolumbar ligaments. As you move onto your back leg, pull the client's ilium back with you slightly. As you scoop into the tissue, push the client's ilium toward your working hand. This brings the erectors into slack and allows for deeper work.

2. The second line of strokes begins at the L5 area, approximately 1 inch inferior to the first line. Perform another series of 1-inch scooping strokes in the superior direction. Continue your series of strokes to the ilium. Rock your entire body and your client's body as you perform your strokes. If you find fibrotic tissue, your strokes may become more brisk, but always maintain the rocking movement. Cover the entire area between L4–L5 and the ilium.

▓ *Study Guide*

Lumbosacral Spine, Level I
1. List the names of the muscles in the seven layers of the back, from superficial to deep.
2. Describe the basic origins and insertions of the erector spinae, the psoas, and the QL.

3. Describe the difference between the signs and the symptoms of muscle strain, facet syndrome, disc degeneration, and disc herniation.
4. Describe the MET that is used for acute LBP.
5. Describe the positional dysfunction of the erector spinae and psoas and the directions of a therapist's strokes.
6. What is the stroke direction for the sacrotuberous and sacrospinous ligaments?
7. Explain the clinical uses of MET and how to perform MET to release the hypertonic lumbar extensors, piriformis, and QL.
8. What muscles are tight and what muscles are weak in the lower (pelvic) crossed syndrome?
9. List the three major factors that predispose a person to an episode of acute LBP.
10. List what functional factors predispose to LBP.

Lumbosacral Spine, Level II

1. Describe the basic origins and insertions of the piriformis, gluteals, and multifidus muscle.
2. Describe the main muscles that are responsible for an increased lumbar curve and for a decreased lumbar curve.
3. Describe the length assessment test and PIR MET for the iliopsoas.
4. List the attachments on the crest of the ilium, from superficial to deep.
5. List three factors that affect the diameter of the IVF.
6. List what attaches to the sacral base, from superficial to deep.
7. Describe the direction of a stroke to release the multifidi and rotatores.
8. Explain how abnormal muscle function can predispose a person to an episode of LBP.
9. Describe the two types of referral of pain and their causes.
10. Describe the SLR test. What are the implications of a positive test?

References

1. Kaul M, Herring SA. Rehabilitation of lumbar spine injuries. In Kibler WB, Herring SA, Press JM (eds): Functional Rehabilitation of Sports and Musculoskeletal Injuries. Gaithersburg, MD: Aspen, 1998, pp 188–215.
2. Porterfield JA, DeRosa C. Mechanical Low Back Pain. Philadelphia: WB Saunders, 1991.
3. Mooney V. Sacroiliac joint dysfunction. In Vleeming A, Mooney V, Dorman T, Snijders CJ, Stoeckart R (eds): Movement, Stability, and Low Back Pain. New York: Churchill Livingstone, 1997, pp 37–52.
4. Swenson R. A medical approach to the differential diagnosis of low back pain. J Neuromusculoskeletal Syst 1998;6:100–113.
5. Kirkaldy-Willis WH, Bernard TN Jr. Managing Low Back Pain, 4th ed. New York: Churchill Livingstone, 1999.
6. Cherkin DC, Sherman KJ, Deyo RA, Shekelle PG. A review of the evidence for the effectiveness, safety, and cost of acupuncture, massage therapy, and spinal manipulation for back pain. Ann Intern Med 2003;138 (11):898–906.
7. Cailliet R. Low Back Pain Syndrome. Philadelphia: FA Davis, 1995.
8. Willard FH. The muscular, ligamentous and neural structure of the low back and its relation to low back pain. In Vleeming A, Mooney V, Dorman T, Snijders CJ, Stoeckart R (eds): Movement, Stability, and Low Back Pain. New York: Churchill Livingstone, 1997, pp 3–35.
9. Freeman MA, Dean MR, Hanham IW. The etiology and prevention of functional instability of the foot. J Bone Joint Surg Br 1965;47:678–685.
10. Bogduk N, Twomey L. Clinical Anatomy of the Lumbar Spine, 3rd ed. London: Churchill Livingstone, 1998.
11. Brukner P, Khan K. Clinical Sports Medicine, 3rd ed. Sydney: McGraw-Hill, 2006.
12. Calais-Germain B. Anatomy of Movement. Seattle: Eastland Press, 1991.
13. Jull GA, Janda V. Muscles and motor control in low back pain: Assessment and management. In Twomey L, Taylor JR (eds): Physical Therapy of the Low Back. New York: Churchill Livingstone, 1987, pp 253–278.
14. Greenman PE. Principles of Manual Medicine, 2nd ed. Baltimore: Williams & Wilkins, 1996.

Suggested Readings

Chaitow L. Muscle Energy Techniques, 3rd ed. New York: Churchill Livingstone, 2006.

Clemente C. Anatomy: A Regional Atlas of the Human Body, 4th ed. Baltimore: Williams & Wilkins, 1997.

Corrigan B, Maitland GD. Practical Orthopaedic Medicine. London: Butterworths, 1983.

Hertling D, Kessler R. Management of Common Musculoskeletal Disorders, 4th ed. Baltimore: Lippincott Williams & Wilkins, 2006.

Kendall F, McCreary E, Provance P, Rogers M, Romani W. Muscles: Testing and Function, 5th ed. Baltimore: Williams & Wilkins, 2005.

Levangie P, Norkin C. Joint Structure and Function, 3rd ed. Philadelphia: FA Davis, 2001.

Lewit K. Manipulative Therapy in Rehabilitation on the Locomotor System, 3rd ed. Oxford, UK: Butterworth Heinemann, 1999.

Liebenson C. Rehabilitation of the Spine, 2nd ed. Baltimore: Lippincott Williams & Wilkins, 2007.

Magee D. Orthopedic Physical Assessment, 3rd ed. Philadelphia: WB Saunders, 1997.

Oatis CA. Kinesiology: The Mechanics and Pathomechanics of Human Movement. Philadelphia: Lippincott Williams & Wilkins, 2004.

Platzer W. Locomotor System, vol 1, 5th ed. New York: Thieme Medical, 2004.

Reid DC. Sports Injury and Assessment. New York: Churchill Livingstone, 1992.

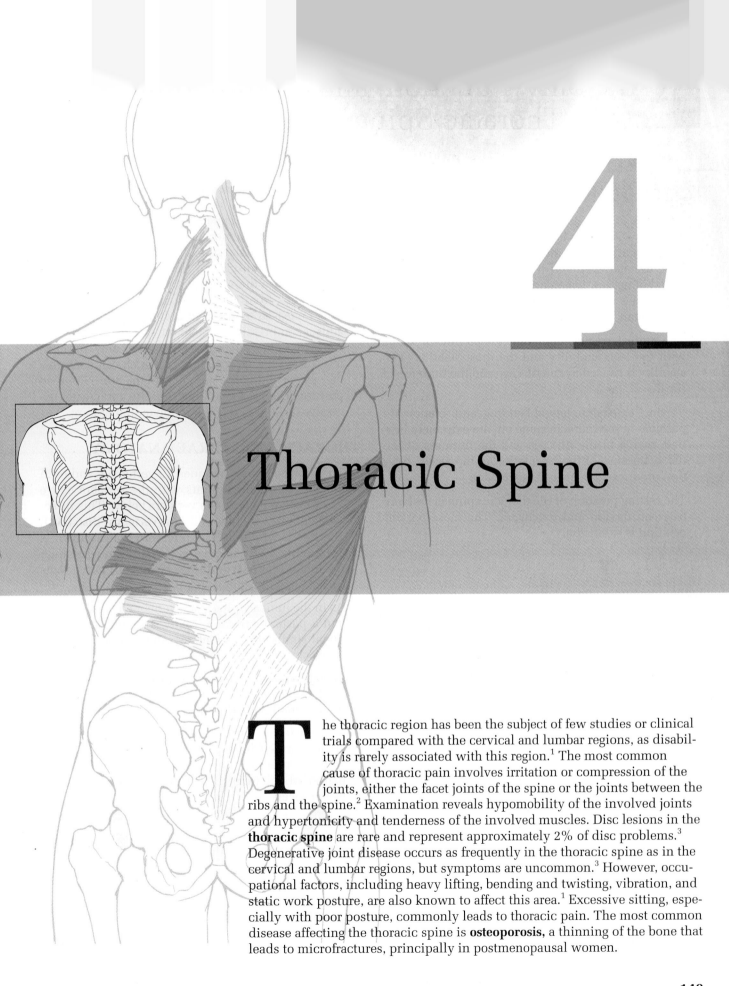

Thoracic Spine

The thoracic region has been the subject of few studies or clinical trials compared with the cervical and lumbar regions, as disability is rarely associated with this region.[1] The most common cause of thoracic pain involves irritation or compression of the joints, either the facet joints of the spine or the joints between the ribs and the spine.[2] Examination reveals hypomobility of the involved joints and hypertonicity and tenderness of the involved muscles. Disc lesions in the **thoracic spine** are rare and represent approximately 2% of disc problems.[3] Degenerative joint disease occurs as frequently in the thoracic spine as in the cervical and lumbar regions, but symptoms are uncommon.[3] However, occupational factors, including heavy lifting, bending and twisting, vibration, and static work posture, are also known to affect this area.[1] Excessive sitting, especially with poor posture, commonly leads to thoracic pain. The most common disease affecting the thoracic spine is **osteoporosis,** a thinning of the bone that leads to microfractures, principally in postmenopausal women.

Anatomy, Function, and Dysfunction of the Thoracic Spine

GENERAL OVERVIEW

■ The thoracic region consists of 12 vertebrae and intervertebral discs, 12 ribs and their associated cartilage, the sternum, and the scapula; it is also composed of nerves, ligaments, muscles, and associated soft tissues (Fig. 4-1). The scapula is considered in more detail in Chapter 6, "The Shoulder."

■ The thoracic region is the longest part of the spine with the least mobility and the most stability. The stability is caused by the rib cage and the thinness of the discs.

■ Flexion, extension, lateral bending, and rotation are possible in the thoracic spine but are extremely limited, owing to the rib cage and the thinness of the discs. Because of the orientation of the facets, rotation produces the greatest movement.

■ The resting position of the thoracic spine is midway between flexion and extension. The close-packed position is extension.

THORACIC CURVE

The thoracic spine normally has a mild, smooth posterior curve, called thoracic kyphosis. This curve is primarily determined by the shape of the thoracic vertebral bodies. However, as Grieve[3] points out, the degree of thoracic curve can vary greatly. The interscapular region may be flat with a normal X-ray.

POSTURE

■ The curve in the thoracic spine is affected by the position of the head, pelvis, and lower back, just as the position of the head and neck are influenced by the thoracic spine. An increased lumbar curve causes an increase in the thoracic and cervical curves. A common postural fault is a rounded-shoulder, forward-head posture (FHP), which also creates an increase in the thoracic curve, further contributing to an increase in the cervical curve.

■ **Dysfunction and injury:** With a rounded-shoulder, FHP, the thoracic spine goes into flexion, compressing the discs, potentially leading to early degenera-

tion (Fig. 4-2). The facets are held in a flexed position, losing their ability to move into extension. The joint capsules have an increased load in the flexed position and develop abnormal crosslinks and adhesions, leading to loss of normal joint motion. The tension in the extensor muscles of the upper thoracic spine must increase dramatically to prevent the head and upper back from falling forward because of gravity. This increased tension not only is fatiguing but also adds a compressive force to the facets. Compression can also occur in the space above and below the clavicle, called the *thoracic outlet*, which can compress the nerves and blood supply into the arm. Slumped posture decreases vital lung capacity and creates excessive tension in the temporomandibular joint.

THORACIC VERTEBRAE ANATOMY

■ The thoracic spine includes 12 vertebrae, and each vertebra forms three joints with the vertebra above and three joints with the vertebra below. This three-joint complex includes an **intervertebral disc (IVD)** and two **facet joints.** The **intervertebral foramen** is an opening between two vertebrae through which the motor (ventral) and sensory (dorsal) nerve roots travel along the spine.

■ As in the lumbar spine, each vertebra has an anterior and a posterior portion. Many structural and functional similarities as well as some important differences exist.

■ The **anterior portion** consists of a vertebral **body** and an **IVD,** which forms a fibrocartilaginous joint with the vertebral body (Fig. 4-3).

■ The **posterior portion** consists of two vertebral arches formed by a pedicle and lamina, a central spinous process, two transverse processes, and paired articulations, called the **inferior** and the **superior facets,** which form synovial joints.

■ A unique feature of the thoracic vertebrae is that the body and transverse processes have synovial joints for articulation with the ribs. These joints are called **costovertebral joints** and are discussed in the section "Costovertebral Joints."

VERTEBRAL BODY

■ Unlike the cervical and the lumbar spine, the thoracic vertebral bodies are shorter anteriorly than

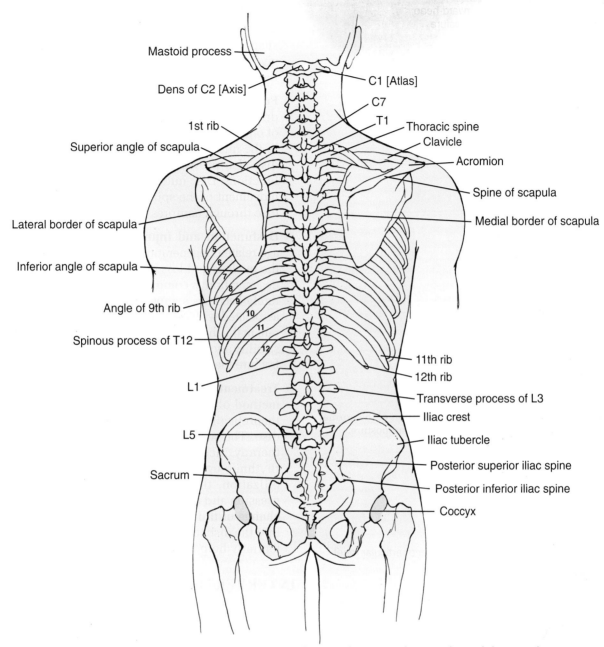

Figure 4-1. Posterior view of the thoracic region showing the 12 vertebra, 12 ribs, and the scapulae overlying the rib cage.

posteriorly, giving this area its normal thoracic kyphosis. As in the lumbar and cervical regions, a fibrocartilage joint is located between the two vertebral bodies and the disc.

▨ **Dysfunction and injury:** The vertebral body is the site of pathologic fractures secondary to **osteoporosis,** which are most common in the midthoracic region.[1] Calcium deficiency, estrogen loss, and lack of weight-bearing exercise cause a thinning of the bone and create wedge-shaped vertebrae due to

these microfractures. Because the weight is placed on the anterior part of the vertebrae, a round back called *senile kyphosis* may occur, especially in the elderly.

INTERVERTEBRAL DISC

▨ **Structure:** The IVD is composed of a **nucleus** and an **annulus.** The nucleus is a colloidal gel contained within a fibrous wall that is 80% to 90% water.

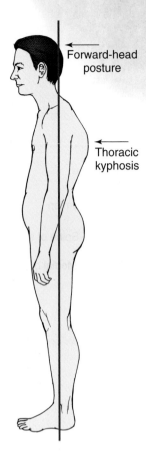

Figure 4-2. Thoracic kyphosis is an exaggeration of the normal thoracic curve and contributes to a forward-head posture.

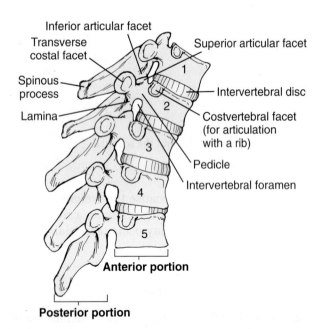

Figure 4-3. Anterior and posterior portions of the thoracic vertebra.

Concentric layers of interwoven fibrocartilaginous fibers form the annulus. The thoracic discs are proportionally smaller than the cervical or lumbar discs, and the disc height is symmetric rather than wedge-shaped as in the other two regions. Therefore, discs give the cervical and lumbar regions their curves, and the vertebral body shape defines the thoracic curve.

- **Function:** The discs provide a shock-absorbing hydraulic system that permits a rocker-like movement of one vertebra upon the other, owing to a fluid shift in the nucleus and an elasticity of the annulus. The disc also provides proprioceptive and nociceptive functions. Disc nutrition into the annulus occurs by movement of the spine, which pumps fluid into the disc through compression and decompression.

- **Dysfunction and injury:** The IVD is susceptible to age-related degeneration that involves loss of fluid in the nucleus and loss of elasticity of the annulus. Disc degeneration is common in the thoracic region, but it rarely becomes symptomatic, other than the stiffness associated with decreased mobility.[3] Disc herniation is rare in the thoracic spine because of the protection and stability afforded by the rib cage. Compression injuries fracture the vertebra before they injure the disc.[1]

- **Treatment implications:** This text introduces a new method of treatment called *wave mobilization* that theoretically helps promote fluid exchange to the disc. The wave mobilization method of soft tissue therapy incorporates joint mobilization. Through rhythmic cycles of posterior-to-anterior (P–A) mobilization, the author postulates that these compression and decompression cycles promote the exchange of fluids deep within the joint, pump fluid into the disc to keep the disc well hydrated, and potentially help to rehydrate a degenerated disc.

INTERVERTEBRAL FACETS

- **Structure:** The **superior and inferior vertebral facets** are synovial joints between two vertebrae (see Fig. 4-3). As in the lumbar and cervical regions, joint capsules that are highly innervated with mechanoreceptors and pain receptors surround these facet joints. They also contain fibrocartilage meniscoid structures.[3]

- **Function:** The facets determine the range and direction of movement. The mechanoreceptors and nociceptors have reflexive (automatic) communication to the surrounding muscles, creating reflex hypertonicity or inhibition in the surrounding muscles in predictable patterns (see below). They are designed to slide on each other in the healthy state. Extension closes the facets, and flexion opens them. For facets to maintain a healthy state, it is necessary for them to be moved through their full range of motion regularly. Stretching programs, such as yoga, are extremely beneficial to the spinal facets.

Dysfunction and injury

☐ **Hypomobility:** Restricted motion at the thoracic facets implies a loss of the normal gliding motion on the cartilage surfaces. This restriction is called a **fixation** and may be caused by poor posture (such as forward-head posture), injury, sustained muscle tension, entrapment of the articular meniscoid, or roughened articular surfaces because of degeneration. Hypomobility leads to fibrosis of the joint capsule, resulting in decreased nutrition to the disc and articular cartilage. Poor posture causes adaptive changes in the connective tissue, shortening the tissue in the front of the spine. Clients lose thoracic extension and rotation. This pattern is associated with hip flexion contractures. Restricted motion of the facets results in a reflex that typically creates hypertonicity of the muscles at the same vertebral level.

☐ **Degeneration:** Degeneration is the loss or thinning of the cartilage on the surface of the facet, in which the cartilage has lost some or all of its lubricating and shock-absorbing functions. This loss of synovial fluid causes the joint to "dry out." Advanced degeneration is called osteoarthritis, arthrosis or degenerative joint disease. Degeneration can be caused by prior injury, repetitive stresses, hypomobility, and muscle or movement imbalances. Sustained contraction of the paraspinal muscles (muscles on either side of the spine) increases the compression to the facets, reducing their mobility and, therefore, reducing their nutritional exchange, which depends on movement. This compression and the consequent decreased lubrication of the facets accelerate their degeneration. This is common in the thoracic spine and causes an inhibition of the normal gliding characteristics of the facets, creating stiffness, called **hypomobility syndrome.** In the thoracic spine, the most hypomobile areas are C7–T1 and T12–L1. High stress occurs in these two areas where the curves change direction.

☐ **Irritation and injury:** Injury to the facet joint affects the cartilage and joint capsule. It can be a minor irritation or cracking/tearing of these structures. Without treatment, the area becomes fibrotic and degenerates. When the thoracic joints are irritated as a result of acute injury or cumulative stress, they produce local pain and may refer pain into the anterior chest.[4] The pain is described as a deep, dull ache.

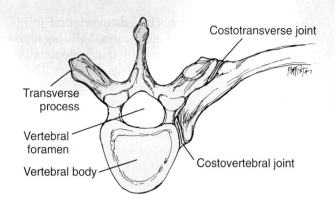

Figure 4-4. Costovertebral joints. Each rib forms a joint with the thoracic vertebra at two places: the vertebral body and the transverse process.

Treatment implications:
Dysfunction and injury to the facets are best treated with muscle energy technique (MET), soft tissue mobilization of the hypertonic thoracic extensor muscles, and P–A mobilization of the joints. Unlike the cervical and lumbar spine, the thoracic spine is rarely unstable. Rather, it typically becomes too stiff and requires increased movement, especially extension.

COSTOVERTEBRAL JOINTS

Structure:
The **costovertebral joints** are synovial joints on the bodies and transverse processes of the thoracic vertebrae that articulate with the ribs (Fig. 4-4). The articulation between the rib and the transverse process is also called the **costotransverse joint.**

☐ Except for T1, which has only one joint at the body, each vertebra has two joints on the body and one on the transverse process for articulation with the rib. Each articulation is a synovial joint with a joint capsule and articular meniscoid, supported by numerous ligaments. The center of the head of the rib is attached to the intervertebral disc by interarticular ligaments.

☐ The costovertebral joints are highly innervated with pain fibers and mechanoreceptors. A powerful reflex creating hypertonicity in the muscles overlying the joint can be caused by irritation of these nerves.[3]

Function:
In the healthy state, the ribs have considerable movement at their articulation with the transverse processes and vertebral body.[5] The primary motion of the ribs is elevation and depression in response to respiration. Respiration, bending and twisting of the thoracic cage, and reaching with the arm all generate movement at the costovertebral joints.

■ **Dysfunction and injury:** The costovertebral joints are susceptible to loss of their normal gliding characteristics due to injury, sustained muscle tension, meniscoid entrapment, and degeneration. Using the arms influences these joints because of the attachments of the powerful arm muscles. Polishing or scrubbing; repetitive reaching, especially overhead; or reaching with a twisting motion, such as reaching into the backseat of a car, can create irritation to the costovertebral joints. Injury may also be caused by a cough or sneeze. Injury to the costovertebral joint may sprain the joint capsule and cause a subluxation (partial dislocation) or fixation of the joint. Fixation of the costovertebral or costotransverse joints decreases respiratory function. If acute, it potentially causes a "catch," or sharp pain, on inspiration. This catch may be felt a few inches lateral to the spinous process (SP), along the lateral portion of the chest wall, or in the anterior chest.[5] A common dysfunction involves the T1 rib. Because of forward-head posture and rounded shoulders, the rib fixates in an elevated position, narrowing the thoracic outlet through which the nerves travel into the arm. The client has tightness in the scalenes and pectoralis minor. Symptoms include local pain at the C7–T1 area and aching pain referred into the arm, especially the ulnar border.

■ **Treatment implications:** Soft tissue mobilization and MET help to reduce muscle hypertonicity in the paraspinal and intercostal muscles and diaphragm and increase movement to the joints. P–A mobilization of the costovertebral joints stimulates the secretion of synovial fluid and helps to reintroduce normal gliding characteristics. If your client has a catch in the thoracic spine with inspiration and your treatment does not resolve it, refer the client to a chiropractor or an osteopath for manipulation.

SPINOUS PROCESS

The SPs slope inferiorly and overlap the SP of the inferior vertebra. They are frequently asymmetric. It is fruitless to try to determine dysfunction merely by the position of the SP.

STERNUM

The sternum is divided into three parts: the **manubrium, body,** and **xiphoid** (Fig. 4-5). The manubrium articulates with the clavicle and first rib at its superior-lateral aspect and with the second rib at its inferior-lateral aspect. The sternum protects the heart, lungs, and other vital structures in the thoracic cavity.

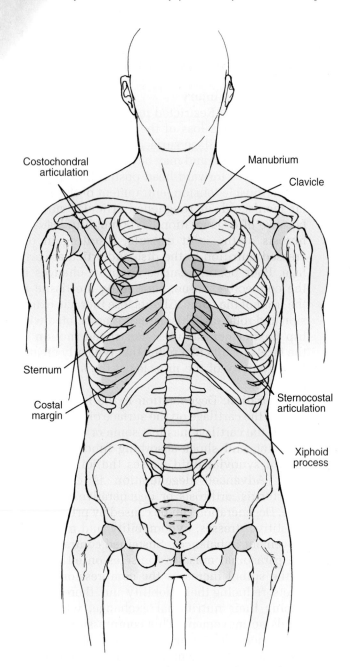

Figure 4-5. Anterior view of the rib cage, showing the costochondral and sternocostal joints.

STERNOCOSTAL AND COSTOCHONDRAL JOINTS

■ **Structure:** The **sternocostal joints** are synovial articulations between the costal (rib) cartilages and the sternum (see Fig. 4-5). At the first rib, the articulation is cartilaginous, not synovial.

■ The **costochondral joints** are the articulations of the bony portion of the T1–T7 ribs with cartilage. They are located 1 to 2 inches lateral to the sternocostal joints. Costochondral joints are cartilaginous joints (synchondrosis) in which cartilage and bone are bound together by periosteum.

▨ **Dysfunction and injury:** Excessive weight training of the pectoral muscles or repetitive pushing or pulling can irritate or injure these joints. Acute trauma, such as falling on an outstretched arm, a blunt sports injury, or the impact of the shoulder harness during a car accident, can create an acute inflammation that typically manifests as a localized, painful swelling, called *costochondritis* or *Tietze's syndrome.*

RIB CAGE

▨ **Structure:** There are 12 ribs on each side (see Fig. 4-5). The first seven are called "true ribs" because they attach directly to the sternum. Ribs 8 to 10 articulate below the sternum through cartilage, and the last two ribs, 11 and 12, are called "floating ribs" because they have no attachment to the sternum.

☐ Twenty muscles that attach to the rib cage provide stability and movement to the trunk, pelvis, head, neck, and arms and assist in respiration.

☐ An intercostal nerve travels between the ribs and can be irritated with injury to the ribs or from the synovial joints of the spine and ribs (Fig. 4-6).

▨ **Function:** The rib cage serves as protection to the heart and lungs and as attachment sites for the muscles. Its movement increases thoracic volume for respiration. The rib cage is resilient in the normal state; this springing quality is essential to maintain full respiratory capacity.

☐ Movement of the rib cage is primarily concerned with respiration. The chest can expand in three directions: vertically, owing to the contraction of the diaphragm, and in the transverse and anterior-to-posterior directions due to the movement of the ribs.[1] The lateral aspect of the ribs elevates during inspiration, then lowers on expiration.

▨ **Dysfunction and injury:** The most common dysfunction of the rib cage is hypomobility that leads to stiffness and rigidity. This loss of movement contributes to hypomobility of the facet joints of the thoracic spine and of the costovertebral joints, decreasing respiratory function. Causes include adhesions as the result of trauma, respiratory diseases such as emphysema or asthma, chronic shallow breathing from emotional depression, or depression of the anterior rib cage caused by rounded shoulders.

☐ Weakness of the extensors of the upper thoracic spine and the middle and lower trapezii prevents straightening of the upper back and decreases the ability of the chest to expand.[6]

INTERVERTEBRAL FORAMEN

▨ **Structure:** The IVF is an opening (foramen) formed by:

1. Two pedicles from the superior and inferior vertebrae that form the roof and floor;
2. The disc, posterior longitudinal ligament, and vertebral body anteriorly;
3. The facets, anterior capsule, and ligamentum flavum posteriorly.

▨ **Function:** The IVF provides an opening for the motor and sensory nerve roots that originate at the spinal cord.

▨ **Dysfunction and injury:** The IVF of the thoracic spine is large; bone spurs seldom decrease the opening. Unlike in the lumbar spine, the IVF is posterior to the vertebral body rather than the disc, and therefore thoracic disc lesions do not affect the IVF. Also, because of restriction from the ribcage, the movements of the thoracic spine are much smaller than those of the cervical and lumbar regions. Therefore, the nerve roots, which lie in the IVF, have much less movement, and consequently the risk of irritation is not as great.[7]

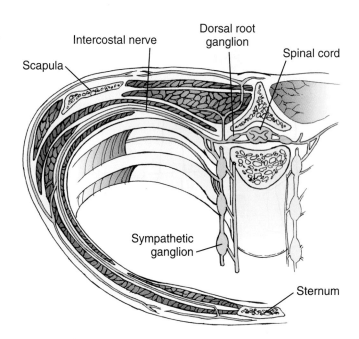

Figure 4-6. Nerves of the thoracic region, showing the intercostal nerves, spinal cord, dorsal root ganglion, and sympathetic ganglion.

Labels: Scapula; Intercostal nerve; Dorsal root ganglion; Spinal cord; Sympathetic ganglion; Sternum

NERVES OF THE THORACIC REGION

▨ **Structure:** As in the other areas of the spine, the **thoracic nerves** are mixed nerves formed from the union of **motor (ventral)** and **sensory (dorsal) roots** that emerge from the spinal cord. The roots merge to become the **spinal nerve.**

- □ **Sclerotomes:** No sclerotomes are in the thoracic spine.
- □ **Myotomes:** There are no myotomes in the thoracic region, except T1, which innervates the intrinsic muscles of the hand and controls abduction and adduction of the fingers.
- □ **Dermatomes:** Dermatomes are segmentally arranged, correspond to the level of the vertebrae, and follow the ribs. Note that the T1 dermatome covers the inner arm to the medial wrist and that the T2 covers the pectoral, scapular, and axillary regions.

- **Dysfunction and injury:** Except for T1 and T2, the thoracic spine is not generally involved in radicular (nerve root) pain, which would refer sharp, well-localized pain into the arm.[1] However, when the upper half of the thoracic spine is involved, diffuse, achy pain in the upper arm and axillary region may be greater than thoracic pain.[7]

- Irritation of the thoracic spinal nerve roots may also simulate visceral disease. For example, pain over the stomach or pancreas can be produced by T6–T7; pain over the gallbladder by T7–T8; and pain in the kidney by T9.

SYMPATHETIC NERVOUS SYSTEM

- **Structure and function:** Fibers from the **sympathetic nervous system** emerge from the spinal cord from T1–L2 and innervate the cardiac, respiratory, and digestive systems. Sympathetic nerves mediate neurological reflexes, called *viscerosomatic* and *somatovisceral reflexes,* between the internal organs and the somatic structures such as the muscles, ligaments, and joint capsules.

- **Dysfunction and injury:** Pain may be referred into the thoracic region from irritation of the abdominal organs (Fig. 4-7). For example, gallbladder irritation can refer pain to the right scapular region. The pain can vary from mild to severe and is not well localized. Pain in the thoracic somatic structures may create increased sympathetic nerve impulses to the internal organs, creating pain and decreased function.[3]

MUSCLES OF THE THORACIC REGION

- **Structure:** As was mentioned in Chapter 3, the muscles of the trunk can be divided into posterior, anterior, and lateral muscles. The muscles of the back, or posterior region, can be divided into seven fascial layers (see Table 3-2 and Figs. 3-8, 3-9, and 3-10) and two groups: the superficial (extrinsic) group, which

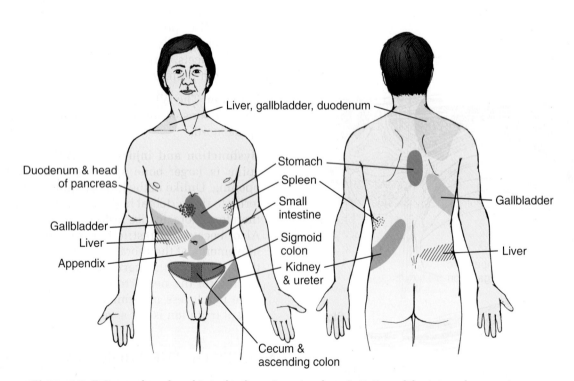

Figure 4-7. Pain may be referred into the thoracic region from irritation of the internal organs in predictable patterns.

affect the movement of the trunk, arm, and respiration, and the deep (intrinsic) group, which move the trunk, maintain posture, and stabilize the spine.

▨ Superficial back muscles: trapezius, latissimus dorsi, levator scapula, rhomboids, serratus posterior superior and inferior, and splenius capitus and cervicus.

▨ Deep back muscles can be further divided into three groups: erector spinae group (sacrospinalis), including the iliocostalis, longissimus, and spinalis; transversospinalis group, including the semispinalis, multifidus, and rotatores; and the deepest layer, consisting of the interspinalis and intertransversarii. Bogduk[8] has further divided the erector spinae into a superficial or costal portion and a deep or vertebral portion. The deep portion is not described in most texts but can be palpated by experienced therapists. It consists of lumbar fibers of the iliocostalis and longissimus (see Fig. 3-52).

▨ The anterior muscles include the flexors of the lumbosacral spine, which include the abdominals and the iliopsoas. The abdominals consist of four muscles: the rectus abdominus, internal oblique, external oblique, and transverse abdominus.

▨ The lateral muscle of the lumbosacral spine is the quadratus lumborum. It is a lateral flexor and a significant stabilizer of the spine.

▨ **Intrinsic muscles of the thorax:** The serratus posterior superior and inferior, the internal and external intercostals, and the diaphragm, are unique to the thoracic region. The spinalis group of the erector spinae, the most medial group, is found only in the thoracic and cervical region.

▨ **Function:** Muscles not only provide a dynamic stabilizing force to the thoracic region for posture and movement of the arms but also create the movement of breath (the diaphragm). Muscles also unconsciously (reflexively) communicate with the ligaments and joint capsule. Remember that muscles of the shoulder complex have a profound influence on thoracic function. Muscle contraction is often a primary source of thoracic stiffness, and restoration of proper muscle function is essential to an upright posture and normal mobility of the spine.

▨ **Dysfunction**
  □ Muscular imbalance in the thoracic spine is most commonly caused by poor posture. The client typically has a forward head, rounded shoulders, and increased thoracic curve (kyphosis).
  □ As the connective tissue of the fascia, muscle coverings, ligaments, and joint capsules adapt to faulty posture, shortening occurs in the upper chest, the

thoracic outlet regions of the supraclavicular and infraclavicular spaces, the anterior shoulder, and the posterior cervical region. Reciprocal lengthening and weakening occur in the scapular muscles, erector spinae, and lower trapezius.
  □ As in the lumbar spine, the deep stabilizers, including the multifidi and rotatores, become hypertonic with acute irritation or injury and weak with chronic problems.
  □ **Paradoxical breathing** is a common breathing dysfunction caused by stress, anxiety, and weakness of the diaphragm. On inspiration, the chest expands, but the abdomen flattens as the diaphragm is pulled up into the thoracic cavity.[9] In the author's opinion, sustained tension in the diaphragm and paradoxical breathing are primary causes of hiatal hernia.

As was mentioned, Janda[6] has identified predictable patterns of muscle imbalance. The thoracic region is susceptible to **upper crossed syndrome,** because the tight pectoralis and upper trapezius and the weak deep neck flexors, rhomboids, and middle and lower trapezius form a cross (Fig. 4-8).

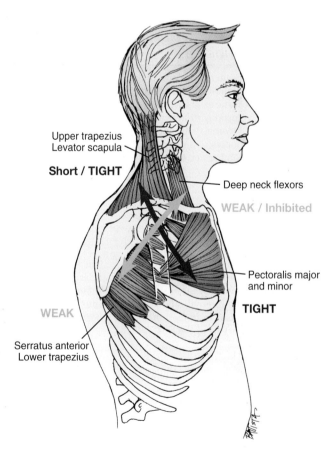

Figure 4-8. Upper crossed syndrome, a typical pattern of muscle imbalance. The upper trapezius and levator scapula are usually short and tight, and the deep neck flexors and the serratus anterior are typically weak and inhibited.

Muscle Imbalances of the Thoracic Region

▨ Muscle imbalances in the thoracic region can be caused by muscles that are weak and inhibited or by muscles that are tight and short.

  ☐ **Muscles that tend to be weak and inhibited:** The middle and lower trapezius, rhomboids, serratus anterior, deep neck flexors, multifidi and rotatores in chronic conditions, and scalenes.

  ☐ **Muscles that tend to be tight and short:** The upper trapezius and levator scapula, thoracic extensors, pectoralis major and minor, neck extensors, multifidi and rotatores in acute and subacute conditions, and diaphragm.

▨ Although the erector spinae of the thoracic region typically palpates as tight, these muscles are usually in a lengthened contraction and often test weak. This weakness is called a *stretch weakness,* as a muscle loses strength in its most lengthened position. Although the rhomboids are weak in the rounded-shoulder posture, they are often short and tight in the client with retracted and elevated shoulders. The scalenes may be either weak and long or short and tight. With a decreased cervical curve, the deep neck flexors are short and tight.

Positional Dysfunction of the Thoracic Spine Muscles

▨ Thoracic spine muscles can have the following dysfunctions of position:

  ☐ The thoracic and cervical extensors are pulled toward the midline into a medial torsion.

  ☐ The levator scapula rolls into an inferior torsion as the scapula protracts and rotates upward.

  ☐ The diaphragm is pulled toward the midline.

  ☐ The pectorals and anterior deltoid roll into an anterior and medial torsion.

▨ **Treatment implications:** In treating muscle imbalances anywhere in the body, it is important to release the short and tight muscles first, then

| Table 4-1 | Muscles of the Thoracic Spine that are Not Listed in Chapter 3 |

Muscle	Origin	Insertion	Action	Dysfunction
Diaphragm	From the dorsum of the xiphoid process, inner surfaces of the lower six costal cartilages and lower six ribs and the bodies of the upper lumbar vertebrae	Into a central tendon in the middle of the muscle	The principal muscle of respiration. During inspiration, the diaphragm contracts and descends. During expiration, the muscle relaxes, and the elastic recoil of the lungs moves the air out. The diaphragm is often held in a sustained tension, shortening its fibers and pulling the anterior-inferior portion of the rib cage toward the spine. This tension reduces full inhalation.	In the author's clinical experience, the sustained tension in the diaphragm is also an underlying cause of reflux and many conditions that have been diagnosed as hiatal hernia. The tension pulls the stomach up slightly.
External and internal intercostals	The external intercostal arises from the lower border of the ribs, and the internal intercostal arises from the inner surface of the ribs	The external and internal intercostals insert into the superior border of the ribs	These muscles elevate the ribs and expand the chest. They play an important role in respiration and posture, as they stabilize and maintain the shape of the rib cage.	When the chest is depressed, as in the rounded-shoulders posture (a kyphotic spine) or because of adhesions after injury, there is a decreased ability to expand the chest.
Levator costarum	The transverse processes of C7 and the upper 11 thoracic vertebrae	Onto the rib immediately below each vertebra	Elevates and abducts the ribs and assists in inspiration.	
Serratus anterior (See Chapter 6: The Shoulder.)				

strengthen the weak and inhibited muscles. This release may be accomplished with MET or manual techniques. For example, first release the thoracic and cervical extensors, levator, pectorals, upper trapezius, and diaphragm. Next, facilitate and strengthen the lower and middle trapezii, rhomboids, abdominals, and deep neck flexors. A typical session may involve postural assessment and correction before table work as well as after the session.

ANATOMY OF THE THORACIC REGION MUSCLES

Table 4-1 lists muscles of the thoracic spine that are not listed in Chapter: Lumbosacral Spine.

Thoracic Region Dysfunction and Injury

FACTORS PREDISPOSING TO DYSFUNCTION AND PAIN IN THE THORACIC REGION

- Poor posture
- Excessive sitting
- Joint dysfunction
- Muscle imbalances
- Deconditioning
- Fatigue
- Altered movement patterns
- Emotional tension

TYPICAL REGIONS OF DYSFUNCTION IN THE THORACIC SPINE

The junctions between the cervical spine and the thoracic spine and between the thoracic spine and the lumbar spine are two common areas of increased functional disturbances and are areas of high incidence of degenerative changes in the facet joints. This increased vulnerability has several causes.

CERVICOTHORACIC JUNCTION

- A change occurs in the orientation of the facets between C7 and T1, creating increased mechanical stress.

- This junction represents the point in the curves where the highly mobile cervical spine meets the relatively immobile thoracic spine.

- It is an area of attachment for many scapular muscles and muscles that support the weight of the head. FHP causes a drastic increase in tension to the muscles that attach in this area.

THORACOLUMBAR JUNCTION

- The orientation of the facets changes in this area from the coronal-facing facets of T12 to the mostly sagittal-facing facets at L1.

- This area often becomes hypertonic and hypomobile to compensate for a hypermobile and unstable lumbosacral junction.

- It is a high-stress area because it is where the curves change direction.

- It is prone to rotational injury.[1]

TYPICAL POSTURAL FAULTS IN THE THORACIC SPINE

KYPHOSIS

- A **kyphotic thoracic spine** is an increase in the normal posterior curve. A common cause is slouching (poor posture), which presents as the forward-head, rounded-shoulder appearance. Congenital factors, a localized healed fracture, osteoporosis, or degeneration of the vertebrae may cause also a kyphotic thoracic spine.

- If the increased curve is a result of postural changes, the following muscle imbalances typically occur:

☐ Short upper trapezius and levator scapula and weak middle and lower trapezii causing elevation and protraction of the shoulders.

☐ Tight thoracic erector spinae and weak lower trapezius causing FHP.

☐ Short and tight pectorals, especially pectoralis minor causing rounded shoulders and tight and short internal rotators creating an internally rotated humerus with a short anterior joint capsule.

☐ Weak serratus anterior causing winging of the scapula.

☐ **A flat upper thoracic spine** may be a normal variant, with completely normal X-rays and good motion characteristics, as determined by motion palpation. However, a flattened thoracic curve is often an area of painful stiffness. Postural changes and muscle imbalances with a flat thoracic spine are as follows:

☐ Decreased thoracic curve, depressed scapula and clavicle, and decreased curve in the cervical spine (military spine).

☐ Muscle imbalances such as tight erector spinae, tight scapula retractors (rhomboids and middle and lower trapezii), and decreased scapulothoracic mobility.

SCOLIOSIS

▨ **Definition: Scoliosis** is defined as one or more lateral curves in the spine (Fig. 4-9). The abnormal curve is caused by the rotation of the body of a thoracic vertebra to the side of convexity. The curve is described to the side of convexity. For example, a left thoracic scoliosis has the body of the thoracic vertbra rotated left, moving the left transverse process and left rib posteriorly on the left, creating a convexity or high side of the curve to the left.

▨ **Causes:** There are many known causes of scoliosis that are the result of disease or injury. However, 70% to 80% of cases are classified as idiopathic; that is, there is no known cause.[10] Although there is a genetic predisposition, with 25% to 33% of cases occurring among relatives of those with scoliosis, Lauren Berry, RPT, believed that scoliosis often begins as a mechanical disorder. The situation begins when a young child has a hard fall, which creates muscle hypertonicity and a vertebral fixation or subluxation in the lumbosacral region. When left untreated, this muscle hypertonicity and fixation or subluxation cause an unleveling of the pelvis, and the spine grows unevenly. This situation is based on the Heuter-Volkman theory, which states that increased pressure across an epiphyseal (growth) plate inhibits growth, whereas decreased pressure accelerates growth.[11]

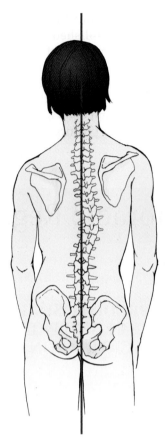

Figure 4-9. Scoliosis is a lateral deviation of the spine. View of a right thoracic scoliosis as the convexity of the curve is to the right.

▨ The paraspinal muscles have been implicated as a major causative factor in the production and progression of adolescent idiopathic scoliosis.[12] Paradoxically, some studies show greater electrical activity in the muscles at the apex of the convex side, suggesting that a deep muscle contracture of the multifidus on the convex side can create scoliosis.[12]

▨ There are two types of scoliosis: functional and structural.

☐ **Functional:** Functional scoliosis disappears with forward flexion of the trunk. It is caused by muscle imbalances, postural imbalances, or leg-length differences. The functional curve is believed to be the precursor of the structural curve.[12]

☐ **Structural:** The lateral curve does not straighten with forward or lateral flexion of the spine. The vertebrae have a fixed rotation of the body toward the convexity. Since the ribs rotate with the vertebrae, there is a prominence of the ribs posteriorly on the side of vertebral body rotation. This prominence is the result of bony deformity or soft tissue changes in the discs, ligaments, joint capsules, and muscles. Structural scoliosis is classified into two major types: irreversible and reversible.[11]

☐ **Irreversible:** Structural scoliosis that is irreversible is caused by structural deformity within, between, or around the vertebrae. The soft tissue changes are the same as those described below under reversible.

☐ **Reversible:** Structural scoliosis that is reversible is caused by structural changes that are the result of possible reversible ligament shortening or chronic muscular hypertonicity.[11] The joint capsules shorten on the concave side. The intertransversarii, erector spinae, quadratus lumborum, psoas major, and oblique abdominals all shorten on the concave side, limiting lateral flexion toward the convex side.[10]

▨ **Muscle imbalances related to scoliosis:** A complex pattern of imbalance affects the pelvis. The erectors are typically short on the concave side and weak on the convex side. In addition, there is sustained contraction in the multifidi at the apex of the convex curve.

▨ **Treatment implications:** As Kendall and colleagues[13] point out, scoliosis is a problem of asymmetry. Because muscle imbalances play an important role in the development of scoliosis, assess the length of the iliopsoas, adductors, quadratus lumborum, hamstrings, thoracolumbar fascia, iliotibial band, and latissimus. Assess the strength of the back extensors, abdominals, hip extensors, hip abductors, and lower trapezius. Also release the diaphragm, as it is typically short and tight. Soft tissue mobilization (STM) and contract-relax (CR) MET on the tight muscles and MET to help facilitate the weak muscles provide a valuable contribution. It is essential that the client receive proper exercise instruction and maintain a home program that involves stretching the tight areas and strengthening the weak areas.

DIFFERENTIATION OF THORACIC PAIN

▨ The thoracic spine and chest wall are common sites of referral from conditions other than the neuromusculoskeletal system, including inflammation and diseases of the heart, lungs, and abdominal organs. Dysfunction and injury to the thoracic spine and costovertebral joints can also mimic symptoms of diseases from these organs. These symptoms can generate a lot of anxiety because of the concern about heart disease. Refer to the section titled "Contraindications to Massage Therapy: Red Flags" in Chapter 2 for information on when a massage therapist should refer a client to a doctor. Here it is assumed that your client is under the care of a doctor for any persistent pain in the thoracic region.

▨ The vast majority of mid-back pain is caused by a mechanical disorder. The most common disorders include sustained muscle tension, hypomobility of the thoracic intervertebral and costovertebral facets, and acute fixation of those facets.

▨ Hypertonicity of the thoracic muscles is typically caused by poor posture or emotional tension, which can create a diffuse, dull ache in the mid-back and stiffness in the upper trapezius region. It is worse at the end of the day and better with rest.

▨ Corrigan and Maitland[4] state that the most common cause of chest pain is a referral from irritation of the thoracic or lower cervical facet joints. The thoracic vertebral facets produce both local and referred pain.[14] The pain is typically described as a deep, dull ache, worse with extension and rotation toward the side of pain and better with rest. With an acute episode of joint fixation and capsular inflammation, the symptoms can be sharp and well localized. If the client does not gain symptom resolution after a brief trial of therapy, refer him or her to a chiropractor or an osteopath for a trial of manipulation.

▨ Except for T1 and T2, the thoracic spine is generally not involved in radicular (nerve root) pain that would refer sharp well-localized pain into the arm.[1] However, when the upper half of the thoracic spine is involved, pain in the upper arm and axillary region may be greater than that of the thoracic region.[2]

▨ Fixation of the costovertebral or costotransverse joints often causes a "catch" or sharp pain on inspiration that may be felt posteriorly along the lateral portion of the chest wall, in the anterior chest, or through the chest.[1]

▨ Degeneration of the intervertebral facets (osteoarthrosis) or degeneration of the intervertebral disc (spondylosis) create a dull, achy stiffness in the mid-back region. The symptoms are typically worse in the morning and at the end of the day.

▨ A cervical disc lesion or injury to the lower cervical spine is a common cause of pain in the upper thoracic spine.[7] The scapular region is innervated primarily by cervical nerves and is often a referral site for cervical injury.

▓ The pain from pathologic fractures of the vertebral body, secondary to osteoporosis, is most common in the midthoracic region and is described as a persistent ache, even at rest. Remember that osteoporosis may be asymptomatic.[1]

COMMON TYPES OF DYSFUNCTION AND INJURY OF THE THORACIC REGION

THORACIC MUSCLE STRAIN (UPPER TRAPEZIUS MOST COMMON)

▓ **Causes:** Forward head, rounded-shoulders posture; emotional or psychological stress; prolonged sitting; or injury, such as a whiplash.

▓ **Symptoms:** Dull, diffuse, achy pain or stiffness—typically located in the posterior neck and upper scapular region with trapezius involvement, and in the upper back and mid-back with rhomboid hypertonicity—or sustained contraction of the lower attachments of the cervical erectors. Pain is made worse with neck movements, especially cervical flexion, or sitting, and it is relieved with rest. The suboccipital nerves are often entrapped in the fascia and muscle of the trapezius attachment to the occiput, creating an occipital headache.

▓ **Signs:** Upper trapezius, rhomboids, levator scapula, and cervical extensors are taut and tender to palpation; postural slumping; and weakness in the deep neck flexors.

▓ **Treatment:** The primary intention in treating **acute** injuries is to reduce pain, swelling, and muscle spasms. Perform the Level I series of strokes, beginning on the non-involved side. Gentle, rhythmic rocking of the body in the side-lying position is deeply relaxing. Perform reciprocal inhibition (RI) or CR MET on the tight and tender muscles, interspersed with your massage strokes. For **chronic** conditions, the intention is to identify short, tight muscles; fibrous tissue; weak muscles; and hypomobile joints. Perform both Level I and Level II strokes. Perform CR MET for the thoracic extensors (MET #4), scan the other muscles while performing the soft tissue work, and perform METs as needed. Identify weak muscles, and perform CR MET to help recruit them. The wave mobilization strokes are now performed more deeply to dissolve adhesions, and the P–A mobilization of the spine is performed more deeply to increase the motion to the joints. Depending on the severity of the injury, an acute strain resolves in 1 to 4 weeks. Strengthening exercise for the lower trapezius and scapular stabilizers, postural training, and stress management are often indicated for self-care.

ARTHROSIS (ARTHRITIS) OR SPONDYLOSIS

▓ **Causes:** Degeneration of the facet joints, often caused by adaptive shortening from poor postural habits or prior trauma, that leads to fibrosis of the joint capsules. Spondylosis is a degeneration of the intervertebral disc. In the early stages, this condition begins as hypomobility of the vertebral facets.

▓ **Symptoms:** Dull, diffuse, achy pain located in the middle of the back; usually feels stiff but can get sharp with certain movements; pain is worse in the morning and at the end of the day.

▓ **Signs:** Client often presents with forward-head and rounded-shoulder posture, with increased kyphosis. Active range of motion is limited, especially extension and lateral flexion and rotation to the painful side. Passive motion of the spine reveals a stiffened or hardened spine, with a capsular or bony-end feel. Palpation reveals thick, fibrous soft tissue.

▓ **Treatment:** The primary goal of treatment is to rehydrate the joints, lengthen capsular tissues, and reduce excessive tension in the multifidi muscles, which interweave with the joint capsules. Perform MET #4 to reduce thoracic hypertonicity and increase extensibility of the capsular tissues and MET #9 for the transversospinalis group. Perform Level I strokes, concentrating on the first series, and the first series in Level II for the multifidi. Perform strong P–A mobilization with the strokes, mobilizing the facets to rehydrate the joints. As you perform the Level I strokes, identify areas of tightness and perform MET as indicated. Clients who have degeneration need to move, such as brisk walking, and they need to stretch. Some discomfort accompanies increased movement, but it is a necessary discomfort to recover function in the joint. The general rule is that the client should be able to completely relax into the discomfort of moving the involved area.

FIXATION OR SUBLUXATION OF THE VERTEBRAL FACETS

▓ **Cause:** Injury, poor posture, muscle imbalances, and emotional or psychological tension leading to muscle hypertonicity, fatigue, and deconditioning all predispose to altered joint movement and potential fixation of the facets.

Symptoms: An acute episode involves sharp, local pain, often radiating laterally. The upper thoracic spine can cause arm pain, and the lower thoracic spine can refer pain to the lumbar spine, iliac crest, buttock, and anterior groin.

Signs: Loss of joint play at the involved joint; hypertonic and tender muscles at the fixated segment.

Treatment: Clients with **acute** thoracic pain are most comfortable in the side-lying fetal position with a pillow between the knees. Begin the Level I series of strokes on the non-involved side, with gentle rocking to induce relaxation. Perform a scanning palpation of the thoracic and lumbar regions to assess areas of tenderness and spasticity. Perform CR and RI MET for the lumbar and thoracic erectors. Perform wave mobilization strokes with a slow rhythm and light pressure until a comfortable depth has been established. The P–A mobilization to the facets will help to reduce swelling, reduce hypertonicity, and induce normal mobility to the facets. If your client does not show significant improvement after four treatments, refer to a chiropractor or osteopath to assess the need for spinal manipulation. **Chronic** fixations are hypomobile joints, and the primary intention of the treatment is to mobilize the restricted segment. Identify the hypomobility with motion palpation. Begin with the Level I series of strokes, scan the body for areas of hypertonicity, and use MET on those muscles. Perform Level II strokes, especially the first series of strokes to release the multifidi and to mobilize capsular adhesions, which will allow for greater movement at the facets. When performing the wave mobilization strokes, sink deeply into the tissue within patient tolerance to induce deep P–A mobilization on the restricted segments.

SCOLIOSIS

Cause: Some 70% to 80% of cases are classified as idiopathic, having no known cause. 25% to 30% of cases may be genetic and occur among relatives. See p. 160 for further discussion.

Symptoms: Stiff, achy back, often localized to one side. May be asymptomatic, but if the curve is noticeable, it often creates embarrassment and emotional distress.

Signs: Adam's test is positive. Client stands with feet together and with palms together, then bends over as if to place her fingertips between her feet. A positive test reveals a rib hump on the side of spinal rotation, indicating a structural scoliosis. In functional scoliosis, the curve is evident in standing and straightens in forward bending.

Treatment: In **acute** cases of thoracic pain with scoliosis, the first aim of treatment is to reduce the swelling and hypertonicity in the spinal muscles. This is accomplished through MET and Level I series of soft tissue mobilization. For chronic conditions, the client typically presents with tight and short spinal erectors on the side of concavity. The quadratus lumborum will be tight on the side of the high ilium, the iliopsoas will be tight on the side of lumbar body rotation, and the adductors will be tight on the side of the high ilium. Use postisometric relaxation (PIR) MET to lengthen the tight and shortened muscles. The gluteus medius will be weak on the side of the high ilium. Use CR MET to strengthen the gluteus medius. P–A mobilization and rib compression-decompression techniques from Level I protocol are performed for hypomobile spinal segments. The treatment goals are to reduce hypertonicity, dissolve fibrosis near the facet joints, increase mobility in restricted joints, and strengthen weak muscles. Check for leg-length imbalances and pronated ankles, as the pelvis is typically unleveled. Functional curves may be improved with manual therapy. Treatment goals for structural scoliosis are to decrease pain, hypertonicity, and maintain mobility in the joints. Treatment recommendations for acute pain are weekly treatments for six weeks, with a reevaluation. **Chronic** scoliosis protocol is based on the level of discomfort. Patients would benefit from proper exercise instruction and manipulation by a chiropractic or an osteopathic doctor.

COSTOVERTEBRAL JOINT FIXATION

Cause: The costovertebral joints are susceptible to loss of their normal gliding characteristics due to injury; muscle spasm; meniscoid entrapment; reaching, twisting, and lifting with an outstretched arm; and degeneration.

Symptoms: Localized pain, typically a few inches lateral to the SP, and when the upper ribs are involved, a dull ache in the scapular area. Often refers pain to the lateral and anterior chest. Pain can be sharp, stabbing, burning, or aching. Client may report a pain through the chest.[5] The first rib is commonly involved; symptoms include a dull, nagging ache in the lower neck with occasional burning pain in the upper trapezius.[3]

Signs: Increase in pain on deep inspiration; localized areas of extreme sensitivity to pressure at the transverse processes and rib angles; muscular spasm in the interscapular area. With first rib involvement, decreased cervical rotation to the side of fixation occurs; increased pain occurs with cervical extension.

▨ **Treatment:** For **acute** conditions, scan the muscles of the spine with gentle Level I thoracic strokes. Keep your hands soft and your P–A movements slow and shallow. Identify areas of tenderness and hypertonicity. Perform METs #1 and #4 to release the erector spinae, MET #9 to release the transversospinalis group, and MET #8 for the diaphragm and intercostals. Return to the Level I spinal strokes, and gently compress the rib cage while performing the strokes to help restore normal passive glide in the costovertebral joints. (See the note after first series of Level I strokes.) For **chronic** conditions, the same techniques described above are applied with greater depth in the strokes and stronger force with the METs. Level II strokes are applied to dissolve fibrosis in the capsular tissues of the spinal facets and costovertebral joints. PIR MET for the latissimus and thoracolumbar fascia (MET #2) is used to place traction to increase mobility. As the scalenes, serratus anterior, and subclavius all attach to the first rib, manual release and MET to those areas will help to release the fixation. (See Chapter 5, "Cervical Spine," and Chapter 6, "The Shoulder.")

OSTEOPOROSIS

▨ **Cause:** Calcium deficiency, estrogen loss, and lack of weight-bearing exercise cause a thinning of the bone and wedge-shaped vertebrae due to microfractures. Because the weight is placed on the anterior part of the vertebrae, a round back called *senile kyphosis* may occur.

▨ **Symptoms:** Osteoporosis can be asymptomatic even with a pronounced kyphotic spine. Typically, a persistent ache in the thoracic spine and a lower backache are present.

▨ **Signs:** Observation reveals either a rounded kyphosis or a sharp angulation if there is a localized collapse of a vertebra.

▨ **Treatment:** Level I thoracic and lumbar strokes are performed for **acute** pain in osteoporosis to reduce pain and swelling and induce relaxation in the muscles. Gentle CR and RI MET are performed for the thoracic and lumbar spine. Gentle P–A mobilization with the spinal strokes for the thoracic and lumbar spine helps to maintain joint movement. For **chronic** conditions, caution must be applied to all techniques. The soft tissue and joint mobilizations and METs must be pain-free. The therapist needs to exercise great caution to avoid deep pressure with the P–A spinal mobilization. Patients need weight-bearing exercise, such as walking, postural education, dietary advice, and calcium and vitamin D supplements.

Assessment

BACKGROUND

Once you have ruled out the "red flags" (see Chapter 2, "Assessment and Technique") that may indicate a serious pathology and the need for an immediate referral to a doctor, the primary intention of assessment of the thoracic spine for the massage therapist is to differentiate between three broad categories of complaints: simple conditions such as muscle tension that arise during periods of high stress, an acute episode of pain in the normally healthy client, and complaints that arise from chronic conditions in this area. The first group of clients respond well to treatment but might require advice in stress management or good posture. The second group require short-term inter-

vention to bring an injured area back to full function; and the third group respond well to long-term treatment if the client is willing to pursue active care. A few simple questions will help to differentiate between complaints arising from simple muscle tension, injury, and inflammation and chronic conditions, such as degeneration.

HISTORY QUESTIONS FOR CLIENTS WHO HAVE THORACIC PAIN

The information gathered from the history questions and examination will help you to determine (1) the appropriate depth of your massage strokes, (2) the appropriate amount of joint mobilization, (3) the strength of the pressure used in MET, (4) the necessity of referring your client to a doctor for further evaluation, and (5) the recommendations for follow-up treatments. Refer to the section "Subjective Examination: Taking a History" in Chapter 2 for more information.

Clients typically use words such as *tightness*, *stiffness*, or *aching* when describing their complaints in the thoracic region. It is important to differentiate between muscle tension problems that arise during periods of high stress, an acute episode of pain, and chronic conditions in this area. The thoracic spine is a classic area where chronic poor posture, underlying degeneration, hypomobility in the spine, or a combination of the foregoing may be underlying causes. It can be frustrating for both therapist and client to have the client return week after week with the same tension, even after a great massage therapy treatment. A few simple questions will help to differentiate complaints arising from poor posture and degeneration from simple muscle tension.

▦ How long has this area been troubling you?
  ☐ Obviously, the longer the area has been problematic, the more you suspect an underlying postural or degenerative condition. The assessment can differentiate between these two causes.

▦ Is your discomfort (pain, stiffness) better or worse in the morning?
  ☐ Muscle tension is typically better after a night's rest. Clients who have degenerative arthritis and hypomobility syndromes are stiffer or ache more in the morning and at the end of the day.

▦ Is the pain sharp and well localized or dull and achy?
  ☐ Sharp pain in the thoracic spine typically indicates a joint fixation, either at the vertebrae or at the articulation of the rib to the vertebrae. A fixation of the rib and vertebrae is often painful with breathing. Sharp pain in the spine in the elderly may also be an indication of microfractures from osteoporosis. If the client can lie comfortably on the table without pain, proceed with the massage. After the massage, refer the client who has sharp local pain to a chiropractor or an osteopath for further assessment and treatment.

OBSERVATION: CLIENT STANDING

POSTERIOR VIEW

▦ Observe the skin for any redness or swelling that may indicate inflammation and the need for much lighter pressure in your strokes. Also, notice any

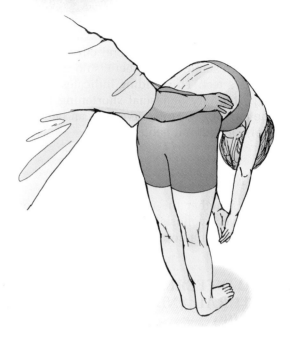

Figure 4-10. Adam's test. The therapist observes the thoracic spine to see whether the ribs deviate or form a hump to one side, a sign of structural scoliosis.

scars that may indicate a previous serious injury or surgery.

▦ Observe any asymmetry in the level of the client's shoulders and iliac crests (see Chapter 3: Lumbosacral Spine, "Observation: Client Standing," p. 122).

ADAM'S TEST

▦ The Adam's test is performed to detect whether the client has scoliosis (Fig. 4-10).
  ☐ **Position:** Have the client stand with feet and palms together, in front of you.
  ☐ **Action:** Instruct the client to bend forward until her spine is parallel to the floor. Have the client relax her arms and head, pointing the fingertips midway between the feet.
  ☐ **Observation:** Bend down so that your eyes are level with the spine. This is called the "skyline view." Note whether there is a rib hump on one side of the rib cage. The rib hump indicates that the bodies of the vertebrae have rotated to the side of the hump and that the client has structural scoliosis. If you noticed a curvature in the spine when the client was standing and the curve straightens out with performance of Adam's test, the client has functional scoliosis.
  ☐ **Structural scoliosis:** Client has a rib hump when performing Adam's test. This indicates a

dysfunction or growth deformity in the spinal body, joint structure, or both.

☐ **Functional scoliosis:** Lateral curve in the spine noted in standing, but there is no rib hump with Adam's test. This finding indicates that muscle hypertonicity or fascial shortening has caused the curvature. This curvature can be a result of work or postural habits.

SIDE VIEW

▤ Observe whether the client has an increased thoracic curve (kyphosis), a decreased curve (flat thoracic spine), or a normal curve.

TEST TO DIFFERENTIATE BETWEEN A STRUCTURAL AND A FUNCTIONAL KYPHOSIS

▤ **Position:** Have the client stand, with feet shoulder width apart. Stand to the client's side (Fig. 4-11).

▤ **Action:** Instruct the client to bend forward, arms hanging, until the spine is approximately parallel to the floor.

▤ **Observation:** Note whether the spine has a smooth, even curve or whether it has a sharp bend in the thoracic region. A sharp bend in the thoracic spine is indicative of structural kyphosis.

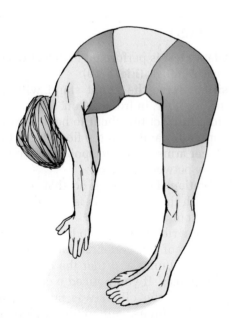

Figure 4-11. Side view of normal thoracic curve. Notice the smooth bend to the spine, rather than a sharp angle that would indicate a kyphotic spine.

MOTION ASSESSMENT

ACTIVE MOTION

▤ Active motion assessment of the thoracic spine is considered part of the motion assessment of the lumbosacral spine (see p. 121).

TEST TO CONFIRM A STRUCTURAL KYPHOSIS

▤ **Position:** Have the client lie prone on the massage table, with arms at the sides. Stand at the side of the table.

▤ **Action:** Have the client slowly lift his or her head and chest off the table to the comfortable limit.

▤ **Observation:** Note whether the kyphosis changes as the client lifts into extension. Structural kyphosis remains on active extension. A structural kyphosis is caused by bone distortion, fixation in the joints, or ligamentous shortening. A functional kyphosis is caused by sustained muscular imbalances, most commonly in the erector spinae, iliopsoas, quadratus lumborum, and diaphragm.

PALPATION

SCANNING EXAMINATION

▤ Most of the soft tissue palpation is done while performing the strokes. As you perform each stroke, feel for temperature, texture, tenderness, and tone.

MOTION PALPATION OF THE JOINTS AND PARASPINAL SOFT TISSUE

▤ **Intention:** Motion palpation is used to assess the condition of the soft tissue and joints of the thoracic region. The goal is to detect loss of joint play (hypomobility) in the intervertebral and costovertebral joints, and hypertonicity in the muscles. An experienced practitioner can differentiate stiffness in the joints from tightness in the muscle.

▤ **Position:** Have the client lie in the fetal position, with a pillow between the knees and the arms and hands folded together in the "prayer position."

▤ **Action:** Using the supported-thumb position, first perform a series of slow, medial-to-lateral scooping strokes into the medial portion of the erector spinae muscles, from approximately T12 to C7. Next, using a soft fist, press into the SPs of the thoracic spine in a P–A direction, performing a series of rhythmic P–A mobilizations on the intervertebral joints. Finally, using a double-thumb technique, perform P–A mobilizations on the costovertebral joints about 1 to 2 inches from the midline (see Fig. 4-45 later in the chapter).

▧ **Observation:** The mobilization and palpation strokes should feel relaxing and completely pain-free in the healthy spine. Healthy muscles are relaxed, pliable, and resilient. Inflamed tissue is painful. The degree of pain indicates the level of inflammation. Hypertonic muscles have a tight, springy resistance to pressure. Fibrous, chronic tension in the muscles feels thick and gristly. Healthy facet joints of the thoracic spine and cos-

tovertebral joints are resilient and bend with your pressure. Thickened ligaments and capsular tissue have a thick, "leathery" resistance to your P–A mobilization. A localized degeneration has a hard resistance to movement, while more diffuse degeneration also has this hard resistance but in a broader area.

SPECIFIC MUSCLE PALPATION

▧ Specific muscle palpation is performed in the context of doing the strokes. As you perform each stroke, feel for temperature, texture, tenderness, and tone. Through soft tissue mobilization, you can assess not only the quality of the soft tissue but also the mobility of the joints (see Chapter 2, "Assessment and Technique").

Techniques

GUIDELINES TO APPLYING TECHNIQUES

A thorough discussion of "Treatment Guidelines" can be found on p. 86 in Chapter 2: Assessment and Technique In the method of treatment described in this text, we make two underlying assumptions: that pain or dysfunction in one localized area affects the entire region, so we assess and treat an entire region rather than localized pain, and that pain that localizes in one tissue affects all of the structures in the region. Thoracic pain, for example, typically involves muscles, tendons, ligaments, joints capsules, facet joints, and intervertebral discs. This is called *somatic dysfunction*, a term developed by osteopaths that is defined as "*impaired or altered function of related components of the somatic (body framework) system; skeletal, arthrodial (joint), and myofascial structures; and related vascular, lymphatic, and neural elements.*"[15] A simple upper trapezius strain, for example, is not an isolated condition but adds compressive load to the joints of the cervical spine; affects the nerves by inhibiting the lower trapezius; affects other muscles compensating for the strain, such as a shortening of the suboccipitals; and affects the vascular and lymphatic systems. The treatment described in this text addresses all the components of somatic dysfunction through three techniques: MET, soft

tissue mobilization, and joint mobilization. These techniques can be applied to every type of thoracic pain, but the "dose" of the technique varies greatly from slow movements and light pressures for acute conditions to stronger pressures and deeper-amplitude mobilizations for chronic problems. Each aspect of the treatment is also an assessment to determine pain, tenderness, hypertonicity, weakness, and hypomobility or hypermobility. We use the philosophy of treating what we find when we find it. Remember that the goal of treatment is to heal the body, mind, and emotions. Keep your hands soft, keep your touch nurturing, and work only within the comfortable limits of your client so that he or she can completely relax into the treatment.

THE INTENTIONS OF TREATMENT FOR ACUTE CONDITIONS ARE AS FOLLOWS

▧ To stimulate the movement of fluids to reduce edema, increase oxygenation and nutrition, and eliminate waste products.

▧ To maintain as much pain-free joint motion as possible to prevent adhesions and maintain the health of the cartilage, which is dependent on movement for its nutrition.

▧ To provide mechanical stimulation to help align healing fibers and stimulate cellular synthesis.

▓ To provide neurological input to minimize muscular inhibition and help maintain proprioceptive function.

 *CAUTION: Stretching is **contraindicated** in acute conditions*

THE INTENTIONS OF TREATMENT FOR CHRONIC CONDITIONS ARE AS FOLLOWS

▓ To dissolve adhesions and restore flexibility, length, and alignment to the myofascia.

▓ To dissolve fibrosis in the ligaments and capsular tissues surrounding the joints.

▓ To rehydrate the cartilage and restore mobility and range of motion to the joints.

▓ To eliminate hypertonicity in short, tight muscles; strengthen weakened muscles; and reestablish the normal firing pattern in dysfunctioning muscles.

▓ To restore neurological function by increasing sensory awareness and proprioception.

Clinical examples are described below under "Soft Tissue Mobilization."

MUSCLE ENERGY TECHNIQUES

THERAPEUTIC INTENTION OF MUSCLE ENERGY TECHNIQUE (MET)

A thorough discussion of the clinical application of MET can be found on p. 76. The MET techniques described below are organized into one section for teaching purposes. In the clinical setting, the METs and soft tissue mobilization techniques are interspersed throughout the session. METs are used for assessment and treatment. A healthy muscle or group of muscles is strong and pain-free when isometrically challenged. MET will be painful if there is ischemia or inflammation in the muscles or their associated joints. The muscle will be weak and painless if the muscle is inhibited or the nerve is compromised. During treatment, MET is used as needed. For example, when you find tight and tender rhomboids, use CR MET to reduce the hypertonicity and tenderness. If it is painful while contracting, perform an RI MET, which contracts the pectoralis, inducing a neurological relaxation to the rhomboids.

MET is very effective for an acute, painful midback, but the pressure that is applied must be very light, so as not to induce pain. Gentle, pain-free contraction and relaxation of the thoracic extensors and related muscles provide a pumping action to reduce swelling, promoting the flow of oxygen and nutrition and eliminating waste products.

THE BASIC THERAPEUTIC INTENTIONS OF MET FOR ACUTE CONDITIONS ARE AS FOLLOWS

▓ To provide a gentle pumping action to reduce pain and swelling, promote oxygenation of the tissue, and remove waste products

▓ To reduce muscle spasms

▓ To provide neurological input to mimimize muscular inhibition.

▓ To help maintain as much pain-free joint motion as possible.

THE BASIC THERAPEUTIC INTENTIONS OF MET FOR CHRONIC CONDITONS ARE AS FOLLOWS

▓ To decrease excessive muscle tension

▓ To strengthen muscles

▓ To lengthen connective tissue

▓ To increase joint movement and increase lubrication to the joints

▓ To restore neurological function.

The MET section below shows techniques that may be used for most clients, including acute, painful conditions, but three technique (METs #2, #7, and #11) are designed for chronic conditions only.

Remember that MET should not be painful. Mild discomfort as the client resists the pressure is normal if the area is irritated or inflamed. Refer to Chapters 3 and 5 for METs for the lumbar spine and the cervical spine, respectively.

MUSCLE ENERGY TECHNIQUE FOR ACUTE THORACIC PAIN

1. Contract-Relax Muscle Energy Technique for the Thoracic Extensors

▓ **Intention:** To help reduce hypertonicity in the thoracic extensors. This MET is particularly indicated for clients who are in acute pain (Fig. 4-12).

▓ **Position:** Client is in the side-lying position, with the chin tucked slightly to lengthen the cervical

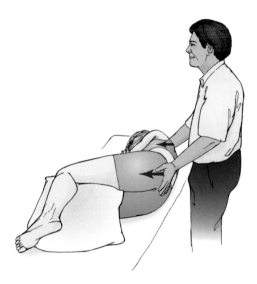

Figure 4-12. CR MET for acute thoracic pain.

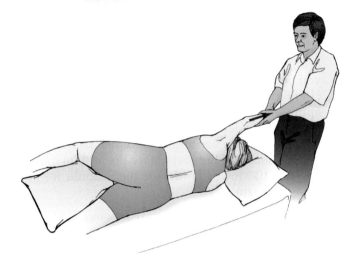

Figure 4-13. PIR MET for the latissimus dorsi and thoracolumbar fascia.

extensors. Place one hand on the occiput and your other hand on the sacrum.

▓ **Action:** Have your client resist as you press P–A with both hands. This resistance engages the client's extensors. To reciprocally inhibit the thoracic extensors, place one hand on the anterior humerus and one hand on the anterior superior iliac spine and have the client resist as you attempt to pull posteriorly.

MUSCLE ENERGY TECHNIQUES TO RELEASE HYPERTONIC MUSCLES IN THE THORACIC REGION

2. *Postisometric Relaxation Muscle Energy Technique for the Latissimus Dorsi, Lower Trapezius, and Thoracolumbar Fascia*

▓ **Intention:** To reduce muscle hypertonicity, lengthen the latissimus dorsi, and reduce tension in the thoracolumbar fascia (Fig. 4-13).

▓ **Position:** The client is in the side-lying position, and the top arm is overhead. The knees are tucked to flatten the lower back, which stretches the latissimus. Hold the distal forearm with both hands.

▓ **Action:** Have the client resist from the pelvic attachment of the latissimus as you attempt to pull the arm further overhead. Have the client relax, and as she is relaxing, pull the arm until you reach a new resistance barrier. Have the client resist as you attempt to pull again, and repeat this CR–lengthen cycle several times. Reciprocally inhibit the muscles by having the client make a fist and resist as you push on the fist toward her body.

3. *Contract-Relax Muscle Energy Technique and Sensory Awareness for the Middle and Lower Trapezii*

▓ **Intention:** To increase sensory awareness and strengthen the middle and lower trapezii. The lower trapezius is typically weak, which allows the scapula to migrate headward, losing essential stability in the shoulder complex. This MET helps the client learn to use this muscle effectively, bringing strength and sensory awareness to the muscle (Fig. 4-14).

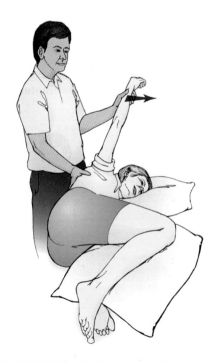

Figure 4-14. CR MET for the lower trapezius.

- **Position:** The client is side-lying. Client lifts her arm into two different positions. First, have the client lift her arm in a "T" position, that is, reaching toward the ceiling, for the middle trapezius. After you perform MET on the middle trapezius, have the client lift her arm in the "Y" position, that is, approximately 135° of abduction, with the palm facing the client's ear. Place one hand on the client's distal forearm and the other hand on the middle border of the scapula for the middle trapezius and the lower border of the scapula for the lower trapezius.

- **Action:** Have the client resist as you attempt to press the arm anteriorly for approximately 5 seconds. Tap on the muscle fibers and say, "Feel this muscle working," to bring sensory awareness to the muscle. Perform both the "T" and "Y" positions. Reciprocal inhibition (RI) is having the client resist as you attempt to pull the arm back toward you for approximately 5 seconds.

4. Contract-Relax Muscle Energy Technique to Reduce Hypertonicity in the Thoracic Erector Spinae

- **Intention:** To reduce the hypertonicity of the thoracic erector spinae and release tension in the thoracolumbar fascia.

- **Position:** The client is in the side-lying position, and the top arm is overhead in the "I" position, with palms facing the floor (Fig. 4-15). The knees are tucked to flatten the lower back, which stretches the erector spinae and thoracolumbar fascia. Place one hand on the distal forearm and the other hand on the erector spinae.

- **Action:** Instruct the client to resist as you attempt to press the arm forward for approximately 5 seconds.

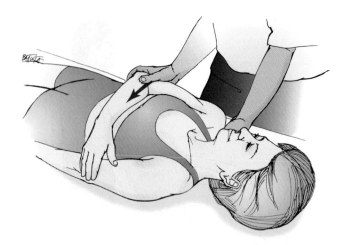

Figure 4-16. CR and PIR MET for the rhomboids.

Do not allow the client to arch the lower back as she resists you.

5. Contract-Relax and Postisometric Muscle Energy Technique for the Rhomboids

- **Intention:** To reduce hypertonicity and lengthen the rhomboids and to stretch the posterior joint capsule of the shoulder (Fig. 4-16).

- **Position:** Client is supine, with arm resting on the chest. Place one hand on the elbow and the other hand on the rhomboids.

- **Action:** Instruct the client to resist as you attempt to push the arm across her chest. Push for 5 seconds, have the client relax, and either repeat in the same position or, while the client is relaxing, stretch the rhomboids by moving the arm further across the chest, protracting the scapula. After the client relaxes, use your fingertips to scoop the rhomboids headward as you push the elbow toward the pelvis, approximately 1 inch. To reciprocally inhibit the rhomboids, after performing the PIR, have the client resist as you attempt to pull the arm laterally. This engages the pectoralis muscles and inhibits the rhomboids.

6. Contract-Relax Muscle Energy Technique for the Muscles Attaching to the Scapula

- **Intention:** To reduce the hypertonicity of the muscles attaching to the scapula (Fig. 4-17).

- **Position:** Client is in the side-lying fetal position. Place both hands on the scapula.

- **Action:** Have the client resist for approximately 5 seconds in four directions: (1) client resists as you

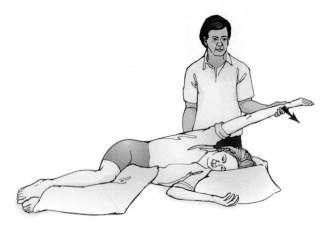

Figure 4-15. CR MET to reduce the hypertonicity in the thoracic extensor muscles.

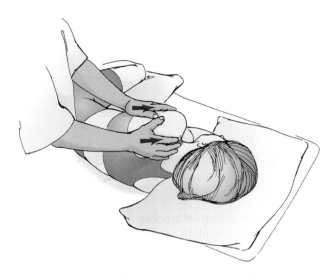

Figure 4-17. CR MET for muscles attaching to the scapula.

attempt to push the scapula headward to reduce lower trapezius hypertonicity; (2) client resists as you attempt to pull the scapula inferiorly to help release the upper trapezius and levator scapula; (3) client resists as you push the scapula anteriorly to release the middle trapezius and rhomboids; and (4) client resists as you attempt to pull the scapula posteriorly for the pectoralis minor and major. After performing the MET, mobilize the scapula in a circular motion.

7. Postisometric Relaxation Muscle Energy Technique for the Levator Scapula

▒ **Intention:** To reduce hypertonicity and lengthen the levator scapula (Fig. 4-18).

▒ **Position:** Client is in the side-lying fetal position. Place one hand over the acromion and one hand on the mastoid process.

▒ **Action:** Ask your client to rotate her head slightly toward the pillow. Next, pull the shoulder caudally until the slack in the tissue is taken out. Then ask the client to resist as you attempt to push her head into the pillow. Have the client hold for 5 seconds, then relax, and after the client relaxes for a few seconds, pull the scapula away from the head. Repeat the CR–stretch cycle several times.

8. Contract-Relax Muscle Energy Technique for the Diaphragm and Intercostals and Mobilization of the Rib Cage

▒ **Intention:** To reduce hypertonicity in the diaphragm and intercostals and to increase respiratory capacity. The diaphragm elevates the lower ribs, increasing both the anterior-to-posterior and medial-to-lateral dimensions of the thorax (Fig. 4-19).

▒ **Position:** Place the client in the supine position, with knees up and feet on the table. Facing 45° headward, place both hands on the lateral aspect of the lower ribs, with your fingers in the intercostal spaces.

▒ **Action:** Gently compress the rib cage and offer slight resistance as you ask the client to inhale slowly and fully, expanding the rib cage. As the client is inhaling, cock your wrists into ulnar deviation to elevate the anterior portion of the ribs,

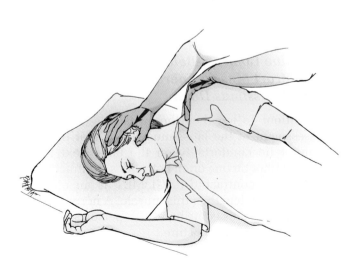

Figure 4-18. PIR MET for the levator scapula in the side-lying position.

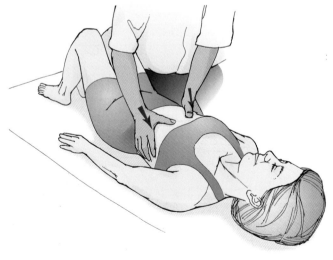

Figure 4-19. CR MET for the diaphragm and intercostal muscles and mobilization of the rib cage.

reproducing the pump-handle motion of the ribs. Tell the client to relax, and as she exhales, gently compress the rib cage to squeeze the air out and mobilize the ribs. Repeat this several times. For chronic dysfunction, after three or four resisted cyles, as the client is in the middle of an inhale, quickly release your hands to help restore the normal recoil.

▨ **Alternative Position:** A simple variation of this technique is to perform resisted inhalation with the client in the side-lying position. The therapist places one hand on the posterior rib cage and the other hand on the anterolateral rib cage. Resist the movement of the ribs as the client inhales into your hands, and gently squeeze the rib cage on the exhalation. Ulnar deviation is not required in this position.

9. Contract-Relax Muscle Energy Technique for the Transversospinalis Group

▨ **Intention:** To reduce hypertonicity in the transversospinalis group, especially the multifidi.

▨ **Position:** The client is in the fetal side-lying position. Place one hand on the upper back and one hand on the lower back (Fig. 4-20).

▨ **Action:** Have the client rotate her trunk posteriorly. Press on the client's back and resist as the client rotates into your hands for approximately 5 seconds. The multifidi are more easily engaged if the client rotates into the therapists hands rather than

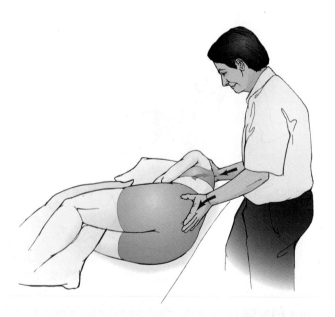

Figure 4-20. CR MET for the transversospinalis group.

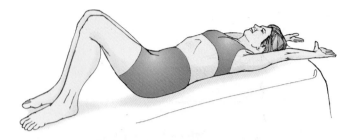

Figure 4-21. Assessment of the length of the latissimus dorsi.

resisting the therapist's pressure. Have client relax, and repeat several times. To reciprocally inhibit these muscles, place one hand on the anterior portion of the head of the humerus and the other hand on the anterior superior iliac spine. Have the client roll forward slightly and resist as you attempt to rotate her posteriorly.

10. Assessment of the Length of the Latissimus Dorsi

▨ **Intention:** To assess the length of the latissimus dorsi. The latissimus is often short, contributing to a rounded-shoulder posture, which also contributes to the humerus being internally rotated.

▨ **Position:** The client is supine, with arms at the sides, hips and knees flexed, and feet on the table (Fig. 4-21).

▨ **Action:** Have the client do a pelvic tilt to bring the lower back flat on the table. Then have the client raise her arms overhead, keeping them as close to the head as possible. Tightness in the latissimus prevents the arms from lying flat on the table when they are in an elevated position. A tight pectoralis minor pulls the scapula forward and also prevents the arms from lying flat on the table.

11. Supine Contract-Relax-Antagonist-Contract Muscle Energy Technique for the Latissimus Dorsi

▨ **Intention:** To lengthen the latissimus dorsi. If the assessment of the latissimus shows that the arms cannot lie comfortably on the table next to the head, either on one or on both sides, contract-relax-antagonist-contract (CRAC) MET is an effective technique to lengthen this muscle. A normal length in the latissimus contributes to a person's ability to assume an upright posture.

▨ **Position:** The client is supine, with the hips and knees flexed, feet on the table, and arms overhead to their comfortable limit. Hold the distal forearm

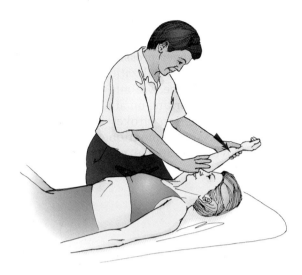

Figure 4-22. Supine CRAC MET for the latissimus dorsi.

with one hand, and stabilize the arm with the other hand (Fig. 4-22).

▨ **Action:** Instruct the client to tighten the abdominals, which flattens the lower back and thus lengthens the lower attachment of the latissimus. Next, have the client resist as you attempt to press the client's distal forearm toward the table. Press for 5 seconds. Have the client relax, then have her pull the distal arm back toward the table to the new limit. Relax, and have the client resist as you again press the distal forearm toward the table. Repeat this CRAC cycle several times. CRAC may be performed simultaneously on both arms.

SOFT TISSUE MOBILIZATION

BACKGROUND

A thorough discussion of the clinical application of soft tissue mobilization can be found on p. 68. In the Hendrickson Method of therapy described in this text, the soft tissue mobilization movements are called *wave mobilization* and are a combination of joint mobilization and soft tissue mobilization performed in rhythmic oscillations with a frequency of 50 to 70 cycles per minute, except in performing brisk transverse friction massage strokes, which can be two to four cycles per second, or if a person is in extreme distress, when the rhythm might be slower than 50 cycle per minute. These mobilizations are presented in a specific sequence, which has been found to achieve the most efficient and effective results. This allows the therapist to "scan" the body to determine areas of tenderness, hypertonicity, and decreased mo-

bility. It is important to "follow the recipe" until you have mastered this work. The techniques described below are divided into two sequences: Level I and Level II. Level I strokes are designed for every client, from acute injury to chronic degeneration, to enhance health and bring the body to optimum performance. Level II strokes are typically applied after Level I strokes and are designed for chronic conditions. Guidelines for treating acute and chronic conditions are listed below.

GUIDELINES FOR THE THERAPIST

▨ **Acute:** The primary intention of treatment is to decrease pain and swelling as quickly as possible, maintain as much pain-free joint motion as possible, and induce relaxation. In this method of treatment, the soft tissue is compressed and decompressed in rhythmic cycles. This provides a pumping action that helps to promote fluid exchange, reducing swelling. We perform the strokes for the thoracic spine in the side-lying position, which keeps the joints in their open position. This is the resting position for the spine and the most pain-free position. The strokes that are applied to the client in acute pain need to be performed with a gentle touch, slow rhythm, and small amplitude. There is no uniform "dose" or depth of treatment. The depth of treatment is based on the client's level of pain. If the soft tissue does not begin to relax, return to gently rocking the body and then use more METs, especially METs #1, #4, and #9, to help reduce muscle guarding. As was mentioned previously, intersperse your soft tissue mobilization work with MET. Remember that **stretching is contraindicated** in acute conditions.

▨ **Chronic:** The typical exam findings in clients with complaints in the thoracic region are short and tight upper trapezius, levator scapula, and pectoralis major and minor and weakness in the anterior neck and scapular stabilizers (the upper crossed syndrome). The erector spinae and diaphragm are typically hypertonic. The joints are typically hypomobile, with thick, fibrotic ligaments and capsular tissues. Some patients demonstrate the opposite: hypermobility in the joints; weak, deconditioned muscles; and atrophy in the ligaments and capsular tissues. This latter condition is described as *instability*. The primary goals of treatment depend on the patient. For patients who are hypomobile, the treatment goals are to reduce the hypertonicity of the muscles; promote mobility and extensibility in the connective tissue by dissolving the adhesions in the muscles, tendons, ligaments, and capsular tissues surrounding the joints; rehydrate the cartilage of the facet joints and discs; establish normal joint play and range of motion in the joints; and restore normal neurological function by stimulating the proprioceptors and reestablishing the normal firing patterns in the muscles. Patients who are unstable need exercise rehabilitation. Our treatments can support their stability by reducing tension in the tight muscles and performing MET to the weak muscles to help reestablish normal firing patterns and to rehabilitate the proprioceptors. With chronic thoracic conditions, it is also important to treat tightness in the lumbar and cervical spine. With chronic conditions, we use stronger pressure on the soft tissue and more vigorous mobilizations on the joints. In the Level II sequence, we add deeper soft tissue work, as well as working on attachment points, using transverse friction strokes if we find fibrosis (thickening). As was mentioned in the "Acute" section above, intersperse your soft tissue work with METs.

Clinical Example: Acute

Subjective: AM is a 37-year-old acupuncturist who presented with pain in her low back and thoracic region and severe pain in her anterior chest, especially the sternum, after being thrown from a horse one week previously. She was taken to the emergency room, where X-rays were performed, and they were negative for fracture. She described the worst pain as a deep ache in the chest with occasional intense, sharp pain, especially if she tried to lie down. Consequently, she was sleeping sitting up. She denied any referral of pain into the arms or legs.

Objective: Examination revealed that active range of motion of the trunk was severely limited owing to pain in the chest. Palpation revealed severely tender anterior chest, especially at the sternum, and spastic and tender lumbar and thoracic muscles. Gentle P–A motion palpation of her spine revealed dramatic guarding.

Assessment: Inflammation of the sternocostal and costochondral joints (costochondritis) and spasticity and inflammation of the erector spinae.

Treatment (Action): The treatment began with the patient in the side-lying position with a pillow between the knees and another in front of her chest to support her arm. I began with slow, gentle rocking of the whole body to induce a relaxation response. I began Level I wave mobilization strokes in the thoracic region slowly and gently, using very little pressure. The intention was to assess the level of muscle guarding. The tissue was very tight and mildly tender, but if I pressed slightly too deep, she felt pain in the chest. I performed very gentle CR and RI METs (MET #1) for the thoracic extensors several times. This reduced hypertonicity and provided a pumping action for the lymph and blood, reducing intramuscular edema and promoting reoxygenation of the tissue. The muscles were much less tender after three to four MET cycles. The treatment continued with the Level I series of strokes for the erector spinae. I used METs #3 and #6 to induce relaxation in the trapezius and muscles attaching to the scapula. I performed the RI MET for #6 with extremely light pressure to begin to engage the anterior chest muscles. Although they were tender to light contraction, she could relax into the MET. I performed the wave mobilization strokes over the thoracic spine again for several minutes. The muscles began to relax, and the movement of the spine and ribs became more comfortable. I applied the same treatment to her other side. Next, I asked her to lie on her back and supported her neck with several pillows. Palpation revealed a very tender anterior chest. A series of very gentle METs (#6 shoulder) were used for pectoralis major, which attaches to the sternum. I then used an extremely gentle MET for the rib cage (MET #8 thoracic). She was able to provide only the most minimal inspiration against my hands holding her rib cage. The session ended with gentle work on her cervical spine. She reported feeling much better after the session. She was able to breathe more easily and move about the treatment room with much less discomfort.

Plan: I recommended weekly visits for four weeks. The same treatment techniques described above were repeated. At the sessions progressed, she was able to relax into deeper pressures with the P–A mobilization, which helped to normalize motion of the spine and rib cage. At the time of her fourth visit, she reported feeling much better and that she was able to sleep much more comfortably and perform her other daily activities with much less pain. She was now beginning exercises. I recommended four additional treatments over the next two months. At the time of her last visit, examination demonstrated full and pain-free range of motion and normal motion in the soft tissue and joints. We were able to mobilize the rib cage and spine without pain. She reported that she was able to perform her daily activities without pain. She was discharged from active care but elected to return in one month for wellness care.

Clinical Example: Chronic

Subjective: NB is a 66-year-old professor who presented to my office complaining of chronic "enormous tightness" in his mid-back, which affected his breathing, especially while swimming. His history includes a laminectomy and spinal fusion for a herniation of the L4–L5 disc. He denied a prior injury to the thoracic region.

Objective: Examination revealed a significant loss of thoracic extension and significant loss of passive motion of the intervertebral and costovertebral joints. The ribs had very little resilience. The erector muscles, rhomboids, and levator scapula were thick and dense, and the lower trapezius was weak.

Assessment: Hypomobility of the costovertebral and intervertebral joints, with adhesions in the soft tissues.

Treatment: I began with gentle rocking of his whole body in the side-lying position to induce a relaxation response. Because his erector spinae was thick and tight, I used MET #4 to reduce the hypertonicity in the erectors, and MET #2 to lengthen the latissimus and thoracolumbar fascia. I began wave mobilization strokes, emphasizing the P–A mobilization of the vertebral and costovertebral facets. In the beginning, the joints felt rigid and resistant to movement. I performed MET #2 several more times to lengthen the fascia and decompress the joints. His muscles began to relax and allow greater amplitude with the wave mobilization strokes. I next concentrated on the diaphragm and intercostals, performing both MET #8 and the fifth series of Level I soft tissue mobilization strokes in the side-lying position. The diaphragm attachments on the posterior aspect of the anterior rib cage were thick and tender. The rib cage was rigid as we began the MET and soft tissue work but began to gain more "spring" as we worked. I performed the same treatment on the other side and then began to work with him supine. His pectoralis muscles were tight, and I used MET #6 from Chapter 6, "The Shoulder." I ended the treatment with him supine and performed a series of METs and Level I cervical strokes. He was in a profound state of relaxation at the end of our session and noticed that his breathing was much easier.

Plan: I recommended a series of weekly visits for one month. I performed the strokes with deeper pressure and a stronger P–A component to help induce increased lubrication and joint play in both the intervertebral and costovertebral joints. I repeated the same basic treatment each visit, concentrating on areas of fibrosis, hypertonicity, and hypomobility. As I penetrated deeper into the tissue, I used shorter, more brisk transverse friction strokes on the multifidi and joint capsules (Level II, series 1). I interspersed the soft tissue work with MET #9 to release the transversospinalis group. He reported less stiffness in his mid-back and that his breathing was greatly improved with his usual swimming exercise. Upon examination, there was a significant decrease in muscular tension, and there was better glide and greater range of motion to the facets joints. I recommended another series of weekly visits for one month to help resolve the deep level of adhesions. After that series, I recommended treatments once a month to help improve his functional status. At that time, we began working on his low back and neck, which both had limited motion but were not symptomatic.

Table 4-2	Essentials of Treatment

- Rock the client's body while performing the strokes.
- Shift your weight while performing the strokes.
- Perform the strokes rhythmically, about 50 to 70 cycles per minute.
- Keep your hands and whole body relaxed.

Table 4-2 lists some essentials of treatment.

LEVEL I: THORACIC

1. *Release of the Thoracolumbar Fascia, Latissimus, Trapezius, and Erector Spinae*

- **Anatomy:** Thoracolumbar fascia, latissimus, trapezius (Fig. 4-23), erector spinae (see Fig. 3-9).

- **Dysfunction:** The erector spinae tends to pull toward the midline and needs to be moved in a medial-to-lateral direction. The fascia and ligaments thicken with chronic tension, a common cause of hypomobility in the thoracic spine.

Position

- **Therapist Position (TP):** Standing, facing 45° headward for longitudinal strokes and 90° toward the client for transverse strokes.

- **Client Position (CP):** Side-lying.

Strokes

The strokes have two directions in three lines. The first line is along the SP, the second line is approximately 1 to 2 inches laterally over the area of the costotransverse joint, and the third is on the ribs approximately 2 to 4 inches laterally. These strokes also promote hydration of the joints through gentle mobilization in P–A glide.

1. Perform MET for the trapezius, latissimus, thoracolumbar fascia, and erector spinae (see Figs. 4-13 to 4-15).
2. Using the supported-thumb technique, perform a series of short, scooping strokes, in an inferior to superior direction, approximately 1 inch in length, beginning at T12 and continuing to C7 on the areas outlined above, covering all three lines (Fig. 4-24). Superficially, these strokes release the thoracolumbar fascia, the latissimus dorsi, and the trapezius. More deeply, these strokes release the erector spinae.
3. Perform a series of strokes, in a medial to lateral direction, approximately 1 inch in length. Begin at

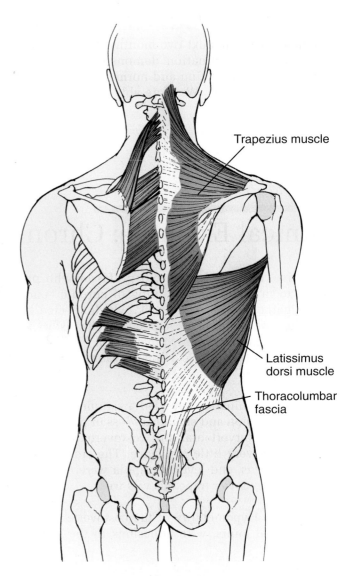

Figure 4-23. Thoracolumbar fascia, latissimus dorsi, and trapezius.

T12, just lateral to the SP (Fig. 4-25). Move to the C7 area inch by inch. Begin a second line approximately 1 inch laterally, from T12 to C7. Repeat a third series on the soft tissue over the ribs from T12 to C7.

Clinical Reminder: To assist in the effectiveness of these strokes, gently compress the rib cage with the supporting hand as you sink into the tissue with the working hand. This brings the tissue into slack, helps to turn off the muscle spindle cells, and mobilizes the ribs and the vertebral facets. Pull the rib cage back as you move onto your back leg, then gently compress the rib cage as you move onto your front leg with the stroke. If a client is particularly tense, it is important

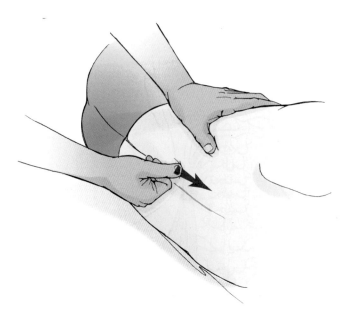

Figure 4-24. Supported-thumb technique for inferior-to-superior release of the thoracolumbar fascia, latissimus dorsi, trapezius, and erector spinae.

to slow your strokes down and work on the client's exhale, as this also enhances relaxation.

2. *Transverse Release of Rhomboids*

▨ **Anatomy:** Rhomboid major and minor (Fig. 4-26).

▨ **Dysfunction:** These muscles tend to shorten from chronic stress or become weak, allowing the scapula to protract away from the spine. In the weakened position, there is a decreased scapular

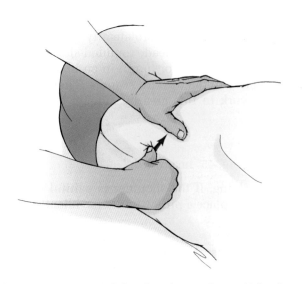

Figure 4-25. Supported-thumb technique for medial-to-lateral release of the medial line of soft tissue next to the spinous process.

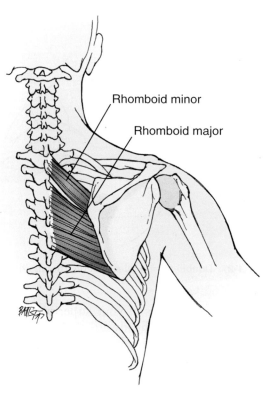

Figure 4-26. Rhomboid major and minor.

stabilization and an increased likelihood of glenohumeral impingement, as the acromion overhangs the head of the humerus.

Position
▨ **TP:** Standing, facing 45° headward.

▨ **CP:** Side-lying.

Strokes
1. Perform CR MET on the muscles that attach to the scapula (see Fig. 4-17, p. 171).
2. Using a supported-thumb, double-thumb, or fingertips technique, perform 1-inch, inferior-to-superior, scooping strokes on the rhomboids (Fig. 4-27). Begin next to the SP of C7 and perform a series of strokes between C7 and the vertebral border of the scapula. Begin the next line of strokes about 1 inch inferior at T1, and perform inferior-to-superior strokes between T1 and the scapula. Work the entire area from the T5 to C7 SPs to the vertebral border of the scapula. The strokes are performed as rhythmic oscillations. Your supporting hand is on the scapula and moves it headward, coordinated with the movement of each stroke.
3. Another way to release the rhomboids is with shearing strokes. Beginning on the vertebral border at the superior angle of the scapula, use the supported

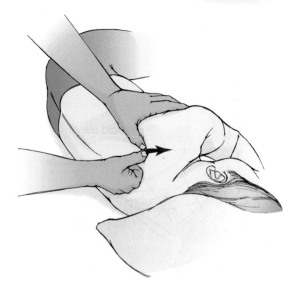

Figure 4-27. Double-thumb release of the rhomboids.

thumb or fingertips of your superior hand to perform short, lifting, headward strokes on the rhomboids as your inferior hand cups the head of the humerus and pulls the scapula in an inferior direction (Fig. 4-28). Continue to the inferior angle. These strokes are more staccato and more quickly paced. Rotate your entire body from the waist as you perform the strokes. The shearing technique brings the deeper fibers up to the surface, where they can then be released.

3. Release of the Levator Scapula at the Superior Angle of the Scapula

▨ **Anatomy:** Levator scapula (Fig. 4-29).

▨ **Dysfunction:** The superior angle of the scapula is a critical stress point due to the strain on the levator

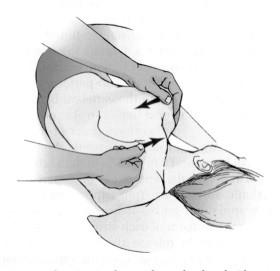

Figure 4-28. Shearing stroke to release the rhomboids.

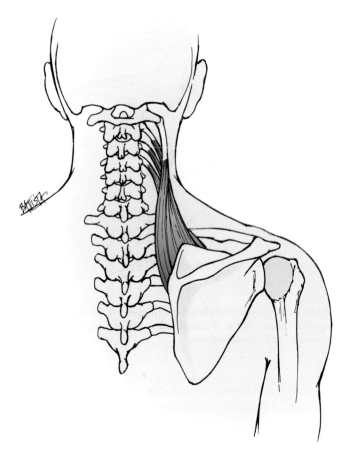

Figure 4-29. Levator scapula.

as it holds the head in an upright position. The levator tends to drop into an inferior-medial torsion relative to the superior angle of the scapula and must be lifted in a 45° headward direction. This might seem paradoxical, but Lauren Berry, RPT, taught that the typical pattern of dysfunction is for the scapula to rotate anterolaterally around the rib cage in the forward-head, rounded-shoulder posture and for the levator to roll in an inferior direction relative to the upward scapula. Therefore, finish the work in this area by moving the scapula down.

Position

▨ **TP:** Standing, 45° headward.

▨ **CP:** Side-lying. If the shoulder is painful or especially tight, place a pillow under the client's arm.

Strokes

1. To help release a short and tight levator scapula, perform PIR MET (see Fig. 4-18, p. 171).
2. Perform 1-inch, scooping strokes on the levator scapula in a 45° headward direction, using fingertips, single-thumb, or supported-thumb technique

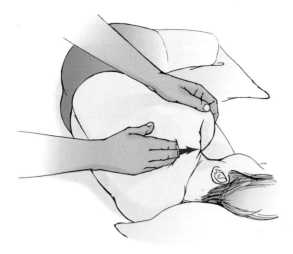

Figure 4-30. Fingertip release of the levator scapula.

with your superior hand (Fig. 4-30). Begin at the superior angle of the scapula, and continue your strokes to the cervical spine. The strokes are performed as rhythmic oscillations. Your supporting hand is on the scapula and moves it headward, coordinated with the movement of each stroke.

3. Perform shearing strokes on the levator scapula (Fig. 4-31). Using the thumb or fingertips of your superior hand, perform short, scooping strokes in a 45° headward direction. Your supporting hand cups the head of the humerus and draws it toward you, moving the scapula inferiorly. Coordinate the movement of the two hands in a rhythmic oscillation.

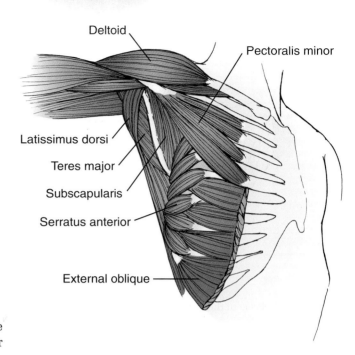

Figure 4-32. Latissimus dorsi, external abdominal oblique, serratus anterior, and pectoralis minor.

4. Release of the Lateral Rib Cage and the Anterior Surface of the Scapula

▨ **Anatomy:** Latissimus dorsi, pectoralis minor, serratus anterior, external obliques (Fig. 4-32).

▨ **Dysfunction:** The scapulothoracic joint can become hypomobile owing to chronic tension or adhesions at the inferior angle caused by tension in the latissimus or a short serratus anterior. It can also become hypermobile owing to a weak serratus, rhomboid, and trapezius; when strong, these muscles provide scapular stabilization. These strokes are for hypomobility and adhesions.

Position

▨ **TP:** Standing, 45° or 90° to the client.

▨ **CP:** Side-lying.

Strokes

1. Have the client rest his or her arm on a pillow. Facing 45° headward, use a fingertips-next-to-thumb technique, and perform anterior-to-posterior scooping strokes on the lateral rib cage, following the contour of the bone, to release the latissimus dorsi and serratus anterior. Proceed to the hairline of the axilla (Fig. 4-33).

2. Place the client's arm in 90° flexion, 90° internal rotation, and 90° elbow flexion. Face 45° headward and use your fingertips to perform short, scooping strokes in a lateral-to-medial direction on the anterior rib cage for the pectoralis minor (Fig. 4-34).

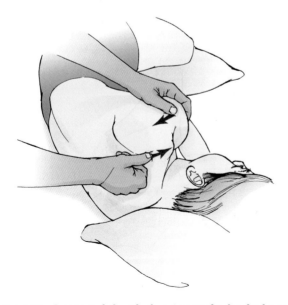

Figure 4-31. Supported-thumb shearing stroke for the levator scapula. Pull the scapula back with one hand as you scoop the levator 45° headward.

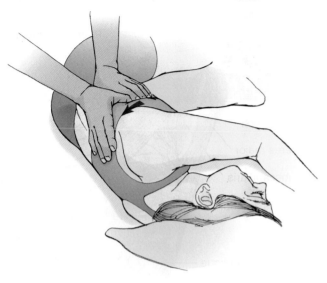

Figure 4-33. Release of the lateral and anterior rib cage using fingertips and thumb.

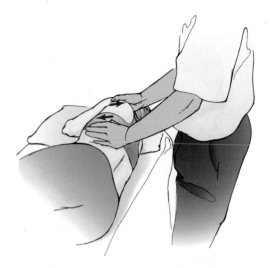

Figure 4-35. Thumb release of the inferior angle of the scapula.

3. Facing 90° to the table, release the latissimus from the inferior angle of the scapula by using the thumb of the inferior hand to push the latissimus anteriorly while using the superior hand to cup the humerus and pull the scapula posteriorly (Fig. 4-35). This is a back-and-forth shearing stroke to dissolve the adhesions.

4. Facing 45° headward, place the client's arm on the lateral aspect of his or her rib cage. Stabilize the client's arm by placing your forearm next to his or her arm, cupping the head of the humerus. Cup the fingertips of your superior hand under the vertebral border of the scapula to touch the attachments of the serratus anterior. Scoop headward with your fingertips in 1-inch strokes as you mobilize the client's arm and scapula headward (Fig. 4-36). If

you cannot place your fingertips under the scapula, have the client roll backward slightly and place his or her arm behind the back, as this position wings the scapula and exposes the undersurface.

5. *Release of the Diaphragm*

■ **Anatomy:** Diaphragm (Fig. 4-37).

■ **Dysfunction:** The diaphragm attachments tend to thicken with chronic tension, which is often due to rounded-shoulders posture, lack of aerobic exercise, shallow breathing from emotional tension, disease processes that cause difficulty breathing, such as asthma, or chronic hypomobility of the

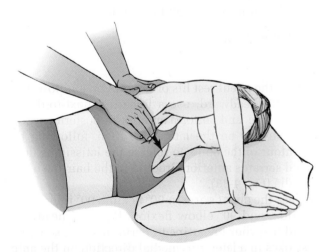

Figure 4-34. Fingertip release of the pectoralis minor.

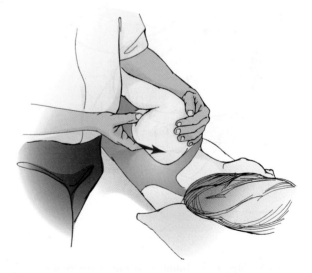

Figure 4-36. Fingertip release of the attachments of the serratus anterior on the anterior surface of the scapula.

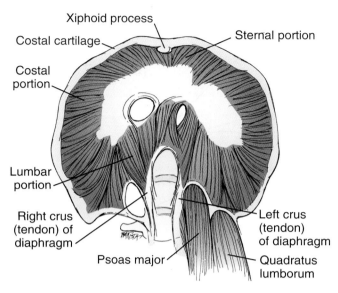

Figure 4-37. The diaphragm, showing its attachments to the inner surface of the rib cage.

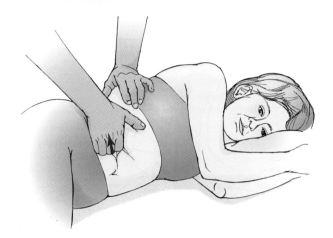

Figure 4-38. Side-lying release of the diaphragm.

costovertebral joints. Chronic tension in the diaphragm adds significantly to the hypomobility of the spine and to thoracic kyphosis. Tension in the diaphragm pulls the muscle fibers toward the midline and pulls the thoracic cage forward. The diaphragm attaches to the lumbar vertebrae by means of a powerful tendon called the crus. Persistent coughing or even a sneeze can severely irritate the lumbar discs.

Position
▨ **TP:** Standing.

▨ **CP:** Side-lying position; or, supine, with knees up.

Strokes
1. Perform MET for the diaphragm (see Fig. 4-19, p. 171).
2. Place your client in the side-lying position (Fig. 4-38). Place your working hand on the lateral aspect of the rib cage such that your flexed fingertips are approximately 1 inch inferior to the ribs. As the client exhales, use your stabilizing hand to compress the lateral rib cage gently into your working hand to give some slack to the tissue. Tuck your fingertips under the rib cage, then stroke on the posterior surface of the ribs in a medial to lateral direction. Proceed in 1-inch segments to the midline.
3. With the client supine, stand in the 45° headward position, opposite the side being worked on (Fig. 4-39). Beginning on the most lateral aspect of the anterior rib cage, place your thumb or braced thumb approximately 1 inch below the ribs. This hand placement allows some slack in the tissue.

On the client's exhale, gently press under the ribs and flex your thumb onto the posterior surface of the ribs, then scoop in a medial-to-lateral direction. Perform a series of slow, gentle, scooping strokes on the inner surface of the ribs in 1-inch segments, continuing to almost 1 inch lateral to the xiphoid process at the midline. Tell the client that there might be some sensitivity in this area if there are adhesions of the diaphragm to the rib cage, including a burning or biting pain. Remember to mention to the client that she should be able to completely relax. Releasing this area may elicit an emotional response. Proceed slowly and with sensitivity.

LEVEL II: THORACIC

1. *Release of the Transversospinalis Group*

▨ **Anatomy:** Semispinalis thoracis, cervicis, multifidus, rotatores (Fig. 4-40).

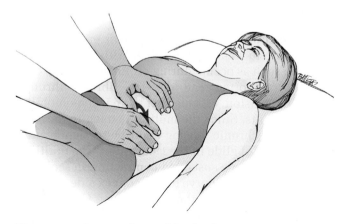

Figure 4-39. Supine release of the diaphragm.

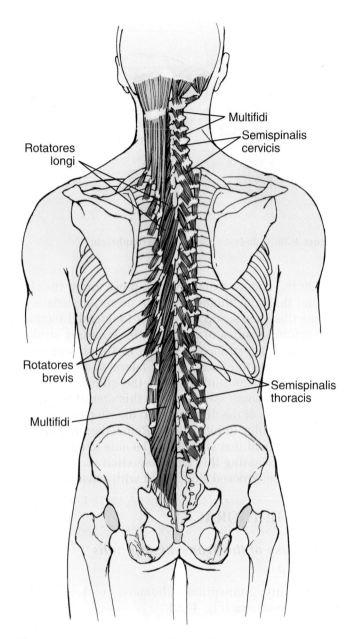

Figure 4-40. Transversospinalis muscle group.

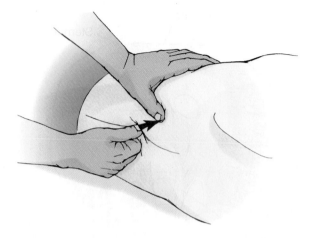

Figure 4-41. Supported-thumb release of the transversospinalis group.

Position

■ **TP:** Standing, facing 45° headward.

■ **CP:** Side-lying.

Strokes

1. Perform CR MET on the transversospinalis group (see Fig. 4-20, p. 172).

2. Using a supported-thumb or a braced-thumb technique, perform a series of scooping strokes in a 45° headward direction (Fig. 4-41). Place your thumb next to the SP, and slide it along the SP, tucking your thumb under the erector spinae to release the multifidi and semispinalis group in the area between the SP and the transverse processes. The stabilizing hand presses into the rib cage with a gentle compressing force with each stroke. This gives some slack to the erector spinae, allowing an easier access to the deeper transversospinalis group. It also mobilizes the ribs and costovertebral joints. Perform these strokes from T12 to C7, 1 inch at a time. This series can be done many times to dissolve the adhesions in the connective tissue layers of the muscles and to mobilize the spine.

2. *Release of the Attachments to the Spinous Processes*

■ **Anatomy:** Trapezius, thoracolumbar fascia, supraspinous ligament, rhomboid major, splenius cervicis, spinalis, multifidus, and rotatores (Fig. 4-42).

■ **Dysfunction:** The tenoperiosteal junctions on the SPs are an interweaving of the fascia, the supraspinous ligament, and the fascial expansions of the muscles. Attachments thicken as the result of previous injury or chronic dysfunction, such as poor posture. Extended periods of sitting, especially in a slumped posture, create a tethering or pulling

■ **Dysfunction:** The transversospinalis group of muscles help to stabilize the spine. With lack of movement, such as occurs during prolonged sitting, they tend to shorten and develop fibrosis through chronic tension, especially if there is hypomobility in the joints. Since the multifidi attach to the joint capsules, chronic tension contributes significantly to the lack of glide in the facet joints. The multifidi may also be in a sustained contraction in scoliosis, at the apex of the curve on the convex side. Pay particular attention to the T12–L1 and C7–T1 junctions, as these are the most common areas of facet degeneration.

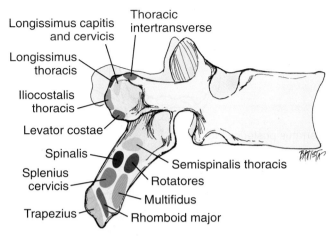

Figure 4-42. Muscle attachments to thoracic spinous processes.

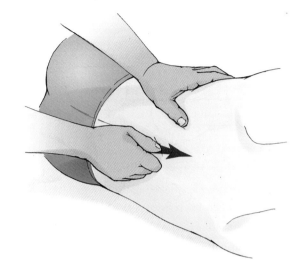

Figure 4-43. Supported-thumb technique to release attachments to the thoracic spinous processes.

force on the SPs. Over time, the tissue thickens and becomes ischemic and tender. This treatment is for chronic conditions only.

Position

▨ **TP:** Standing, facing 45° headward.

▨ **CP:** Side-lying.

Strokes

Note that the midthoracic SPs are angled steeply in an inferior direction, whereas the upper thoracic SPs are almost straight posterior. Your intention is to clean the bone, as a healthy bone has a smooth and glistening feel to it.

1. Beginning at the SP of T12, use a supported-thumb technique to perform short, back-and-forth strokes in the inferior to superior plane on the SP of each of the thoracic vertebrae (Fig. 4-43). Your flexed index finger rests on the other side of the SP. You may use a slight pinching grasp of the SP to stabilize your thumb. Use your supporting hand to compress the rib cage gently as you are working, thus bringing the overlying soft tissue into slack. Rock the entire body as you work. If the soft tissue attachments to the SP feel fibrous, you may use brisk, back-and-forth strokes.

3. *Release of the Soft Tissue at the Transverse Processes*

▨ **Anatomy:** Longissimus thoracis, cervicis, and capitis; semispinalis thoracis, cervicis, and capitis; iliocostalis thoracis and intertransverse; multifidus; and levator costarum (Fig. 4-44).

▨ **Dysfunction:** The area in the region of the transverse process is clinically significant for two

main reasons. First, there are significant muscle attachments on the transverse processes between the mid-back and the neck and head. These muscles become chronically taut in a FHP. Second, hypertonicity in the muscles attaching to the transverse process can create compression in the rib joints, owing to the interweaving of the muscles, fascia, and ligaments. This would decrease the mobility of the ribs. Hypertonicity may also be caused by a loss of normal joint play at the costovertebral joint (the rib is "out"), which leads to irritation of the joint. A reflex to the surrounding muscles, called an *arthrokinetic reflex,* creates hypertonicity.

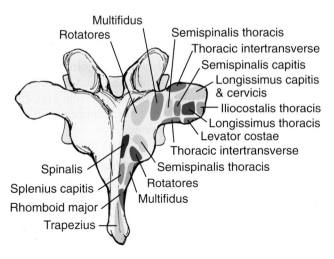

Figure 4-44. Muscle attachments to thoracic transverse processes.

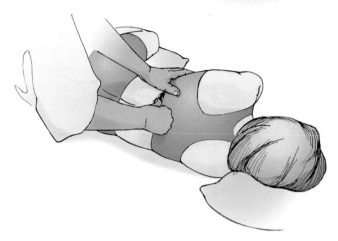

Figure 4-45. Supported-thumb release of attachments to the thoracic transverse processes and mobilization of the costotransverse joints.

Position

▧ **TP:** Standing, 90° to the line of the fiber.

▧ **CP:** Side-lying.

Strokes

1. Using a supported-thumb or braced-thumb technique, begin a series of strokes on the muscle attachments to the transverse processes and on the muscle attachments to the ribs at the area of the T12 vertebra approximately 1 to 2 inches lateral to the SP (Fig. 4-45). First, perform short, slow, scooping strokes, and then perform brisk transverse strokes where you find areas of fibrosis. You are "looking" with your hands for a feeling of hypertonicity or thickening and fibrosis. The direction of the strokes may be slightly inferior, slightly superior, 45° headward, or 90° to the midline. As you perform the slow, scooping strokes, you are pressing P–A into the area of the costotransverse joint. Identify areas of hypomobility, and repeat the strokes many times in those areas. Emphasize the P–A mobilization in your strokes to help restore normal mobility to these joints.

2. Continue this series of strokes to the C7 vertebra. Perform several strokes in the area of one vertebra, then move approximately 1 inch higher and perform another series of strokes.

4. *Release of the Iliocostalis Thoracis, Cervicis, Serratus Posterior Superior*

▧ **Anatomy:** Iliocostalis thoracis, cervicis, serratus posterior superior (Fig. 4-46).

▧ **Dysfunction:** The iliocostalis thoracis and cervicis are often hypertonic as a result of FHP or an injury to the neck. The iliocostalis develops an eccentric

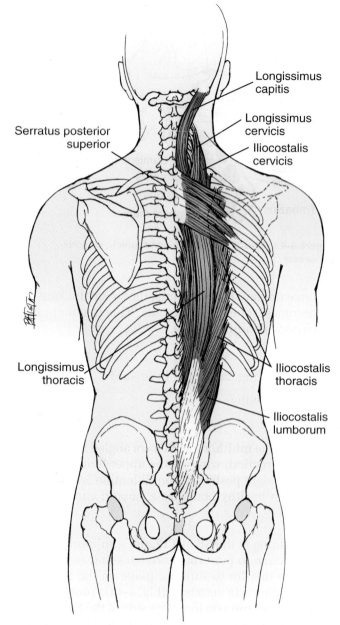

Figure 4-46. Iliocostalis thoracis and cervicis and serratus posterior superior.

contraction with FHP that leads to tenderness under the scapulae. These muscles tend to develop fibrosis under chronic tension. The serratus posterior superior acts like a retinaculum holding down the erector spinae and can also assist in elevating the ribs. As this muscle is attached to ribs 2 to 5, it is often hypertonic and can develop a tender thickening, especially with fixation of the upper ribs.

Position

▧ **TP:** Standing, 90° to the line of fiber.

▧ **CP:** Side-lying and supine.

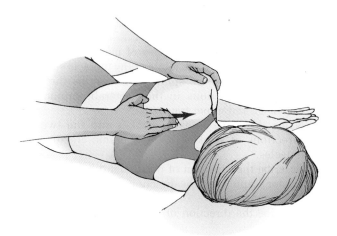

Figure 4-47. Fingertip release of serratus posterior superior.

Strokes

Locate the serratus posterior superior under the rhomboids and the trapezius. The serratus feels flat and fibrous, like a tuck in a sheet over the ribs, not fleshy like the rhomboids. To palpate the difference, move the scapula toward the spine. As the rhomboids attach to the scapula, they slacken and feel fleshy at the vertebral border of the scapula. The serratus remains flat against the ribs. If you press deeply over the ribs in a 45° headward direction, you feel the serratus "strum" under your fingers.

1. Using a supported-thumb or fingertips technique, perform a series of 45° headward, scooping strokes through the rhomboids on the serratus posterior superior. Cover the entire muscle from its attachments at the SPs of C7 and upper two or three thoracic vertebrae to its attachments to ribs 2 to 5 under the scapula (Fig. 4-47).
2. Using a supported-thumb, fingertips, or double-thumb technique, perform short, scooping strokes in a medial-to-lateral direction to release the iliocostalis thoracis and cervicis (Fig. 4-48). They are

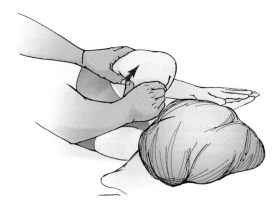

Figure 4-48. Double-thumb release of the iliocostalis thoracis and cervicis.

running underneath the vertebral border of the scapula. With your supporting hand, move the scapula laterally as you stroke, coordinating the two hands in a rhythmic oscillation. Cover the entire area under the scapula.

3. An alternative position for releasing the iliocostalis is to first have the client lie on her back. Place the client's forearm on her chest, and grasp the elbow with your inferior hand. Place the fingertips of your superior hand on the iliocostalis, and perform a series of medial-to-lateral scooping strokes as you move the client's arm across the chest.

5. *Release of the Posterior Scalene and Iliocostalis Cervicis at the Upper Ribs*

▨ **Anatomy:** Posterior scalene, iliocostalis cervicis (Fig. 4-49).

▨ **Dysfunction:** These muscles are eccentrically contracted under an excessive load from a FHP. They can also develop a sustained contraction after a neck injury such as a whiplash. Attachment points tend to thicken.

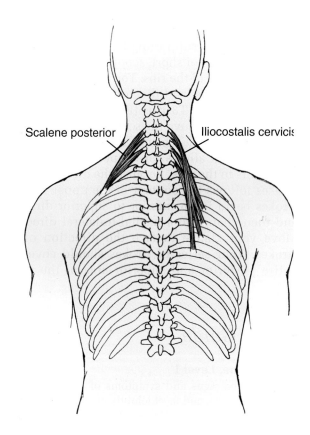

Figure 4-49. Posterior scalene and iliocostalis cervicis.

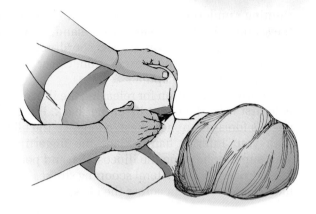

Figure 4-50. Fingertip release of posterior scalene and iliocostalis attachments to the T1 to T3 ribs.

Position
▓ **TP:** Standing, facing your stroke.

▓ **CP:** Side-lying or supine.

Strokes
Use short, scooping strokes in the P–A plane or brisk transverse friction strokes at the attachment points if fibrosis is found.

1. Place the fingertips of your superior hand above the superior angle of the scapula on the upper ribs. Place your supporting hand on the scapula. Perform a series of short, scooping strokes following the contour of the ribs. You are working on the posterior scalene, and iliocostalis cervicis attachments on the T1–T3 ribs (Fig. 4-50). As you are working, gently move the scapula in the direction of your stroke. This brings the superficial tissue into slack and allows for deeper work on the attachments to the ribs. Because the direction of the strokes follows the contour of the upper ribs, the strokes begin in an inferior to superior direction and then change to a medial-to-lateral direction. Move your stance to face the direction of the strokes. Your series of strokes should cover the entire posterior and superior area of the upper ribs.

▓ *Study Guide*

Thoracic Spine, Level I
1. Describe the signs and symptoms of thoracic muscle strain, arthrosis, and facet joint fixation.
2. Describe the upper crossed syndrome. List the muscles that tend to be weak and the muscles that tend to be tight.
3. Name three factors that predispose to dysfunction and pain in the thoracic region.
4. Describe how the first series of massage strokes promotes hydration of the joints of the thoracic spine.
5. Describe a kyphotic spine, and describe the typical muscle dysfunctions in the pectoralis minor, lower trapezius, and upper trapezius.
6. Name the three lines of strokes and the two basic directions of strokes in the thoracic erector spinae muscles.
7. Describe the direction of positional dysfunction of the levator scapula and the direction of our stroke to correct it.
8. Describe the direction of our stroke to release the diaphragm.
9. Describe what scoliosis is, and describe Lauren Berry's theory of its origin.
10. List the three most common mechanical disorders that cause mid-back pain.

Thoracic Spine, Level II
1. Describe the MET for acute thoracic pain and for the lower trapezius.
2. Describe the signs and symptoms of osteoporosis, scoliosis, and a costovertebral fixation.
3. Describe the muscular imbalances of a kyphotic spine.
4. How do we palpate the serratus posterior superior and differentiate it from the rhomboids?
5. Describe the palpation findings in a healthy thoracic spine and in a degenerated spine.
6. List the stroke direction for the multifidus and iliocostalis cervicis.
7. Describe the Adam's test, and describe how you differentiate between a structural and a functional scoliosis.
8. Describe how you would differentiate between a functional and a structural kyphosis.
9. Describe the MET to release the rhomboids and to increase respiratory function.
10. Describe why the area of C7–T1 is often thick and fibrotic to palpation.

▓ *References*

1. Hayek R, Henderson C, Hayek A. Unique features of the thoracic spine: Impact on chiropractic management. Top Clin Chiro 1999;6:69–78.
2. Blair JM. Examination of the thoracic spine. In Grieve GP (ed): Modern Manual Therapy of the Vertebral Column. New York: Churchill Livingstone, 1986, pp536–546.
3. Grieve G. Common Vertebral Joint Problems. Edinburgh: Churchill Livingstone, 1981.
4. Corrigan B, Maitland GD. Practical Orthopaedic Medicine. London: Butterworths, 1983.
5. Triano J, Erwin M, Hansen D. Costovertebral and costotransverse joint pain: A commonly overlooked pain generator. Top Clin Chiro 1999;6:79–92.
6. Janda V. Evaluation of muscular imbalance. In Liebenson C. Rehabilitation of the Spine, 2nd ed. Baltimore: Williams & Wilkins, 2007, pp 203–225.

7. Kessler R, Hertling D. Management of Common Musculoskeletal Disorders, 4th ed. Baltimore: Williams & Wilkins, 2006.

8. Bogduk N, Twomey L. Clinical Anatomy of the Lumbar Spine, 3rd ed. London: Churchill Livingstone, 1998.

9. Oatis CA. Kinesiology: The Mechanics and Pathomechanics of Human Movement. Philadelphia: Lippincott Williams & Wilkins, 2004.

10. Faraday JA. Current principles in the nonoperative management of structural adolescent idiopathic scoliosis. Phys Ther 1983;66:512–523.

11. Schafer RC. Clinical Biomechanics. Baltimore: Williams & Wilkins, 1983.

12. Ford DM, Bagnall KM, McFadden KD, et al. Paraspinal muscle imbalance in adolescent idiopathic scoliosis. Spine 1984;9:373–376.

13. Kendall F, McCreary E, Provance P, Rogers M, Romani W. Muscles: Testing and Function, 5th ed. Baltimore: Lippincott Williams & Wilkins, 2005.

14. Dreyfuss P, Tibiletti C, Dreyer S. Thoracic zygapophyseal joint patterns. Spine 1994;19:807–811.

15. Greenman PE. Principles of Manual Medicine, 2nd ed. Baltimore: Williams & Wilkins, 1996.

■ *Suggested Readings*

Brukner P, Khan K. Clinical Sports Medicine, 3rd ed. Sydney: McGraw-Hill, 2006.

Calais-Germain B. Anatomy of Movement. Seattle: Eastland Press, 1991.

Chaitow L. Muscle Energy Techniques. New York: Churchill Livingstone, 1996.

Clemente C. Anatomy: A Regional Atlas of the Human Body, 4th ed. Baltimore: Williams & Wilkins, 1997.

Corrigan B, Maitland GD. Practical Orthopaedic Medicine. London: Butterworths, 1983.

Lewit K. Manipulative Therapy in Rehabilitation on the Locomotor System, 3rd ed. Oxford: Butterworth Heinemann, 1999.

Magee D. Orthopedic Physical Assessment, 3rd ed. Philadelphia: WB Saunders, 1997.

Norkin C, Levangie P. Joint Structure and Function, 3rd ed. Philadelphia: FA Davis, 2001.

Platzer W. Locomotor System, vol 1, 5th ed. New York: Thieme Medical, 2004.

Reid DC. Sports Injury and Assessment. New York: Churchill Livingstone, 1992.

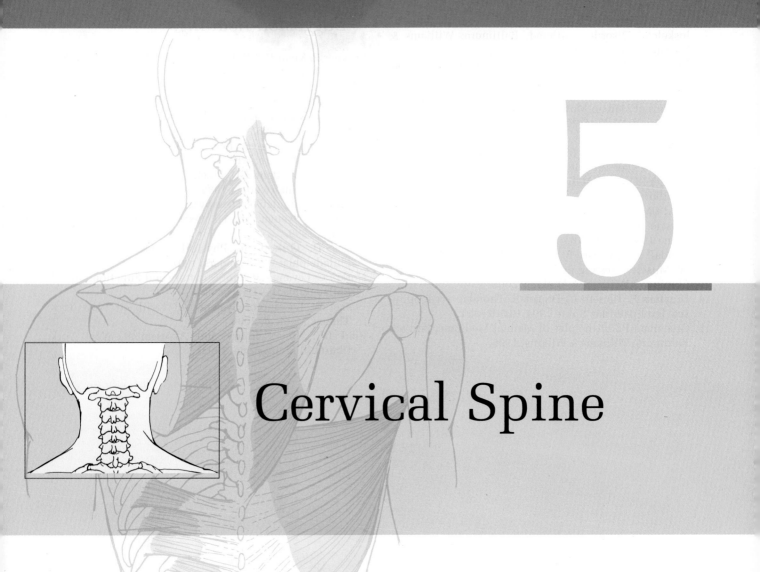

Cervical Spine

5

Neck pain is one of the most common complaints presented to a massage therapist. The causes of neck pain are diverse but include injuries from sports or motor vehicle accidents, cumulative stress from poor posture, and emotional and psychological tension. The structures that typically cause neck pain are the muscles, ligaments, facet joints, discs, and nerve roots. Approximately one-third of the population has experienced neck pain within the past year, and nearly 14% of the population experiences chronic neck pain.[1] Outside of injury, the most common cause of neck ache is postural strain. Studies suggest that in 87% of patients with neck pain from injuries, the soft tissue is the source of pain.[2]

Anatomy, Function, and Dysfunction of the Cervical Spine

GENERAL OVERVIEW

▨ **Seven vertebrae** form the cervical spine (Fig. 5-1). They are numbered from the vertebra under the skull, called C1, or the atlas, to C7, also called the vertebra prominens, because the spinous process (SP) is significantly longer than the SPs of the other cervical vertebrae. C2 is also called the axis. The occipital portion of the skull is included in the cervical spine, because it forms a joint with the atlas, the occipitoatlantal joint (Occ–C1).

▨ These seven vertebrae may be divided into two segments on the basis of their anatomy.

▨ The lower segment includes C3–C7 and consists of typical vertebrae.

▨ The upper segment includes C1–C2 and the occiput, as they are atypical.

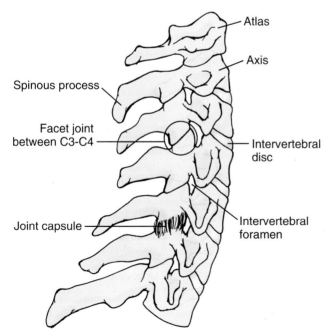

Figure 5-1. Lateral view of the anterior and the posterior portions of the cervical spine showing the vertebral body, intervertebral disc, facet, intervertebral foramen, transverse process, and transverse foramen.

Labels: Atlas, Axis, Spinous process, Facet joint between C3-C4, Intervertebral disc, Joint capsule, Intervertebral foramen

CERVICAL CURVE

▨ The cervical spine has a normal lordotic curve (i.e., the curve is convex anteriorly). Lordosis is a position of stability, maintained by the ligaments, muscles, facets, and shape of the discs.

▨ The apex of the forward cervical curve occurs at C5–C6. The greatest amount of flexion, extension, and rotation in the lower cervical spine occurs here. This great mobility makes the area susceptible to injury.

▨ The curve may be increased or decreased by many factors. Essentially, muscle tone is the primary factor in determining the degree of spinal curves.[3]

▨ With an increase in the curve, as in a **forward-head posture (FHP),** the facets are excessively compressed.

▨ A decrease of the curve places an excessive compressive force on the intervertebral discs.[4] This loss of curvature may be caused by previous trauma and consequent shortening of the anterior ligaments or by sustained muscle contraction of the deep cervical flexors.

POSTURE

▨ Grieve[5] states that "Head posture governs body posture." This is an important insight because it emphasizes the critical importance of the position of the head. How a person carries the head is also an expression of the person's self-image and self-esteem.

▨ There are three major factors that influence posture: heredity, prior injury, and acquired habit.[3] As Cailliet[3] points out, since postural habits develop in childhood, slumped posture may be the result of family or peer pressure or of anxiety, insecurity, fear, anger, or depression.

▨ In normal posture, to balance the head on the neck requires contraction of the extensor muscles because the weight of the head in front of the center of gravity. This explains why the head falls forward when you fall asleep while sitting.

▨ The upper cervical connective tissue, including the joint capsules and ligaments, contains an extremely dense concentration of proprioceptive nerves that serve as an important sense organ for posture.[6] The muscles of the suboccipital triangle are some of the most finely controlled muscles in the body. They have approximately one motor nerve per four to five muscle fibers, the same ratio as the muscle moving the eyes, compared with one motor nerve for every 1600 muscle fibers in the gastrocnemius. The proper function of the upper cervical area is critical to our sense of balance, coordination, and finely tuned movements of the head in response to visual and auditory cues.

■ **Dysfunction and injury:** FHP is one of the most common causes of neck pain. With a rounded shoulder and FHP, the cervical spine goes into extension, which increases the cervical curve, closes the intervertebral foramen (IVF) slightly, and potentially leads to nerve root pressure. The facets are compressed, which creates increased weight bearing on the cartilage, decreasing its lubrication and nutrition and leading to early degeneration. The joint capsules shorten and develop abnormal crosslinks, leading to loss of normal joint motion. The tension in the extensor muscles of the cervical spine and upper thoracic spine must increases dramatically to hold the weight of the head. This not only is fatiguing but also adds a compressive force on the facets and disc and further closes the IVF. The space above and below the clavicle, called the *thoracic outlet,* is compromised, which can compress the nerves and blood supply into the arm. There is decreased thoracic extension and decreased range of motion (ROM) in the shoulders. Slumped posture also decreases vital lung capacity and creates excessive tension in the temporomandibular joint (TMJ).

■ FHP compromises the blood flow through the vertebral artery, which is deep within the suboccipital triangle. The artery travels over the superior surface of the atlas and under the occiput before it enters the foramen magnum and travels to the brain. Lauren Berry, RPT, theorized that sustained FHP could compress the vertebral artery and could be a major contributing factor to early senility. This compression is caused by the narrowing of the space between the occiput and the atlas due to the posterior rotation of the occiput and extension of the cervical spine that occurs during FHP.

GENERAL ANATOMY OF CERVICAL VERTEBRAE

■ As in the lumbar spine and the thoracic spine, there is an anterior and a posterior portion to each of the vertebra. There are many similar structural and functional similarities and some important differences.

■ The anterior portion consists of a vertebral body and an intervertebral disc (IVD) that forms a fibrocartilaginous joint with the vertebral body (see Fig. 5-1). The two upper joints, Occ–C1 and C1–C2, do not have discs, and C1 does not have a body.

■ The posterior portion consists of two vertebral arches formed by a pedicle and lamina; two transverse processes; a central SP; and paired articulations—the inferior and superior facets—which form synovial joints. The atlas does not have an SP. Instead it has a posterior tubercle that is generally not palpable.

UNIQUE ANATOMY OF CERVICAL VERTEBRAE

■ *Transverse processes* are bony processes that project from both sides of the body of each vertebra. They are unique in the cervical spine (Fig. 5-2). Transverse processes have two distinct portions, the anterior and posterior portions, with an opening in the middle for the vertebral artery, called the **transverse foramen.** At the most lateral projections of the transverse process are the anterior and posterior tubercles, which serve as attachment points for nine muscles in the lower segment and six muscles in the upper segment. The transverse process also has a groove or sulcus in its superior surface on which the spinal nerve travels.

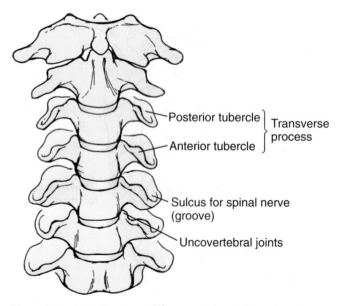

Figure 5-2. Anterior view of the cervical vertebrae showing the uncinate process, the anterior and posterior tubercle of the transverse process, and the groove or sulcus for the spinal nerve.

UNIQUE ANATOMY OF LOWER CERVICAL VERTEBRAE

■ The *vertebral bodies* are much smaller than the thoracic or the lumbar bodies. The increased size that would have afforded stability has been exchanged for the increased mobility allowed by the smaller size.[2] The vertebral bodies are also unique in that the anterior portion has a lip that projects downward slightly in front of the IVD, which contributes greater protection to the disc.

■ *The spinous processes* (SPs) are the bony prominences that project posteriorly and can be palpated on the back of the neck. They increase in length from C3 to C7. The axis (C2) has the first SP that you can palpate under the skull. C4–C6 have bifid SPs, or SPs that have two parts, that may be asymmetric.

■ The *uncinate processes* are elevated edges on the posterolateral rim of the superior surfaces of the body of C3–C7 (see Fig. 5-2). They articulate with a beveled edge of the lower border of the vertebra above. These articulations are called uncovertebral joints or joints of von Luschka. Grieve[5] describes them as synovial joints, lined with hyaline cartilage and surrounded by a joint capsule. They are bordered by the IVD. These joints add stability to the region by limiting lateral flexion and protecting the posterolateral disc. Like other synovial joints, they have a rich supply of proprioceptors and nociceptors.[7]

■ **Dysfunction and injury:** It is important to realize that you cannot assess the function of the vertebrae by the position of the SPs. The SPs should not be tender to palpation. Pain with digital pressure on the SPs should alert the therapist to a dysfunction or injury to the vertebrae. The uncovertebral joints are especially susceptible to degenerative changes, as shearing occurs at these joints with flexion and extension. There often develop thickened soft tissue and bony outgrowths that can irritate the neighboring nerve root and vertebral artery.[5] Because of their location, these processes minimize lateral bending. As they are the first areas to degenerate in the cervical spine, a chronic loss of lateral flexion is a clinical sign of cervical degeneration.

UNIQUE ANATOMY OF UPPER CERVICAL VERTEBRAE

■ The *atlas (C1)* is the first cervical vertebra. The superior aspect of the atlas forms a synovial joint with the occipital portion of the skull, called the Occ–C1 joint. The atlas is shaped like a ring and does not

have a body or an SP. It is like a "washer" between the skull and the axis.[8]

■ The *axis (C2)* is the second cervical vertebra. It has a unique vertical projection from the anterior body called the dens or the odontoid process. The anterior portion of the dens forms a synovial joint with the posterior portion of the arch of the atlas, forming the atlantoaxial joint. The posterior tip of the dens abuts the anterior aspect of the brainstem and upper spinal cord.

■ **Function:** Fifty percent of flexion and extension of the entire cervical spine occurs at the Occ–C1 joint, and 50% of cervical rotation occurs at the atlantoaxial (C1–C2) joint. C1–C2 is the most mobile joint in the spine.[8] Both of these joints do not have discs between them and therefore lack the tight fit offered by the IVDs. These joints are consequently less stable. Their stability relies on a dense network of ligaments and the surrounding muscles and fascia.

■ **Dysfunction and injury:** The upper segment of the cervical spine is one of the most common sources of dysfunction and injury in the body. Because of the lack of stability in this region, it is susceptible to strains from falls, whether from sports or daily life or car accidents. It is also commonly strained by postural stresses in the common FHP. When the head is held in this forward posture, it has to rotate posteriorly on the atlas to keep the eyes on the horizon, thus shortening the suboccipital muscles. This can lead to tension headaches from the entrapment of the first and second cervical nerves. Diseases that weaken the connective tissue, such as rheumatoid arthritis, can create further instability and require extreme caution from the therapist. It is **contraindicated** to introduce vigorous movement in the upper cervical spine.

INTERVERTEBRAL DISC

As was mentioned, there are IVDs between each of the vertebrae except the occiput and the atlas and the atlas and the axis.

■ **Structure:** A nucleus and an annulus compose the IVD.

  ☐ **Nucleus:** The nucleus is a colloidal gel that is 80% to 90% water contained within a fibrous wall. In the cervical spine, it is located in the anterior portion of the disc, compared with the central location in the lumbar spine. The disc is wedge shaped, with its anterior height two times greater than its posterior height, and contributes to the normal cervical lordosis. In the lumbar spine, the discs are parallel.

☐ **Annulus:** Concentric layers of interwoven fibro-cartilaginous fibers form the annulus.

▥ **Function:** The IVD provides a shock absorbing hydraulic system that permits a rocker-like movement of one vertebra upon the other due to a fluid shift in the nucleus and the elasticity of the annulus. The disc also provides proprioceptive and nociceptive functions. Disc nutrition into the annulus occurs by movement of the spine, which pumps fluids into the disc through compression and decompression.

▥ **Dysfunction and injury:** Two major lesions occur in the IVD: degeneration and herniation. Sustained muscular contraction creates compressive forces that can lead to disc degeneration and, according to Cailliet,[3] may cause disc herniation.

☐ **Disc herniation** may be due to either acute injury or cumulative stresses. Stresses or injury can cause an **internal disruption** due to small tears of the annulus. The annulus may become lax because of these tears, creating bulges around the circumference of the disc. This is called a **disc bulge.** The bulge could develop into a **herniated disc,** which is a displacement of disc material. Disc injuries can create local neck pain and referred pain. An internal disruption to the disc creates neck pain and referral of pain to the interscapular area. If the disc has herniated, it can compress the nerve roots in the IVF, creating ischemia. Most nerve root irritations occur at C5–C6 and at C6–C7. Pain is referred into the arm in specific myotomes (muscles supplied by motor roots of spinal nerves) and dermatomes (areas of skin supplied by the spinal nerve sensory root), which are described in the section "Cervical Spine Nerves."

☐ Disc herniation is not as common in the neck as in the lumbar spine because of the protection afforded by the uncovertebral joints, the more anterior location of the nucleus, and the much stronger posterior longitudinal ligament. The posterior longitudinal ligament is double-layered in the neck and completely surrounds the disc, whereas in the lower back, it is thin and narrow.

☐ Some authors consider **disc degeneration** to be an age-related condition, but others believe that it is the result of prior injury or repetitive stresses. The disc loses its water-binding capacity and therefore its shock-absorbing capacity, and as a result, the annular rings weaken and break down. Degeneration affects other tissues of the cervical spine. For example, as the disc loses height, it compresses the facets, leading to degeneration of the articular cartilage of these joints.

☐ Symptoms of a cervical disc degeneration are achy neck pain, stiffness upon awakening, loss of motion, especially lateral flexion, and possible referred pain into the shoulders. As the condition worsens, symptoms may include pain and weakness in the arms.

▥ **Treatment implications:** Clients who have a disc herniation are approached with special precaution. Some of the muscle tension in the neck is providing stability to the disc, and deep massage is **contraindicated.** Disc herniations are treated with contract-relax (CR) muscle energy technique (MET) with a neutral spine. Gentle soft tissue mobilization (STM) is performed, but posterior-to-anterior (P–A) joint mobilization of the spine is minimized. The intention of these techniques is to reduce inflammatory edema, which creates venous congestion and ischemia around the nerve roots, as well as to decompress the disc by reducing muscle hypertonicity. The chronic, degenerated disc is treated with CR MET, joint mobilization, and STM to help rehydrate the disc.

FACET JOINTS

▥ **Definition:** The facet (see Fig. 5-1), or apophyseal joint, is a synovial joint surrounded by a connective tissue joint capsule, fat tissue pads, and a fibromeniscus. As in the lumbar and thoracic spine, the vertebrae articulate at two superior and two inferior facet joints.

▥ **Structure**
☐ **Articular surface:** In the healthy state, the articular surface of the facets is covered by hyaline cartilage that is lubricated with synovial fluid. As in the other regions of the body, the nutrition to the articular cartilage depends on cycles of compression and decompression that arise from movement.

☐ **Joint capsule:** An inner synovial layer and a thick and dense outer fibrous layer compose the joint capsule. In the cervical spine, the capsule is loose and elastic, which allows the cervical spine to have the greatest mobility of all the regions in the spine. The capsule also has fibromenisci infoldings, which allow the joint to bear a greater load.

▥ **Function**
☐ The facets determine the range and direction of movement and have some weight-bearing capacity. In the healthy state, they are designed to slide on each other. The closed-packed position of the cervical facets is extension and lateral flexion, and the open position is flexion.

☐ The joint capsule (capsular ligament) functions to passively stabilize the facet joints. The capsules are highly innervated and serve as receptors for proprioception or position sense, movement and pressure through mechanoreceptors, and pain through pain fibers (nociceptors). Proprioception in the cervical spine is more refined than that in the lumbar spine, as a higher concentration of proprioceptors exists in the facet joint capsules.[4]

Dysfunction and injury: The facets are susceptible to cumulative stresses and acute injury. The facets can be a source of both local and referred pain, including headaches. The most common causes are as follows:

☐ **Forward-head posture:** This posture places the facets in a sustained extension, the closed-packed position, compressing the joints, decreasing the joint lubrication, and leading to early degeneration.

☐ **Muscle imbalances:** There are predictable patterns of muscle imbalances in the cervical spine, called *upper crossed syndrome.* See the section below entitled "Cervical Region Muscle Imbalances."

☐ **Hypomobility:** The facets can lose their normal gliding characteristics owing to muscular tension, FHP, ligamentous and capsular thickening, joint fixation, degeneration or herniation of the disc, or arthritic changes.

☐ **Degeneration:** Many factors cause facet degeneration. Muscle imbalances generate abnormal stresses to the cartilage, creating instability in the joint. Sustained muscle contraction decreases joint motion, creating hypomobility, and adds a compressive load to the cartilage. Degeneration of the cartilage of the facets is a source of local and referred pain. Clients describe it as a dull, achy pain that can be felt in the neck, shoulder, or interscapular area. Eventually, the cartilage can form osteophytes that can encroach into the IVF and lead to nerve root irritation, which would manifest as pain, numbing, tingling, or weakness in the arm, hand, or both.

☐ **Injury:** The cartilage is susceptible to acute injury (e.g., a sports injury, a fall, a blow to the head or neck), to the cumulative stresses of sustained muscular contraction or FHP.

☐ **Acute facet syndrome:** A common complaint is a "crick" in the neck, in which the client in unable to turn the neck. As was mentioned, theoretically, this is caused by a fixation of the articular cartilage surfaces or an entrapment of the fibromenisci between the facets.

☐ **Joint capsule injury:** Because the capsule is highly innervated, a sprain is painful, potentially causing local and referred pain in the arm. Injury also affects the mechanoreceptors, resulting in dysfunctions of coordination and balance, altered movement patterns, and altered reflexes to the muscles, creating either weakness or hypertonicity.

☐ Pain in the neck is often caused by limited joint movement and capsular thickening.[5] Restricted motion of the facets results in a reflex that typically creates hypertonicity of the muscles at the same vertebral level.

Treatment implications

☐ Examination of acute facet conditions reveals loss of cervical lateral flexion and extension with localized pain at the involved facet at the end range, tenderness and loss of passive glide at the involved facet, and hypertonic and tender muscles. Examination of chronic facet involvement reveals hypertonic muscles; muscle length and strength imbalances; thickened, fibrous tissue, especially in the multifidi and capsular ligaments; and loss of normal joint play at the facets. As motion in the joint creates lubrication, decreased motion means decreased lubrication and, consequently, increased friction and wear and tear of the joint surfaces.

☐ Many clients tell the therapist that "the doctor says I have arthritis in my neck, and that I just have to live with the pain." They are afraid to move their necks or, worse, have been instructed not to move their necks if it is uncomfortable. It is important to realize, as Cailliet[3] notes, that "There is little or no correlation found between the degree of pain felt in the neck and the degree of arthritic changes found on X-ray." In the author's clinical experience, most of these patients can have a dramatic reduction in pain and improvement of function with manual therapy and instruction in proper posture and exercise.

☐ The basic treatment protocol is to release the hypertonicity in the short and tight muscles, broaden the fibers in the capsular ligaments, facilitate the weak muscles through CR MET, rehydrate the cartilage through compression and decompression, and reintroduce the normal gliding characteristics in the facets with gentle mobilization.

☐ It is important to instruct the client in proper posture. Postural strain is one of the major sources of neck pain.

☐ Some clients, on the other hand, are unstable and weak in their cervical muscles because of previous injury. They need proper instruction in strengthening exercises to help stabilize the cervical spine. This typically requires a referral to a physical therapist or personal trainer. Finally, because of the high concentration of proprioceptors in the neck, balance exercises are important to rehabilitate the function of these nerves.

☐ Acute facet syndrome requires a referral to a chiropractor or an osteopath for manipulation.

INTERVERTEBRAL FORAMEN

▓ **Structure:** The IVF is narrow in the cervical spine and relatively wide in the thoracic and lumbar regions (see Fig. 5-1). The IVDs form a much smaller part of the boundary of the IVF here than in the lumbar region. Most cases of narrowing of the IVF caused by bony spurs are in the cervical spine, but more than 90% of the disc protrusions in the spine are in the lumbar region.[3]

▓ **Function:** The IVF provides an opening for the sensory and motor nerve roots and for the blood vessels. The IVF opens on flexion and closes slightly on extension.

▓ **Dysfunction and injury:** Narrowing of the IVF can cause compression of the nerve roots creating pain, numbing and tingling, and weakness in the arms or hands. The IVF can be narrowed because of disc degeneration, disc herniation, osteophytes or spurs, facet inflammation, sustained muscle contraction, thickening and fibrosis of the ligamentum flavum and joint capsule, malposition of the facets, osteoarthritis of the facets or uncovertebral joints, or increased lordosis caused by FHP. Significant narrowing of the IVF is called **foraminal encroachment** and can lead to nerve root irritation.

CERVICAL SPINE NERVES

▓ As in the other areas of the spine, the cervical nerves are mixed nerves from the union of **motor (ventral)** and **sensory (dorsal)** roots that have emerged from the spinal cord. The roots merge to become the spinal nerve. The motor nerve has intimate contact with the uncovertebral joints, and the sensory root lies close to the facet joint and capsule.

▓ The C1, C2, and C3 nerves innervate the head and face. These first three cervical nerves travel through the muscles at the base of the skull and are sensitive to irritation from sustained muscle contraction

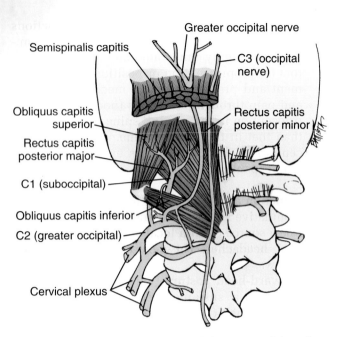

Figure 5-3. Suboccipital muscles and the nerves of the suboccipital region showing the C1–C3 nerves.

(Fig. 5-3). The medial branch of C2 is also called the greater occipital nerve and travels through the semispinalis capitis and pierces the scalp as it travels onto the back of the skull. C3 extends forward to the area above the eye and, if irritated, can feel like sinus pain.[3]

▓ The **spinal cord** occupies four-fifths of the spinal canal, and as the neck flexes, the nerve roots are pulled taut and have a pulling or tethering effect on the spinal cord. Normally, there is enough slack in the roots and the cord, but many factors can compromise their free movement.

Dorsal Root Ganglion

▓ **The dorsal root ganglion** is a cluster of cell bodies of the sensory nerves and has been postulated to be a major site of pain, called radicular (which means root) pain. Dorsal root ganglion irritation elicits a sharp pain, numbing, and tingling in the dermatome corresponding to the root. A **dermatome** is an area of skin that is supplied by the sensory root of a spinal nerve (Fig. 5-4).

Ventral (Motor) Root

▓ The ventral (motor) root is a cluster of cell bodies of the motor nerves. A **myotome** is a group of muscles that are supplied by the motor (ventral) root(s) of the spinal nerve(s). Irritation of the motor root

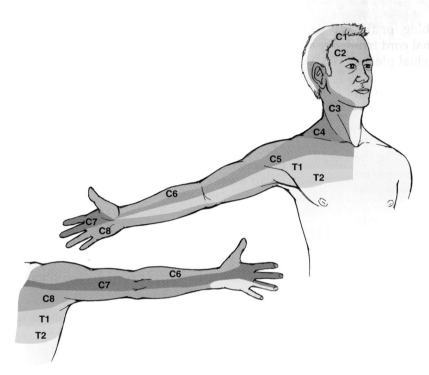

Figure 5-4. Dermatomes of the cervical spine, which cover the head, neck, shoulder, arm, and hand.

elicits deep, boring pain; muscle weakness; and potential atrophy in the muscle supplied by that root. The corresponding myotomes of the cervical nerve roots are C1–C2, neck flexion; C3, side flexion of the neck; C4, shoulder elevation; C5, shoulder abduction; C6, elbow flexion and wrist extension; C7, elbow and finger extension and wrist flexion; C8, thumb extension; and T1, abduction of the fingers.

Brachial Plexus

▨ The anterior portion of C5–C8 and T1 nerves forms the brachial plexus (Fig. 5-5), which becomes the ulnar, median, and radial nerves of the arm. They emerge from the transverse processes and travel between the anterior and middle scalenes, under the clavicle and subclavius, under the pectoralis minor, and then into the arm. The covering of the nerve, called the epineurium, of C4–C6 is partially anchored to the scalene muscle group, and sustained contraction of these muscles could irritate these nerves.

▨ **Dysfunction and Injury**
   ☐ The nerve roots and spinal cord can become inflamed, compressed, or stretched (tethered) near the IVF because of disc herniations, thickening of the ligamentum flavum, osteophytes (bone spurs), or degeneration and hypertrophy (bone deposits) of the facets.

☐ The current model of nerve root irritation describes the cause of symptoms as venous stasis due to swelling. The swelling causes ischemia (low oxygen), which causes the nerve roots to become extremely sensitive.[7,9]

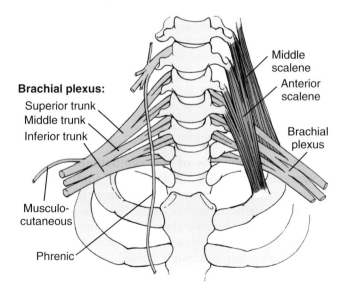

Brachial plexus:
Superior trunk
Middle trunk
Inferior trunk

Musculo-
cutaneous

Phrenic

Middle
scalene
Anterior
scalene

Brachial
plexus

Figure 5-5. Brachial plexus and the scalenes muscle. The brachial plexus travels in between the anterior and the middle scalenes, under the clavicle, under the pectoralis minor, and into the arm.

☐ Three types of referred pain, numbing, or tingling into the extremities occur: spinal cord irritation, nerve root irritation, and brachial plexus peripheral irritation.

☐ Irritation from the spinal cord is a condition called **cervical myelopathy.** This cord compression often affects the elderly and causes gait disturbances, impaired fine hand movements, lower-extremity weakness, and numbness in the trunk.[3] Passive neck flexion that causes lower-extremity numbness is a sign of cord compression.

☐ Nerve root pain is also called **radicular pain** and results from irritation of the cervical nerve roots in the region of the IVF. If the sensory root is irritated, it creates pain, numbing, and tingling that is localized to a specific area, called the dermatome, rather than to a diffuse region. The pain varies from a deep aching to sharp. If the motor root is irritated, it causes deep and boring pain in the muscles supplied by that root and weakness. The cause of the pain is often hard to differentiate.

☐ The third source of referred pain comes from the brachial plexus, which may also become compressed by sustained contraction in the anterior and middle scalenes, under the pectoralis minor or subclavius, or by thickened fascia in the area above or below the clavicle. These conditions are broadly defined as thoracic outlet syndrome. Thoracic outlet syndrome is often caused by slumped posture but may be the consequence of injury or overuse from work or recreational habits.

▨ **Treatment implications:** MET, STM, and joint mobilization provide a gentle pumping action around the nerve roots to decrease swelling, increase oxygen, and induce normal movement to the soft tissue and joints.

Sympathetic Nerves

▨ Major components of the sympathetic nervous system are located in the neck, including the three sympathetic ganglia in the anterior neck. The sympathetic nerves travel through the longus colli and are susceptible to irritation with sustained muscle contracture or may be irritated from an excessive stretch caused by a hyperextension injury.

▨ **Dysfunction and injury:** Whiplash injuries can damage the cervical sympathetic nerves.[10] Irritation of these nerves can lead to headache, vertigo, tinnitus, nasal disturbance, facial pain, facial flushing, and pharyngeal paresthesias, nausea, and blurred vision.[3]

▨ **Treatment implications:** Manual therapy has been found to be clinically effective in many cases to reduce or relieve symptoms of sympathetic irritation with MET and STM of the deep cervical flexors. All clients who have these symptoms should also be under the care of a chiropractor or an osteopath to evaluate and treat potential joint fixations.

LIGAMENTS

▨ The stability of Occ–C1 and C1–C2 is provided primarily by dense ligaments, principally the cruciate, alar, and apical ligaments.

▨ The principal ligaments of the lower segment include the following:
☐ An **anterior longitudinal ligament,** which is thin in the cervical spine and thick in the lumbar spine.
☐ A **posterior longitudinal ligament,** which is wide and thick in the neck and narrow in the lumbar spine. Posterior longitudinal ligament thickness offers protection from a posterior protrusion of the disc.
☐ A **ligamentum flavum,** which blends with the joint capsule.
☐ A **supraspinous ligament** and its broad expansion called the ligamentum nuchae, which extends from C7 to T1 to the external occipital protuberance. As the center of the mass of the head lies anterior to the center of gravity, the ligamentum nuchae and extensor muscles are designed to resist this forward pull.
☐ A **capsular ligament** of the facet joints (see the discussion of joint capsule above).

▨ **Dysfunction and injury:** Cervical spine degeneration has the potential to contribute to narrowing of the spinal canal and to cause folds in the ligamentum flavum, which can buckle during extension.[2] Because the ligamentum flavum blends with the joint capsule, sprains of the joint can create hypertrophy to the capsule and ligamentum flavum, decreasing the space of the IVF, causing encroachment of the nerve roots. Diseases that weaken the connective tissue, such as rheumatoid arthritis, can severely affect the stability of the upper cervical spine.

▨ **Treatment implications**
☐ Because many clients who have chronic neck pain have fibrotic capsular ligaments, the intention

of massage therapy is to gently and gradually broaden these fibers and rehydrate these tissues through manual techniques. Thick and dense capsular ligaments prevent the normal gliding of the vertebral facets and contribute to joint degeneration.

☐ Clients who have a history of rheumatoid arthritis or acute neck injury need protection from vigorous mobilization. If a client tests weak in the cervical muscles, then treatment is geared toward stabilization through CR MET with the client in a neutral position. These clients are referred to a physical therapist for rehabilitation exercises to strengthen the muscles and increase the density of the ligaments.

CERVICAL FASCIA

▨ **Structure:** Fascia is a sheet of dense connective tissue. In addition to the fascia that surrounds each muscle, there are six layers of fascia in the cervical spine. The **prevertebral fascia,** which completely surrounds each vertebra, is continuous with the thoracolumbar fascia.[2]

▨ **Function:** Fascia plays an important role in transmitting the forces generated by the muscles and in giving shape to the body. The fascia forms muscle compartments that allow for the precise direction of muscle contraction.

▨ **Dysfunction and injury:** Injury or irritation thickens the fascia through abnormal crosslinks and collagen deposition (adhesions). This fascial thickening restricts the normal muscle movement within the fascial compartments and decreases the ROM of the joints.

CERVICAL REGION MUSCLES

▨ **Structure:** The muscles of the cervical spine may be divided into four functional groups: superficial posterior, deep posterior, superficial anterior, and deep anterior.[7] The superficial posterior group includes the trapezius, levator scapula, and splenius cervicis and capitis. They serve to hold the head up against gravity and extend the head and neck. The deep posterior group includes the longissimus cervicis and capitis, iliocostalis cervicis, semispinalis cervicis and capitis, multifidi, and suboccipital muscles. The superficial anterior muscles include the sternocleidomastoid (SCM), scalenes, and hyoid muscles. The deep flexors are the longus colli and longus capitis.

▨ A further division may be made between muscles that move the head, which Cailliet[3] calls the capital muscles, and those that move the cervical spine. In addition to the suboccipital group, the muscles that move the head are the longissimus capitis; semispinalis capitis; splenius capitis; deep flexors of the cranium, including the rectus capitis anterior and lateralis; and suprahyoid muscles, which, because of their attachment to the mandible, assist in flexing the head. These two categories also describe a functional differentiation in that the occiput, atlas, and axis can be moved independently of the lower cervical spine.[2] This independent movement allows for stability in the lower segment and fine-tuned movements in the upper segment for sight and hearing.

▨ **Function:** Muscles of the cervical spine provide dynamic stabilization, mobility, and proprioceptive feedback that are essential to our balance and fine postural control. In the lumbopelvic region, the essential function of the muscles and associated fascia is to promote stability for lifting and carrying activities. In the cervical spine, mobility is as essential as stability. Adequate mobility allows us to be able to move the eyes and ears quickly and efficiently. Stability from the muscles provides balance and control of the forces moving through the joints and discs and also acts as a shock absorber to prevent excessive movement from damaging the joints and discs. The muscles that are most essential to this stabilization are the multifidi, suboccipitals, and deep flexors. These cervical muscles are unique because they attach to the bone not by tendons but by myofascial tissue, and they contain a tremendous number of mechanoreceptors. These receptors in the muscles play an essential role in position and movement of the head and neck. There are also vast reflex connections between the organs of balance, called the vestibular apparatus, the muscles of the eyes, and the musculature of the head and neck.[2]

▨ An intimate relationship exists between the jaw and the muscles of the cervical spine. Swallowing, chewing, and vocalization all involve the hyoid muscles. For the jaw to open, the occiput must be stabilized.

▨ **Dysfunction and injury**
  ☐ **Muscle tightness:** Muscle tightness usually develops from postural faults or from psychological and emotional stress. As in the lumbar spine, it is typical for the extensor muscles of the cervical spine to be held in a sustained contraction. With a FHP, the extensors shorten, increasing the

lordosis of the cervical spine and placing the facets in the closed-packed position. These postural changes result in compression of the facet joints and disc, contributing to neck pain and headaches and to early degeneration of these structures.[4]

☐ **Anterior scalene syndrome:** The brachial plexus and subclavian artery travel in between the anterior and middle scalenes. With sustained contraction of these muscles, pain, numbing, and tingling can manifest, especially along the ulnar border of the hand. This is called *anterior scalene syndrome* (or *scalenus anticus syndrome*). This condition is part of a constellation of similar lesions that fall under the broad category of thoracic outlet syndrome.

☐ **Hypertonicity of muscles of TMJ:** The hyoid muscles and muscles of the TMJ may also be held in a sustained contraction because of injury or FHP. As the head tilts posteriorly to keep the eyes level in FHP, the mandible is pulled down and posteriorly, which means that the masseter and temporalis must increase their tension to bring the TMJ back into its resting position.[2,4]

☐ **Headaches:** Headaches have diverse causes, including the cervical facets (and capsule) and the muscles. According to Kendall and colleagues,[4] two types of headaches are associated with muscle tension: the occipital headache and the tension headache. The occipital headache develops from sustained contraction of the semispinalis capitis. The semispinalis capitis can entrap the greater occipital nerve, leading to pain, numbness, and burning from the occipital region to the top of the head. Tension headaches, on the other hand, are caused by faulty posture and emotional or psychological stress that lead to sustained tension in the posterior neck muscles. Periods of increased stress increase the tension. The rectus capitis posterior minor is also implicated in tension headaches, as it attaches to the covering of the brain called the dura, and sustained contraction creates a tethering or pulling force on the dura, creating a headache.

☐ **Muscle injury:** Muscle strain is often associated with an acute injury but may develop from minor repetitive strains. The SCM is the most commonly injured muscle in rear-end auto accidents, followed by the longus colli. If the SCM is held in a sustained contraction, it pulls the head forward. Typically, the longus colli, a deep flexor of the neck, is weak after injury, which allows an increase in the cervical curve. However, the longus colli may be short and tight as a result of

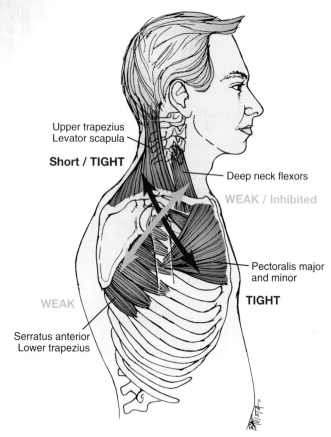

Figure 5-6. Upper crossed syndrome is characterized by short and tight suboccipitals, cervical extensors, upper trapezii, levator scapulae, and pectoral muscles and by weak and inhibited deep cervical flexors, middle and lower trapezii, and serratus anterior. This syndrome is characterized by forward-head posture, rounded shoulders, hyperextension of the head, elevated shoulders, and an increased cervical curve.

injury, which would contribute to a decreased cervical curve.

☐ As was mentioned previously, Janda describes predictable patterns of muscle dysfunction. In the upper body, this dysfunction is called the **upper crossed syndrome** (Fig. 5-6), because the muscles that are typically tight form one arm of the cross and those that are typically weak form the other arm of the cross. The postural signs of the upper cross syndrome are listed in Table 5-1.

Cervical Region Muscle Imbalances

▨ **Muscles that tend to be tight and short:** Levator scapula; upper trapezius; SCM; suboccipitals; scalenes; cervical extensors, including the splenius capitis and the semispinalis capitis; temporalis; masseter; and pectoralis minor.

Table 5-1	Postural Signs of the Upper Crossed Syndrome	

Postural Finding	*Dysfunction*
Rounded shoulders	Short pectoralis minor
Forward head	Kyphotic thoracic spine
Hyperextension of head	Short suboccipital muscles
Elevated shoulders	Short upper trapezius and levator
Winging of scapula	Weak serratus anterior
Increased cervical lordosis	Short cervical extensors, weak deep flexors

- **Muscles that tend to be weak and inhibited:** Deep neck flexors, including longus colli and capitis; middle and lower trapezius; rhomboids; and serratus anterior.

- These patterns have common variations. For example, the scalenes may be either tight and short or weak and inhibited.

Positional Dysfunction of the Cervical Spine Muscles

- Cervical extensors develop a medial torsion.

- Scalenes and SCM tend to develop an anterior torsion.

Muscular Relations to the Balance of the Head and Neck

- Muscles that increase the cervical curve:
  - Semispinalis cervicis and capitis.

- Muscles that decrease the cervical curve:
  - Longus colli and capitis.

- Muscular imbalances that contribute to FHP:
  - Short and tight SCM.

- Weak cervical extensors, lower trapezius, and abdominals.

- **Treatment implications**
  - The foundation of treatment for the muscles of the cervical spine is to correct faulty posture. The only exception is the client who is in acute pain, who will adopt compensatory postures because of the pain. Exercises are recommended to strengthen the deep cervical flexors, lower trapezius, and latissimus to help correct postural faults. Kendall and colleagues[4] provide exercise guidelines.
  - *The primary intention in treating the acute client* is to apply gentle reciprocal inhibition (RI) MET or CR MET, which helps to disperse excess fluids, restore proper nutrition, and provide gentle stress to the collagen to promote healing of the fibers in their proper alignment. The strained muscles will be swollen, boggy, and tight to palpation, with a thin-membraned rigidity caused by the swelling.
  - *The primary intention in treating the subacute or chronic client* is to reduce muscle hypertonicity, lengthen shortened muscles and their associated fascia, and promote mobility in the cervical spine. CR MET and postisometric relaxation (PIR) MET are used to promote strength and stability. Finally, balance exercises are recommended to restore proper function of the proprioceptors.

ANATOMY OF THE CERVICAL SPINE MUSCLES

Muscles cited in Table 5-2 are in addition to those listed in Chapter 3.

MUSCULAR ACTIONS OF THE NECK

See Table 5-3 for a comprehensive listing of the muscles responsible for neck movement, including flexion, extension, lateral flexion, rotation, and circumduction.

Table 5-2	Anatomy of the Muscles of the Cervical Spine[a]			
Muscle	*Origin*	*Insertion*	*Action*	*Dysfunction*
Anterolateral Neck Muscles *(see Fig. 5-7)*				
Scalenus anterior (anticus) *(see Fig. 5-7B)*	Anterior tubercle of the transverse processes of C3–C6	Superior surface of first rib	Lateral flexion and stabilizer of the cervical spine	Scalenes tend to be short and tight with forward-head posture. Sustained contraction can entrap the brachial plexus, creating pain, numbing, and tingling in the hands, especially the ulnar border. Because the scalenes act as guy wires to help stabilize the cervical spine, sustained tightness can lead to weakness and instability.
Scalenus medius *(Fig. 5-7B)* **Clinical Note:** The brachial plexus travels between the anterior and the medial scalenes, under the clavicle, under the pectoralis minor, and into the arm.	Anterior tubercle of transverse processes C3–C7	Superior surface of first rib	Lateral flexion stabilizer of the cervical spine	
Scalenus posterior *(Fig. 5-7B)*	Posterior tubercle of transverse process of C3–C7	Posterior-lateral portion of the second rib, anterior to levator scapula	Lateral flexion of the cervical spine	
Sternocleidom-astoid (SCM) muscle *(Fig. 5-7A)*	Sternal head—anterior surface of manubrium of sternum Clavicular head—superior surface of the medial one-third of the clavicle	Into the lateral surface of the mastoid process of the temporal bone and the lateral two-thirds of the superior nuchal line	Acting bilaterally, flexion of the head. Unilaterally, lateral bending of the head to side of contraction and rotation to opposite side.	The SCM muscle is the most commonly injured muscles after whiplash. Pain commonly refers into the head. Because one of the functions of the SCM is to pull the head and neck forward, a tight SCM leads to forward-head posture.
Suboccipital Muscles *(see Fig. 5-3)*				
Rectus capitis posterior major	Lateral and superior half of the SP of the axis (C2)	Lateral half of the inferior nuchal line	Bilaterally, extension of the head on the atlas. Unilaterally, rotation to the same side with some lateral bending	Suboccipital muscles tend to be tight and short, ofter due to forward-head posture. Sustained tightness may lead to proprioceptive deficits, such as loss of balance, as suboccipital muscles have large populations of mechanoreceptors. Because the rectus capitus posterior minor interweaves with the dura of the brain, sustained tension is implicated in tension headaches.
Rectus capitis posterior minor	Tuberosity on posterior arch of atlas	Medial one-third of the inferior nuchal line	Posture and stabilization of occipital–first cervical (OCC–C1) junction	
Obliquus capitis superior	Thick tendinous fibers from the posterior corner and lateral segment of the transverse process of C1	Superior to the lateral one-third of the inferior nuchal line	Bilaterally, extension of the head on the atlas. Unilaterally, lateral bending of the head to the same side.	
Obliquus capitis inferior	Lateral surface of the apex of the SP and the arch of the axis (C2)	Inferior and posterior surface of the transverse process of the atlas (C1)	Rotation of the head to the same side	

Table 5-2	Anatomy of the Muscles of the Cervical Spine[a] (*Continued*)			
Muscle	*Origin*	*Insertion*	*Action*	*Dysfunction*
Suprahyoid Muscles *(see Fig. 5-8)*				
Digastric	Two bellies united by a rounded tendon—extends from mastoid to chin. Posterior belly attaches in mastoid notch of temporal bone and passes downward and forward.	Anterior belly attaches to digastric fossa on the base of the mandible; the two bellies meet in an intermediate tendon, which perforates the stylohyoid muscle	Depresses the mandible and can elevate the hyoid bone	Forward-head posture places the occiput into extension and creates a pulling force on the hyoid muscles. The mandible is pulled down and back, which then requires continuous contraction of the masseter and temporalis muscles to keep the mouth closed. This tension may also pull the tongue into an abnormal resting position behind the lower teeth, rather than in its normal resting position behind the upper teeth.
Stylohyoid	Arises by a small tendon from the posterior surface of the styloid process	Into the body of the hyoid at its junction with the greater cornu	Elevates and draws back the hyoid	
Mylohyoid	Forms the muscular floor of the mouth. It is a flat, triangular sheet attached to the entire length of the mylohyoid line of the mandible.	Passes medially and downward to the anterior medial body of the hyoid	Elevates the floor of the mouth in the first stage of swallowing; elevates the hyoid bone or depresses the mandible	
Hyoglossus	Form the greater horn of the hyoid bone	Passes superiorly to the aponeurosis of the tongue	The hyoglossus moves the tongue in concert with the genioglossus and the styloglossus	
Infrahyoid Muscles *(see Fig. 5-8)*				
Sternohyoid	Arises from the posterior surface of the medial end of the clavicle, the posterior sternoclavicular ligament, and the superior-posterior surface of the sternum	Lower border of the most medial part of the body of the hyoid	Depresses the hyoid after swallowing	Forward-head posture places the occiput into extension and creates a pulling force on the hyoid muscles. The mandible is pulled down and back, which then requires continuous contraction of the masseter and temporalis muscles to keep the mouth closed. This tension may also pull the tongue into an abnormal resting position behind the lower teeth, rather than in its normal resting position behind the upper teeth.
Sternothyroid	Shorter and wider than above muscle and deep to it. Arises from the posterior surface of the manubrium below the origin of the sternohyoid.	Oblique line on lamina of thyroid cartilage	Draws larynx down after it has been elevated in swallowing or vocalization	
Thyrohyoid	Oblique line on lamina of thyroid cartilage.	Lower border of greater cornu and adjacent part of hyoid underneath the sternohyoid and omohyoid	Depresses the hyoid or raises the larynx	
Omohyoid	Arises from upper border of the scapula near the scapular notch. Consists of two fleshy bellies united by an intermediate tendon.	Lower border of hyoid bone body, lateral to insertion of sternohyoid	Depresses the hyoid after it has been elevated	

(continued)

| Table 5-2 | Anatomy of the Muscles of the Cervical Spine[a] (Continued) |

Prevertebral Neck Muscles (see Fig. 5-9)

Muscle	Origin	Insertion	Action	Dysfunction
Rectus capitis lateralis	The transverse process of the atlas.	Inferior surface of the occipital bone lateral to the occipital condyle	Bends the head to same side and stabilizes the head	The prevertebral muscles tend to be weak, which leads to instability of the cervical spine and forward-head posture. If the SCM is tight and the deep prevertebral muscles are weak, the chin and head juts forward. These muscles may also be tight and manifest tightness-weakness. The longus colli and longus capitus help to stabilize the head and neck to prevent extension, as the posterior muscles, such as the upper trapezius, elevate the shoulders. Whiplash injuries or other injuries involving forceful hyperextension of the head, commonly overstretch and tear the longus muscles. This manifests as the patient's inability to elevate the shoulders or lift the head off the pillow without pain. The longus muscles also tend to be weak, leading to forward-head posture, and tightness of the extensors
Rectus capitis anterior	Anterior surface of the lateral mass of the atlas and the transverse process	Inferior surface of the occipital bone in front of the occipital condyle	Flexes the head	
Longus capitis	Anterior tubercles of the transverse processes of C3–C6	Inferior surface of the basilar part of the occipital bone	Flexes the head when acting bilaterally and straightens the upper cervical spine; side bends the head when acting unilaterally. Helps to stabilize head and neck	
Longus colli—inferior oblique	From anterior bodies of T1–T3	Anterior tubercles of transverse processes of C5 and C6	Flexes and straightens the upper cervical spine when acting bilaterally; unilaterally, it assists in side bending and rotation of the neck to the same side. Helps to stabilize the neck.	
Longus colli—superior oblique	Anterior tubercles of C3 and C5	Anterior tubercle of atlas		
Longus colli—medial (intermediate) fibers	Anterior bodies of upper three thoracic and lower three cervical vertebrae	Anterior bodies of upper three cervical vertebrae		

[a]In addition to those listed in Chapter 3, pp. 106–113.

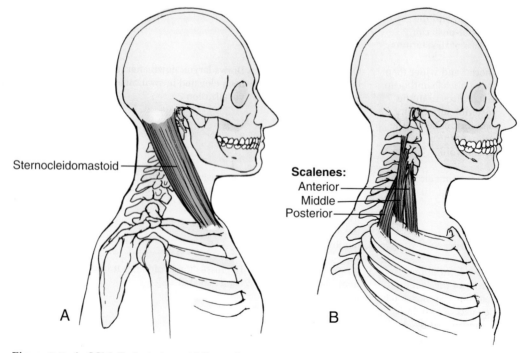

Figure 5-7. A. SCM. **B.** Anterior, middle, and posterior scalenes.

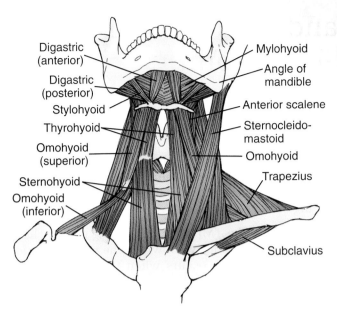

Figure 5-8. Superficial anterior muscles of the neck are the suprahyoid and infrahyoid muscles.

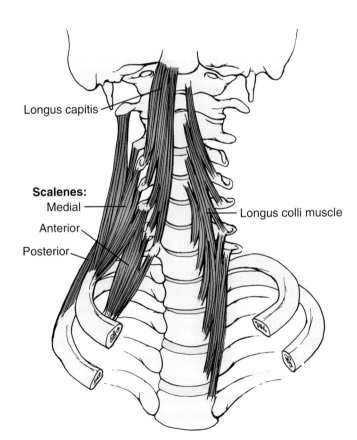

Figure 5-9. Muscles on the deepest aspect of the anterior neck are called the prevertebral muscles.

Table 5-3	Muscular Actions of the Neck

The neck is capable of the same movements as the trunk (i.e., flexion, extension, right and left rotation, right and left lateral flexion, and circumduction).

Flexion

- SCM—contributes to neck flexion when acting bilaterally and to lateral flexion and rotation to the opposite side when acting unilaterally
- Scalenes (anterior, medial, and posterior)—assist in forward flexion when acting bilaterally, and when acting unilaterally, assist in lateral flexion
- Longus colli—bends the neck forward, and when acting unilaterally, assists in lateral flexion to the same side and rotation to the opposite side
- Longus capitis—flexes the head forward
- Rectus capitis anterior—flexes the head forward

Extension

- Erector spinae
- Semispinalis capitis—extends the neck and head when acting bilaterally, bending the head backwards, and draws the head to the opposite side when acting unilaterally
- Semispinalis cervicis—extension, lateral flexion, and rotation to the opposite side
- Splenius capitis—extends the head and neck; lateral flexion and rotation of the head to the same side when acting unilaterally
- Splenius cervicis—same as splenius capitis
- Multifidus—extends the neck when acting bilaterally and provides lateral flexion and rotation of the neck to the opposite side when acting unilaterally

Lateral Flexion

- Splenius capitis
- Splenius cervicis
- SCM
- Scalenes
- Semispinalis capitis
- Semispinalis cervicis
- Erector spinae
- Multifidus
- Levator scapulae

Rotation

- SCM—rotates to opposite side
- Semispinalis cervicis and capitis—rotate to opposite side
- Multifidus—rotates to opposite side
- Splenius cervicis and capitis—rotate to same side
- Erector spinae—rotates to same side

Circumduction

As with the trunk, neck circumduction is the combination of flexion, lateral flexion, and hyperextension in a sequential movement.

Anatomy, Function, and Dysfunction of the Temporomandibular Joint

The TMJ is part of what is called the stomatognathic system, which includes the muscles of chewing (the mandibular and cervical muscles); the tongue; the TMJ; the occlusion of the teeth; and the associated ligaments, muscles, nerves and vessels.[11] The TMJ is probably used more than any other joint in the body, as it is involved in eating, chewing, speaking, and swallowing.

TEMPOROMANDIBULAR JOINT ANATOMY

▨ **Structure:** The TMJ is a synovial joint formed by the articulation of the horseshoe-shaped mandible and the two temporal bones of the skull (Fig. 5-10). An intervening disc separates the two bones, essentially creating an upper and a lower joint.[12] The mandible is composed of a body and right and left rami. The articulating region of the mandible is called the *mandibular condyle*; it is a rounded projection of bone that sits in the concave portion of the temporal bone called the *mandibular fossa*. On the anterior portion of each ramus is another bony protuberance, called the *coronoid process*, which serve as the attachment site for the temporalis and masseter muscles. The TMJ is located immediately anterior to the opening of the ear.

▨ **Function:** The TMJ functions during eating, chewing, speaking, and swallowing. The *resting position of the mandible* occurs when the teeth are held slightly apart, and in this position, there is minimal muscular effort.[13] The *resting position of the tongue* occurs when the superior portion of the tongue is resting lightly against the palate and the anterior tip is lightly touching the back of the upper front teeth.[11]

There is a functional relationship among the cervical spine, the TMJ, and the occlusion or articulation of the teeth. A change in head position affects the way the mandible closes, the resting position of the mandible, and the way the teeth make contact.[13] The TMJ is capable of five motions: opening the mouth, closing the mouth, jutting the chin forward (protrusion), sliding the jaw backward (retrusion), and lateral deviation of the mandible.

ARTICULAR DISC OR MENISCUS

▨ **Structure:** The meniscus is a fibrocartilage structure in the TMJ. Portions of the disc are highly innervated.

▨ **Function:** The meniscus functions to add congruency to the articulating surfaces throughout their ROM and to distribute the compressive forces.[12] The disc essentially follows the movement of the condyles of the mandible and moves anteriorly as the mouth opens and posteriorly as it closes.[13] The lateral pterygoid muscle attaches to the disc and pulls the condyle and the disc forward.

▨ **Dysfunction and injury:** The disc is susceptible to both acute injury and repetitive stresses. It can misalign, called subluxation, and create an inability to open and close the jaw properly. The disc can be cracked or torn owing to grinding the teeth or an injury (i.e., a blow to the jaw). Symptoms include

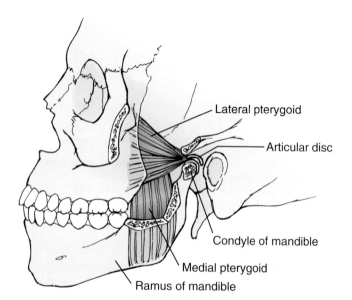

Lateral pterygoid

Articular disc

Condyle of mandible

Medial pterygoid

Ramus of mandible

Figure 5-10. Temporomandibular joint and the medial and lateral pterygoid muscles.

local pain, potential referral of pain to the head and ear, and a popping sensation.

LIGAMENTS

- The TMJ ligaments are the capsular ligaments, the stylomandibular ligament, the sphenomandibular ligament, and the temporomandibular ligament, which is a thickening of the joint capsule.

TEMPOROMANDIBULAR JOINT MUSCLES

- The mandible has eight muscles attached to it, and five of the eight muscles are essential to the movement of the TMJ: the temporalis, masseter, lateral pterygoid, medial pterygoid, and digastric muscles (Fig. 5-11 and see Fig. 3-10).

- The primary muscles that open the jaw are the lateral pterygoids and the digastrics. The suprahyoid muscles assist in mandibular opening, as the hyoid bone is fixed by the infrahyoid muscles.[13]

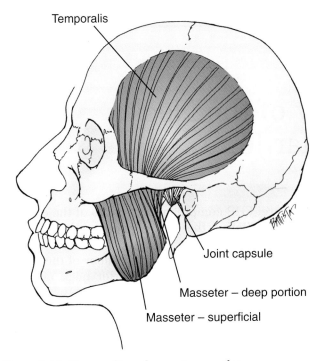

Figure 5-11. Temporalis and masseter muscles.

- The temporalis, masseter, and medial pterygoid muscles close the jaw.

- The masseter and the medial and lateral pterygoids provide protrusion.

- The posterior fibers of the temporalis perform retrusion, which is also called *retraction*.

- The medial and lateral pterygoids on one side and the contralateral temporalis provide lateral movement of the mandible. The muscles of the cervical spine stabilize the head, allowing for efficient mandible movements.

- **Dysfunction and injury:** Head posture has a significant and immediate effect on the resting position of the mandible.[12,13] In the FHP, as the cranium rotates posteriorly, the position of the tongue changes from the normal resting position behind the upper teeth to a position of dysfunction behind the lower teeth. This contributes to tightness in the suprahyoid muscles and anterior neck muscles.[11] Sustained tension in the masseter muscles is often associated with emotional or psychological stress and contributes to teeth grinding (bruxism). TMJ injury is common and results from incidents such as a blow or fall, or an acceleration force such as a car accident. Osteoarthritis of the TMJ is common and manifests as a painful reduction of the ability to open the mandible. Osteoarthritis develops from previous injury, cumulative stress of chronic tension, or imbalanced forces through the joint caused by malocclusion of the teeth or muscle imbalances.

- **Treatment implications:** Postural correction is the first treatment goal. Second, if sustained muscle tension is palpated in the client who has chronic pain or dysfunction, encourage stress management, such as aerobic exercise, yoga, meditation, or biofeedback. The easiest way to reduce sustained hypertonicity and balance the muscles of the TMJ is by application of CR MET (METs #10, #11, and #12). These techniques are performed in the resting position of the mandible to help stabilize the joint in neutral. Perform PIR MET to increase the joint ROM.

TEMPOROMANDIBULAR JOINT MUSCLE ANATOMY

See Figures 5-10 and 5-11. See Table 5-4 for a comprehensive listing of TMJ muscles and their origin, insertion, and action.

Table 5-4	Anatomy of the Muscles of Temporomandibular Joint		
Muscle	**Origin**	**Insertion**	**Action**
Temporalis	Entire temporal fossa; tendon passes through the gap between the zygomatic arch and the side of the skull	Medial surface, tip and front and back borders of coronoid process and front border of the ramus of the mandible	Elevates the mandible and so closes the mouth. Important muscle in chewing and biting.
Lateral pterygoid	Superior head from the infratemporal surface of the greater wing of the sphenoid and inferior head from the lateral pterygoid of the sphenoid	Inferior head into the neck of the mandible and pterygoid fovea and the superior head to the articular capsule and disc of the TMJ	Assists the mouth in opening by pulling the condyle and disc forward (protrusion). In closing the mouth, backward gliding of the disc and condyle are controlled by its slow relaxation.
Medial pterygoid	Thick, quadrilateral muscle attached to the medial surface of the lateral pterygoid plate of the sphenoid and the palatine bone	Passes down, laterally and backward and is attached to the inner surface of the mandibular ramus	Assists in elevating the mandible and with the lateral pterygoids, helps to protrude it.
Masseter	Consists of three superimposed layers: ■ The zygomatic process of the maxilla and the anterior two-thirds of the zygomatic arch ■ The deep surface of the front two-thirds of the zygomatic arch and the lower border of the posterior one-third of the arch ■ The deep surface of the zygomatic arch	■ The angle and lower half of the lateral surface of the mandibular ramus ■ The middle of the ramus of the mandible ■ The upper part of the ramus and into the coronoid process	Elevates the mandible to occlude the teeth in chewing

Dysfunction and Injury of the Neck and Temporomandibular Joint

FACTORS PREDISPOSING TO NECK AND TEMPOROMANDIBULAR JOINT DYSFUNCTION AND PAIN

■ **Injury:** An acceleration-deceleration strain of the neck, called *whiplash*, can result from a motor vehicle accident, sports injury, or fall. This whipping or jerking of the neck and jaw can damage ligaments as well as the joint capsule, muscles, cartilage, and nervous system.

■ **Posture:** FHP compresses the facets of the cervical spine, irritating the joint capsule, and causes the extensor muscles to be tight and short. It also causes increased tension in the floor of the mouth and the suprahyoid and anterior neck muscles. This leads to fatigue in the soft tissue, which predisposes it to injury.

■ **Emotional and psychological stress:** Tension, stress, anxiety, fear, resentment, uncertainty, and depression cause local areas of vasoconstriction and sustained contraction in the muscles of the neck and jaw, which leads to muscle fatigue. These changes result in altered patterns of muscle contraction and movement.

▨ **Abnormal function of the muscles:** Abnormal function of the muscles creates abnormal movement patterns and excessive stresses on the facets and disc. The result of these changes is that movement of the neck, jaw, or both becomes restricted and painful, leading to fibrosis around the joints.

▨ **Joint dysfunction:** Excessive mobility or loss of mobility in the joints of the cervical spine or TMJ predisposes the area to injury. The loss of normal gliding characteristics has reflexive changes in the surrounding muscles, setting up a continuing cycle of muscle and joint dysfunction.

▨ **Deconditioning or inactivity:** As the muscles dynamically stabilize the spine, if there is generalized muscle weakness caused by immobilization, lack of exercise, or previous injury, the lack of stability creates excessive movement to the joints, irritating the cartilage and capsular tissues.

▨ **Fatigue:** Factors that lead to fatigue include overuse, illness, and emotional and psychological stress, which lead to either sustained muscle contraction or weakness. A muscle that is held in constant tension develops ischemia and pain, whereas a weak muscle creates instability.

▨ **Aging:** The connective tissue becomes less resilient and less lubricated as a result of aging, and the soft tissues lose some of their shock-absorbing capacity.

▨ **Degeneration:** Aging and prior injury typically lead to loss of cartilage in the articular surfaces (facets), IVD, and disc of the TMJ. This degeneration is also referred to as osteoarthritis.

DIFFERENTIATION OF NECK, ARM, AND TEMPOROMANDIBULAR JOINT PAIN

▨ Neck pain and TMJ pain can be caused by many conditions, but we will assume that the following discussion applies to benign conditions (i.e., conditions that are not disease processes). For guidelines in ruling out pathologies, refer to Chapter 2, "Assessment and Technique"; see the section "Contraindications to Massage Therapy: Red Flags."

▨ The vast majority of neck pain is caused by a mechanical disorder, that is, a problem of function and not pathology. The precise cause of mechanical neck pain can be difficult to determine. Sometimes it is a case of a frank injury, but more often, there is an underlying hypomobility or degeneration of the facets, chronic muscle imbalance, poor posture, or emotional stress. Assuming that the client's pain is caused by a mechanical disorder, there are three broad categories of symptoms in the neck:

☐ **Tight, stiff:** An acute presentation of these symptoms typically implicates a muscle strain; chronic stiffness is a common symptom of a degenerated disc and joint.

☐ **Ache:** An acute, mild to moderate ache can be muscle, ligament, or joint strain/sprain complex; a severe ache implicates the disc or an inflammatory condition due to injury.

☐ **Sharp:** A sharp pain in the neck indicates a joint involvement, including the joint capsule. It can be a mild irritation, moderate inflammation, or severe damage to the cartilage and capsular tissues.

▨ Muscle injury is clinically evaluated by the presence of swelling, heat, spasm, tenderness to palpation, and pain elicited by isometric contraction. Muscle dysfunction will demonstrate predictable patterns of sustained tightness/weakness (upper crossed syndrome).

▨ Ligament injuries are extremely difficult to assess. Acute ligament sprain will demonstrate pain with passive motion. The pain is sharper and more localized than muscle pain. Chronic ligament involvement palpates as thickened tissue and restricted joint play (accessory motion) with a leathery end feel. There is pain with passive cervical rotation or passive opening of the jaw, but if the pain is at the end range, it could be a result of stretching an irritated muscle. It takes ligaments much longer to heal than muscles, and if recovery from a neck or TMJ injury has not occurred in several weeks, one possibility is that there has been ligament damage in addition to other structures that might be involved.

▨ The facet joints (zygapophyseal joints) are also a source of neck pain and of referral of pain into the head, shoulder, scapular region, and anterior chest wall and arm. Active motion often elicits a sharp, local pain during the acute phase. This is referred to by many names, such as *wry neck* and *acute facet syndrome*. In the chronic condition, the facets typically degenerate. The pain then becomes a more diffuse ache, and the neck is stiff in the morning. Assessment reveals loss of passive glide at the involved facets.

There are two fundamental types of pain that refer into the arm(s): sclerotomal and radicular. The two types are differentiated by the quality of pain. These two types of referral are important to distinguish, because it helps you to differentiate a simple mechanical disorder from a serious condition, such as a herniated disc.

■ **Sclerotomal pain,** the first type of referred pain, is caused by an injury to the paraspinal muscle, ligament, facet joint capsule, disc, or dura mater and can manifest locally and be referred to an extremity. Internal disc derangement in the cervical spine refers a deep, boring pain into the back of the neck and interscapular region. Pain from a muscle strain in the cervical region may be felt as a pain in the shoulder and arm as well as the neck. Usually, the sclerotomal referred pain is described as *deep, aching, and diffuse.*

■ **Radicular pain,** the second type of referred pain, is caused by an irritation of the spinal nerve root. The most common cause of nerve root irritation is disc herniation. If the sensory (dorsal) root is irritated, *sharp pain, numbing, or tingling that is well localized* in dermatomes occurs. If there is compression of the motor (ventral) nerve root in addition to the deep, boring pain, there may be a weakness in the muscles supplied by that nerve root (myotome) and a decrease in the response in the corresponding reflex. Nerve root pain is much more serious and requires an assessment by a chiropractor or osteopath.

COMMON TYPES OF DYSFUNCTION AND INJURY TO THE CERVICAL SPINE AND TEMPOROMANDIBULAR JOINT

MUSCLE STRAIN

■ **Causes:** Forward-head posture; emotional or psychological stress; repetitive strains, resulting from the dynamic movement of the neck in activities such as dance, gymnastics, martial arts, and sports; prolonged abnormal posture, such as cycling or working at the computer; or injury from a specific trauma, such as a car accident.

■ **Symptoms:** Muscle strains typically manifest as diffuse, dull, achy pain, or as tight areas or lines of stiffness in the neck, across the shoulders, or in the suboccipital region. The involved muscles are worsened with active motion. Moderate and severe muscle strain can manifest as sharp, local pain. Muscle strains are usually better with rest.

■ **Signs:** Involved muscles palpate as tight and tender. There may be a thickened texture with chronicity. With an active inflammation, the muscles are painful with isometric testing. There may be loss of active ROM, eliciting discomfort in the muscles.

■ **Treatment:** The primary intention in treating **acute** injuries is to reduce pain, swelling, and muscle spasms. Perform the Level I series of strokes, beginning on the non-involved side. Gentle, rhythmic rocking of the body in the side-lying position is deeply relaxing. Perform RI or CR MET on the tight and tender muscles, interspersed with your massage strokes. For **chronic** conditions, the intention is to identify short, tight muscles; fibrous tissue; weak muscles; and hypomobile joints. Perform both Level I and Level II strokes. Perform CR and eccentric MET for the cervical extensors (METs #1 and #8), and contract-relax-antagonist-contract (CRAC) MET (MET #9) to increase cervical rotation. Perform the cervical flexion test to determine whether the deep flexors are weak, and perform CR MET to help recruit them. The wave mobilization strokes are now performed more deeply to dissolve adhesions, and the P–A mobilization of the spine is performed more deeply to increase motion to the joints. It is important to instruct your client in good posture. Depending on the severity of the injury, an acute strain resolves in one to four weeks.

WHIPLASH SYNDROME (CERVICAL ACCELERATION/DECELERATION INJURY)

■ **Causes:** A common cause of whiplash is a rear-end auto collision, but any jolt to the head and neck—from a fall off a bike or horse, a ski accident, or a fall down stairs—can be considered a whiplash. A mild whiplash is essentially an injury of the soft tissue and would be diagnosed as a cervical sprain or strain injury. A moderate to severe whiplash may cause serious injuries to the muscles; ligaments; cartilage of the facets; disc; and nerves, including the brain. The main cause of the injury in a rear-end collision is the acceleration of the tissues, not necessarily the speed of the vehicles. When the car is hit, the head and neck accelerate at 250 milliseconds, overwhelming the integrity of the soft tissues.

■ **Symptoms:** Whiplash can have a wide possibility of symptoms, and there is often a delay of symptoms due to the gradual swelling and accumulation of waste products.
  □ *Neck pain and stiffness:* For neck pain, clients usually describe muscles that are sore, tight, and achy. There is often interscapular pain, from local strains and referred pain from the neck. The

muscles most commonly involved are the SCM, longus colli, and scalenes.

☐ *Decreased ROM in the neck:* The degree of lost motion often predicts the degree of injury. Severe loss of motion due to muscle splinting is a poor prognosis. Certain movements may elicit acute, sharp pain, which implicates joint involvement of the capsular ligaments, the cartilage, or both.

☐ *Headache:* May result from a variety of causes. Loss of short-term memory may occur if there is *minimal traumatic brain injury* (MTBI).

☐ *Referral of pain,* numbing, or tingling into the shoulders, arms, and hands may occur.

☐ *Vertigo,* dizziness, tinnitus, and visual disturbances from irritation of the cervical sympathetic nerves may occur.

☐ *Emotional distress* such as irritability and depression may be experienced.

▨ **Signs:** Hypertonic and tender musculature, which is often due to an acute reflex contraction caused by damaged fibers, may occur. Superficial and deep anterior and posterior muscles of the neck will be painful. Swelling in the soft tissues; painful restriction of motion; and neurologic signs, such as loss of reflexes and muscle weakness, may occur.

▨ **Treatment:** RI MET and CR MET (METs # 1, #2, and #3) are used in the **acute** phase, always within comfort, to reduce swelling and pain and relax hypertonic muscles. Next perform MET #5 from Chapter 4 ("Thoracic Spine") for the rhomboids, as this will help to release the muscles attaching to the cervicothoracic junction. Perform Level I STM strokes, minimizing the rocking. Next, perform gentle figure-eight joint mobilization, even if only as micromovements, to reduce inflammatory edema. Edema impedes venous flow around the nerve roots and facets, leading to poor repair. It is helpful to instruct the client in isometric exercises for a home program, with the METs for self-care. Active cervical and thoracic rotation is encouraged, as is movement of the arms, even if it is slightly uncomfortable, as long as the client can relax into the mild discomfort. One of the unfortunate outcomes the author has been treating for years is the degeneration and subsequent loss of motion in the cervical spine after improper treatment of a neck injury. In the author's opinion, this sequela is associated with the adhesions that have deposited owing to the lack of movement in the initial phases after a whiplash injury. For **chronic** conditions, use palpation and isometric testing to identify short, tight muscles; weak muscles; fibrous tissue, especially the joint capsules; and hypomobile joints. Typically, the SCM, scalenes, extensors, and suboccipitals are

short and tight, and the longus colli and multifidi are weak. Perform the Level I and Level II strokes, and treat what you find. Intersperse MET with your strokes when you identify tight or weak muscles. Perform CR and eccentric MET for the cervical extensors (METs #1 and #8), and CRAC MET (#9) to increase cervical rotation. If there is a loss of the cervical curve, it is contraindicated to stretch the cervical extensors. Instead, strengthen the multifidi to help restore the normal curve and stabilize the neck. See MET #5 to strengthen the multifidi. The wave mobilization strokes are now performed more deeply to dissolve adhesions, and the figure-eight mobilization of the spine is performed with greater amplitude to increase motion to the joints, unless the client is hypermobile, in which case small-amplitude mobilizations are continued. It is important to instruct your client in good posture and to encourage your client to be as active as possible.

FIXATION OR INJURY TO VERTEBRAL FACETS

▨ **Cause:** Trauma, sustained muscle contraction, and postural faults.

▨ **Symptoms:** A fixation or subluxation is a loss of joint play and may be completely asymptomatic. The fixation needs to be corrected; otherwise, it leads to degeneration. Facet syndrome (acute locking, or "wry neck") describes an acute episode of a sudden onset of sharp pain with a certain movement or upon awakening. Pain is usually well-localized, but pain, numbing, and tingling may radiate to the arm and hand.

▨ **Signs:** There is significant loss of motion in certain directions, especially rotation, lateral bending, and extension. Passive motion is restricted and elicits pain at the involved facet. Joint-play assessment identifies loss of normal passive glide of the involved facet. Palpation reveals tender muscle spasms, which have a thin-membraned rigidity due to acute spasticity.

▨ **Treatment:** Clients with **acute** neck pain are most comfortable in the side-lying fetal position with a pillow between the knees. Begin the Level I series of strokes on the non-involved side, with gentle rocking to induce relaxation. Perform a scanning palpation of the thoracic and cervical regions to assess areas of tenderness and spasticity. Perform wave mobilization strokes with a slow rhythm and light pressure until a comfortable depth has been established. The P–A mobilization to the facets will help to reduce swelling, reduce hypertonicity, and induce normal mobility to the facets. Perform

CR and RI MET (METs #1, #2, and #3), always within comfort, to reduce swelling and pain and relax hypertonic muscles. Next perform MET #5 from Chapter 4 ("Thoracic Spine") for the rhomboids, as this will help to release the muscles attaching to the C7 vertebra. Next, perform Level II, fifth series: the figure-eight mobilization of the cervical spine. If your client does not show significant improvement after four treatments, refer the client to a chiropractor or osteopath to assess the need for spinal manipulation. **Chronic** fixations are hypomobile joints, and the primary intention of the treatment is to mobilize the restricted segment. Identify hypomobility with motion palpation. Begin with Level I series of strokes, scanning the body for areas of hypertonicity, and use MET on those hypertonic muscles. Perform Level II strokes, especially the first series to release the multifidi and to mobilize capsular adhesions, which will allow for greater movement at the facets. When performing the wave mobilization strokes, sink deeply into the tissue within patient's tolerance to induce deep P–A mobilization on the restricted segments. It is important to remember that fixations or subluxations can be completely asymptomatic. Fixations in the vertebrae are common, and in the author's opinion, a chiropractor or an osteopath should assess patients who have any dysfunction in the cervical region.

ARTHROSIS (ARTHRITIS)— DEGENERATION OF VERTEBRAL FACETS

■ **Causes:** Previous trauma, FHP, and sustained muscle contraction. The degeneration begins as restriction of the joint capsule.[6] The articular cartilage needs movement to maintain lubrication on the surface. It also needs cycles of decompression that are inherent in moving the joint to allow the cartilage to imbibe its nutrition.

■ **Symptoms:** Arthrosis may be asymptomatic. Gradual onset of dull, achy neck, shoulder. or interscapular pain might occur. The neck is typically stiff and achy in the morning, feels better after it warms up with movement, and then worsens again at the end of the day, owing to fatigue. Extension and lateral bending aggravate the stiffness and pain.

■ **Signs:** Signs of arthritis are a loss of active motion in lateral bending and extension or a more complete loss of all motions except flexion with more serious degeneration in multiple joints. There is also a loss of passive motion (joint play) in the involved facets with a capsular or bony end feel.

■ **Treatment:** The primary goal of treatment is to rehydrate the joints, lengthen capsular tissues, and re-

duce excessive tension in the multifidi muscles, which interweave with the joint capsules. Use palpation and isometric testing to identify short, tight muscles; fibrous tissue; weak muscles; and hypomobile joints. Perform Level I and Level II strokes, with emphasis on the fourth series in Level II for the multifidi and joint capsule. Perform METs #5 and #9 to reduce hypertonicity in the multifidi and semispinalis capitus and to increase extensibility of the capsular tissues. These METs are intended to increase rotation, as this provides the greatest change in the client's function in daily activities. Perform strong P–A mobilization with the strokes, mobilizing the facets to rehydrate the joints. As you perform the strokes, identify areas of tightness, and perform MET as indicated. Clients who have degeneration need to move, such as brisk walking and simple ROM exercises for the neck. Some discomfort accompanies increased movement, but it is a necessary discomfort to recover function in the joint. The general rule is that the client should be able to completely relax into the discomfort of moving the involved area.

SPONDYLOSIS—DISC DEGENERATION

■ **Causes:** Whether the degeneration is a natural aging process or the result of previous trauma, sustained muscle contraction, or faulty posture is controversial.

■ **Symptoms:** Disc degeneration may be painless, or there may be a dull and achy neck pain, worsened by sudden movements. Diffuse neck stiffness and decreased ROM are also possible, as are headache and arm pain. Typically, the pain is worse in the morning.

■ **Signs:** When there is disc degeneration, the deep musculature of the neck is usually thick and has a fibrous feel. Ligaments and joint capsules are also thickened and gristly. Active ROM and passive ROM are limited in most directions, especially lateral bending and extension.

■ **Treatment:** Disc degeneration and degeneration of the facets are intimately related, and the treatments for the two conditions are identical. Follow the protocol for arthrosis, described above. Disc and facet degeneration will often lead to upper crossed syndrome, described earlier in the chapter. As you perform the Level I and Level II strokes, identify areas of tightness by palpation and areas of weakness with MET. Release the tight muscles first, then use CR MET to help strengthen the weak muscles. A stretching program, such as yoga, is helpful. In addition, clients should walk briskly for 20 minutes or more per day. Traction on a slant board may be performed to promote fluid uptake in the disc. Instruct the client in good posture.

CERVICAL DISC HERNIATION

- **Cause:** Traumatic injury, cumulative stresses caused by postural strain, sustained muscle contraction, joint dysfunction caused by fixation of the facets, adhesions of the ligaments or stresses through the region caused by muscle imbalance. It is typical in middle-aged adults and most common in the lower cervical spine (C4–C7).

- **Symptoms:** Disc herniation has two categories: internal herniation or derangement, which would cause constant deep, gripping pain in the neck or interscapular region, and external herniation, also called a disc bulge or protrusion. This protrusion typically compresses or stretches the nerve roots, causing pain that is sharp or gripping as well as numbing and tingling into the arms and hands, in a dermatomal and myotomal distribution. The pain, numbing, and tingling worsen with movements of the neck, especially extension and lateral flexion. Typically, the neck is painful even with rest and disturbs sleep. The pain is eased with positions that decrease the nerve root tension, such as the arm cradled or resting overhead.

- **Signs:** Cervical disc herniation painfully limits most movements, especially lateral flexion and extension. If the motor root of the nerve is affected, it leads to loss of muscle strength in the affected myotome. A positive foraminal compression test elicits pain, numbing, and tingling into the arms.

- **Treatment:** The goal of treatment is to reduce the pain and inflammation as quickly as possible. Place the client in side-lying fetal position, which is the position of greatest comfort for acute neck pain. Perform RI MET and CR MET (METs #1, #2, and #3) to reduce swelling and muscle spasms. Although reflex muscle guarding typically accompanies an acute disc problem, it is important to realize that the goal of treatment is to reduce *excessive* tension in the muscles. Deep release of the muscles is **contraindicated,** as it can destabilize the spine. Perform Level I strokes with a gentle, light pressure and slow, small rocking motions. Palpate the muscles as you perform the strokes, and perform CR MET on the tight muscles, typically the cervical extensors, SCM, and scalenes. Next perform MET #5 from Chapter 4 ("Thoracic Spine") for the rhomboids, as this will help to release the muscles attaching to the C7 vertebra. As the client improves, deeper P–A mobilization may be applied with the wave mobilization strokes to restore normal passive motion to the facets. Work under the supervision of a doctor (chiropractic, osteopathic, or medical). Treatment should include strengthening, stabilizing, and proprioceptive reeducation.

SCALENUS ANTICUS SYNDROME (ANTERIOR SCALENE SYNDROME)

- **Causes:** Previous strain to the scalenes, such as whiplash or other cervical trauma; FHP, which shortens the anterior scalene; or a dysfunctional respiratory pattern of chest breathing in which the scalenes are overused, which is associated with periods of emotional and psychological stress.

- **Symptoms:** Pain, numbness, and tingling may occur, usually on the ulnar side of the hand but may affect the entire hand.

- **Signs:** Anterior scalene syndrome elicits pain that is often brought on with arm elevation, the *elevated-arm stress test.* Digital pressure on scalenes may produce pain, numbing, or tingling that radiates to the ulnar border of the hand.

- **Treatment:** The primary intention of treatment is to reduce sustained muscle tension in the scalenes and correct posture. Use palpation and isometric testing (MET) to identify short, tight muscles; fibrous tissue; weak muscles; and hypomobile joints. It is important to remember that a condition such as anterior scalene syndrome is not isolated to one muscle group but involves the entire body. In the approach described in this text, it is recommended to perform the entire Level I spinal work described in Chapter 3 ("Lumbosacral Spine") and Chapter 4 ("Thoracic Spine") to identify tight and tender tissue and treat what you find. Next, perform the Level I cervical series of strokes, with emphasis on the fifth series for the scalenes. Perform RI or CR MET #4 for the scalenes, interpersed with your strokes. For **chronic** conditions, perform both Level I and Level II strokes. Perform PIR MET for the upper trapezius, levator, and scalenes (METs #6 and #7). The STM strokes are now performed more deeply to dissolve adhesions, and the P–A mobilization of the spine is performed more deeply to increase the motion to the joints. It is important to instruct your client in good posture and abdominal breathing.

TEMPOROMANDIBULAR JOINT DYSFUNCTION

- **Causes:** FHP; emotional stress creating sustained contraction of the muscles that close the jaw; malocclusion of the teeth; trauma, such as a whiplash.

- **Symptoms:** Decreased motion of the jaw and insidious onset of dull, aching pain in the area of the

TMJ, often radiating to the face, head, neck, and shoulders are indicators of TMJ dysfunction (TMJD). Temporomandibular joint dysfunction can lead to osteoarthritis in the elderly.

Signs: Muscle tenderness, especially the masseter; decreased ROM in the ability to open the jaw; deviation in the mandible while opening; and clicking in the joint while opening and closing, which typically indicates derangement of the disc, may occur.[12]

Treatment: For **acute** TMJ pain, perform METs #10, #11, and #12. This will help to reduce pain, swelling, and muscle spasms. Perform Level I cervical strokes and Level II, fifth series, for the TMJ. For **chronic** conditions, use soft tissue palpation, motion palpation of the joints, and isometric testing to identify short, tight muscles; fibrous tissue; weak muscles; and hypomobile joints. Use MET, STM, and joint mobilization to treat what you find. Instruct the client in good posture.

Assessment

BACKGROUND

One of the primary intentions of assessment of the cervical spine for massage therapists is to differentiate an acute disc injury from injuries and dysfunctions to the muscles, ligaments, and joints. The details from your client's history regarding symptoms and onset will guide your examination. A deep, gripping pain in the arm that is not associated with an injury to the arm and is not worsened by arm motion is an indication that a cervical disc might be involved. The physical exam will rule in or rule out an acute disc injury as distinguished from other dysfunctions and injuries. This objective is accomplished primarily through active ROM. A herniated disc will severely limit cervical ROM, and will manifest as arm pain that is greater than neck pain. The second goal is to assess the passive ROM of the intervertebral joints. The third goal is to assess the soft tissue through isometric testing and palpation. One clinical use of MET is to assess the muscles for pain and strength. Assessment through palpation is accomplished primarily through performing the strokes.

HISTORY QUESTIONS FOR NECK PAIN CLIENTS

Do you have neck pain that is worse at night?
☐ Localized, constant, gripping neck pain that is worse at night is a symptom that need immediate referral to a doctor. This pain could indicate a tumor, as the cervical spine is a common site for metastatic tumors from the breast, lung, and prostate.[2] Pain can be worse at night with significant inflammation as a result of the pooling of inflammatory waste products, but it typically is not localized, constant, or gripping.

Is the pain, stiffness, or ache better or worse in the morning?
☐ Pain that is worse in the morning or at night implies inflammation. These clients typically take longer to respond to treatment, as there is a chemical, not just a mechanical, basis to their pain, and that requires a longer healing time.
☐ Chronic morning stiffness implies a degenerative condition. These clients need postural and exercise instruction, including stretching of the muscles of the spine, in addition to manual therapy.
☐ Pain that is better in the morning and worsens during the day implies fatigue as a contributing factor. This fatigue could result from postural stresses, tension from emotional stress, or a functional problem with a soft tissue basis.

Do you have pain, numbing, or tingling in the arm(s) or hand(s)?
☐ If the client has arm or hand pain that is sharp and localized in a dermatome, it could be a result of a nerve root irritation in the neck. Perform the foraminal compression test (see "Foraminal Compression Test" below) and the active ROM tests to the area of referral and isometric muscles tests to the area of pain. If the pain is referred, the ROM of the extremity is full and pain free. It is not uncommon for a client to present with arm or hand pain that is worse than the neck pain, indicating a nerve root irritation. If the client can lie comfortably on the table, proceed with your

massage, but strokes should be light, and rocking should be gentle. Pain-free CR for the hypertonic muscles may also be performed.

▨ **Do you have headaches, blurred vision, or dizziness?**
  ☐ Headaches may be caused by muscle tension or an upper cervical facet syndrome, which is usually responsive to treatment. If the client has throbbing headaches, unrelated to activity, associated with blurred vision and nausea, refer the client to a doctor. As was mentioned previously, symptoms of nausea, blurred vision, tinnitus, and dizziness after a neck injury are often associated with an irritation of the sympathetic nervous system.

OBSERVATION: CLIENT STANDING

▨ Notice any signs of inflammation such as redness or swelling or signs of previous trauma or surgery such as bruising or scars, in all views described below.

FRONT VIEW

▨ Is head held in a tilted or rotated position? A neck or head that is held in a sustained, painless rotation, flexion, or lateral flexion may be caused by muscle imbalances, fixation of a vertebral facet, or degenerative joint disease. If the neck is painful, the pain may be due to a herniated disc, entrapped fibromeniscus in the joint, or an acute spasm caused by soft tissue injury.

SIDE VIEW

▨ Does the client stand in a forward-head, rounded-shoulder posture? As was mentioned in the beginning of this chapter, this posture is a major source of neck pain because of the excessive demand on the soft tissues.
  ☐ Correct the client's posture in the standing position as described in Chapter 3, p. 123, by first correcting the lumbar curve and then bringing the head back so that the opening of the ear is in line with the upright acromion.

OBSERVATION: CLIENT SITTING

SIDE VIEW

▨ Observe the client's posture when seated (Fig. 5-12). With correct posture, the opening of the ear

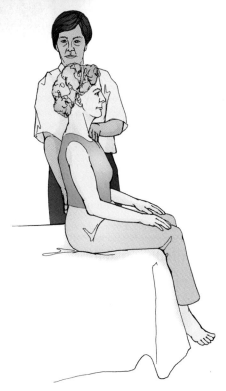

Figure 5-12. If the client has slumped posture, instruct her in the correct posture by first introducing a slight curve in the lumbar spine. Next, have her lift her sternum and then bring the head upright so that the opening of the ear is over the acromion.

should be over the upright shoulder. If the client is slumping, instruct the client in correct posture by first introducing the normal lumbar curve, and then bring the head so that the opening of the ear is in line with the upright acromion.

MOTION ASSESSMENT

To assess **active movements,** stand, facing the seated client. Note the ROM, and ask the client whether the movement is painful, where it is painful, and the quality of pain. Perform the most painful movements last, as movement into pain may irritate the other structures.

ROTATION

▨ **Action:** Ask the client to turn the head as far as is comfortable in one direction and then in the other.

▨ **Observation:** The range of rotation is approximately 70°, that is, not quite to the plane of the shoulder (Figs. 5-13 and 5-14). A line or area of tension indicates muscle hypertonicity. A diffuse

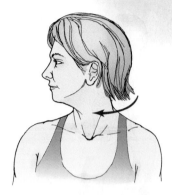

Figure 5-13. Active cervical rotation to the right.

area of pain indicates soft tissue irritation or in-flammation. A sharp, local pain indicates a facet syndrome, including irritation of the joint capsule.

EXTENSION

- **Action:** Ask the client to look up as far as is comfortable.

- **Observation:** In active cervical extension, the client should be able to look at the ceiling comfortably (Fig. 5-15). Extension closes the facet joints and the IVF and elicits a sharp, local pain in the neck if there is a fixation of the facet or irritation of the joint capsule. This motion often elicits a soreness or pain in the suboccipital region due to compression of tight suboccipital muscles or a pain in the front of the neck if there has been injury to the anterior neck muscles. Sometimes this movement elicits suboccipital pain and pain in the front of the neck. A referral of pain to the top of the shoulder or scapular area indicates irritation of the joint, and referral of a sharp dermatomal pain into the arm or hand indicates a nerve root problem.

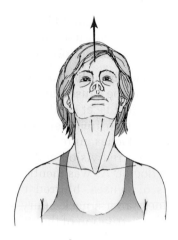

Figure 5-15. Active cervical extension.

FLEXION

- **Action:** Ask the client to bend the head toward the chest as far as is comfortable.

- **Observation:** In active cervical flexion, two finger-tips' distance between the chin and the chest is within normal limits (Fig. 5-16). Flexion opens the vertebral facets and provides relief for joint problems. However, this motion stretches the muscles of the back of the neck and shoulders, including the cervical extensors and trapezius, and often elicits a pulling sensation or pain in the scapular region caused by muscle injury or hypertonicity.

LATERAL FLEXION

- **Action:** Ask the client to bring the ear toward the shoulder to the comfortable limit (Figs. 5-17 and 5-18).

- **Observation:** The normal range is approximately 45°, that is, approximately halfway to the shoulder. A spot of pain on the side of bending usually indicates a joint problem. A line of pain or tension on

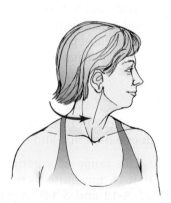

Figure 5-14. Active cervical rotation to the left.

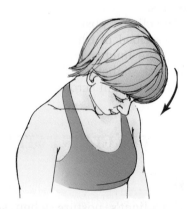

Figure 5-16. Active cervical flexion.

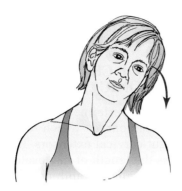

Figure 5-17. Active side bending to the left.

the opposite side usually indicates muscle injury or hypertonicity. Lateral bending closes the facets and the IVF on that side. It may elicit a diffuse referral of pain to the top of the shoulder or to the scapular region with joint irritation; or it might elicit sharp dermatomal pain, numbing, or tingling into the arm or hand with nerve root irritation. Chronic limited side bending is indicative of capsular fibrosis or degenerative joint disease.

SPECIAL TESTS: CLIENT SITTING

FORAMINAL COMPRESSION TEST

▓ **Intention:** The foraminal compression test is performed if there is referral of pain, numbing, or tingling into the shoulder or arm. The intention is to determine whether the injury is a joint problem or nerve root irritation (Fig. 5-19).

▓ **Action:** The client laterally flexes the head to one side, and the therapist carefully pushes straight down onto head. Do not proceed with this test if positioning the neck in lateral flexion elicits sharp,

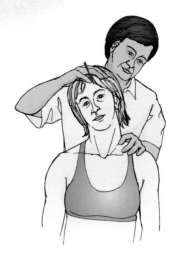

Figure 5-19. Foraminal compression test. The client laterally flexes neck to the painful side. Press down gently into the crown of the head. Localized pain in the neck usually indicates a joint problem. Referral of pain, numbing, or tingling into the arm indicates irritation of the nerve root.

local pain or referral of symptoms into the shoulder or arm.

▓ **Observation:** This test closes the IVF, compresses the facets, and reproduces the client's symptoms if the joint is injured or the nerve root is irritated. If pain, numbing, or tingling radiates into the arm or hand or there is increased radiation in a dermatomal pattern, it indicates a nerve root irritation. A diffuse referral of pain into the top of the shoulder or scapular region indicates a facet joint irritation. A sharp pain local to the neck could indicate a subluxation or fixation of the facet.

ELEVATED ARM STRESS TEST

▓ **Intention:** The elevated-arm stress test test is performed if there is numbing or tingling in the hand(s). The intention is to determine whether the client has compression of the neurovascular bundle in the area of the thoracic outlet.

▓ **Action:** Have the client sit. Flex the client's elbows to 90°, and abduct and externally rotate the client's shoulders to 90°. Have the client open and close her hands for 3 minutes (Fig. 5-20).

▓ **Observation:** This test stretches the neurovascular bundle that travels under the clavicle. If the brachial plexus, artery, or vein is compressed, the client will feel numbing, tingling, coldness, or weakness in the hands. This compression may be due to injury; postural stresses; or muscle hypertonicity of the scalenes, subclavius, or pectoralis minor. Weakness in the arms manifests as unconscious lowering of the arm as the client performs the test.

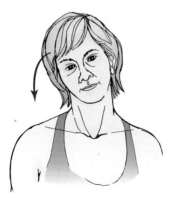

Figure 5-18. Active side bending to the right.

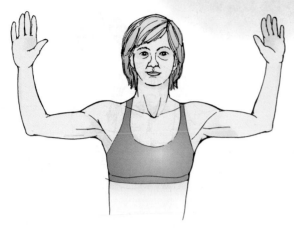

Figure 5-20. Elevated-arm stress test. This helps to determine whether the client has compression of the neurovascular bundle in the area of the thoracic outlet.

ASSESSMENT OF THE TEMPOROMANDIBULAR JOINT RANGE OF MOTION

▨ **Action:** Have the client open the mouth to the comfortable limit. Ask the client to place three fingers between the front teeth (Fig. 5-21).

▨ **Observation:** Limited motion or pain is an indication of TMJ dysfunction. A person should be able to place the width of three fingers in the opening of the mouth. Loss of motion may be caused by pain, muscle hypertonicity, disc derangement, or osteoarthritis. Notice whether there are deviations of the mandible to the side when the client opens the jaw. Deviations may be caused by muscle hypertonicity, subluxation of the TMJ, or disc derangement.

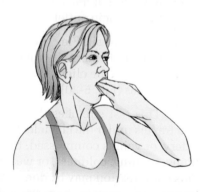

Figure 5-21. To determine whether the client has a normal opening of the jaw, ask the client to place three fingers into the opening of the mouth. Limited motion or pain is an indication of temporomandibular dysfunction.

SPECIAL TESTS: CLIENT SUPINE

ASSESSMENT OF CERVICAL EXTENSORS LENGTH (CHRONIC ONLY)

▨ **Intention:** This is performed if the client has an increased cervical curve, which would indicated short and tight cervical extensors. It is also important to assess the length of the levator scapula, upper trapzeus, scalenes, and pectoralis major in chronic conditions. These techniques are shown in the MET section below.

▨ **Action:** Gently lift client's head, and passively flex it toward the client's chest to the resistance barrier (Fig. 5-22).

▨ **Observation:** Performing an assessment of the cervical extensor muscle length is **contraindicated** for the client who is in acute pain. The client's chin should be able to touch the area above the sternum. Perform PIR for cervical extensors if there is a limitation of motion (see Fig. 5-32 later in the chapter).

CERVICAL FLEXION TEST TO ASSESS THE DEEP CERVICAL FLEXOR STRENGTH (CHRONIC ONLY)

▨ **Intention:** The cervical flexors are typically weak after injury or chronic dysfunction. The intention is to test their strength and instruct the client in a home exercise if they are weak.

▨ **Action:** Ask your client to bend her knees, and bring her feet flat on the table. Ask her to raise her head off the table to look toward her feet (Fig. 5-23).

▨ **Observation:** Watch to see whether the head is extending on the neck, that is, whether the chin is

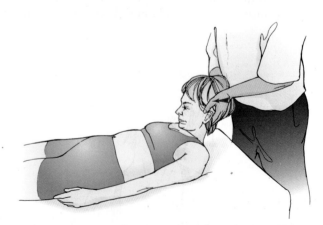

Figure 5-22. Assessment of the cervical extensor muscles length. Slowly lift the head toward the sternum. It is **contraindicated** to perform this on a client in acute pain.

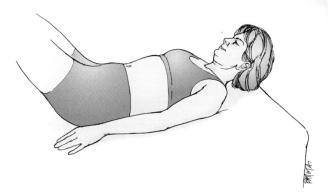

Figure 5-23. Cervical flexion test. In clients who have weak deep cervical flexor muscles, the chin juts away from the throat.

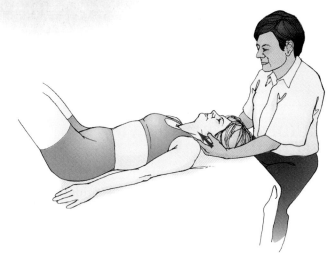

Figure 5-24. Joint play to assess the passive mobility of the vertebral facets. This is an assessment and a treatment.

jutting away from the throat or the head is being flexed with the neck and the chin moves closer to the throat. If the deep neck flexors are of normal strength, the chin moves toward the throat and not up to the ceiling. If the deep cervical flexors are weak, the SCM and scalenes substitute, extending the head, jutting the chin toward the ceiling. A home exercise to recruit the deep flexors is the head nod exercise.[7] Have the client lie on her back on a mat on the floor. Tell her to tuck her chin and curl the neck to slowly lift the head off the mat. Repeat ten times. If there is pain, have the client place a small pillow under her head. Place a small rolled towel under the neck to support the normal lordosis.

PALPATION

SOFT TISSUE PALPATION

▨ Perform a brief scan of the soft tissue as part of the assessment, and perform a much more precise palpation in the context of the strokes. Palpate the soft tissue on either side of the vertebrae, in the suboccipital region, and on the superior border of the scapulae. Assess temperature, texture, tenderness, and tone. Ask the client whether it hurts and whether there is referral of pain. If it is painful, ask whether the pain is mild, moderate, or severe. If the pain is severe, refer the client to a chiropractor or osteopath.

VERTEBRAE PALPATION

▨ Put the fingertips of one hand on each SP from C7 to C2, and push P–A to assess joint play and tenderness of the vertebrae. To induce P–A joint play,

add a slight posterior cranial rotation as you press on each vertebra.

ASSESSMENT OF VERTEBRAL FACET JOINT MOBILITY

▨ Passive glide in a joint is called *joint play,* and to function properly, each joint in the spine needs to have this play (Fig. 5-24).

▨ **Intention:** The intention is to induce a passive glide gently into the vertebral facets from C7 to C2, one joint at a time, to assess ROM.

▨ **Action:** Find the vertebral facets 1 inch lateral to the SP, over the muscle bundle. Place your fingertips on the facets, and press in a medial direction, one side at a time. Move up to the next vertebra, and perform this motion in rhythmic oscillations.

▨ **Observation:** A normal, painless gliding motion is present in a healthy joint. Localized restriction indicates a fixation of the facet joint or localized degeneration. Diffuse hypomobility indicates more generalized degeneration. Localized pain or local pain that refers to the scapular region indicates irritation or inflammation of the vertebral facet.

ISOMETRIC TESTS

▨ Isometric tests are performed to determine whether muscles are strong and pain free, weak, or painful. Isometric tests of the cervical spine and CR MET are performed simultaneously. The muscles should be strong and pain free with isometric challenge. Ask the client whether the resisted motion is painful. If it is painful, ask the client the location and quality of the pain.

Techniques

GUIDELINES TO APPLYING TECHNIQUES

A thorough discussion of treatment guidelines can be found on p. 86 in Chapter 2. In the method of treatment described in this text, we make two underlying assumptions: that pain or dysfunction in one localized area affects the entire region, and so we assess and treat an entire region rather than localized pain, and that pain that localizes in one tissue affects all of the structures in the region. Neck pain, for example, typically involves muscles, tendons, ligaments, joints capsules, facet joints, and IVDs. This is called *somatic dysfunction*, a term developed by osteopaths that is defined as "*impaired or altered function of related components of the somatic (body framework) system; skeletal, arthrodial (joint), and myofascial structures; and related vascular, lymphatic, and neural elements.*"[14] A simple muscle strain, for example, is not an isolated condition but affects the associated joints, nerves, and muscles that are compensating for the strain, as well as the vascular and lymphatic systems. The treatments described in this text address all the components of somatic dysfunction through three techniques: muscle energy technique (MET), soft tissue mobilization (STM), and joint mobilization. These techniques can be applied to every type of neck pain, but the "dose" of the technique varies greatly from slow movements and light pressures for acute conditions to stronger pressures and deeper-amplitude mobilizations for chronic problems. Each aspect of the treatment is also an assessment to determine pain, tenderness, hypertonicity, weakness, and hypomobility or hypermobility. We use the philosophy of treating what we find when we find it. Remember that the goal of treatment is to heal the body, mind, and emotions. Keep your hands soft, keep your touch nurturing, and work only within the comfortable limits of your client so that he or she can completely relax into the treatment.

THE INTENTIONS OF TREATMENT FOR ACUTE CONDITIONS ARE AS FOLLOWS

▓ To stimulate the movement of fluids to reduce edema, increase oxygenation and nutrition, and eliminate waste products.

▓ To maintain as much pain-free joint motion as possible to prevent adhesions and maintain the health of the cartilage, which is dependent on movement for its nutrition.

▓ To provide mechanical stimulation to help align healing fibers and stimulate cellular synthesis.

▓ To provide neurological input to minimize muscular inhibition and help maintain proprioceptive function

 CAUTION: *Stretching is* **contraindicated** *in acute conditions*

THE INTENTIONS OF TREATMENT FOR CHRONIC CONDITIONS ARE AS FOLLOWS

▓ To dissolve adhesions and restore flexibility, length, and alignment to the myofascia.

▓ To dissolve fibrosis in the ligaments and capsular tissues surrounding the joints.

▓ To rehydrate the cartilage, and restore mobility and ROM to the joints.

▓ To eliminate hypertonicity in short, tight muscles; strengthen weakened muscles; and reestablish the normal firing pattern in dysfunctioning muscles.

▓ To restore neurological function by increasing sensory awareness and proprioception.

Clinical examples are described below under "Soft Tissue Mobilization."

MUSCLE ENERGY TECHNIQUE

THERAPEUTIC GOALS OF MUSCLE ENERGY TECHNIQUE

A thorough discussion of the clinical application of MET can be found on p. 76. The MET techniques described below are organized into one section for teaching purposes. In the clinical setting, the METs and STM techniques are interspersed throughout the session. METs are used for assessment and treatment.

A healthy muscle or group of muscles is strong and pain free when isometrically challenged. MET will be painful if there is ischemia or inflammation in the muscles or their associated joints. The muscle will be weak and painless if the muscle is inhibited or the nerve is compromised. During treatment, MET is used as needed. For example, when you find a tight and tender SCM, use CR MET to reduce the hypertonicity and tenderness. If the SCM is painful while contracting, perform a RI MET for the SCM, which contracts the posterolateral extensors, inducing a neurological relaxation to the SCM. If the deep cervical flexors are weak and inhibited, first release the tight cervical extensors (MET #1), and then use isotonic MET to recruit and strengthen the deep cervical flexors.

MET is very effective for an acute, painful neck, but the pressure that is applied must be very light so as not to induce pain. Gentle, pain-free contraction and relaxation of the cervical extensors and related muscles provide a pumping action to reduce swelling, promote the flow of oxygen and nutrition, and eliminate waste products.

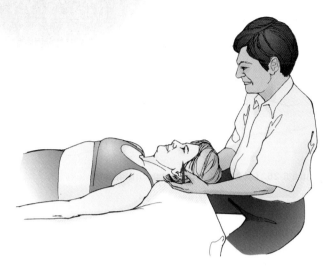

Figure 5-25. CR MET for the cervical extensors.

THE BASIC THERAPEUTIC INTENTIONS OF MET FOR ACUTE CONDITIONS ARE AS FOLLOWS

▨ To provide a gentle pumping action to reduce pain and swelling, promote oxygenation of the tissue, and remove waste products.

▨ To reduce muscle spasms.

▨ To provide neurological input to mimimize muscular inhibition.

THE BASIC THERAPEUTIC INTENTIONS OF MET FOR CHRONIC CONDITONS ARE AS FOLLOWS

▨ To decrease excessive muscle tension.

▨ To strengthen muscles.

▨ To lengthen connective tissue.

▨ To increase joint movement and increase lubrication to the joints.

▨ To restore neurological function.

The MET section below shows techniques that are used for most clients, but three techniques (METs #1, #2, and #3) are designed especially for acute, painful conditions. PIR METs that lengthens muscles and fascia are **contraindicated** for acute conditions.

Remember that MET should not be painful. Mild discomfort as the client resists the pressure is normal if the area is irritated or inflamed. Refer to Chapter 6 for METs for the shoulder.

MUSCLE ENERGY TECHNIQUE FOR ACUTE NECK PAIN

1. Contract-Relax Muscle Energy Technique for the Cervical Extensors

▨ **Intention:** To release the cervical extensors. Cervical extensors are typically hypertonic in acute neck pain.

▨ **Position:** Client is supine. If the client is in acute distress, a pillow may be placed under the head to give it extra support. Place both your hands under the skull (Fig. 5-25).

▨ **Action:** Instruct the client to resist as you gently attempt to lift the head straight off the table for approximately 5 seconds.

2. Contract-Relax Muscle Energy Technique for the Suboccipital Muscles

▨ **Intention:** To perform CR MET to release the suboccipital muscles. The suboccipital muscles are typically short and tight, owing to FHP. If these muscles are injured, the client might feel suboccipital pain and posterior cranium pain. In addition, injuries to these muscles can contribute to disturbances in balance and position sense (proprioception).

▨ **Position:** Hold the base of the client's head (occipital bone), and ask the client to rotate the head backward approximately 1 inch, as if looking overhead (Fig. 5-26).

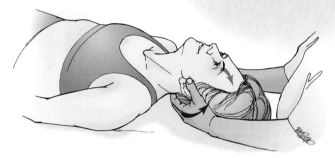

Figure 5-26. CR MET for the suboccipital muscles.

▨ **Action:** Instruct the client to resist as you attempt to roll the head back into flexion.

3. *Contract-Relax Muscle Energy Technique for the Lateral Flexors*

▨ **Intention:** To perform CR MET to release the lateral flexors. Lateral flexors are typically short and tight.

▨ **Position:** Client is supine, with the head in neutral. Place the palm of your hand on the mastoid processes, with your index and ring fingers behind the ears (Fig. 5-27).

▨ **Action:** Instruct the client to resist as you press gently into the side of the head. Hold for 5 seconds, and repeat on the opposite side. This cycle of CR on one side and then the other is repeated three to five times.

MUSCLE ENERGY TECHNIQUE FOR SUBACUTE AND CHRONIC NECK PAIN

4. *Contract-Relax Muscle Energy Technique for the Cervical Flexors*

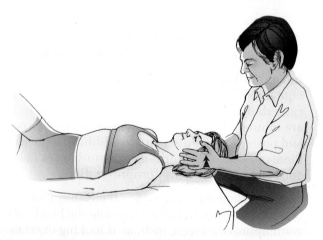

Figure 5-27. CR MET for the lateral flexors.

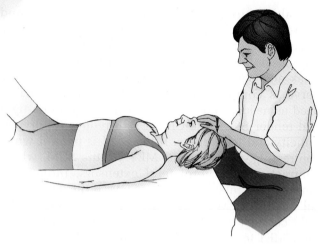

Figure 5-28. CR MET for the cervical flexors.

 CAUTION: This motion might be painful after a cervical strain. Do not perform this movement if it is painful.

▨ **Intention:** To perform light CR of the flexors to help normalize cervical flexor function and also to create greater relaxation by reciprocally inhibiting hypertonic extensors. Cervical flexors are often injured in cervical trauma. They are typically weak as a result of chronic dysfunction and pain owing to injury.

▨ **Position:** Tuck one hand under the skull, and place the other hand on the forehead to stabilize the head (Fig. 5-28).

▨ **Action:** Lift the client's head 1 or 2 inches off the table, and rotate the cranium slightly to move the chin toward the throat. If this position is not painful, have the client resist as you attempt to press the head back to the table.

5. *Contract-Relax Muscle Energy Technique for the Anterolateral Flexors and the Posterolateral Extensors*

▨ **Intention:** To perform CR MET for the anterolateral flexors, especially the SCM, and the posterolateral extensors, including the multifidi and semispinalis capitis. The SCM is one of the most commonly injured muscles. It is typically short and tight and contributes to FHP. The multifidi interweave with the joint capsule and may interfere with normal joint function.

▨ **Position:** Hold the client's head at the mastoid processes (Fig. 5-29).

▨ **Action:** Lift the client's head, and rotate it to one side. Have the client resist as you attempt to press the

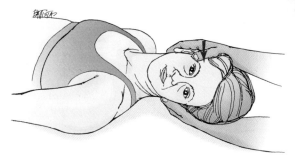

Figure 5-29. CR MET for the anterolateral flexors and the posterolateral extensors.

head back toward the table. Hold for approximately 5 seconds. Next, have the client resist as you attempt to lift the head up while it is in a rotated position. This engages the multifidi and reciprocally inhibits the SCM. Repeat on both sides. This MET may be given as a home exercise to strengthen the multifidi, stabilize the neck, and restore the normal lordosis.

6. *Postisometric Relaxation Muscle Energy Technique for the Upper Trapezius and the Levator Scapula*

▧ **Intention:** To relax and lengthen the more lateral fibers of the levator scapula and upper trapezius. The upper trapezius and levator are typically short and tight.

▧ **Position:** Tuck one hand under the skull, and place the fingers of one hand on the mastoid bone behind the ear. Place the other hand on top of the shoulder (Fig. 5-30).

▧ **Action:** Instruct the client to resist as you attempt to pull the head and shoulder apart. Hold for 5 seconds, relax, and then move the head toward the opposite shoulder until a resistance barrier is felt. Have the client resist as you attempt to pull the head and shoulder away from each other again. Re-

peat this CR–lengthen cycle several times, and then perform on the other side.

7. *Variations in Postisometric Muscle Energy Technique for the Upper Trapezius, Levator Scapula, and Scalenes*

▧ **Intention:** The scalenes, levator scapula, and upper trapezius are typically short and tight and need to be lengthened. The intention is to use PIR MET to isolate these muscles more specifically.

▧ **Position:** For the left levator, lift the client's head into cervical flexion with your left hand, and stabilize the shoulder with your right hand. Have client rotate the head to the right (Fig. 5-31). For left trapezius and middle scalenes, keep the client's face toward the ceiling. For the left anterior scalenes, have client rotate the head toward the left shoulder.

▧ **Action:** Instruct the client to resist as you pull the client's head into greater flexion and to the right; that is, away from the shoulder. Hold for 5 seconds, relax for a couple of seconds, and move the head away from the held shoulder until a new resistance barrier is felt. Repeat several times, and perform on the other side.

MUSCLE ENERGY TECHNIQUE FOR CHRONIC NECK PAIN OR LOSS OF RANGE OF MOTION

8. *Eccentric Muscle Energy Technique to Increase the Length of the Cervical Extensors*

▧ **Intention:** To use eccentric MET to lengthen the cervical extensors. The cervical extensor muscles

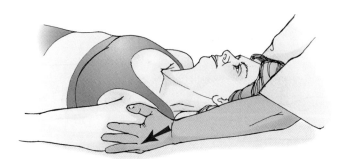

Figure 5-30. PIR for the upper trapezius and the levator scapula. This MET is used to relax and lengthen the more lateral fibers of the upper trapezius and the levator scapula.

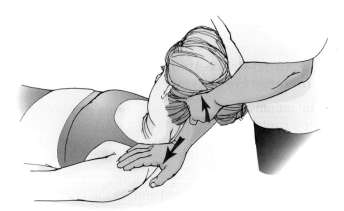

Figure 5-31. Variations in PIR MET for the upper trapezius, the levator scapula, and the scalenes. This MET is used to isolate the muscles more specifically. This figure shows the head turned away from the stabilizing hand for the levator scapula.

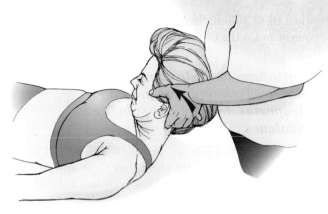

Figure 5-32. Eccentric MET to lengthen the cervical extensors. It is common for the extensors to shorten in chronic neck problems. This MET effectively lengthens the connective tissue of the extensors.

are typically short and tight, owing to chronic forward-head posture or as a consequence of prior injury (Fig. 5-32).

 CAUTION: *This should not be performed if the client has lost the normal cervical curve.*

▨ **Position:** Place both hands under the client's skull.

▨ **Action:** Ask the client to resist as you attempt to lift the head off the table. After approximately 5 seconds, instruct the client to allow you to lift the head toward the chest while offering some resistance. "Let me win as you press into my hands" is a good cue. Continue lifting, rolling the chin toward the throat until pain or a resistance barrier is felt. After you have reached the comfortable limit, place one hand on the client's forehead and have the client resist as you attempt to push the head back toward the table. This "sets" the extensors at their new length. Repeat several times.

9. *Contract-Relax-Antagonist-Contract to Increase the Cervical Spine Rotation*

▨ **Intention:** To use CRAC MET to increase cervical spine rotation. Cervical rotation is typically limited because of chronic muscular or ligamentous problems or degeneration of the joints (Fig. 5-33).

▨ **Position:** For increasing cervical spine rotation to the right, place the right hand on the client's right mastoid process and the left hand over the client's left ear.

▨ **Action:** Have the client rotate the head to the right to the comfortable limit. Have the client resist as

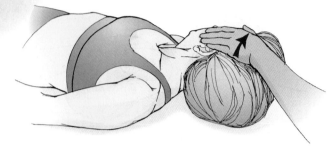

Figure 5-33. CRAC MET to increase the rotation of the cervical spine. Rotation is often limited, owing to shortening of the connective tissue in the muscles and joint capsules.

you attempt to lift the head further off the table. As the client is resisting, have her rotate the head further to the right. Have the client relax, and after a few seconds, have the client resist as you attempt to rotate further to the right. Repeat this CRAC cycle several times. Repeat in the other direction.

MUSCLE ENERGY TECHNIQUE FOR THE TEMPOROMANDIBULAR JOINT MUSCLES

10. *Contract-Relax Muscle Energy Technique to Release the Muscles Primarily Responsible for Opening of the Jaw (Digastrics and Lateral Pterygoids)*

▨ **Intention:** The digastrics and the lateral pterygoids—the muscles that are chiefly responsible for opening the jaw—can be released with CR MET (Fig. 5-34).

▨ **Position:** Place the fingertips under the client's mandible. Have the client open the jaw to its resting position, approximately one finger width.

▨ **Action:** Instruct the client to resist as you gently attempt to close the jaw. Hold for approximately 5 seconds. Relax, and perform the next two METs in

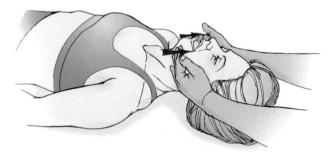

Figure 5-34. CR MET to release the muscles that are primarily responsible for opening the jaw, the digastrics, and the lateral pterygoids.

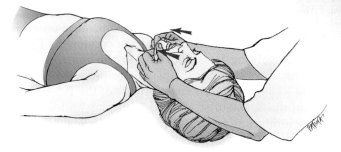

Figure 5-35. CR MET to release the muscles that are primarily responsible for closing the jaw, the masseter, the temporalis, and the medial pterygoid.

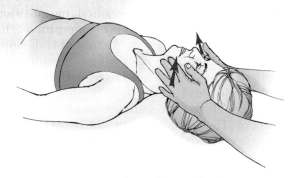

Figure 5-36. CR MET to release the muscles that are primarily responsible for lateral movement of the jaw and the medial and lateral pterygoids.

the jaw sequence. Repeat this cycle several times, and instruct the client in how to do this at home.

11. *Contract-Relax Muscle Energy Technique to Release the Muscles Primarily Responsible for Closing the Jaw (Masseter, Temporalis, Medial Pterygoid)*

▓ **Intention:** The masseter, temporalis, and medial pterygoid—the muscles that are chiefly responsible for closing the jaw—can be released with CR MET (Fig. 5-35).

▓ **Position:** Place the shaft of both thumbs on the anterior aspect of the client's mandible, with the tips of your thumbs nearly touching under the client's lower lip.

▓ **Action:** Instruct the client to keep the jaw open approximately one finger width into the resting position of the TMJ and to resist as you attempt to open the jaw further.

12. *Contract-Relax Muscle Energy Technique to Release the Muscles Primarily Responsible for Lateral Movement of the Jaw (Medial and Lateral Pterygoids)*

▓ **Intention:** The medial and the lateral pterygoids—the muscles that are chiefly responsible for lateral jaw movement—can be released with CR MET (Fig. 5-36).

▓ **Position:** Place the palm and fingertips on the lateral side of the client's mandible.

▓ **Action:** Instruct the client to open the jaw slightly into the resting position and to resist as you press into one side of the jaw. Make sure the client keeps the jaw in neutral and does not jut it to one side. Repeat on the opposite side.

SOFT TISSUE MOBILIZATION

BACKGROUND

A thorough discussion of the clinical application of STM can be found on p. 68. In the Hendrickson Method of therapy described in this text, the STM movements are called *wave mobilization* and are a combination of joint mobilization and STM performed in rhythmic oscillations with a frequency of 50 to 70 cycles per minute, except in performing brisk transverse friction massage strokes, which can be two to four cycles per second. These mobilizations are presented in a specific sequence, which has been found to achieve the most efficient and effective results. This allows the therapist to "scan" the body to determine areas of tenderness, hypertonicity, and decreased mobility. It is important to "follow the recipe" until you have mastered this work. The techniques described below are divided into two sequences: Level I and Level II. Level I strokes are designed for every client, from acute injury to chronic degeneration, to enhance health and bring the body to optimum performance. Level II strokes are typically applied after Level I strokes and are designed for chronic conditions. Guidelines for treating acute and chronic conditions are listed below.

GUIDELINES FOR THE THERAPIST

▓ **Acute:** The primary intention of treatment is to decrease pain and swelling as quickly as possible, maintain as much pain-free joint motion as possible, and induce relaxation. In this method of treatment, the soft tissue is compressed and decompressed in rhythmic cycles. This provides a pumping action that helps to promote fluid exchange and reducing swelling. We begin our work for the cervical spine in the side-lying position, which keeps the joints in their open position. This is the resting position for the spine and is the most pain-free position. The strokes that are applied to the client in acute pain need to be performed with a very gentle touch, a very slow rhythm, and small amplitude. There is no uniform "dose" or depth of treatment. The depth of treatment is based on the client's level of pain. If the soft tissue does not begin to relax, return to gently rocking the body, and then use more METs to help reduce muscle guarding. As mentioned previously, intersperse your STM work with MET. Remember that **stretching is contraindicated** in acute conditions.

Chronic: The typical exam findings in clients with chronic neck problems are short and tight cervical extensors, suboccipitals, and pectoralis minor and weakness in the deep cervical flexors and scapular stabilizers (the upper crossed syndrome). The joints are typically hypomobile, with thick, fibrotic ligaments and capsular tissues. Some patients demonstrate the opposite: hypermobility in the joints; weak, deconditioned muscles; and atrophy in the ligaments and capsular tissues. This latter condition is described as *instability*. The primary goals of treatment depend on the patient. For patients who are hypomobile, the treatment goals are to reduce the hypertonicity of the muscles; promote mobility and extensibility in the connective tissue by dissolving the adhesions in the muscles, tendons, ligaments, and capsular tissues surrounding the joints; rehydrate the cartilage of the facet joints and discs; establish normal joint play and ROM in the joints; and restore normal neurological function by stimulating the proprioceptors and reestablishing the normal firing patterns in the muscles. Patients who are unstable need exercise rehabilitation. Our treatments can support their stability by reducing tension in the tight muscles and by performing MET to the weak muscles to help reestablish normal firing patterns and rehabilitate the proprioceptors. With chronic neck conditions, it is also important to treat tightness in the levator scapula, the rhomboids, and the internal rotators of the shoulder. With chronic conditions, we use stronger pressure on the soft tissue and more vigorous mobilizations on the joints. In the Level II sequence, we add deeper soft tissue work and work on attachment points, using transverse friction strokes if we find fibrosis (thickening). As was mentioned in the "Acute" section above, intersperse your soft tissue work with METs.

Clinical Example: Acute

Subjective: AP is a 54-year-old schoolteacher who presented with acute neck and upper back pain and headaches, which developed immediately after her car was rear-ended the morning of her evaluation and treatment. She reported that she also had tingling in the fingers 3, 4, and 5 on the left side and that she was exhausted and unable to concentrate.

Objective: Examination revealed FHP and an elevation of the left shoulder. Active ROM was 75% of normal in extension, right rotation, and right lateral flexion and that these motions elicited a pain at the cervicothoracic junction. There was a positive foraminal compression test eliciting pain in the neck. Palpation revealed spastic and tender cervical muscles, especially the SCM, levator scapula, upper trapezius, and suboccipitals. There was also fixation of normal glide at the C1–C3 vertebrae on the left.

Assessment: Spastic and tender cervical and upper thoracic muscles with a loss of normal ROM and restrictions of passive cervical motion (joint play).

Treatment (Action): The treatment began with the patient in the side-lying position and a pillow between the knees. I began with slow, gentle rocking of the whole body to determine the level of guarding and pain and to induce a relaxation response. I began Level I STM strokes in the lumbar and thoracic regions slowly and gently, using very little pressure. The intention was to induce gentle motion in the entire spine. Next, I performed Level I STM for the cervical spine. The intention was to provide gentle movement to the soft tissue and joints, to reduce swelling, to promote cellular synthesis, and to realign the healing fibers. Palpation revealed that she was quite tight and tender in the rhomboids, levator, upper trapezius, and cervical extensors. Very gentle MET was used for the muscles attaching to the scapula (thoracic MET #6). After treatment of the other side in the side-lying position, the client was asked to lie on her back. METs #1, #2, and #3 were used to treat the cervical extensors, lateral flexors, and suboccipitals. This helped to reduce hypertonicity and provided a pumping action for the lymph and blood, reducing intramuscular edema and promoting reoxygenation of the tissue. The muscles were much less tender after three to four MET cycles. The treatment continued with the Level I series of strokes for the SCM, scalenes, extensors, and suboccipitals. The treatment ended with very gentle figure-eight joint mobilization for the cervical spine, concentrating on the upper vertebrae on the left. She was very relaxed and calm after the treatment and reported feeling much better.

Plan: I recommended weekly visits for six weeks, with a reevaluation at that time. On her next visit, she reported feeling less pain and that the headaches were subsiding. She said that she continued to feel "spacey." She stated that she had seen her regular doctor who had referred her to a neurologist. The same basic treatment described above was repeated on the subsequent visits. With each visit, the most tender and hypertonic muscles were treated. At the time of her sixth visit, she reported feeling much less pain but that she still had cognitive deficits and occasional tingling in her left hand. The cognitive deficits are typical of minimal traumatic brain injury, and these injuries typically heal within a year. Examination demonstrated some restrictions of cervical extension and right lateral flexion and rotation. The cervical soft tissue continued to have some hypertonicity and tenderness to palpation. There were slight fixations of normal glide at the upper cervical vertebrae. I recommended an additional six weekly visits. After the additional six visits, she reported feeling 90% better. I continue to see her on a monthly basis, six months after her injury.

Clinical Example: Chronic

Subjective: YR is a 45-year-old female designer who presented to my office complaining of neck pain that radiated to the left scapular region. The pain had begun insidiously three years prior to our first visit. She denied any prior injury to her neck.

Objective: Examination on the first visit revealed that cervical ROM was 75% of normal in left rotation and lateral flexion with discomfort in the left cervical spine. Isometric testing was normal for her cervical spine. To palpation, she had spastic and tender cervical and upper thoracic musculature; thick, fibrotic tissue near the facet joints of C7–T1; and a loss of normal joint play at the left C7 and C1 regions.

Assessment: Hypomobility and loss of motion of the cervical spine with muscle spasms and adhesions in the soft tissues.

Treatment: I placed the client on her side and began gentle rocking of her whole body to induce a relaxation response and to determine the level of resilience in the whole spine. I began with lumbar and thoracic strokes and palpated thick, dense muscles in the upper thoracic region. I performed MET and STM to release the upper thoracic region. I began the first series of Level I cervical strokes and palpated thick and fibrous tissue at the cervicothoracic junction. I treated both sides in the side-lying position and then had her lie supine. I began with MET to help induce deeper relaxation in the cervical muscles. I then used PIR MET: METs #6–9 to lengthen the levator, upper trapezius, and extensors, as well as to increase lateral bending and rotation. I ended with the figure-eight mobilization.

The second treatment also began with her in the side lying position. I performed the wave mobilization strokes with deep pressure and a strong P–A component to help induce increased lubrication in the joints and greater joint play. In the supine position, I concentrated on thoracic MET #5 for the rhomboids, as it induces such a profound release of the soft tissue attaching to the C7–T1 vertebrae. I then repeated the METs that were used in the first treatment but with greater pressure, to induce a deep release of the adhesions. I ended the treatment once again with figure-eight mobilization.

Plan: I recommended a series of weekly visits for one month. I repeated the same basic treatment at each visit. As I penetrated deeper into the tissue, I used shorter, more brisk transverse friction strokes on the multifidi and joint capsules (Level II, first series). She reported feeling much less pain in the neck and that the pain in the scapula region was resolved. Upon examination, there was normal ROM, and there was a significant decrease in muscular tension. The tissue around the C7–T1 junction was more pliable and less fibrotic, but there was still a thickened feel to the pariarticular tissue. Although there was better glide in the facet joints, there was still restrictions to full passive glide at the C7 vertebra. I recommended another series of weekly visits for one month.

Table 5-5	Essentials of Treatment
■ Rock the client's body while performing the strokes ■ Shift your weight while performing the strokes ■ Perform the strokes rhythmically ■ Perform the strokes about 50 to 70 cycles per minute ■ Keep your hands and whole body relaxed	

Table 5-5 lists some essentials of treatment.

LEVEL I: CERVICAL SPINE

1. *Release of the Soft Tissue Between the Spinous and Transverse Processes*

■ **Anatomy:** Splenius capitis and cervicis, erector spinae, semispinalis cervicis and capitis, rotatores, multifidi (Figs. 5-37A and 5-37B).

■ **Dysfunction:** Extensor muscles of the cervical spine, except the suboccipitals, tend to contract eccentrically with FHP, becoming taut (i.e., tight and long). With FHP, the suboccipital muscles become tight and short, and the extensor muscles develop an abnormal medial torsion and need to be stroked away from the SPs.

Position

■ **Therapist Position (TP):** Standing, facing headward for longitudinal strokes, facing the table for transverse strokes.

■ **Client Position (CP):** Side-lying, with the chin tucked and the shoulder near the therapist at the edge of the table.

Strokes

Your supporting hand is on the scapula. Move the scapula in the direction of your stroke, as this brings the superficial tissue into slack.

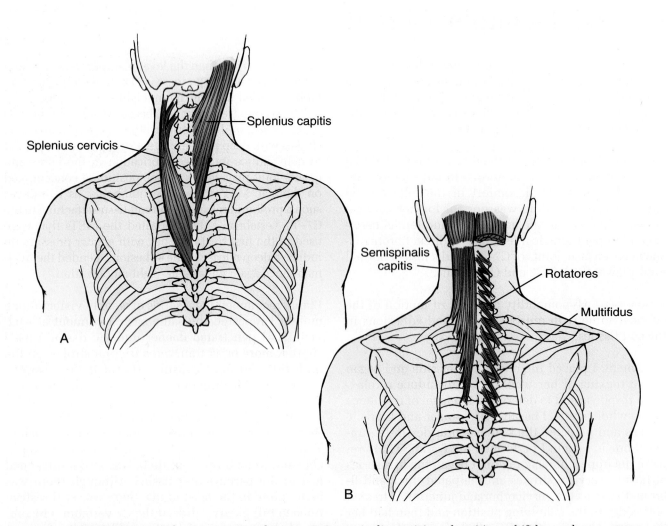

Figure 5-37. **A.** Splenius cervicis and capitis. **B.** Semispinalis cervicis and capitis, multifidus, and rotatores.

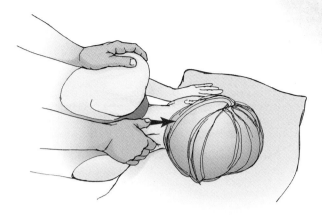

Figure 5-38. Thumb release of the cervical soft tissue in an inferior-to-superior direction. Keep your wrist in neutral, and gently squeeze the neck with each stroke.

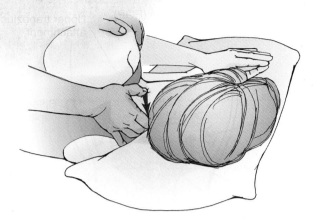

Figure 5-40. Thumb release of the soft tissue from the area of the posterior surface of the transverse process.

1. With your body facing 45° headward, use a single-thumb technique to perform short, scooping inferior-to-superior (I–S) strokes from C7 to C2 (Fig. 5-38). Your fingertips are placed underneath the neck. Gently squeeze the neck with each stroke; this is nurturing, adds stability, and disperses the pressure throughout the entire hand. Perform this stroke in three lines: at the SP, at the lamina groove 1 inch laterally, and on the posterior surface of the transverse process, approximately 1 inch lateral to the second line. Be cautious at C1, approximately one finger's breadth under the skull, as direct pressure on this vertebra may sublux it (shift its position) and cause headaches.

2. With your body facing perpendicular to the table, use your thumb to perform short, scooping strokes in the P–A and medial-to-lateral (M–L) direction (Fig. 5-39). Begin at the SPs and proceed in 1-inch segments from C7 to C2. The same stroke is repeated in a second line in the area of the lamina groove beginning approximately 1 inch lateral to the SPs.

3. Turn your body to face 45° headward again. The transverse processes are found in a line between the ear and the shoulder. Using a single-thumb technique, feel for the bony protuberance of the transverse process, then slide your thumb to its posterior surface (Fig. 5-40). Perform a series of 1-inch scooping strokes in an anterior to posterior (A–P) direction over the transverse process. This is an unwinding stroke, rolling the soft tissue posteriorly and toward the table. Begin at C7, and proceed inch by inch to C2. Keep an even, smooth rhythm. Do not slide over the skin.

2. Release of the Muscle Attachments on the Base of the Skull

- **Anatomy:** Trapezius, longissimus capitis, semispinalis and splenius capitis, rectus capitis posterior minor and major, SCM, obliquus capitis superior, greater occipital nerve (Fig. 5-41).

- **Dysfunction:** Muscle attachments on the skull tend to thicken and become fibrotic with sustained tension in the cervical extensors and suboccipital muscles. This is commonly caused by FHP, previous injury, or emotional tension. This sustained muscle tension can lead to tension headaches. The rectus capitis posterior minor interweaves with the fibrous covering of the brain (the dura), and special attention to this muscle is indicated. The greater occipital nerve can become entrapped in the semispinalis capitis fascia.

Position

- **TP:** Standing, facing headward.

- **CP:** Side lying, neck flexed.

Strokes

Use short, scooping strokes with the thumb or braced thumb from the mastoid to the midline. Move the

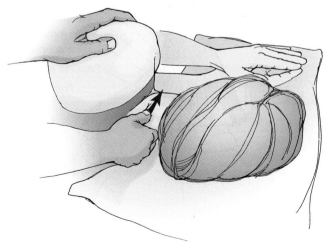

Figure 5-39. Thumb release in the medial to lateral direction.

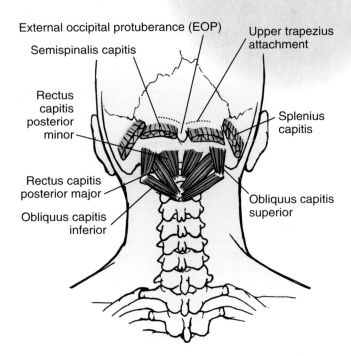

Figure 5-41. Muscle attachments to the base of the skull.

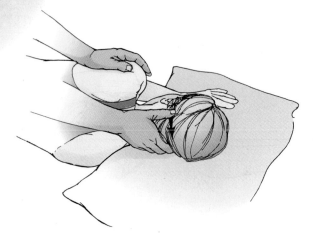

Figure 5-42. Release of the muscle attachments in the area of the superior nuchal line.

scapula with the inferior hand in a superior motion to feed the area. It is important not to dig into the skull. Rather, take the tissue into tension, and using the bone as a guide, scoop it medially. Gently pull the skin back 1 inch, scoop in, and move approximately 1 inch. When you encounter an area of thickening in the soft tissue, you may use strokes that are shorter and more brisk. Three lines of strokes are described below. Remember that for attachment points, it is not necessary to be concerned with positional correction; rather, be concerned with dissolving fibrosis, and therefore, use transverse strokes in both directions.

1. Locate the external occipital protuberance in the center of the posterior skull at the level of the top of the ear. The area from the external occipital protuberance to the top of the ear is called the *superior nuchal line*. Release the attachments of the SCM on the mastoid and the trapezius in the midline of the occiput on this superior nuchal line. These muscles have thin, flat tendons at their attachments (Fig. 5-42).
2. Working on the mastoid 1 inch inferior to your previous series in the area of the middle nuchal line, release the splenius capitis and longissimus capitis. Continue a series more medially on the occiput for the obliquus capitis superior and the semispinalis capitis.
3. As you follow the contour of the bone of the skull, turn your thumb to face superiorly, and perform a third line of strokes. Begin approximately 1 inch inferior to the previous series on the medial third

of the inferior nuchal line to release the rectus capitis posterior minor and major.

3. *Release of Soft Tissue Between the Clavicle and the Supraspinous Fossa of the Scapula and Between the Posterior Scapula and Spine*

■ **Anatomy:** Scalenus anterior, medius, and posterior; levator scapula; upper trapezius; supraspinatus; rhomboids; and serratus posterior superior (Fig. 5-43).

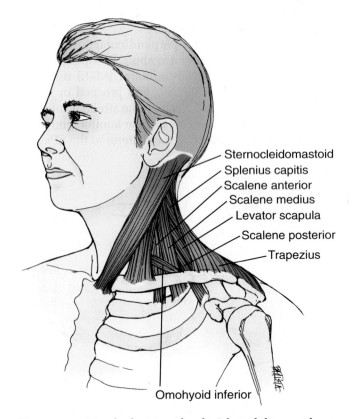

Figure 5-43. Muscles between the clavicle and the scapula.

▩ **Dysfunction:** These muscles tend to develop torsion as they roll forward and shorten with FHP or as a result of spinal trauma. In the client with rounded shoulders, this soft tissue shortens and thickens. The rhomboids, levator, and upper trapezius are commonly short and tight, owing to emotional tension or FHP.

Position

▩ **TP:** Standing, facing table.

▩ **CP:** Supine.

Strokes

1. In this stroke, we have two intentions: to unwind the abnormal torsion and release adhesions in the scalenes, levator scapula, trapezius, and supraspinatus and to release the tension in the rhomboids
   □ Begin by placing the client's flexed elbow on the chest so that the arm rests across the chest (Fig. 5-44).
   □ With your inferior hand, grasp just above the client's elbow, and gently impulse the arm headward and posteriorly toward the superior hand.
   □ At the same time, with the thumb of your superior hand, perform 1-inch scooping strokes in the A–P direction in the area between the clavicle and the scapula.
   □ To repeat the stroke and return to the starting position, release the thumb of your superior hand, and lift the scapula and the arm anteriorly and inferiorly. Reposition the thumb of your superior hand to a new position, and scoop as you pulse the arm headward and posteriorly.

2. Perform the MET for the rhomboids (see Fig. 4-16, p. 170).

3. Release the soft tissue between the upper third of the scapula and the spine. Your inferior hand remains in the same position. The fingertips of your working hand scoop the soft tissue headward, coordinating it with the upward movement of the client's arm in short, brisk, oscillatory strokes. Begin at the superior angle of the scapula, and perform the next stroke 1 inch closer to the spine. Cover the entire area between the vertebral border of the upper third of the scapula and the SPs of the upper thoracic and lower cervical vertebrae.

4. *Release of the Sternocleidomastoid Muscle*

▩ **Anatomy:** SCM (Fig. 5-45).

▩ **Dysfunction:** The SCM is one of the most commonly injured muscles in the cervical region, especially with whiplash injuries. The SCM is typically short and tight and pulls the head into an FHP. It can be a source of headaches and chronic neck tension.

Position

▩ **TP:** Seated at the head of the table.

▩ **CP:** Supine.

Strokes

To identify the SCM, have the client rotate the head to one side and begin the motion of lifting the ear toward the ceiling. The SCM will protrude from the side of the neck. Have the client bring the head back to

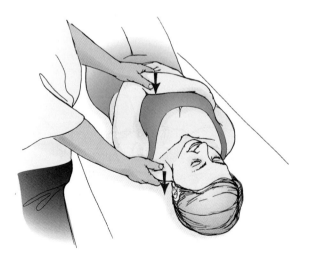

Figure 5-44. Thumb release of the soft tissue between the clavicle and the supraspinous fossa of the scapula. Move the arm in an oscillating rhythm coordinated with the strokes. Each stroke works in a slightly different area.

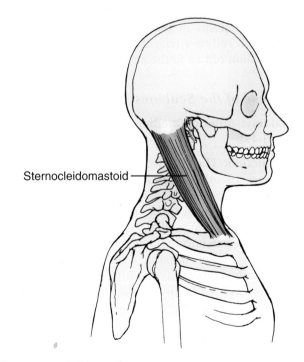

Sternocleidomastoid

Figure 5-45. SCM muscle.

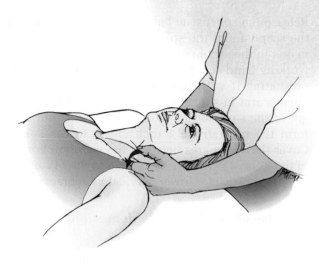

Figure 5-46. Release of the SCM. Gently squeeze the muscle between your thumb and flexed index finger, and unwind the muscle laterally.

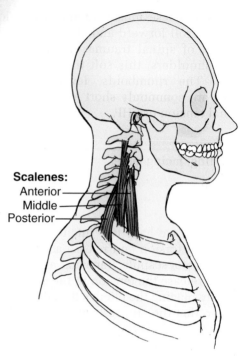

Figure 5-47. Anterior, middle, and posterior scalenes.

neutral and then rotate it slightly toward the side on which you will be working.

1. Place your thumb on top of the SCM and your flexed fingers underneath (Fig. 5-46). Gently squeeze the SCM, and perform a 1-inch stroke from anterior to posterior and from superior to inferior, inducing a subtle spiral from medial to lateral as you perform the stroke. Rock your whole body forward and laterally with the stroke. Place the nonworking hand under the opposite mastoid, cupping the head, and roll the head slightly with the stroke.

Note: If this stroke refers pain to the head, it can indicate a trigger point in the SCM. As has been mentioned, MET relieves trigger points, so perform CR MET, and then return to the strokes.

5. *Release of the Scalenes*

- **Anatomy:** Anterior, medial, and posterior scalenes (Fig. 5-47).

- **Dysfunction:** These muscles often contract after a whiplash or other spinal trauma or with chronic tension and tend to develop an anterior and medial torsion. They need to be moved from anterior to posterior and from medial to lateral. This sustained contracture can entrap the brachial plexus and axillary artery, causing pain, numbing, and tingling into the arm, especially the ulnar side of the hand. This is called *scalenus anticus syndrome.*

Position
- **TP:** Seated at client's head.

- **CP:** Supine.

Strokes
There are three lines of strokes, one each for the anterior, medial, and posterior scalenes.

1. Place the flat surface of the shaft of your thumb on the scalenes by tucking it under the SCM and finding the lateral aspect of the posterior surfaces of the transverse processes (Fig. 5-48). Perform gentle 1-inch scooping strokes in a medial to lateral, anterior to posterior direction, transverse to the line of fiber. This is also an unwinding stroke, like moving around a cylinder. Gently supinate your forearm with the stroke. Start near the attachments on the transverse processes of C2, and work down to the

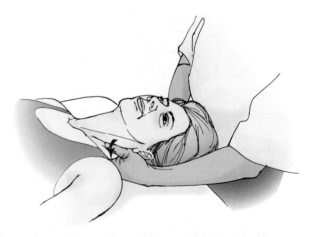

Figure 5-48. Release of the scalenes. Place your flat thumb posterior to the SCM, and gently scoop the muscles posteriorly. This should be a nurturing stroke.

area above the clavicle. Roll the client's head toward the side you are working with each stroke. Roll it back to center on release. Rock your entire body laterally as you stroke. Your fingertips rest underneath the client's neck. Gently squeeze the neck as you are stroking. This stroke should feel nurturing.

2. To release the anterior scalenes, perform the same strokes described above but on the anterior surface of the cervical transverse processes. To contact the anterior scalenes and bring them into slack, rotate and laterally bend the client's head slightly toward your working hand. Gently tuck the pad of your thumb under the SCM, and place it on the anterior surface of the cervical transverse processes. Perform slow, gentle scooping strokes in the A–P and M–L planes, unwinding the tissue transverse to the line of the fiber of the anterior scalene. Proceed inch by inch down the neck, covering the area from the muscle's origin at C3 to the first rib area under the clavicle.

3. To release the lower portion of the scalenes, place your fingertips on the most lateral portion of the

area above the clavicle, and perform gentle 1-inch strokes in the M–L direction. After several strokes, move your fingertips more medially, and perform the same M–L strokes. Cover the entire supraclavicular fossa. Rock your body with each stroke in the same direction as your stroke.

Note: Mention to the client that it is normal for some people to feel a slight tingling in the arm while they undergo this treatment. It indicates that the nerves are under tension and that the area needs release. This sensation is relieved a few minutes after the strokes. Do not work more than 1 minute in this area if there is a referral of pain, numbing, or tingling into the extremity.

6. *Transverse Release of the Cervical Soft Tissue*

▨ **Anatomy:** Posterior cervical muscles (Fig. 5-49) and the suboccipital muscles at C1 to C2 and at the occiput (see Fig. 5-41).

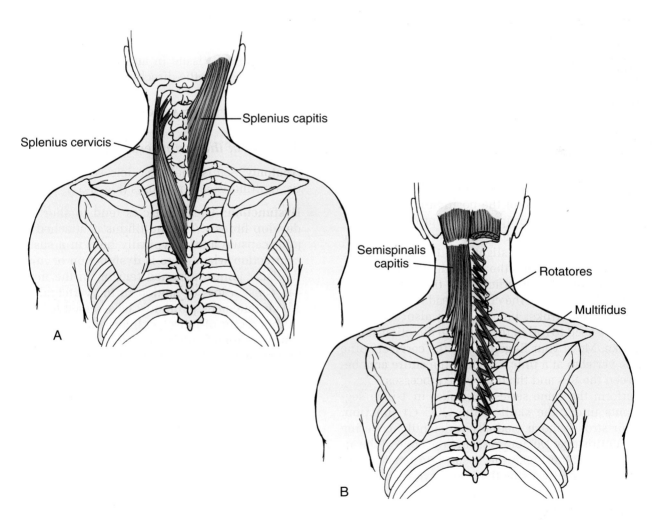

Figure 5-49. A. Splenius cervicis and capitis. **B.** Semispinalis cervicis and capitis, multifidus, and rotatores.

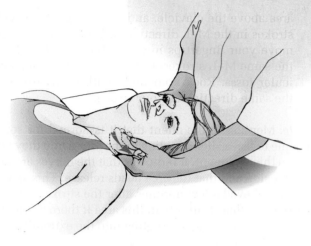

Figure 5-50. Fingertip release of the soft tissue in the posterior neck. This position places the superficial tissue into slack and allows for work on the deeper layers. This is also the best position for work on the area of the atlas-occipital region.

▨ **Dysfunction:** The posterior cervical muscles, including the suboccipital muscles, are typically short and tight. They thicken and become fibrotic because of chronic irritation caused by poor posture, emotional tension, or inflammation from injury.

Position

▨ **TP:** Seated, at client's head.

▨ **CP:** Supine.

Strokes

1. With the fingertips of one hand on the lateral side of the SP, scoop 1 inch laterally to clear any residual tension that was not released in prior work (Fig. 5-50). Because of the position of function of your hand, the fingertips scoop approximately 45° headward. Treat one side of the neck at a time. Rotate the client's head slightly to the side you are working on, and bend the head slightly laterally, as this will put the superficial soft tissue into slack. Typically, you rock the client's head into the direction of the stroke, but you may also allow the client's head to roll in the opposite direction as you stroke. Move your fingertips up the cervical spine one vertebra at a time, covering the entire area between the SPs and the transverse processes.
2. Perform the same series of strokes in 1-inch segments under the skull at the OCC–C1 junction. Your strokes move medially to laterally, covering the entire area. Do not press into the bone of the atlas (C1). Rather, take the tissue into tension and scoop it laterally, using the bone as your guide.
3. Perform the same series of strokes on the three nuchal lines described in the second stroke of Level I. Lift the skull with one hand, and rotate it to the side of the working hand. Using fingertips,

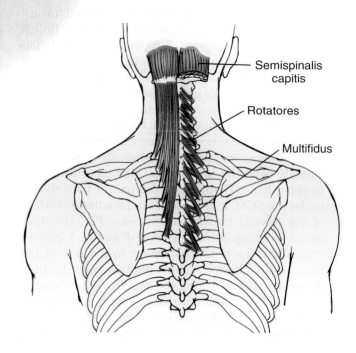

Figure 5-51. Semispinalis capitis, rotatores, and multifidus.

scoop the soft tissue in an M–L direction as you rock the head in the direction of the stroke.

LEVEL II: CERVICAL SPINE

1. *Release of the Transversospinalis Group*

▨ **Anatomy:** Semispinalis cervicis, semispinalis capitis, multifidus, and rotatores (Fig. 5-51).

▨ **Dysfunction:** These muscles tend to shorten and develop fibrosis. The multifidus is attached to the joint capsule and is typically held in a sustained contraction when there is dysfunction or injury to the facet joint. Sustained tension in the multifidi can cause a loss of motion in the vertebral facets. All chronic neck pain must be assessed for fibrosis in this group of muscles. Injuries to the neck can cause eventual fibrosis and thickening of the capsular ligaments, which interweave with the multifidi.

Position

▨ **TP:** Standing.

▨ **CP:** Side-lying, neck propped on a pillow to allow some slack in the tissue.

Strokes

1. Use a single-thumb technique to perform 1-inch, scooping strokes in an M–L, 45° headward direction (Fig. 5-52). Tuck the thumb under the erectors to contact the underlying transversospinalis group.

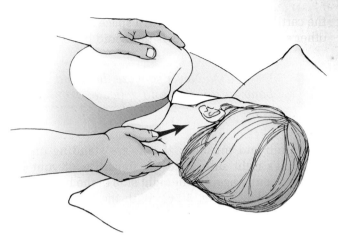

Figure 5-52. Release of the transversospinalis group. Tuck your thumb under the more superficial erector spinae group. Direct your stroke 45° headward, perpendicular to the line of the fiber of these muscles.

Begin your strokes next to the SP of the C7 vertebrae, and work to C2. Use your inferior hand to cup the scapula, and gently move it headward while you are stroking to help bring the tissue into slack.

2. Release of Joint Capsule and Muscle Attachments on the Posterior Cervical Spine

▓ **Anatomy:** *Spinous process attachments* from superficial to deep—trapezius, spinalis cervicis, rhomboids, semispinalis cervicis insertion, splenius cervicis and capitis, and multifidus insertion; *transverse process attachments* from superficial to deep—levator scapula, semispinalis capitis origin, iliocostalis cervicis insertion, multifidus origin, longissimus cervicis and capitis origins, and joint capsule (capsular ligaments) (Fig. 5-53).

▓ **Dysfunction:** These attachment sites tend to thicken as the result of previous inflammation or because of chronic dysfunction, such as FHP. As was mentioned in the description of the previous stroke, the fascia of the deepest layers of the cervical muscles interweave with the capsular ligaments. These areas of the tenoperiosteal insertions are thick and fibrotic in nearly all patients who have chronic neck pain or loss of motion.

Position
▓ **TP:** Standing, facing headward.

▓ **CP:** Side-lying.

Strokes
Hold the neck with your fingertips, and gently squeeze the neck to support it while your thumb is performing the following strokes.

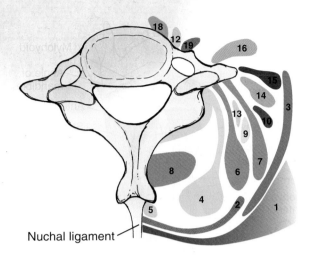

Figure 5-53. Muscle attachments to the posterior cervical spine. 1: Trapezius m, 2: Splenius capitis m, 3: Sternocleidomastoid m, 4: Semispinalis capitis m, 5: Interspinalis cervicis m, 6: Longissimus capitis m, 7: Levator scapulae m, 8: Semispinalis cervicis m, 9: Longissimus cervicis m, 10: Splenius cervicis m, 11: Multifidus m, 12: Rotatores muscles, 13: Iliocostalis cervicis m, 14: Scalene posterior m, 15: Scalene medius m, 16: Scalene anterior m, 17: Longus capitis m, 18: Longus colli m.

1. Spinous processes: Beginning at the C7 SP, use the fleshy pad of your thumb to perform gentle back-and-forth strokes in the I–S plane on the lateral side of the SPs (Fig. 5-54). If the tissue is fibrous, perform a series of gentle, transverse friction strokes. Work on each SP from C7 to C2. The supporting hand moves the shoulder headward with your strokes.

2. Lamina groove: Using the fleshy pad of your thumb, begin a series of gentle, back-and-forth strokes on the area of the lamina–pedicle junction. Begin at C7, and work on one vertebra at a time

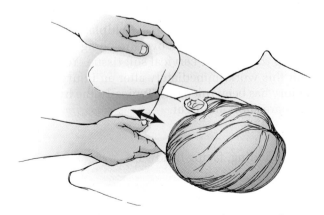

Figure 5-54. Release of the soft tissue attachments in three areas: the SP, the lamina groove, and the transverse process. These are gentle, deep, back-and-forth strokes to release any fibrosis at the attachments to the periosteum covering the bone.

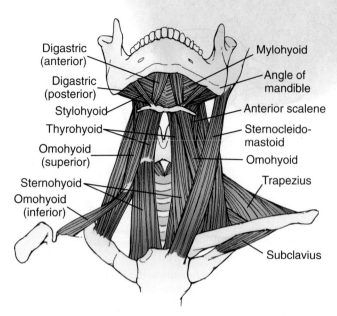

Figure 5-55. Superficial anterior muscles of the neck are the suprahyoid and the infrahyoid muscles.

from C7 to C2. Work in the P–A and I–S planes. Try to identify the line of the fiber, and work transverse to it. When you are perpendicular to the fiber, you will feel the fibers "strum" under your fingers as you cross them.

3. Transverse processes: Using either fingertips or thumb, perform a series of gentle back-and-forth strokes in the I–S plane on the posterior surface of the transverse processes. Begin at C7 and proceed to C2.

3. *Release of the Superficial Muscles of the Anterior Neck*

▧ **Anatomy:** *Suprahyoids*—digastric, mylohyoid, stylohyoid, geniohyoid; *Infrahyoids*—thyrohyoid, sternothyroid, sternohyoid, omohyoid (Fig. 5-55).

▧ **Dysfunction:** Typically, in a whiplash injury, the head is hyperextended, overstretching and traumatizing the anterior cervical soft tissue. You may begin this work immediately after an injury if severe injury has been ruled out. Typically, the hyoid muscles are short and tight.

Position

▧ **TP:** Standing, facing headward.

▧ **CP:** Supine.

Strokes

Find the hyoid bone by first placing your thumb and index finger on the thyroid cartilage in the center of the anterior neck. As you gently walk your fingers up

the cartilage, you will come to a space and then to another solid structure. This is the hyoid bone.

> ❗ *CAUTION: Never squeeze the hyoid bone, as it is thin and delicate.*

1. Suprahyoid muscles: If you are standing on the client's right side, hold the fingertips of your left hand gently against the right side of the hyoid bone to stabilize it (Fig. 5-56). With the index finger of your right hand, gently perform back-and-forth strokes on the superior surface of the left side of the hyoid bone to release the stylohyoid and the mylohyoid on the anterior-medial surface. Perform a series of strokes until you reach the midline.

2. Infrahyoid muscles: Place the index finger of your right hand on the inferior lateral surface of the client's left hyoid bone. Perform gentle back-and-forth strokes to release the sternohyoid and the omohyoid superficially and the thyrohyoid more deeply.

3. Muscles over the thyroid cartilage: Place the fingertips of your left hand on the lateral surface of the right thyroid cartilage to stabilize it. With the fingertips of your right hand, perform gentle back-and-forth strokes to release the sternohyoid superficially and the sternothyroid and thyrohyoid more deeply on the anterior surface of the left thyroid cartilage. Gently stroke across the thyroid cartilage; however, be careful not to press down into the throat. You might elicit the coughing reflex if you press too hard or if the area is particularly tense. If the client remains comfortable, you may proceed, but be more gentle.

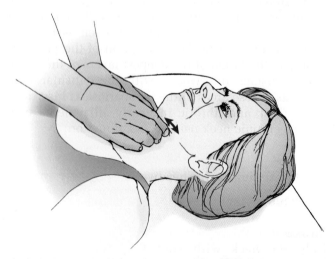

Figure 5-56. Fingertip release of the superficial muscles of the anterior neck.

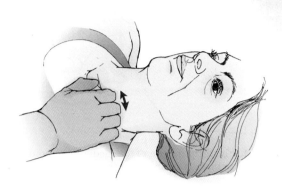

Figure 5-57. Fingertip release of the attachments to the clavicle and sternum.

4. Muscles attaching to the sternum: Move your body to the opposite side of the table, facing 45° headward (Fig. 5-57). Cupping your fingertips around the top surface of the sternum, release the lower attachment points of the sternohyoid and the sternothyroid by performing back-and-forth strokes in the M–L plane.

4. *Release of Deep Anterior Cervical Musculature*

▨ **Anatomy:** Longus capitis, longus colli, and cervical sympathetic nerves (Fig. 5-58).

▨ **Dysfunction:** These muscles tend to shorten after spinal trauma, causing a loss of cervical curve, called "military neck." This can lead to entrapment of the sympathetic nerves that travel through these muscles, producing various symptoms, including tinnitus, dizziness, blurry vision, and nausea.

Position
▨ **TP:** Standing, facing headward.

▨ **CP:** Supine.

Strokes
1. Stand on the right side of the table. Gently grasp the trachea with your right thumb and index finger, and move it toward you to give some slack to the soft tissue (Fig. 5-59). Place the index finger of your left hand next to your right thumb. Move the trachea to the client's left so that your index finger is nearly at the midline. Slowly and gently press posteriorly, superiorly, and medially with your left index finger until you make contact with the muscles on the anterior surface of the cervical vertebrae. The carotid artery will be lateral to your fingertips; remember, never put pressure on a pulse. Gently move your finger and thumb as a unit, back and

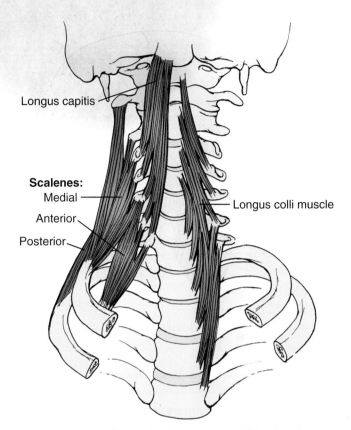

Figure 5-58. Muscles on the deepest aspect of the anterior neck are called the prevertebral muscles.

forth, transverse to the midline. Release the pressure on the fingers, move inferiorly 1 inch, and repeat the same strokes. Continue in 1-inch segments until approximately 2 inches above the clavicle. Repeat on the other side.

5. *Release of Temporomandibular Joint*

▨ **Anatomy:** Masseter, temporalis, medial pterygoid, lateral pterygoid, joint capsule (Fig. 5-60).

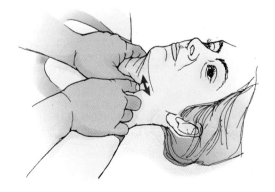

Figure 5-59. Fingertip release of the deep anterior neck muscles.

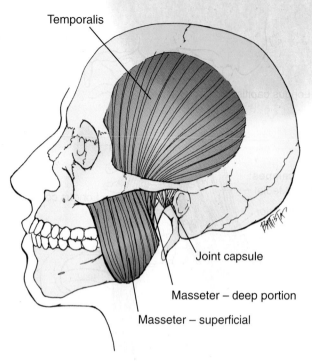

Figure 5-60. Temporalis and masseter muscles.

Dysfunction: These muscles tend to shorten and become fibrotic with chronic tension (e.g., grinding or clenching of the teeth) or with cervical trauma. The jaw moves forward in a whiplash, rolling the masseter and temporalis into an anterior and medial torsion. The masseter and temporalis are typically short and tight. The joint capsule may become inflamed with acute injury or thick and fibrotic with chronic tension of degeneration of the joint.

Position
■ **TP:** Seated.

■ **CP:** Supine.

Strokes
1. To release the masseter, use your fingertips to perform a series of 1-inch, scooping strokes, in the A–P direction in three lines (Fig. 5-61). The first line be-

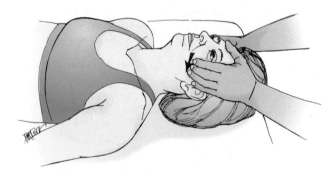

Figure 5-61. Fingertip release of the masseter. Perform gentle scooping strokes in an anterior to posterior direction.

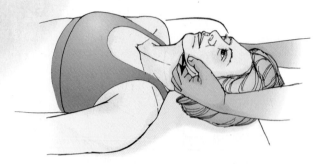

Figure 5-62. Fingertip release of the medial pterygoid, mylohyoid, and proximal attachments of the suprahyoid muscles.

gins under the zygomatic arch, near the ear. The second line is in the mid-belly, 1 inch inferior to the first line, and the third line is on the mandible.
2. To release the joint capsule, use your fingertips to perform a series of short, back and forth strokes, in the A–P plane under the posterior part of the zygomatic arch, which is in front of the ear.
3. To release the temporalis, use single-thumb technique or the fingertips to perform short, scooping strokes in an A–P direction, covering the entire temporal fossa. Concentrate your attention on the tendon immediately superior to the zygomatic arch.
4. Release the medial pterygoid, the mylohyoid, and the proximal attachments of the suprahyoids by cupping your fingertips under the mandible at the angle of the jaw to contact its posterior surface (Fig. 5-62). Perform a series of short, scooping strokes in a posterior direction to release these muscles. Begin each new stroke approximately 1 inch more anteriorly, and scoop posteriorly.

6. *Mobilization of the Cervical Spine*

■ **Anatomy:** The cervical facets are oriented in a plane facing anteromedially (Fig. 5-63).

■ **Dysfunction:** The facets of the cervical spine are often inhibited from their normal gliding characteristics by sustained muscle contraction. This not only can be a source of local pain, but also can cause an arthrokinetic reflex that contracts the musculature further, leading to increased inhibition of the normal motion of the joint.

Position
■ **TP:** Seated.

■ **CP:** Supine.

Strokes
1. Lateral to medial (L–M) mobilization of the cervical vertebrae: Find the vertebral facets by first locating the SPs in the midline. Move slightly laterally to

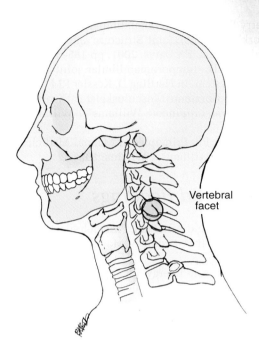

Figure 5-63. Vertebral facets of the cervical spine are located lateral and deep to the soft tissue bundle next to the SPs.

touch the medial extensor muscles. Move your fingertips over that muscle bundle, and you will feel a bony indentation, which is the facet. To assess motion in one vertebra relative to the next, gently push in an L–M direction on one side of the vertebra and then in the same L–M direction on the other side of the same joint (Fig. 5-64). A healthy joint has a resilient end feel. A hypomobile joint has a thickened, dry, stiff or bony-block end feel, depending on the cause of resistance. An analogy that is useful to patients is that joints can

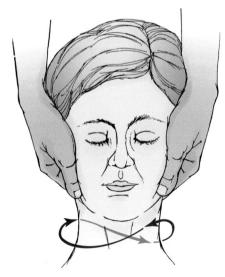

Figure 5-64. Figure-eight mobilization of the cervical facets. For acute conditions, move slowly and gently. For chronic conditions, the ROM of the mobilization may be increased.

become like a rusty hinge and that by moving a joint, we "oil" or lubricate it. Move up to the next joint, and repeat from the C7–T1 to the C1–C2 area.

2. Figure-eight mobilization of the cervical vertebrae: With your fingertips placed at the vertebral facets starting at the C7–T1 area, gently induce a slight movement with the hands in a figure-eight pattern. For example, the client's head is rotated to the right, then side flexed to the left, while the fingertips of your left hand push on the left facets. Then rotate the client's head left, laterally flex it to the right, and so on. This is a slow, extremely gentle procedure, and there should be no pain. For a client with acute injuries, you can perform this mobilization as micromovements, using extremely gentle and small-amplitude movements. Chronic conditions need bigger-amplitude movements.

Study Guide

Cervical Spine, Level I

1. List the four suboccipital muscles.
2. Describe the difference in symptoms between cervical disc degeneration and herniation.
3. Locate the facet joints on a skeleton and on a fellow student.
4. Describe how to perform CR MET for acute neck pain.
5. Describe the possible symptoms of a whiplash injury.
6. Describe the symptoms of anterior scalene syndrome.
7. What is the direction of our stroke for the scalene muscles?
8. List which muscles are tight and which muscles are weak in the upper crossed syndrome.
9. What is the stroke direction for the medial group of erector spinae muscles in the neck?
10. List four factors that predispose a person to developing neck pain.

Cervical Spine, Level II

1. List the suprahyoid, infrahyoid, prevertebral, and TMJ muscles.
2. Describe the basic origins and insertions of the following muscles: scalenes, SCM, suboccipital muscles, longus capitis, longus colli, temporalis, and masseter.
3. What are the ranges of normal motion of the cervical spine?
4. Describe what a positive elevated-arm stress test indicates.
5. Demonstrate PIR MET for the cervical region and CR MET for the TMJ.
6. Describe the two types of headaches that are caused by muscle tension.
7. Describe FHP and its effects on the facet joints.
8. Describe a common site of entrapment of the cervical sympathetic nerves, and describe the massage and MET techniques to release them.

9. Describe the foraminal compression test and its significance.
10. Describe the postural signs of an upper crossed syndrome.

References

1. Bovim G, Schrader H, Sand T. Neck pain in the general population. Spine 1994;19:1307–1309.
2. Porterfield JA, DeRosa C. Mechanical Neck Pain. Philadelphia: WB Saunders, 1995.
3. Cailliet R. Neck and Arm Pain, Philadelphia: FA Davis, 1991.
4. Kendall F, McCreary E, Provance P, Rodgers, M, Romani, W. Muscles: Testing and Function, 5th ed. Baltimore: Lippincott Williams & Wilkins, 2005.
5. Grieve G. Common Vertebral Joint Problems. Edinburgh: Churchill Livingstone, 1981.
6. Richmond FJ, Abrahams VC. What are the proprioceptors of the neck? Prog Brain Res 1979;50:245–254.
7. Hertling D, Blakney M. Cervical spine. In Hertling D, Kessler RM (eds): Management of Common Musculoskeletal Disorders, 4th ed. Baltimore: Lippincott Williams & Wilkins, 2006, pp 707–763.
8. Cole A, Farrell J, Stratton S. Functional rehabilitation of cervical spine athletic injuries. In Kibler WB, Herring S, Press J (eds): Functional Rehabilitation of Sports and Musculoskeletal Injuries. Gaithersburg, MD: Aspen Publication, 1998, pp 127–148.
9. Brukner P, Khan K. Clinical Sports Medicine, 3rd ed. Sydney: McGraw-Hill, 2006.
10. Barnsley L, Lord S, Bogduk N. Critical review: Whiplash injury. Pain 1994;58:283–307.
11. Kraus SL. Influences of the cervical spine on the stomatognathic system. In Donatelli R, Wooden MJ (eds): Orthopedic Physical Therapy, 2nd ed. New York: Churchill Livingstone, 1994, pp 61–76.
12. Perry JF. The temporomandibular joint. In Levangie PK, Norkin CC (eds): Joint Structure and Function, 3rd ed. Philadelphia: FA Davis, 2001, pp 185–195.
13. Hertling D. Temporomandibular joint and stomatognathic system. In Hertling D, Kessler RM (eds): Management of Common Musculoskeletal Disorders, 4th ed. Baltimore: Lippincott Williams & Wilkins, 2006, pp 624–668.
14. Greenman PE. Principles of Manual Medicine, 2nd ed. Baltimore: Williams & Wilkins, 1996.

Suggested Readings

Cailliet R. Neck and Arm Pain. Philadelphia: FA Davis, 1991.

Calais-Germain B. Anatomy of Movement. Seattle: Eastland Press, 1991.

Chaitow L. Muscle Energy Techniques, 3rd ed. New York: Churchill Livingstone, 2006.

Clemente C. Anatomy: A Regional Atlas of the Human Body, 4th ed. Baltimore: Williams & Wilkins, 1997.

Corrigan B, Maitland GD. Practical Orthopaedic Medicine. London: Butterworths, 1983.

Hertling D, Kessler R. Management of Common Musculoskeletal Disorders, 4th ed. Baltimore: Lippincott Williams & Wilkins, 2006.

Kendall F, McCreary E, Provance P, M Rogers, W Romani. Muscles: Testing and Function, 5th ed. Baltimore: Williams & Wilkins, 2005.

Levangie P, Norkin C. Joint Structure and Function, 3rd ed. Philadelphia: FA Davis, 2001.

Magee D. Orthopedic Physical Assessment, 3rd ed. Philadelphia: WB Saunders, 1997.

Platzer W. Locomotor System, vol 1, 5th ed. New York: Thieme Medical, 2004.

Porterfield JA, DeRosa C. Mechanical Neck Pain. Philadelphia: WB Saunders, 1995.

Reid DC. Sports Injury and Assessment. New York: Churchill Livingstone, 1992.

6

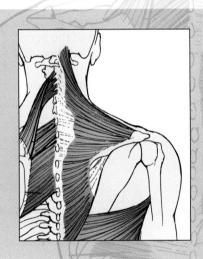

The Shoulder

Pain in the shoulder and shoulder girdle is common in the general population, with a prevalence of 15% to 25% in the 40- to 50-year-old age group.[1] With increasing life expectancy and the aging population remaining active into advancing years, age-related degeneration is a significant factor in rotator cuff injuries.[2] Disorders of the shoulder region account for 30% to 40% of industrial complaints and have increased sixfold in the past decade.[1] Although injuries to the shoulder girdle account for only 5% to 10% of sports injuries, they represent a much higher percentage of physician visits, probably because they are perceived as being serious or disabling by the athlete.[3] In many shoulder disorders, it is the soft tissue, such as the tendons and joint capsule, that is the source of the pain. The shoulder region may also be painful from a referral from the cervical and the thoracic spines and from visceral diseases, such as gallbladder and cardiac problems.[4]

Anatomy, Function, and Dysfunction of the Shoulder Complex

GENERAL OVERVIEW

▨ The bones of the **shoulder complex** includes the bones of the shoulder girdle; the clavicle and scapula; and the humerus, sternum, and rib cage (Fig. 6-1). These bones form **four typical joints**: the glenohumeral (shoulder joint), sternoclavicular, acromioclavicular, and scapulothoracic joints. There is a **fifth functional joint**, the coracoacromial arch, which describes the region where the head of the humerus is covered by the acromion and the coracoacromial ligament. All these joints must be considered together in discussing the shoulder, as any motion of the glenohumeral joint also occurs at each of the other joints. The shoulder is the most mobile joint in the body with the least stability; therefore, it is one of the most frequently injured joints in the body.

▨ The function of the shoulder is influenced by many joints. The function and position of the cervical spine and the thoracic spine influence mobility of the arm. The upper thoracic vertebrae must be able to extend, rotate, and side-bend to accomplish full elevation of the arm.[1] There must also be mobility in the upper ribs as well as mobility in the acromioclavicular and sternoclavicular joints for full range of motion (ROM) in the arm. Stability of the scapula is necessary to allow proper positioning of the head of the humerus in the glenoid fossa of the scapula.

▨ Normal neurological function is necessary for adequate strength and stability. Dysfunction of the nervous system can come from the cervical or thoracic spine, reflex inhition from irritated mechanoreceptors from the joint (arthrokinetic reflex), atrophy due to prior injury, or immobilization.

▨ Most shoulder disorders are not isolated injuries but affect several structures in the region.

BONES AND JOINTS OF THE SHOULDER GIRDLE

SCAPULA

▨ The scapula or shoulder blade is a flat, triangular bone (Fig. 6-2). The resting position of the scapula covers the second to seventh ribs, and the vertebral border is approximately 2 inches from the midline. The posterior aspect has a bony ridge called the *spine of the scapula* that extends laterally as a bulbous enlargement called the *acromion*. The acromion articulates with the clavicle, forming the acromioclavicular (AC) joint. Above the spine is a deep cavity or fossa that contains the supraspinatus muscle belly. Below the spine are the infraspinatus and the teres minor and major. On the anterior surface is a fossa where the subscapularis muscle attaches. There are 15 muscles that attach to the scapula.

▨ On the anterior-superior surface of the scapula is a bony process called the coracoid process, which is a point of attachment for three muscles and three ligaments. The muscles are the pectoralis minor, the short head of the biceps brachii, and the coracobrachialis. The three ligaments are the coracoclavicular, the coracohumeral, and the coracoacromial.

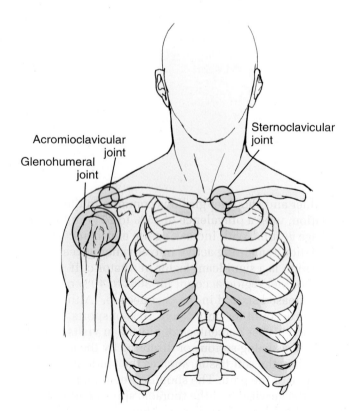

Acromioclavicular joint

Glenohumeral joint

Sternoclavicular joint

Figure 6-1. Anterior view of the bones and joints of the shoulder complex.

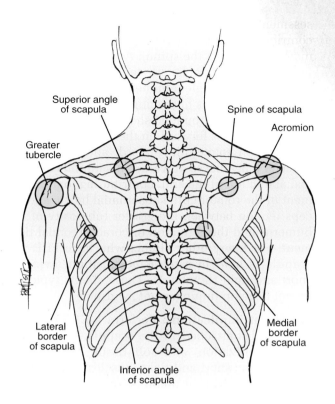

Figure 6-2. Posterior view of the bones and bony landmarks of the shoulder complex.

▓ The glenoid fossa is a shallow cavity on the lateral aspect of the scapula that serves as the articulation for the head of the humerus. In the normal resting position, the glenoid fossa faces laterally, anteriorly, and superiorly. Two body processes lie on the top and bottom of the glenoid fossa: the supra and infraglenoid tubercles for the attachment of the long head of the biceps and triceps, respectively.

CLAVICLE

▓ The clavicle or collarbone is an S-shaped bone, convex anteriorly in the medial two-thirds and concave anteriorly in the lateral one-third. It articulates with the sternum medially, forming the sternoclavicular joint, which connects the upper extremity to the axial skeleton. It articulates with the acromion of the scapula laterally, forming the AC joint. It is the attachment site of six muscles and a number of ligaments.

▓ **Dysfunction and injury:** Fracture of the clavicle is quite common, particularly in sports. Although it heals quickly, it typically heals with the ends overlapping, shortening the clavicle and narrowing the space underneath. The brachial plexus, the group of nerves from the neck that innervates the arm, travels under the clavicle in what is called the **tho-**racic outlet. A broken collarbone or other injuries leading to fibrosis in the fascia attaching to the clavicle or a rounded-shoulder, forward-head posture (FHP) closes down this space and contributes to **thoracic outlet syndrome.**

STERNUM

▓ The sternum or breastbone is a flat bone located in the center of the chest. It is divided into three parts: the manubrium, body, and xiphoid. The manubrium articulates with the clavicle and first rib at its superior-lateral aspect and with the second rib at the inferior-lateral aspect. The body provides an attachment site for the other ribs, forming the sternocostal joint. The xiphoid is the inferior tip. The sternum functions to protect the heart and lungs.

STERNOCLAVICULAR JOINT

▓ The sternoclavicular joint is a synovial joint in which the sternal end of the clavicle articulates with the upper lateral edge of the sternum, as well as the first rib (see Fig. 6-1).

▓ **Structure:** The sternoclavicular joint has a strong joint capsule, an articular disc, and three major ligaments.
  □ The three ligaments of the sternoclavicular joint are the costoclavicular ligament, the interclavicular ligament, and the anterior and posterior sternoclavicular ligaments.
  □ The articular disc, or meniscus, is a fibrocartilage that helps to distribute the forces between the two bones. It is attached to the clavicle, first rib, and sternum.

▓ **Function:** The sternoclavicular joint has five possible motions: elevation, depression, protraction, retraction, and rotation.

▓ **Dysfunction and injury:** The sternoclavicular joint is so strong that the clavicle will break or the AC joint will dislocate before the sternoclavicular joint dislocates.[1]

ACROMIOCLAVICULAR JOINT

▓ The AC joint is a synovial joint in which the lateral aspect of the clavicle articulates with the acromion of the scapula (see Fig. 6-5 on p. 245).

▓ **Structure:** It has a weak joint capsule, a fibrocartilage disc, and two strong ligaments.

▓ The ligaments are the superior and inferior AC ligaments and the coracoclavicular ligament, which is divided into the lateral trapezoid and medial conoid portions. These ligaments function to suspend the scapula from the clavicle and to prevent posterior and medial motion of the scapula, as in falling on an outstretched hand (FOOSH) injury.

■ **Function:** Approximately 30° of rotation of the clavicle can occur at the AC and sternoclavicular joints as the arm is elevated. The clavicle rolls superiorly and posteriorly after approximately 90° of abduction.

  □ The rotation of the scapula, and hence the upward and downward movement of the glenoid fossa, occurs at the AC joint.

■ **Dysfunction and injury:** A fall on the shoulder can tear the AC ligament and cause the clavicle to ride on top of the acromion, which is called a **shoulder separation.** This is visible when observing the client from the anterior view and is called a **step deformity.** The AC joint may degenerate because of repetitive stresses such as heavy lifting or prior injury. Pain is typically felt on the anterior and superior aspects of the shoulder and refers to the anterolateral neck.

SCAPULOTHORACIC JOINT

■ The scapulothoracic joint describes the relationship of the scapula to the rib cage (see Fig. 6-2). It is not a true joint with a synovial capsule, but a functional joint, as the scapula moves on top of the thoracic cage.

■ **Function:** The critical functions of the scapulothoracic joint are to allow for proper positioning of the glenoid fossa for arm motion and to stabilize the scapula for efficient arm motion. The scapula makes approximately a 30° to 45° angle anteriorly as it rests on the thoracic cage. This angle is called the **scapular plane.**

  □ There are six motions of the scapulothoracic joint: elevation, depression, adduction, abduction, and upward and downward rotation, which describes the movement of the inferior angle of the scapula moving away from or toward the vertebral column.

  □ The scapula has static and dynamic stabilizers. The **static stabilizers** are the joint capsule and ligaments, and the principle **dynamic stabilizers** are the rhomboids, trapezius, levator scapula, and serratus anterior. The static and dynamic stabilizers work in concert to provide a stable position of the scapula to allow optimum arm motion.

■ **Dysfunction and injury:** It is common for the dynamic stabilizers of the shoulder to be weak. During our assessment, this is manifested as winging of the scapula and excessive scapular motion when the client does a wall pushup (see "Shoulder As-

sessment," p. 262). Decreased scapular stability contributes to protracted scapula (i.e., the scapula moves away from the spine). As the scapula slides laterally, the optimal length–tension relationship of the muscles of the glenohumeral joint is lost, which results in weakness of the muscles of the arm. This is often caused by rounded shoulders and a FHP. As the scapula rides forward on the rib cage, the superior portion rotates downward, and the glenoid fossa no longer faces upward. This inhibits the normal abduction of the arm, contributing to impingement of the rotator cuff, subacromial bursa, and biceps tendon between the greater tuberosity of the humerus and the acromion or coracoacromial ligament. For many other clients who have FHP, the scapula is held in a retracted position owing to short and tight rhomboids. These clients typically do not develop impingement syndrome.

■ **Treatment implications:** Perform MET to release the muscles attached to the scapula, scapulothoracic mobilization, and soft tissue mobilization (STM) of the short and tight muscles. May require referral to a physical therapist or personal trainer for strength and stabilization training.

BONES AND SOFT TISSUE OF THE GLENOHUMERAL JOINT

GLENOHUMERAL JOINT

■ **Structure:** The glenohumeral joint is a ball-and-socket synovial joint consisting of the shallow glenoid fossa of the scapula and the large, rounded head of the humerus (Fig. 6-3). It contains a joint capsule, a fibrocartilage rim called a *labrum,* and numerous ligaments.

■ **Function:** The glenohumeral joint has the greatest ROM of any joint in the body, but it sacrifices stability for mobility. It is described as an incongruous joint, meaning that the humerus and glenoid fossa barely make contact with each other at rest. In arm motion, only 30% of the head of the humerus is in contact with the glenoid fossa.[2] It is held in the normal resting position by the superior joint capsule and the coracohumeral ligament. This is different from the hip joint, in which two-thirds of the head of the femur is within the acetabulum, and the two articulating surfaces fit closely together.

■ Because the glenohumeral joint is incongruous, the muscles play a dual role of support and motion. The muscles must maintain the proper alignment of the head of the humerus to the glenoid fossa as the arm is moving.[4]

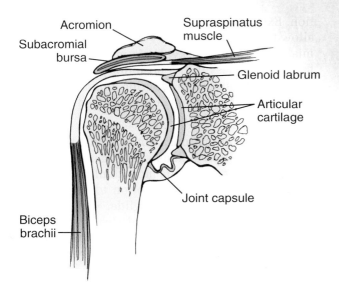

Figure 6-3. Glenohumeral joint showing the articular cartilage, joint capsule, subacromial bursa, supraspinatus, and long head of the biceps.

The glenohumeral joint has six basic motions: flexion, extension, abduction, adduction, and medial and lateral rotation. Abduction is easier in the plane of the scapula, which is 30° to 45° of forward flexion, because the joint capsule is more lax, and the greater tuberosity of the humerus is not abutting against the acromion at this angle.[5] This is the most natural and functional position of abduction. Patients who have shoulder pain typically abduct their arm in this plane.

Elevation of the arm is a combination of rolling and inferior sliding of the humeral head in the glenoid fossa, which requires strength of all the rotator cuff muscles to hold the humeral head stable as the arm is being elevated. As the deltoid muscle abducts the arm, the supraspinatus pulls the head of the humerus into the glenoid fossa, and the infraspinatus, teres minor, and subscapularis contract and pull the humeral head inferiorly. This action creates enough room for the humeral head to slide under the acromion. If the cuff muscles are dysfunctioning and weak, the humeral head migrates superiorly and impinges against the acromion and coracoacromial ligament.

Scapulohumeral rhythm: The first 15° to 30° of arm motion happens solely at the glenohumeral joint. Beginning at 15° to 30° of abduction, the scapula moves to contribute to arm elevation. The relationship of scapular movement to arm motion is called *scapulohumeral rhythm.* For every 10° movement of the humerus, there is 5° of scapular movement. These combined movements allow for 160° of abduction. To achieve 180° of abduction, the upper

thoracic and lower cervical spine bends. Thus, thoracic hypomobility prevents full abduction.[6]

Dysfunction and injury: Because of the poor congruency of the humeral head in the glenoid fossa, this joint is susceptible to dislocation and subluxation (partial dislocation). Acute traumatic dislocation is predominantly an injury of young adults, caused by forced external rotation and extension of the arm, dislocating the humerus in the forward, medial, and inferior direction.[1] Instability of the glenohumeral joint is a common problem, and anterior instability is the most common direction. The instability may be attributable to traumatic dislocation, rotator cuff injury or weakness, or acquired or congenital joint laxity. Acquired instability is caused by prior or recurrent dislocations or by treatment failure of the initial injury.[3] The joint may develop degenerative joint disease, which involves a wearing of the articular cartilage, from prior injury or chronic instability.

Treatment implications: It is important for the massage therapist to appreciate that certain conditions require stabilization and strengthening rather than to assume that all clients need release of muscle tension. If your assessment findings or doctor's diagnosis indicate glenohumeral instability, use contract-relax (CR) muscle energy technique (MET) in the rotator cuff and muscles stabilizing the scapula to help facilitate their normal function. Typically, there is weakness in the supraspinatus and lateral rotators, which allows the head of the humerus to migrate superiorly creating an impingement of the delicate soft tissue structures between the humeral head and the acromion. These clients typically require treatment with a physical therapist or a personal trainer to guide them in proper exercise. Degeneration is treated with STM for the short and tight muscles; joint mobilization to increase accessory motion between the head of the humerus and glenoid fossa and to increase ROM; and MET to release hypertonic muscles and recruit weak, inhibited muscles.

HUMERUS

The humerus or arm bone consists of a body and upper (proximal) and lower (distal) ends. The humeral head forms the upper end. On the anterolateral surface is the greater tubercle, and on the anteromedial surface is the lesser tubercle. Between these two bony prominences is the intertubercular groove, which contains the tendon of the long head of the biceps. The greater tubercle is an attachment site for the supraspinatus, infraspinatus, and teres minor. The lesser tubercle is the attachment site for

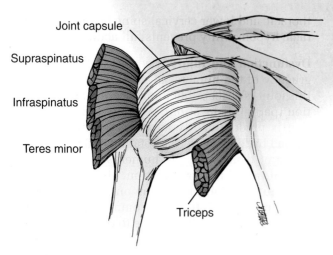

Figure 6-4. Joint capsule, interweaving rotator cuff muscles and long head of the triceps.

the subscapularis. The distal end of the humerus articulates with the radius and ulna to form the elbow.

JOINT CAPSULE

- **Structure:** The joint capsule originates from the glenoid labrum and attaches to the periosteum of the shaft of the humerus (Fig. 6-4). There is a synovial lining throughout the capsule[4] that is reinforced posteriorly and superiorly by the rotator cuff muscles and anteriorly by the subscapularis tendon, pectoralis major, teres major, and the coracohumeral and glenohumeral ligaments. The fibers of the joint capsule have a medial and forward twist with the arm hanging at the side in its resting position.

- **Function:** The twist in the joint capsule is increased with abduction and decreased with flexion. The tension in the capsule in abduction pulls the humerus into external rotation, which allows the greater tubercle of the humerus to clear the coracoacromial arch.[1] The posterior capsule tightens when the arm rotates medially (internally), and the anterior capsule tightens when the arm rotates laterally (externally). The joint capsule is also involved in **instability syndrome** and **rotator cuff tendinitis,** which are addressed later in the chapter (see the sections "Instability Syndrome of the Glenohumeral Joint" and "Rotator Cuff Tendinitis").

- **Dysfunction and injury:** A common problem to the joint capsule is called **frozen shoulder** or **adhesive capsulitis.** The joint capsule becomes fibrotic; the anterior portion of the capsule develops adhesions to the humeral head, and the folds in the capsule can adhere to themselves. This fibrosis and thickening shorten the capsule and prevent external rotation of the shoulder, which, in turn, restricts abduc-

tion. External rotation is necessary in abduction to allow the greater tuberosity to clear the coracoacromial arch. Thoracic kyphosis may be a causative factor.[4] Tightness in the posterior joint capsule results in an anterior superior migration of the humeral head, creating an impingement of the soft tissue under the acromion.

- **Treatment implications:** The treatment of frozen shoulder is a tremendous challenge. Passive traction and MET provide the most comfortable and effective therapy. The first motion to introduce for frozen shoulder is inferior glide, which reduces sustained muscle tension and stretches the joint capsule. Next, perform CR MET to increase external rotation, as this allows the greater tuberosity to roll under the coracoacromial arch for abduction. Finally, perform postisometric relaxation (PIR) or eccentric MET to increase flexion and abduction, first in the sagittal plane, then in the scapular plane, and finally in the coronal plane.

LABRUM

- **Structure:** The labrum is a fibrocartilage lip that surrounds the glenoid fossa (see Fig. 6-3). The outer surface of the labrum is the primary attachment site for the joint capsule and glenohumeral ligaments. The tendon of the long head of the biceps attaches to and reinforces the superior aspect of the labrum, and the long head of the triceps attaches to and reinforces the inferior aspect of the labrum.

- **Function:** The labrum functions to deepen the glenoid cavity, adding stability.

- **Dysfunction and injury:** Injuries to the labrum can result from shearing forces if the humerus is forced through extreme motions, repeated or excessive traction of the long head of the biceps tendon from its attachment, shoulder trauma such as dislocations, falls on an outstreched arm, throwing sports, and overhead work.[2] The two most common tears are the Bankart lesion, which is a tear of the labrum from the anterior glenoid, and the SLAP (superior labral anterior to posterior) lesion, which is a detachment of the superior labrum–long head of the biceps complex. These tears lead to instability of the joint. Clients complain of poorly localized pain over the anterior aspect of the shoulder, exacerbated by elevation of the arm overhead and movement of the arm behind the back. Examination may demonstrate pain at the anterior shoulder with isometric contraction of the long head of the biceps (Speed's test).

- **Treatment implications:** The treatment is to promote strength and stability of the glenohumeral

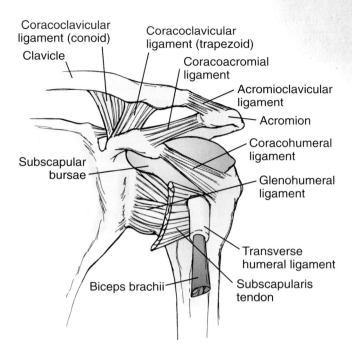

Figure 6-5. Ligaments of the glenohumeral and the acromioclavicular joints and of the subscapular bursa.

joint. MET is applied to help recruit inhibited muscles and reduce excessive tesion in the muscles. Gentle STM to promote circulation is helpful. Patients need exercise rehabilitation.

LIGAMENTS

- The **ligaments** of the glenohumeral joint are the glenohumeral, the coracohumeral, the coracoacromial, and the transverse humeral (Fig. 6-5). The joint capsule thickens in bands that are sometimes referred to as capsular ligaments. As in all joints, there is a reflex from the mechanoreceptors within the joint capsule and ligaments to the muscles surrounding the joint.[7]
  - ☐ The **glenohumeral ligament** lies underneath the coracohumeral ligament, reinforcing the joint anteriorly and tightening on external rotation of the humerus.
  - ☐ The **coracohumeral ligament** is further divided into the superior, middle, and inferior portions. It is a broad band reinforcing and interweaving with the upper part of the joint capsule. It attaches to the lateral border of the coracoid process, passing laterally to blend with the tendon of the supraspinatus, capsule, and transverse humeral ligament.
  - ☐ The **coracoacromial ligament** is a strong triangular band attached to the edge of the acromion just in front of the articular surface for the clavicle and to the entire length of the lateral border of the coracoid process.

- ☐ The **transverse humeral ligament** crosses the intertubercular groove to stabilize the tendon of the long head of the biceps.

CORACOACROMIAL ARCH

- **Structure:** The coracoacromial arch consists of the coracoid process anteriorly, the acromion posteriorly, and the coracoacromial ligament in between them (see Fig. 6-5). In the arch space lie the head of the humerus below; the coracoacromial ligament and acromion above; and the joint capsule, the supraspinatus and infraspinatus tendons, the long head of the biceps, and the subdeltoid bursa in between.

- **Function:** The coracoacromial ligament prevents dislocation of the humeral head superiorly, and along with the acromion and coracoid process, it forms an important protective arch. It also acts as a soft tissue buffer between the rotator cuff and the bony surface of the acromion. The coracoacromial arch may be described as an accessory joint that is lined with the synovial membrane of the synovial bursa.[8]

- **Dysfunction and injury:** The greater tubercle of the head of the humerus may impinge or compress the supraspinatus and infraspinatus tendons, the joint capsule, the bicipital tendon, or the subdeltoid bursa against the coracoacromial ligament and anterior acromion. This is called **impingement syndrome.** The causes of this syndrome are diverse but include postural causes such as thoracic kyphosis or a habitual rounded-shoulder FHP. It may also be caused by muscle weakness from the scapular stabilizers or the rotator cuff muscles and the long head of the biceps, which provide a downward force on the humerus.

- **Treatment implications:** The first intention is to correct the client's posture, if indicated. Next, use CR MET to facilitate and strengthen the external rotators. Then perform transverse massage on the coracoacromial arch to reduce any adhesions and scar tissue in the coracoacromial ligament and to correct any positional dysfunction in the deltoid and rotator cuff muscles.

BURSAE

- **Structure:** A bursa is a synovial-lined sac filled with synovial fluid.

- **Function:** The function of a bursa is to secrete a lubricant to neighboring structures, which decreases friction.

- Of the eight or nine bursae that are about the shoulder, only the subacromial bursa is commonly

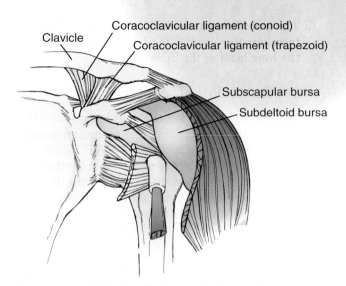

Figure 6-6. Subdeltoid and subscapular bursa.

involved clinically, and two others are occasionally involved.

☐ The **subacromial** or **subdeltoid bursa** lies over the greater tubercle of the humerus and supraspinatus tendon and under the coracoacromial ligament, acromion, and deltoid muscle (Fig. 6-6).

☐ The **subscapular bursa** lies over the anterior joint capsule and under the subscapularis muscle attachment to the lesser tubercle of the humerus.

☐ The **subcoracoid bursa** lies between the coracoid process and the clavicle.

▨ **Dysfunction and injury:** The subacromial bursa can become inflamed due to overuse, postural stresses, or trauma and can become impinged under the acromial arch. Because of its closeness to the supraspinatus tendon, any scarring or calcium deposits in the body of the tendon can irritate this bursa. It is also susceptible to irritation from a type III acromion, also called a *hooked acromion*. This type of acromion has a bony protuberance on the undersurface, which can irritate the supraspinatus tendon that travels underneath it.

▨ The subscapular bursa can become irritated because of increased tension in the pectoralis minor and subscapularis muscles.

▨ The subcoracoid bursa can become irritated because of the forward tipping of the scapula caused by pectoralis minor hypertonicity.

▨ **Treatment implications:** Lauren Berry, RPT, taught that the bursae can be manually drained if they are swollen. They can also be manually pumped to increase their synovial fluids if they are dried out because of adhesions. These techniques are clinically effective for both conditions.

 CAUTION: When treating an acute bursitis, be extremely gentle, or you may aggravate the condition.

NERVES OF THE SHOULDER REGION

▨ Most of the nerve supply of the shoulder and arm arise from the **brachial plexus,** which begins as five nerve roots from C5 to C8 and T1 (Fig. 6-7). As was

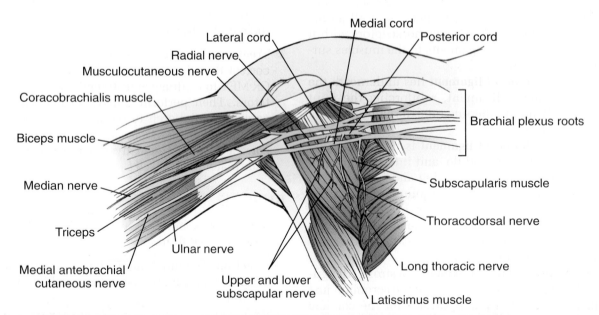

Figure 6-7. Brachial plexus leaves the neck between the anterior and the middle scalenes. It then travels under the clavicle, subclavius, and pectoralis minor and enters the medial arm.

mentioned in Chapter 5, "Cervical Spine," these nerve roots travel through the anterior and the middle scalenes. The roots of the brachial plexus unite just above the clavicle to form the superior, middle, and inferior trunks. The middle part of the clavicle is convex anteriorly, and the axillary artery and vein and brachial plexus pass posterior to this.

▓ The brachial plexus then travels over the first rib and under the clavicle and subclavius muscle. This costoclavicular space can become compromised because of previous trauma, such as a fractured clavicle, or because of postural imbalances, such as rounded shoulders.

▓ The nerves then travel between the pectoralis minor and the rib cage, medial to the coracoid process. At the level of the pectoralis minor, the brachial plexus forms the medial, lateral, and posterior cords. Distal to the pectoralis minor, the three cords divide into many branches, including the radial, median, and ulnar nerves that travel into the arm and down to the hand.

▓ The medial and ulnar nerves travel along the medial arm in the medial bicipital groove, bounded by the biceps and triceps. The radial nerve leaves this groove at the margin of the proximal and middle third of the arm and travels to the posterior surface of the humerus in the radial groove.

▓ In addition to the brachial plexus, there are several peripheral nerves in the shoulder region that we address in the treatment section of this chapter: The **long thoracic nerve** travels on the thoracic wall over the serratus anterior; the **subscapular** and **thoracodorsal** nerves lie on the subscapularis muscle; the **suprascapular** nerve travels through the suprascapular notch of the scapula and supplies the supraspinatus and infraspinatus; the **axillary nerve** travels over the posterior and inferior aspect of the posterior joint capsule to supply the deltoid and teres minor; and the **radial nerve** (see above). These nerves can become entrapped because of shortened fascia or sustained contraction in the muscles.

▓ **Dysfunction and injury:** As was mentioned in Chapter 5, thoracic outlet syndrome is a result of compression or entrapment of the brachial plexus. As Kendall and colleagues[9] point out, the diagnosis of thoracic outlet syndrome is often ambiguous because it includes many similar entities, including costoclavicular, anterior scalene, hyperabduction, and pectoralis minor syndromes.

▓ Nerves become compressed for several reasons: poor posture and faulty alignment of the neck, upper back, and shoulders. A rounded-shoulder FHP, creates a forward depression of the coracoid process, shortening the pectoralis minor and weakening the lower trapezius. This posture also predisposes to an adduction and internal rotation of the shoulder. This leads to compression. Brachial plexus compression may also result from prolonged overhead activities, such as painting, in which the clavicle rotates posteriorly, compressing the nerves between the clavicle and the first rib.

▓ Clinically, the brachial plexus can become compressed at several different sites:
　☐ Between the anterior and middle scalenes.
　☐ Between the clavicle and the first rib, called a *costoclavicular syndrome.* This syndrome is caused by rounded-shoulder posture; thoracic kyphosis; or previous trauma to the clavicle, AC joint, or glenohumeral joint.
　☐ At the pectoralis minor, as the plexus travels between the muscle and the rib cage.

▓ Brachial plexus compression symptoms include a generalized numbing, tingling, and pain. The medial cord, the most inferior part of the brachial plexus, is most vulnerable to compression; therefore, ulnar nerve symptoms along the ulnar border of the forearm and hand are most commonly reported.[4]

▓ **Treatment implications:** Four distinct areas must be released when the therapist considers peripheral entrapment of the brachial plexus: the region of the scalenes, the supraclavicular space, the infraclavicular space, and the pectoralis minor. Refer to Chapter 5 for further discussion of the scalenes.

▓ Begin with instruction in postural awareness. Next, perform CR MET to reduce the hypertonicity in the tight muscles. Then use PIR MET to lengthen the short anterior muscles and fascia, and use CR MET and home exercises to strengthen the weak lower trapezius. Treat the pectoralis minor, pectoralis major, and subscapularis first. After facilitating the lower trapezius, perform manual release on the supraclavicular and infraclavicular spaces.

MUSCLES OF THE SHOULDER REGION

▓ **Structure:** The muscles of the shoulder region may be divided into **two major groups:** muscles that stabilize the scapula and muscles of the rotator cuff.
　☐ Four main **muscles stabilize the scapula:** the rhomboids, trapezius, levator scapula, and serratus anterior (Figs. 6-8 and 6-9). To perform elevation of the arm, these muscles must contract first to stabilize the scapula against the rib cage. Then the rotator cuff muscles and the deltoids contract to elevate the arm.[3]

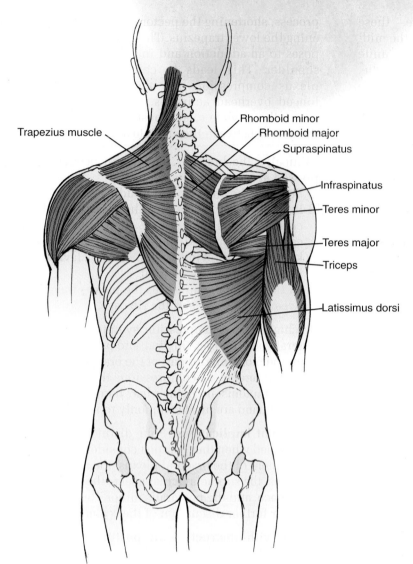

Trapezius muscle

Rhomboid minor
Rhomboid major
Supraspinatus
Infraspinatus
Teres minor
Teres major
Triceps
Latissimus dorsi

Figure 6-8. Muscles of the posterior shoulder region.

☐ The **four muscles of the rotator cuff** are the supraspinatus, infraspinatus, teres minor (Fig. 6-10), and subscapularis (see Fig. 6-9). They attach to the posterior, superior, and anterior head of the humerus as a continuous cuff, not as discrete tendons. The fibers of the cuff blend with the articular joint capsule.

Function: The chief function of the rotator cuff muscles is dynamic stabilization of the glenohumeral joint. In most joints, the close fit of the articulating bones, the ligaments, and joint capsule offers primary stability. As has been mentioned, there is little congruence between the humeral head and the glenoid fossa. When the arm hangs at the side, little contraction of the deltoid or cuff muscles is required, as the superior joint capsule and the coracohumeral ligament provide a reactive tensile force that pulls the humeral head against the glenoid cavity.[6] When the arm is elevated, the superior joint capsule is lax

and no longer stabilizes the joint, so the muscles of the rotator cuff must hold the humerus in proper orientation to the glenoid, playing an essential role in stabilizing the joint. They create joint compression and downward depression, creating a fixed fulcrum so that the deltoid can rotate the arm upward. If the cuff muscles are weak, the contraction of the deltoid causes an abnormal upward movement of the humeral head, causing an impingement of the soft tissue into the coracoacromial arch.

Dysfunction and injury: The rotator cuff is a common site of acute injuries, degenerative conditions, and acute injuries that are the end stage of chronic degeneration caused by cumulative stresses. Rotator cuff injuries may vary from mild irritation and partial strains (tears) to full thickness tears. The most commonly affected muscle is the supraspinatus. The supraspinatus should receive its primary blood supply from the thoracoacromial artery. This

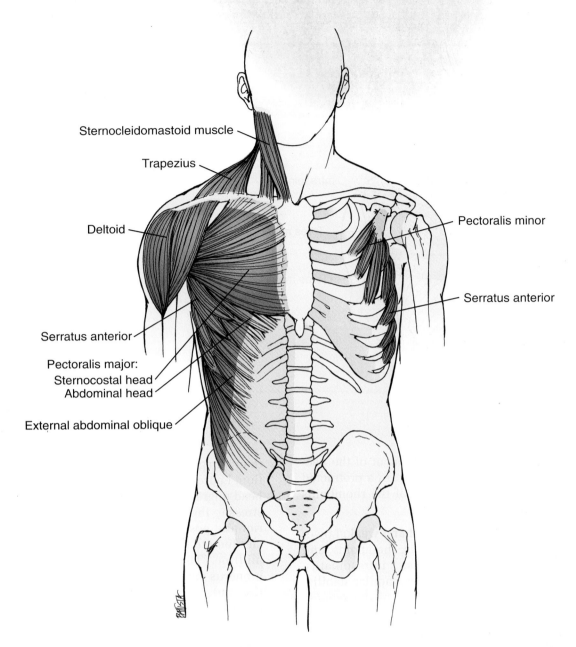

Sternocleidomastoid muscle

Trapezius

Deltoid

Serratus anterior

Pectoralis major:
Sternocostal head
Abdominal head

External abdominal oblique

Pectoralis minor

Serratus anterior

Figure 6-9. Muscles of the anterior shoulder.

artery is frequently absent, leaving the tendon hypovascular.[6] The infraspinatus may also be hypovascular but to a much lesser extent. This decreased blood supply makes the area susceptible to fatigue and degeneration.

☐ Two common conditions decrease the stability of the joint:

☐ Thoracic kyphosis, which causes the tension in the superior joint capsule to be lost, and the rotator cuff muscles must maintain constant contraction to stabilize the arm, making it susceptible to fatigue and degeneration.[6]

☐ Weakness in the scapular stabilizing muscles, especially the serratus anterior and the lower and mid-

dle trapezius. This allows the acromion to migrate forward, into a position of greater impingement.

☐ As was mentioned previously, according to Janda,[10] there are predictable patterns of muscle dysfunction. In the upper body, he describes this as the **upper crossed syndrome.**[10] Below are listed the muscles of the shoulder girdle complex that are typically imbalanced and participate in the upper crossed syndrome.

Muscle Imbalances of the Shoulder Region

▓ **Muscles that tend to be tight and short:** Pectoralis major and minor, upper trapezius, subscapularis,

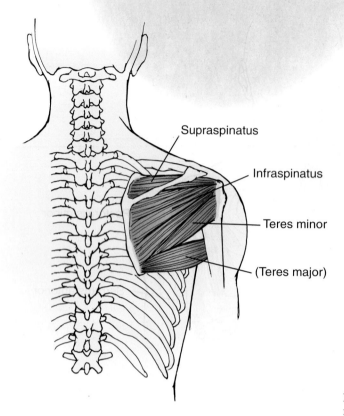

Supraspinatus

Infraspinatus

Teres minor

(Teres major)

Figure 6-10. Supraspinatus, infraspinatus, and teres minor are three of the four rotator cuff muscles.

and levator scapula. Overdevelopment of the pectoralis and the subscapularis result in a protracted scapula and a stretch weakness of the rhomboids and middle trapezius.[11]

- **Muscles that tend to be inhibited and weak:** Lower and middle parts of the trapezius, rhomboids, and serratus anterior, supraspinatus,[12] infraspinatus, and teres minor. Weakness in the scapular stabilizing muscles allows lateral sliding of the scapula and results in anterior motion of the humeral head during abduction and external rotation, stressing the anterior joint and contributing to impingement.

POSITIONAL DYSFUNCTION OF SHOULDER REGION MUSCLES

- ☐ In dysfunction, the shoulder internally rotates and adducts. The humeral head migrates superiorly, leading to impingement. This internally rotated position can cause the bicipital tendon to track abnormally against the medial side of the intertubercular groove, irritating it.[11]
- ☐ The anterior and posterior deltoid, infraspinatus, and teres minor tend to drop into an inferior torsion.

- **Treatment implications:** To treat muscular dysfunction, it is important to treat the short and tight muscles first, as they have an inhibiting effect on

their antagonists. Regarding the positional dysfunction, Lauren Berry, RPT, theorized that the humeral head migrates upward after an injury or cumulative stress to the rotator cuff muscles and that the anterior and posterior deltoid and the rotator cuff muscles tend to roll into an inferior torsion, parting the midline. The treatment implication is that the humerus must be mobilized inferiorly and the anterior and posterior muscles about the head of the humerus must be lifted superiorly. As has been mentioned, it is important to assign home exercises to strengthen the external rotators and thus help depress the humerus. It is also important to strengthen the scapular stabilizers, especially the lower trapezius and the serratus anterior.

SHOULDER MUSCLE ANATOMY

See Table 6-1.

MUSCULAR ACTIONS OF THE SHOULDER

See Table 6-2.

MUSCULAR ACTIONS OF THE SHOULDER GIRDLE

See Table 6-3.

Table 6-1   Anatomy of the Muscles of the Shoulder

Scapular Stabilizing Muscles (see Fig. 6-8)

Muscle	Origin	Insertion	Action	Dysfunction
Trapezius	Medial one-third of superior nuchal line, spinous processes of C7 and all thoracic vertebrae.	Spine and acromion processes of scapula and lateral third of clavicle.	The upper fibers elevate the scapula, the lower fibers depress it, and the middle fibers retract the scapula and have an essential role in stabilizing the scapula.	The upper fibers tend to be tight and short, while the lower fibers tend to be weak and long, allowing the scapula to migrate headward, decreasing stability of the scapula for movement of the arm.
Rhomboid Minor	Spinous processes of C7 and T1	Vertebral border of the scapula, superior to spine of scapula.	Both major and minor draw the scapula upward and medially; holds the scapula to the trunk	Rhomboids tend to be weak, which contributes to a rounded shoulders posture.
Rhomboid Minor	Spinous processes of T2, 3, 4, 5	Vertebral border of the scapula below the spine of the scapula	along with the serratus anterior muscle; retracts the scapula along with the fibers of the middle trapezius.	
Levator Scapula	Posterior tubercles of the transverse processes of C1, 2, 3, 4. This attachment site is significant as there are four major muscles that blend into each other at this point: the splenius cervicis, posterior scalene, longissimus capitis, and the levator.	Superior angle of scapula and to the base of the spine of the scapula.	Pulls the scapula upward and medially (along with the trapezius); if the scapula is fixed, pulls the neck laterally; acts similar to the deep fibers of the erector spinae in helping to prevent forward shear of the cervical spine. Levator acts like a posterior "guy wire" holding up and stabilizing the head and neck along with the scalenes, the anterior "guy wires."	Tends to be short and tight, contributing to rounded shoulders, but is in an eccentric contraction in the forward-head posture(FHP). As levator is active maintaining optimal head and neck posture, FHP will eccentrically load levator.[16]
Serratus Anterior (see Fig. 6-9)	Surface of the upper nine ribs at the side of the chest, and the intercostal muscles in between.	Costal aspect of the whole length of the medial border of the scapula.	It is a major stabilizer of the scapula, holding the scapula against the rib cage. It performs abduction (protraction), i.e., draws the medial border of the scapula away from the vertebrae. Also provides upward rotation. The longer, lower fibers tend to draw the inferior angle of the scapula farther from the vertebrae, thus rotating the scapula upward slightly. It is the antagonist of the rhomboids.	The serratus tends to be weak, demonstated by winging of the scapula during the scapular stabilization (push-up) test. Weakness of the serratus leads to instability of the scapula, contributing to impingement, and impairs the ability to lift the arm overhead with strength.

(continued)

Table 6-1   Anatomy of the Muscles of the Shoulder (Continued)

Rotator Cuff Muscles

Muscle	Origin	Insertion	Action	Dysfunction
Supraspinatus (See Fig. 6-10)	Supraspinous fossa of the scapula.	Superior facet of the greater tubercle of the humerus.	Initiates abduction by compressing the head of the humerus into the glenoid fossa, stabilizing the humerus, so that the deltoid can rotate the arm upward.	The most commonly injured muscle of the shoulder. It is predisposed to degeneration due to hypovascularity. This contributes to a poor repair after an injury, and also predisposes it to fatigue that develops from sustained contraction. This sustained contraction develops from an altered position in the glenohumeral joint from rounded-shoulder posture, or thoracic kyphosis. Tends to be weak, which prevents humeral head from being seated properly in the glenoid fossa during arm movements, leading to instability of the glenohumeral joint.
Infraspinatus	Lower margin of the spine of the scapula, infraspinatus fossa.	Middle facet of the greater tubercle of the humerus.	Lateral rotation; dynamic stabilizer of the glenohumeral joint by compressing and pulling the humeral head down during elevation of the arm. The infraspinatus is more active than the supraspinatus with the arm abducted 120–150°, which explains why it is commonly irritated with excessive overhead activities.	As with the supraspinatus, the infraspinatus has a diminished blood supply relative to the other muscles of the shoulder, and therefore is commonly involved clinically. The infraspinatus tends to be weak either due to irritation or injury, or due to inhibition from the short and tight subscapularis, which allows the humeral head to migrate superiorly, contributing to impingement syndrome.
Teres Minor	Lower portion of the infraspinatus fossa and lateral margin of the scapula.	Lower facet of the greater tubercle of the humerus.	Lateral rotation and adduction; dynamic stabilizer of the glenohumeral joint by compressing and pulling the humeral head down during elevation of the arm.	Tends to be weak, which allows the humeral head to migrate superiorly, contributing to impingement syndrome.
Subscapularis (See Fig. 6-9)	Entire anterior surface of the subscapular fossa.	The lesser tubercle of the humerus, and the joint capsule.	Medial rotation and adduction; dynamic stabilizer of the glenohumeral joint by compressing and pulling the humeral head down during elevation of the arm.	Tends to be short and tight, leading to a sustained adduction and medial rotation of the arm, and contributing to inhibition of the external rotators. Weakness contributes to anterior instability of the glenohumeral joint.

Additional Muscles

Deltoid (see Fig. 6-9)	Outer third of the clavicle, border of the acromion, and lower edge of the spine of the scapula. Divided into three parts, the anterior, middle, and posterior.	Deltoid tubercle on the lateral surface of the humerus.	The deltoid joins with the rotator cuff muscles to act as a force couple during elevation of the arm. The deltoid elevates the humerus, as the infraspinatus, teres minor, and subscapularis pull inward and down. As the origin of the deltoid is on the scapula, which raises during elevation of the arm, this provides an optimal length/tension relationship for the strongest muscle contraction throughout the range of motion. The anterior fibers provide flexion and medial rotation. The posterior fibers provide extension and lateral rotation. The middle fibers provide abduction.	According to Lauren Berry, R.P.T., the fascicles of the deltoid roll into an abnormal anterior and inferior torsion with a rounded-shoulders posture. This posture tends to promote adduction and internal rotation of the humerus, contributing to this torsion.
Biceps Brachii	Short head from the coracoid process; long head from the supraglenoid tubercle above the glenoid cavity, and the superior labrum.	Radial tuberosity of the radius and bicipital aponeurosis, which is a broad sheet of fascia that blends with the deep fascia of the medial forearm.	Primarily a flexor and supinator of the forearm. Long head is involved in abduction, the short head in adduction. The tendon of the long head is fixed, and the humerus moves relative to it. Also acts like a cuff muscle as a dynamic stabilizer of the humeral head during abduction, aiding in humeral depression. In fact, Cailliet states that the greatest downward glide of the humerus has been attributed to the mechanical force of the contracting long head of the biceps.[3]	Long head of the biceps in involved in impingement syndrome, along with supraspinatus. The detachment of the superior labrum-biceps complex is described as a SLAP lesion (superior-labral-anterior-posterior).[2]
Triceps Brachii (See Fig. 6-8)	Three heads: long head from the tubercle below the glenoid; lateral head from the lateral posterosuperior shaft of the humerus; and medial head from the posterior shaft of the humerus.	Olecranon process of the ulna at the elbow.	Primarily an elbow extensor; also extends the arm and adducts it.	

(continued)

Table 6-1   Anatomy of the Muscles of the Shoulder (*Continued*)

Additional Muscles

Muscle	Origin	Insertion	Action	Dysfunction
Teres Major	Lower third and inferior angle of the lateral border of the scapula.	Inner lip of the intertubercular groove of the humerus, and blends with the anterior joint capsule.	Extension—draws the arm from the front horizontal position down to the side. Inward rotation—as it depresses, it rotates the humerus inward. Adduction—draws the arm from the side horizontal position down to the side and rotates inward as it adducts.	Teres major contributes to rounded shoulder posture by pulling scapula into abduction (protraction).
Coracobrachialis	Coracoid process of the scapula.	Medial surface of the humerus, in mid-shaft.	Flexes and adducts arm.	
Pectoralis Major	Medial half of the anterior surface of the clavicle, anterior surface of the costal cartilages of the first six ribs, and adjoining portion of the sternum.	Flat tendon 2" or 3" wide to lateral lip of the intertubercular groove of the humerus, and blends with the anterior joint capsule.	Contraction of both the sternal and clavicular heads produces adduction and medial rotation. Clavicular heads is one of the prime flexors of the shoulder, along with the anterior deltoid.	Pectoralis major tends to be tight, rolling into inferior torsion with FHP and rounded shoulders.
Pectoralis Minor	3rd to 5th ribs	Coracoid process of the scapula.	Depression of shoulder girdle, so that the glenoid cavity faces more inferiorly; abduction and elevation of the scapula—draws the scapula forward and tends to tilt the lower border away from the ribs. Provides downward force on scapula to stabilize it against upward force, such as using arms to get up from a chair.	Tends to be tight and short, leading to rounded-shoulder posture, creating an excessive load on the thoracic extensors, leading to thoracic pain. A short, tight pectoralis minor can also compress the brachial plexus against the rib cage, leading to pain, numbing and tingling down the arm, a type of thoracic outlet syndrome.
Subclavius	From the junction of bone and cartilage of the first rib.	Into the sulcus for the subclavius muscle on the lower surface of the clavicle.	Pulls the clavicle toward the sternum and so stabilizes the sternoclavicular joint.	

Table 6-2	Muscular Actions of the Shoulder

Flexion

- Deltoid (anterior)—also causes abduction and medial rotation
- Pectoralis major (clavicular part)—also causes horizontal flexion, adduction, and medial rotation; and the sternal portion of the pectoralis causes shoulder adduction, horizontal flexion, and medial rotation
- Biceps brachii—short head also assists in horizontal flexion and medial rotation; long head also assists in abduction; and biceps also flexes and supinates the elbow
- Coracobrachialis—also assists in adduction

Extension

- Teres major—also adducts and medially rotates
- Latissimus dorsi—also adducts and medially rotates
- Triceps (long head)—also adducts and extends the elbow
- Deltoid (posterior part)—also abducts and laterally rotates

Horizontal Flexion (Horizontal Adduction)

- Deltoid (anterior)
- Pectoralis major
- Coracobrachialis
- Biceps (short head)

Horizontal Extension (Horizontal Abduction)

- Deltoid (posterior)
- Triceps (long head)
- Latissimus dorsi
- Teres major

Adduction

- Pectoralis major
- Latissimus dorsi
- Teres major
- Triceps brachii (long head)

Abduction

- Deltoid—middle and anterior
- Supraspinatus—may assist in lateral rotation
- Biceps brachii (long head)

The primary muscles of abduction are the middle and anterior deltoid and the supraspinatus. There is debate in the literature as to the function of the supraspinatus. It is easiest to test the supraspinatus at 15° abduction and the deltoid at 90° abduction.

Medial (internal) Rotation

- Subscapularis—also adducts
- Pectoralis major
- Teres major
- Latissimus dorsi

Lateral (external) Rotation

- Infraspinatus—performs greater lateral rotation than the teres minor, deltoid (posterior), and supraspinatus combined
- Teres minor
- Deltoid (posterior)
- Supraspinatus

Table 6-3	Muscular Actions of the Scapula

Elevation

- Levator scapula—also laterally flexes the neck
- Trapezius (upper)
- Rhomboid major—also retracts the shoulder girdle and rotates the scapula downward
- Rhomboid minor—same as the rhomboid major

Depression

- Pectoralis minor—rotates the scapula downward and abducts it
- Serratus anterior (lower)
- Trapezius (lower)

Protraction (Abduction)—Scapula Moves Away from Spine

- Serratus anterior—also rotates the scapula upward
- Pectoralis major and minor

Retraction (Adduction)—Scapula Moves Toward the Spine

- Rhomboid major
- Rhomboid minor
- Trapezius (middle)

Upward Rotation—The Lower Part of the Scapula Moves Away from the Spine, as in Lifting the Arm Overhead

- Serratus anterior
- Trapezius (upper and lower)

Downward Rotation—In the Anatomic Position the Scapula Is Almost to Maximum Downward Rotation

- Levator scapula
- Rhomboid major
- Rhomboid minor

Shoulder Dysfunction and Injury

FACTORS PREDISPOSING TO SHOULDER PAIN

■ Instability of the glenohumeral joint

■ Weakness in the scapular stabilizing muscles

■ Previous injury, including previous dislocation of the glenohumeral joint or separation of the AC joint

■ Hypomobility of the cervical or thoracic spine, which limits full ROM of the glenohumeral joint

■ Postural dysfunction, such as rounded shoulders, FHP, and thoracic kyphosis

■ Muscle imbalances

DIFFERENTIATION OF SHOULDER PAIN

■ Once you have ruled out pathology and pain from visceral diseases such as gallbladder irritation and cardiac problems (see the section "Contraindications to Massage Therapy: Red Flags" in Chapter 2, "Assessment and Technique"), shoulder pain that hurts at night or pain that increases at night indicates that there is an active inflammation. It may be caused by rotator cuff tendinitis, bursitis, capsulitis, or nerve root irritation, called *cervical radiculitis* (meaning "root inflammation").

■ Dysfunctions and injuries of the cervical facets and disc degeneration commonly refer to the interscapular region. Scapular motion rarely increases the pain, but active motion examination of the cervical spine reveals limited motion that may refer pain to the scapular region at the end ranges. As was mentioned in Chapter 5, "The Cervical Spine," irritation of a sensory nerve root elicits sharp pain, numbing, and tingling in a specific area of skin called a *dermatome*. The cervical dermatomes include the shoulder region: C4, top of the shoulder; C5, upper arm and shoulder; and C6, elbow, and the radial side of the forearm and thumb. A myotome includes those muscles innervated by a specific motor nerve. Cervical nerves innervate the shoulder muscles. Irritation of the motor nerve elicits a deep aching in the corresponding muscle and

a weakness in that muscle. The myotomes in the shoulder region are C4, shoulder elevation; C5, shoulder abduction; C6, elbow flexion and wrist extension; and C7, elbow and finger extension and wrist flexion. The shoulder is also a referral site from the fascia, ligaments, and joint capsules in the cervical spine that are innervated by the same segmental nerve. This is called *sclerotomal pain* and is described as deep, aching, and poorly localized.

■ To help differentiate shoulder pain from pain that is being referred from the neck, there are certain guidelines:
  □ Pain originating from the neck is often elicited or increased from neck motion.
  □ Pain originating from the shoulder is typically elicited or increased from active shoulder motion and relieved by rest.
  □ Isometric challenge of the muscles of the shoulder will be painful with a localized lesion in the shoulder.
  □ Often, a painless weakness occurs in the arm and shoulder muscles that have a motor nerve root problem from the cervical spine.

■ Rotator cuff injuries typically manifest as pain at the lateral portion of the upper arm, and a painful limitation when elevating the arm overhead. The involved muscles are identifed by isometric testing.

■ Bicipital tendinitis (long head) manifests as a well-localized pain at the anterior portion of the head of the humerus and aggravation with Speed's test.

■ Stiffness in the shoulder is typically adhesive capsulitis, which presents as a dramatic loss of arm motion, especially external rotation.

■ Impingement manifests as pain over the anterior humerus, with a loss of internal rotation and a painful Neer's impingement test.

■ Instability manifests as clunking in the shoulder with active circumduction and excessive joint play in the passive motion test for the glenohumeral joint.

■ Pain that originates in the glenohumeral joint is rarely felt at the joint, but over the lateral brachial region. This is explained by the concept of sclerotomal pain, because the tissue that is irritated is mainly the joint capsule and interweaving tendons of the rotator cuff, which are innervated by C5–C6 nerves; the lateral brachium is the C5 dermatome.

COMMON DYSFUNCTIONS AND INJURIES OF THE SHOULDER

ROTATOR CUFF TENDINITIS (SUPRASPINATUS TENDINITIS)

Tendinitis of the rotator cuff most commonly involves the supraspinatus tendon and then the infraspinatus.

- **Cause:** Rotator cuff tears are described as partial- or full-thickness tears. They are further categorized as acute tears due to trauma, or chronic tears, which are those that are degenerative and slowly tear over time. The supraspinatus is most commonly involved for many reasons. The supraspinatus tendon has a poor blood supply, and the demands of the muscle can overwhelm the nutritional supply.[6,13] This ischemia, or low oxygen in the tissue, combined with mechanical stress leads to a breakdown of fibrils, which leads to an inflammatory response with consequent scar tissue and potential calcium deposits. The supraspinatus is the only muscle of the rotator cuff that travels through a tunnel, which is formed by the head of the humerus below and the acromion above. Any swelling will compress the tendon because of the confines of the tunnel, compromising the blood supply. This lesion is common in swimmers, tennis players, and baseball pitchers as well as clients who have poor posture. In the rounded-shoulder posture, the supraspinatus is under constant tension, leading to fatigue and degeneration.

- **Symptoms:** Clients experience a generalized, dull, toothache-like pain that refers to the lateral aspect of the humerus and that is often worse at night, with an inability to lay on that shoulder. Calcific tendinitis can cause a hot, burning pain.

- **Signs:** Tendinitis signs are limited, painful elevation; a painful arc, which can be sharp, during active abduction between 60° and 120°; painful resisted abduction at 15°; positive supraspinatus test (empty-can test); and weak external rotators. Palpation reveals tenderness over the supraspinatus tendon proximal to or at its insertion on the greater tuberosity of the humerus.

- **Lesion Sites:** Tendinitis lesions occur at the tenoperiosteal junction and the musculotendinous junction. The tenoperiosteal junction will have the above signs, whereas the musculotendinous lesion will have a painful resisted abduction but will not have a painful arc or impingement test.

- **Treatment:** For **acute** supraspinatus tendinitis perform Level I, second and third shoulder series, with emphasis on releasing the pectoralis minor and major and deltoid to open the area over the supraspinatus tendon. As you perform the strokes, palpate the tissues to assess for hypertonicity, and perform MET and wave mobilization as indicated. Perform CR and reciprocal inhibition (RI) MET for the supraspinatus (MET #9) with light pressure to assess the degree of irritability. Repeat MET with increasing pressure to engage more of the muscle if the technique remains within client's comfort level. Finally, perform Level I, fourth series of STM strokes. Use very gentle touch and slow movements. For **chronic** conditions, first perform PIR MET #10 to lengthen the supraspinatus. Perform transverse friction massage (TFM), Level I, fourth series, at the myotendinous and tenoperiosteal junctions to dissolve adhesions if you palpate any fibrosis. Perform MET for the external rotators to help increase their strength (METs #4 and #5). Perform MET to stretch the posterior capsule and increase medial rotation (METs #4 shoulder, #5 thoracic). Clients need to participate in a strength and stabilization program for the rotator cuff and scapular stabilizers.

INFRASPINATUS TENDINITIS

- **Cause:** Infraspinatus tendinitis commonly occurs in musicians, carpenters, swimmers, tennis players, and others who perform activities that involve sustained abduction, external rotation, and overhead activities. The infraspinatus is more active than the supraspinatus with the arm abducted 120° to 150°, which explains why it is commonly irritated with repetitive overhead activities.[7]

- **Symptoms:** Clients typically experience pain at the insertion over the posterior aspect of the greater tuberosity at the myotendinous junction or anywhere in the belly of the muscle.

- **Signs:** Pain on resisted lateral rotation.

- **Treatment:** For **acute** infraspinatus tendinitis, first perform CR and RI MET (METs #4 and #5) to reduce pain, swelling, and hypertonicity. Next, perform gentle STM (fifth and sixth series) to promote nutritional exchange and cellular synthesis. In **chronic** conditions, the infraspinatus tends to be weak and inhibited and has degenerative fibers rather than inflammation. First perform CR and PIR MET for the subscapularis and other medial rotators (MET #3) to ensure that they are not inhibiting the infraspinatus. Next, perform CR MET to strengthen the infraspinatus (METs #4 and #5). Finally, perform the fifth and sixth series of STM strokes to dissolve any fibrosis and to lift the fibers superiorly, as the fibers are typically in a sustained inferior torsion.

SUBSCAPULARIS TENDINITIS

- **Cause:** Causes of subscapularis tendinitis are activities involving repetitive or excessive internal rotation and adduction, as in carpentry, or cleaning or in throwing or racquet sports.

- **Symptoms:** Clients typically experience pain at the lesser tuberosity.

- **Signs:** Pain on resisted medial rotation is a sign of subscapularis tendinitis, as are painful arc, which is a lesion at upper site of the insertion point, and painful passive horizontal adduction, as it is pinched against the coracoid process.

- **Treatment:** For **acute** subscapularis tendinitis, first perform CR and RI MET (MET #3) to reduce pain, swelling and hypertonicity. Next, perform gentle STM (first series) to promote nutritional exchange and cellular synthesis. In **chronic** conditions, the subscapularis tends to be short and tight. First perform CR MET for the medial rotators (MET #3) to reduce hypertonicity in the subscapularis. Next, perform PIR MET to lengthen the subscapularis and other medial rotators (MET #11). Finally, perform the first series of STM strokes to dissolve any fibrosis.

ADHESIVE CAPSULITIS (FROZEN SHOULDER)

- **Cause:** Adhesive capsulitis begins as an inflammatory lesion of the anterior and inferior portion of the glenohumeral joint capsule that leads to a chronic, degenerative thickening and shortening of the tissue. There is no known cause. It affects women more than men and the middle-aged and elderly more than younger clients. Hertling and Kessler[6] theorize that thoracic kyphosis and the consequent alteration in the scapulohumeral alignment is a predisposing factor.[6]

- **Symptoms:** Adhesive capsulitis symptoms develop in three stages.[2] The **first stage** is the initial freezing stage with an abrupt loss of motion and pain in the shoulder that refers pain to the lateral brachial region with movement. The **second stage** is the frozen stage, which may manifest as a persistent, dull ache, present at night or painful only with movement, and a dramatically reduced ability to elevate the arm. The pain may disturb the client's sleep, especially when the client rolls onto that shoulder, and the pain may radiate to the elbow. The **third** stage, or thawing stage, usually manifests as a slow recovery of motion, which make take one to three years. Muscles of the rotator cuff and scapula stabilizers may atrophy.

- **Signs:** In the **first stage,** active and passive lateral rotation may be limited, but this movement is usually painless. Active and passive abduction is the next most limited motion. A thick, capsular end feel with passive lateral rotation and abduction is present. Resisted movements are not painful. In the **second stage,** active and passive movements may be limited and painful, but resisted movements are painless. In the **third stage,** active and passive motion may be restricted in all planes and painful only at the end ranges of movement.

- **Treatment:** In the **acute** phase, perform inferior glide of the humerus (MET #12), which is helpful in decreasing pain and relieving muscle spasms. Perform CR MET #3 to reduce the hypertonicity in the medial rotators, which interweave with the joint capsule. Next, perform the third series of STM strokes. Emphasize compressing the head of the humerus into the glenoid fossa as you unwind the anterior soft tissue. For the **chronic** phase, first repeat the work described above for the acute phase. After the superficial soft tissue has released, concentrate on lengthening the joint capsule. Perform PIR MET to increase external rotation (MET #13). Finally, PIR or eccentric MET is used to increase elevation (MET #14), first in the sagittal plane, then in the scapular plane, and finally in the coronal plane. If indicated, provide instruction in postural awareness, including retracting and depressing the scapula and engaging the lower and middle trapezius. Encourage the client to use the arm as much as possible within comfortable limits to minimize disuse atrophy.

IMPINGEMENT SYNDROME

- **Cause:** Impingement syndrome is defined as a compromise of the space between the coracoacromial arch and the proximal humerus. The rotator cuff (usually the supraspinatus), subacromial bursa, and biceps tendon are compressed between the humeral head and the acromion or coracoacromial ligament. Impingement may be caused by an acute traumatic impingement from a fall on the shoulder or an outstretched hand. In chronic conditions, impingement syndrome has structural and functional causes. Structural causes include thickening of the rotator cuff tendons, inflamed bursa, and hooked acromion. Functional causes include rotator cuff weakness, scapular instability (weakness of scapular stabilizers), thoracic kyphosis, with either fibrosis and thickening of the posterior joint capsule or a lax capsule. Typically, the client presents with upper crossed syndrome, which includes tight pectoralis minor (which pulls the scapula into a protracted position), upper trapezius, levator scapula, and internal rotators and weakness in the lower trapezius and external rotators. Neer[14] describes three stages: an initial overuse syndrome; the development of thickening and fibrosis; and the development of bony changes, including spurs.

- **Symptoms:** Clients usually experience a gradual onset of pain at the anterior acromion or greater tuberosity, but this pain may refer down the C5–C6 sclerotomes.[6] It also may present as sharp twinges, especially with abduction.

- **Signs:** Painful arc of abduction between 90° and 120° and a positive Neer's impingement test. Internal rotation is the most restricted (opposite the typical capsular pattern), and elevation next, with only a slight loss of external rotation. The posterior capsule is typically thick and fibrotic.

- **Treatment:** The primary goal of assessment is to determine whether the client has instability due to weakness in the rotator cuff and scapular stabilizers and a lax capsule, or rotator cuff thickening and a fibrotic posterior joint capsule. The typical treatment is to release the posterior capsule, and recruit (strengthen) the rotator cuff and scapular stabilizers. In the **acute** phase, perform CR MET to reduce the hypertonicity in the tight muscles and to recruit the weak or inhibited muscles that have been identified by palpation and isometric challenge. The goal is to reduce the swelling in the joint and balance the muscles that stabilize the joint. In **chronic** conditions, the goal of treatment depends on whether the region is deconditioned or thick and hypertonic. For deconditioned muscles and lax capsules, perform CR MET to help recruit the muscles, and refer your client to a physical therapist or personal trainer for strength and stabilization exercises. Emphasis needs to be placed on strengthening the posterior cuff muscles and scapular stabilizers, especially the scapular retractors.[15] For hypertonic muscles and fibrosis in the posterior joint capsule, first perform MET for the hypertonic muscles and Level I, sixth series, and Level II, third series, to release adhesions in the capsule. Perform MET to increase internal rotation (MET #4) and stretch the posterior capsule. Next, perform manual release of any fibrosis that was palpated in the cuff tendons and the coracoacromial ligament.

INSTABILITY SYNDROME OF THE GLENOHUMERAL JOINT

- **Cause:** Instability may result from rotator cuff weakness; lack of scapular stabilization; or damage to the anterior capsule, glenohumeral ligament, and glenoid labrum. Instabilities are classified as trau-matic, nontraumatic, and acquired. Traumatic instability usually involves a history of shoulder dislocation or rotator cuff injury, such as a fall on an outstretched hand. Nontraumatic causes involve rotator cuff weakness and lack of scapular stabilization. Acquired instability describes either congenital laxity in the ligaments or poor treatment outcome after a dislocation.[2]

- **Symptoms:** Clients experience diffuse pain in the shoulder region with the feeling of the shoulder "going out."

- **Signs:** Excessive passive anterior and posterior movement (joint play) of the glenohumeral joint and sulcus sign indicate glenohumeral joint instability syndrome.

- **Treatment:** Instability typically involves sustained contraction in the pectoralis minor and subscapularis and weakness in the external rotators, pulling the humerus forward. First, use palpation and isometric testing to identify the tight and weak patterns of the shoulder. Perform CR MET on the tight muscles first—typically the pectoralis minor and subscapularis—to reduce the hypertonicity. Next, facilitate (strengthen) the external rotators with CR MET. Because the shoulder is too loose, it is important to work selectively on the tighter muscles rather than creating a generalized release in the shoulder region. The client needs exercise instruction to strengthen the rotator cuff muscles and scapular stabilizers.

BICIPITAL TENDINITIS

- **Cause:** Bicipital tendinitis is usually the result of repetitive microtrauma as a result of overhead activities that involve flexion and internal rotation, such as swimming, tennis, or throwing. As the long head attaches to the supraglenoid labrum, an acute or cumulative trauma to the biceps can tear the labrum.

- **Symptoms:** Clients experience pain over the anterior aspect of the humerus at the bicipital groove (tenosynovitis) and at the superior labrum with insertional tendinitis of the long head.

- **Signs:** Pain on resisted forward flexion of the shoulder with the elbow extended and the forearm supinated (Speed's test) and pain on resisted supination.

- **Treatment:** In the **acute** phase, perform CR MET to the biceps. This is accomplished by using the same position as Speed's test. The intention is to reduce pain and swelling and decrease muscle spasms. If light pressure elicits pain, perform RI for the biceps by having the client resist as you attempt to elevate the arm. Perform Level I strokes to gently mobilize the soft tissue and joints. Perform the second series of Level II strokes with light pressure and a slow rhythm to help normalize the position of the tendon in the bicipital groove. In **chronic** bicipital tendinosis (tendinopathy), recent evidence indicates that instead of an inflammatory condition, the tissue is degenerated, with the collagen in disarray and poor blood supply compared with normal tissue.[16] Our intention is to create a micro-inflammatory environment to induce revascularization and remodeling of the tissue. Repeat the treatment protocol described for acute conditions, but use greater pressure with the METs and greater depth with the strokes. The fourth series of Level I strokes and the second series of Level II strokes are emphasized to dissolve adhesions in the rotator cuff and bicipital attachments at the supraglenoid rim and to dissolve adhesions in the bicipital groove and on the bicipital tendon.

SUBACROMIAL (SUBDELTOID) BURSITIS

▨ **Cause:** Excessive overhead activities can irritate the bursa, leading to an acute bursitis in which the bursa swells. This is a rare condition. Typically, the supraspinatus tendon is involved. Over time, calcific deposits from this tendon, which lies under the bursa, may irritate or even rupture the bursa.[6]

▨ **Symptoms:** Clients experience the following symptoms with acute or chronic subacromial bursitis:
  □ **Acute:** Pain can be excruciating, and the patient loses the ability to move the arm.
  □ **Chronic:** Pain can be diffuse and achy over the proximal humerus and is often painful at night.

▨ **Signs:** Acute and chronic subacromial bursitis signs are as follows:

▨ **Acute:** All active ROM is painful. Heat and swelling may be palpable. Resisted abduction is painful. To passive motion testing, there is an empty end feel; that is, the client reports pain, but you do not feel the tension barrier in the tissue.

▨ **Chronic:** A painful arc in the middle of active and passive abduction. Resisted movements are usually painful.

▨ **Treatment:** For **acute** bursitis, perform manual draining of the bursa with Level II, fifth series, but use extreme caution. Students are always surprised at how gentle these strokes are. If the bursitis is **chronic**, assess the rotator cuff muscles. Often, an underlying tendinitis in the supraspinatus is

found, and any fibrosis at the tenoperiosteal junction must be released (Level I, fourth series). You can perform the manual draining of the bursa with greater depth for a chronic bursitis, but always begin with light pressure.

ACROMIOCLAVICULAR LIGAMENT SPRAIN

▨ **Cause:** AC ligament sprain is usually a traumatic event, such as a fall on an outstretched hand or a direct fall onto the shoulder.

▨ **Symptoms:** Clients experience well-localized pain over the AC joint.

▨ **Signs:** Pain at the AC joint from 90° to the end range of active abduction and pain at the AC joint on passive horizontal adduction.

▨ **Treatment:** For **acute** conditions, perform Level I strokes to help normalize the soft tissue of the shoulder. Identify strength/weakness imbalances through palpation and MET, and use MET to reduce hypertonicity in the tight muscles and to strengthen weak muscles. Next, perform very gentle back and forth strokes on the AC ligament (Level II, first series). For **chronic** conditions, repeat the protocol described above but with greater depth, including transverse friction massage to the AC ligaments.

SUPRASCAPULAR NERVE ENTRAPMENT

▨ **Symptoms:** Clients experience poorly localized pain at the posterolateral aspect of the shoulder. The pain may refer to the arm.

▨ **Signs:** Weakness without pain to resisted tests of supraspinatus and infraspinatus, possible pain at the posterolateral aspect of the scapula with overpressure in passive adduction of the arm, and pain after application of digital pressure on the nerve in the suprascapular or the spinoglenoid notch.

▨ **Treatment:** Perform Level I, fifth series, to release the suprascapular nerve.

COSTOCLAVICULAR SYNDROME (PART OF THORACIC OUTLET SYNDROME)

▨ **Cause:** Costoclavicular syndrome is defined as a compromise of the space between the clavicle and the first rib. It may be caused by a rounded-shoulder posture or previous trauma to the clavicle, AC joint, or glenohumeral joint, which lead to fibrous adhesions in the costoclavicular space.

- **Symptoms:** Clients experience a generalized pain, numbing, or tingling down the arm, especially to the ulnar border.

- **Signs:** A positive elevated-arm stress test (see "Assessment" in Chapter 5).

- **Treatment:** For **acute** conditions, perform Level I strokes to help normalize the soft tissue of the shoulder. Identify strength/weakness imbalances through palpation and MET, and use MET to reduce hypertonicity in the tight muscles and to strengthen weak muscles. Next, perform cervical spine Level I, third series (Chapter 5). For **chronic** conditions, repeat the protocol for acute conditions with greater depth, and perform back and forth and transverse friction strokes for the costoclavicular space, Level II, first series. It is important to instruct the client in good posture and provide exercises to strengthen the weak muscles and lengthen the tight muscles. If you are not fluent in exercise rehabilitation, refer your client to a physical therapist or personal trainer.

PECTORALIS MINOR SYNDROME (PART OF THORACIC OUTLET SYNDROME)

- **Cause:** Pectoralis minor syndrome is caused by sustained contraction of the pectoralis minor, which causes forward depression of the coracoid process, narrowing the space between the pectoralis minor and the rib cage, compressing the brachial plexus. The client typically has rounded shoulders, FHP, and the muscle imbalances that are typical of upper crossed syndrome.

- **Symptoms:** Clients experience generalized pain, numbing, or tingling down the arm, especially to the ulnar border.

- **Signs:** Symptoms are elicited with the application of digital pressure over the pectoralis minor and with the elevated-arm stress test (see "Assessment" in Chapter 5).

- **Treatment:** It is important to realize that a tight pectoralis minor is usually only one piece of a more global imbalance, described as upper crossed syndrome. For **acute** conditions, perform Level I strokes of the cervical spine and shoulder to help normalize the soft tissue of the entire neck and shoulder region. Identify strength/weakness imbalances through palpation and MET, and use MET to reduce hypertonicity in the tight muscles and to strengthen weak muscles. Concentrate on the CR and RI for the pectoralis minor. For **chronic** conditions, repeat the protocol described for acute conditions. Perform PIR MET for the pectoralis minor to reduce the hypertonicity and to lengthen it. Remember that the STM for pectoralis minor is performed in a superior direction, as it rolls into a sustained inferior torsion in dysfunction.

Shoulder Assessment

HISTORY QUESTIONS SPECIFIC TO SHOULDER PAIN

- Where is the pain? What is the quality of the pain?
  - ☐ Strains of the rotator cuff usually produce a dull ache that worsens at night, referred to the anterior and lateral shoulder, in the area of the deltoid tuberosity. Shoulder pain from emotional stress or FHP manifests as a dull pain in the upper trapezius and levator muscles. Persistent gripping pain in the arm and elbow—even at rest and especially if there is also numbing and tingling in the hands—could be a nerve root irritation from the cervical spine. An acute onset of throbbing pain that worsens at night can indicate an acute bursitis. Pain with lying on the shoulder is often a rotator cuff tendinitis, adhesive capsulitis, or bursitis. Chronic, severe, gripping pain that worsens at night needs a referral to a doctor.

- Is there a loss of motion in the arm?
  - ☐ Rotator cuff injuries are most inhibited in abduction. Impingement syndrome is reproduced with active flexion with the arm in medial rotation. Adhesive capsulitis can present as a drastic loss of external rotation and abduction, with or without pain. Acute bursitis presents as a drastic loss of motion with pain, especially at night.

OBSERVATION: CLIENT STANDING

ANTERIOR VIEW

▨ Are the clavicles level? Is shoulder height even? The shoulder is often elevated in rotator cuff and frozen shoulder conditions. The shoulder or clavicle is normally lower on the dominant side. Look for redness, swelling, and atrophy.

▨ Notice if there is a smooth contour to the area of the lateral shoulder or if the clavicle lies superior to the acromion at the AC joint. This is called a **step deformity** and indicates a previous AC separation.

▨ Is there a **sulcus sign** (i.e., an indentation below the acromion) resulting from a flattening of the normally round deltoid? This indicates an instability of the glenohumeral joint, a weak deltoid muscle, or an inferior subluxation.

POSTERIOR VIEW

▨ Is there scapular winging? If the inferior angle (or angles) of the scapula juts away from the thoracic wall, there may be a loss of scapular stabilization. Winging of the scapula in the resting position of the arm may be caused by scoliosis. It may also result from muscular injury; inhibition (weakness) of the scapular stabilizers, which are tested below (see "Scapular Stabilization Test"); or a nerve injury.

SIDEVIEW

▨ Are there rounded shoulders and FHP?

MOTION ASSESSMENT

To assess active movements, always begin on the non-involved side to establish a benchmark of normal motion for that client. Observe the ROM on the involved side, and ask the client whether the motion is painful. There may be an arc of pain; that is, there is pain during one part of the movement and then the pain disappears while the client continues the motion. If the motion is painful, ask the client to describe the location and quality of the pain. If the client knows what the painful motions are, ask him or her to perform these motions last. Have the client perform active cervical motions to assess ROM and symmetry between the sides and to see whether cervical motion elicits pain in the shoulder.

SCAPULAR STABILIZATION TEST

▨ **Position:** Have the client stand at arm's distance from the wall and place his or her hands on the

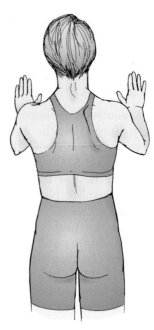

Figure 6-11. Scapular stabilization test. Notice the slight winging of the right scapula, indicating a slight weakness of the serratus anterior.

wall at shoulder level, keeping the elbows straight. Stand behind the client (Fig. 6-11).

▨ **Action:** Ask the client to lean into the wall to perform a push-up against the wall.

▨ **Observation:** When the client is performing the push-up, the scapula should remain stable against the thoracic cage. The inferior angle of the scapula should not wing off of the thoracic cage, and the medial borders of the scapula should not move more than approximately 1 inch. Winging indicates a weak serratus anterior or an injury to the long thoracic nerve. Excessive movement of the scapula indicates weakness of scapular stabilizers, including the serratus anterior, middle trapezius, or rhomboids.

ABDUCTION

▨ **Position:** Client stands with his or her back to you (Fig. 6-12).

▨ **Action:** Instruct the client to rotate his or her arms externally by turning the palms out. Then have the client raise the arms, trying to touch the palms together overhead.

▨ **Observation:** Notice if the top of the shoulder hikes upward at the beginning of the motion. This hiking typically indicates that there is a tight and short upper trapezius and levator scapula and a weak lower trapezius, serratus anterior, and supraspinatus. This muscular imbalance predisposes to impingement syndrome. Also notice if the client needs to

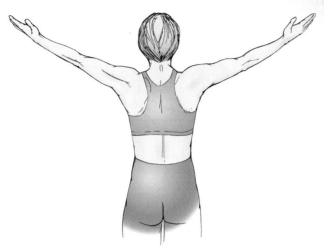

Figure 6-12. Shoulder abduction test. Notice if the top of the shoulder hikes toward the ear as the arm is abducted. This would indicate a tight upper trapezius and a weak lower trapezius.

move in the scapular plane, that is, approximately 30° of forward flexion. This position is assumed with acute and chronic problems. An arc of pain indicates supraspinatus tendinitis, subacromial bursitis, calcific deposits, or an AC joint irritation. Abduction is the best motion to indicate a rotator cuff tear. It may be impossible to perform the motion beyond 90° if there is a significant tear, especially in the supraspinatus.

MEDIAL ROTATION

■ **Position:** Client stands with his or her back to you (Fig. 6-13).

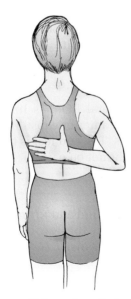

Figure 6-13. Active medial rotation. Notice how far up the spine the client can reach. Compare sides.

■ **Action:** Beginning with the non-involved side, ask the client to reach the hand up the back and try to touch the scapula. Measure the vertebral level that the fingertips or thumb touches. If measuring with the thumb, have the client place the thumb in the "hitchhiking" position. Compare with the other side.

■ **Observation:** It is normal to be able to reach to approximately T5–T10. The client might be able to reach the only greater trochanter or sacrum on one side. This motion elicits pain in the anterior shoulder with an impingement syndrome, as you are forcing the greater tuberosity against the coracoacromial ligament. If the movement is not painful, have the client attempt the "lift-off" test, lifting the hand off the back. This tests the strength of the subscapularis.

FLEXION WITH INTERNAL ROTATION (NEER'S IMPINGEMENT TEST)

■ **Position:** Client faces you and medially rotates the arm so that the thumb faces posteriorly.

■ **Action:** Ask the client to raise the involved arm up to the side of the head. The thumb now faces anteriorly. The therapist then puts overpressure on the elevated arm.

■ **Observation:** The range is normally approximately 170° to 180°. With the arm medially rotated, the supraspinatus, which attaches to the greater tuberosity, needs to slide under the coracoacromial ligament. If there is irritation, swelling, or scarring of the tendon, it impinges against this ligament.

LATERAL ROTATION

■ **Position:** Client faces you (Fig. 6-14).

■ **Action:** There are two actions. Ask the client to clasp his or her hands behind the head, with elbows pulled as far back as possible. If this is difficult, have the client place his or her arms at the sides, with the elbows at 90°, and laterally rotate the arms.

■ **Observation:** The first motion allows for easy comparison of both sides. It combines elevation and external rotation, a position of function for daily activities, such as getting dressed. In the second motion, the normal range is approximately 75° to 90°. Compare both sides. Lateral rotation is the first motion to be lost in adhesive capsulitis.

HORIZONTAL FLEXION (ADDUCTION)

■ **Position:** Client faces you.

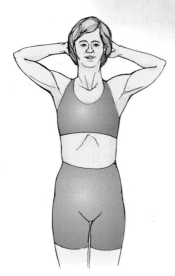

Figure 6-14. Lateral rotation with abduction performed bilaterally is an easy way to compare the ROM of both sides at the same time.

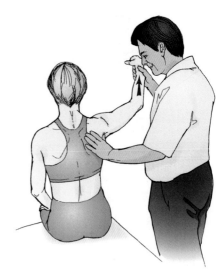

Figure 6-15. Passive abduction. The therapist places one hand on the scapula to detect when it moves. If the scapula moves before approximately 90° of abduction, then adhesion in the joint capsule is indicated.

■ **Action:** Client is instructed to elevate his or her arm to 90° and move the arm across the front of the body, attempting to place the hand on the opposite shoulder.

■ **Observation:** If there is pain at the top of the shoulder, it implicates the AC joint; pain at the posterior shoulder implicates the posterior-inferior capsule; anterior joint pain may be the anterior labrum, subcoracoid bursa, or subscapularis tendon. If there is anterior joint pain, differentiate bursitis from tendinitis by first performing the same movement passively, which would typically be painful with bursitis but not tendinitis. Isometrically challenge the subscapularis, which may be painful with tendinitis but not bursitis.

PASSIVE MOVEMENTS

Passive movements are performed for those movements that do not have full and pain-free active ROM. Note the range, pain, arc of pain, pain with overpressure, and end feel. The following passive shoulder movements are performed with the client sitting.

ABDUCTION

■ **Position:** Stand to one side of the client. Hold the lower scapula with your thumb and index finger with one hand and the distal forearm with your other hand (Fig. 6-15).

■ **Action:** Slowly abduct the client's arm until the resistance barrier is met or until the arm is against the client's head, and feel for when the scapula begins to move.

■ **Observation:** Normally, the range is approximately 170° to 180°. The scapula should not move until 90° of abduction. If there are adhesions of the joint capsule, anchoring the scapula to the humerus, the scapula begins moving before 90°. If there is no pain in passive abduction and active abduction was painful, it indicates a tendinitis of the rotator cuff, typically the supraspinatus. If there is pain in passive abduction before there is tissue tension, this is the "empty" end feel of bursitis, in this case, of the subacromial bursa.

LATERAL ROTATION

■ **Position:** Stand to one side of the client, and place one hand on the client's elbow to stabilize it against the client's body and the other hand on the client's distal forearm, holding it.

■ **Action:** Slowly pull the forearm laterally, which laterally rotates the arm.

■ **Observation:** Lateral ROM is limited in adhesive capsulitis, as the anterior capsule has developed fibrotic adhesions. The end feel is thick and leathery. It might or might not be painful.

CIRCUMDUCTION

■ **Position:** Stand behind and to one side of the client. Place one hand on the top of the glenohumeral joint, and hold the distal forearm with the other hand (Fig. 6-16).

■ **Action:** Slowly draw the arm backward to begin a circumduction motion. Move the arm in a forward circle, like the "crawl" swimming motion.

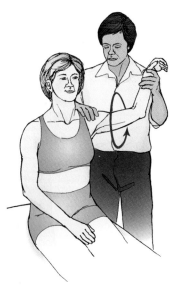

Figure 6-16. Passive circumduction. Lauren Berry, RPT, prefers this method to determine whether the shoulder complaint is muscular, capsular, or articular.

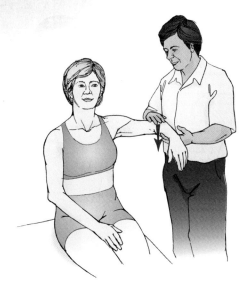

Figure 6-17. Isometric test for the middle deltoid.

▓ **Observation:** Circumduction motion helps to differentiate joint, muscle, and ligament lesions. There will be a loose feel or clunking with joint instability. You will feel crepitus (grinding sounds) with calcific deposits or arthrosis. There is a thickened feel and limited range with capsular lesions. With muscle hypertonicity, fascicular torsion, and soft tissue misalignment, there is a "cogwheel" pattern (i.e., there are resistances and dips in an otherwise smooth motion). Over time, you can learn to feel the subtleties of resistance under your hand.

ISOMETRIC TESTS

The client should be able to provide strong resistance to the following tests. Note if the client has difficulty in providing resistance. Ask whether the resisted action is painful. If it is painful, ask about the location and quality of pain. Remember that the shoulder and arm are common referral sites for neck problems. Painless weakness may be indicative of a nerve root problem. If the client remains weak after treatment, he or she needs a referral to a chiropractor or an osteopath. All of the following muscles are innervated by C5 and C6.

MIDDLE DELTOID

▓ **Position:** The client's arm is placed at 90° of abduction, with the elbow flexed 90° (Fig. 6-17).

▓ **Action:** Instruct the client to resist as you press down on the elbow.

▓ **Observation:** Pain indicates irritation or injury in the middle deltoid.

(EMPTY-CAN TEST)

▓ **Position:** The client's arm is abducted 90°, 30° forward flexion, and maximally internally rotated, that is, with the thumb turned down (Fig. 6-18).

▓ **Action:** Ask the client to resist as you press down on the distal forearm.

▓ **Observation:** The empty-can test isolates the action to the supraspinatus and also challenges the labrum-biceps complex. Pain at the lateral and anterior shoulder indicates irritation, injury, or scarring of the supraspinatus tendon or the biceps–labrum complex.

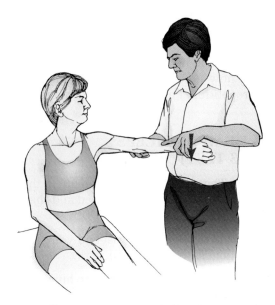

Figure 6-18. The empty-can test to isolate the supraspinatus.

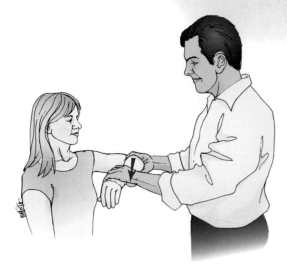

Figure 6-19. Isometric test for lateral rotation.

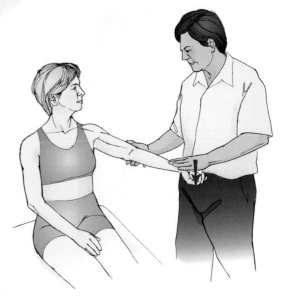

Figure 6-20. Speed's test for the long head of the biceps.

RESISTED LATERAL ROTATION

▓ **Position:** The client's arm is elevated 90° and internally rotated, with the elbow flexed to 90°. Place one hand on the client's elbow to stabilize it and the other at the distal forearm (Fig. 6-19).

▓ **Action:** Instruct the client to resist as you press downward on the client's distal forearm.

▓ **Observation:** The external rotators are typically weak. This weakness may be due to FHP, overuse, or prior injury. Pain at the posterior humerus indicates involvement of the infraspinatus and the teres minor. It is important to instruct the client in a strengthening program for the external rotators if they are weak. One possible home program for strengthening the external rotators is shown in MET #5. Patients are instructed to use a hand weight and lift it to about 70°. Repeat to fatigue. You determine how much weight to use by determining how much weight fatigues them with the tenth repetition. Perform three sets of ten.

LONG HEAD OF BICEPS (SPEED'S TEST)

▓ **Position:** The client's arm is flexed 30° in the scapular plane, with the elbow extended and the forearm supinated (Fig. 6-20).

▓ **Action:** Ask the client to resist and you press down on the client's distal forearm.

▓ **Observation:** Pain in the anterior humerus implicates the long head of the biceps.

ADDITIONAL TEST

MOTION PALPATION AND MOBILIZATION OF THE GLENOHUMERAL JOINT

▓ **Intention:** This test is performed to assess both motion restrictions of the humeral head in the glenoid and to assess excessive motion/instability (Fig. 6-21). The test is shown here for teaching purposes, but in the context of the treatment, it is typically performed after METs and Level I strokes.

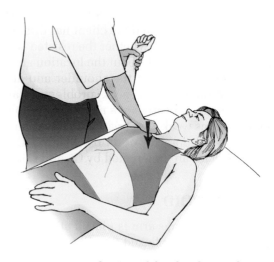

Figure 6-21. Motion palpation of the glenohumeral joint. This test is performed to assess both motion restrictions of the humeral head in the glenoid and to assess excessive motion/instability.

▨ **Position:** The client is supine with the arm at approximately 70° of abduction and elbow flexed to 90°. Hold the distal forearm with one hand, and place the palm of the other hand over the head of the humerus.

▨ **Action:** Gently push the humeral head posteriorly while stabilizing the arm with your other hand. This anterior to posterior mobilization can be repeated several times if the movement of the humeral head feels restricted.

▨ **Observation:** The typical motion restriction and positional dysfunction of the head of the humerus is an anterior fixation. Mobilizing the head of the humerus posteriorly helps to reestablish its normal position and movement. Excessive movement of the humeral head indicates joint instability. Another method to assess instability is to hold the distal forearm as described above and grasp the head of the humerus between your thumb and fingertips. Move the head of the humerus back and forth in an anterior-to-posterior (A–P) direction. An unstable glenohumeral joint will be "sloppy" and loose. Compare to the non-involved side and to other healthy shoulders to get a feeling for what is normal.

Techniques

GUIDELINES TO APPLYING TECHNIQUES

A thorough discussion of treatment guidelines can be found on p. 86 in Chapter 2. In the method of treatment described in this text, we make two underlying assumptions. The first is that an injury or dysfunction in one structure causes compensations in the entire region of the injury, as well as in other areas of the body. A rotator cuff injury, for example, is not isolated to only the fibers of the rotator cuff but typically creates tightening of the pectoralis minor and upper chest muscles, tightening of the extensors of the cervical spine, and weakness of the scapular stabilizers. It is important for the therapist to refer to other chapters to learn the protocol for assessment and treatment in each area involved.

The second assumption is that an injury or dysfunction that localizes in one tissue affects many other tissues in the area. Rotator cuff injury, for example, typically involves not only the muscles of the rotator cuff, but also the ligaments and joints capsule of the shoulder, as well as the alignment and motion of the glenohumeral joint. It is important for the therapist to assess and treat the surrounding muscles, tendons, ligaments, and joints of the shoulder in addition to treating the rotator cuff muscles.

The treatments described in this text address all the structures of the region through three techniques: muscle energy technique (MET), soft tissue mobilization (STM), and joint mobilization. These techniques can be applied to every type of shoulder pain, but the "dose" of the technique varies greatly from slow movements and light pressures for acute conditions to stronger pressures and deeper-amplitude mobilizations for chronic problems. Each aspect of the treatment is also an assessment to determine pain, tenderness, hypertonicity, weakness, and hypomobility or hypermobility. We use the philosophy of treating what we find when we find it. Remember that the goal of treatment is to heal the body, mind, and emotions. Keep your hands soft, keep your touch nurturing, and work only within the comfortable limits of your client so that he or she can completely relax into the treatment.

THE INTENTIONS OF TREATMENT FOR ACUTE CONDITIONS ARE AS FOLLOWS

▨ To stimulate the movement of fluids to reduce edema, increase oxygenation and nutrition, and eliminate waste products.

▨ To maintain as much pain-free joint motion as possible to prevent adhesions and maintain the health of the cartilage, which is dependent on movement for its nutrition.

▨ To provide mechanical stimulation to help align healing fibers and stimulate cellular synthesis.

▨ To provide neurological input to minimize muscular inhibition and help maintain proprioceptive function.

CAUTION: *Stretching is **contraindicated** in acute conditions.*

as not to induce pain. Gentle, pain-free contraction and relaxation of the shoulder flexors and extensors and related muscles provide a pumping action to reduce swelling, promote the flow of oxygen and nutrition, and eliminate waste products.

THE INTENTIONS OF TREATMENT FOR CHRONIC CONDITIONS ARE AS FOLLOWS

▓ To dissolve adhesions and restore flexibility, length and alignment to the myofascia.

▓ To dissolve fibrosis in the ligaments and capsular tissues surrounding the joints.

▓ To rehydrate the cartilage, restore mobility and ROM to the joints.

▓ To eliminate hypertonicity in short, tight muscles; strengthen weakened muscles; and reestablish the normal firing pattern in dysfunctioning muscles.

▓ To restore neurological function by increasing sensory awareness and proprioception.

Clinical examples are described below under "Soft Tissue Mobilization."

MUSCLE ENERGY TECHNIQUE

THERAPEUTIC GOALS OF MUSCLE ENERGY TECHNIQUE (MET)

A thorough discussion of the clinical application of MET can be found on p. 76. The MET techniques described below are organized into one section for teaching purposes. In the clinical setting, the METs and STM techniques are interspersed throughout the session. METs are used for assessment and treatment. A healthy muscle or group of muscles is strong and pain-free when isometrically challenged. MET will be painful if there is ischemia or inflammation in the muscles or their associated joints. The muscle will be weak and painless if the muscle is inhibited or the nerve is compromised. During treatment, MET is used as needed. For example, when you find a tight and tender pectoralis minor, use CR MET to reduce the hypertonicity and tenderness. If the pectoralis minor is painful while contracting, perform an RI MET, inducing a neurological relaxation. If the external rotators are weak and inhibited, first release the tight internal rotators, then use CR MET to recruit and strengthen the external rotators.

MET is very effective for an acute, painful shoulder, but the pressure that is applied must be very light so

THE BASIC THERAPEUTIC INTENTIONS OF MET FOR ACUTE CONDITIONS ARE AS FOLLOWS

▓ Provide a gentle pumping action to reduce pain and swelling, promote oxygenation of the tissue, and remove waste products.

▓ Reduce muscle spasms.

▓ Provide neurological input to mimimize muscular inhibition.

THE BASIC THERAPEUTIC INTENTIONS OF MET FOR CHRONIC CONDITONS ARE AS FOLLOWS

▓ Decrease excessive muscle tension.

▓ Strengthen muscles.

▓ Lengthen connective tissue.

▓ Increase joint movement and increase lubrication to the joints.

▓ Restore neurological function.

The internal rotators are typically short and tight, and the external rotators are typically weak. We will first assess the ROM of internal and external rotation. Next, we will assess and treat the muscles that tend to be tight (described in the upper crossed syndrome of Janda). In the muscles of the shoulder in the upper crossed syndrome, we usually find the pectoralis major and minor and subscapularis (an internal rotator) short and tight. Next, we will assess and facilitate the muscles of the rotator cuff that tend to be weak: the supraspinatus, and the primary external rotators, the infraspinatus, and teres minor.

The MET section below shows techniques that are used for most clients. In acute conditions, use MET #4 to increase external rotation and METs #7 and #8 to release the hypertonicity in the pectoralis major and minor. PIR MET, which lengthens muscles and fascia, is **contraindicated** for acute conditions.

Remember that MET should not be painful. Mild discomfort as the client resists the pressure is normal if the area is irritated or inflamed. Refer to Chapters 4 and 5 for METs for the thoracic spine and the cervical spine.

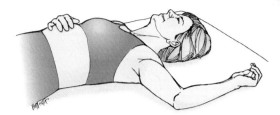

Figure 6-22. Assessment of the ROM of glenohumeral joint in lateral rotation and length of the medial rotators.

ASSESSMENT OF MUSCLE LENGTH OF GLENOHUMERAL JOINT AND PASSIVE RANGE OF MOTION

1. Assessment of the Range of Motion of Lateral Rotation of the Glenohumeral Joint

▨ **Intention:** For full external rotation, there must be normal length in the medial rotators—the pectoralis major, the latissimus, the teres major, and the subscapularis—and the anterior joint capsule (Fig. 6-22).

▨ **Position:** Client is supine, with the knees flexed and the feet on the table and with the low back flat on the table. Client then rests the arm at shoulder level (90° abduction) and lowers the forearm toward the head of the table without lifting the low back off the table.

▨ **Observation:** The normal ROM allows the forearm to lie flat on the table (90° of external rotation). This motion is drastically reduced in frozen shoulder and slightly reduced with shortness of the medial rotators.

2. Assessment of the Range of Motion of Medial Rotation of the Glenohumeral Joint

▨ **Intention:** For full internal rotation, there must be normal length in the lateral rotators—teres minor, infraspinatus, and posterior deltoid—and the posterior joint capsule.

▨ **Position:** Client is supine, with the knees flexed and the feet on the table and with the low back flat on the table. Client then rests the arm at shoulder level (90° abduction) and lowers the forearm toward the foot of the table without lifting the low back off the table.

▨ **Stabilization:** Hold the head of the humerus down to prevent it from moving forward.

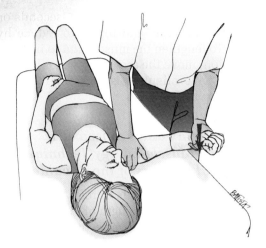

Figure 6-23. CR and PIR MET of the shoulder medial rotators.

▨ **Observation:** The normal range of medial rotation is 70° (i.e., for the forearm to be 20° from the table). This motion may be reduced in impingement syndrome, bicipital tendinitis, supraspinatus tendinitis, and shortening of the posterior joint capsule.

CONTRACT-RELAX AND POSTISOMETRIC RELAXATION TECHNIQUES

3. Contract-Relax and Postisometric Relaxation Muscle Energy Technique for the Medial Rotators of the Shoulder and to Increase External Rotation

▨ **Intention:** The intention is to relax the medial rotators, to increase the strength of the medial rotators if they test weak, to increase their length if they were found short by the previous assessment, and to increase external rotation of the shoulder (Fig. 6-23).

▨ **Position:** Client is supine, with the knees flexed and the feet on the table and with the low back flat on the table. Client then rests the arm at shoulder level (90° abduction) and lowers the forearm into lateral rotation as far to the table as comfortable, without lifting the low back off the table.

▨ **Stabilization:** Hold the head of the humerus down to prevent it from moving forward. As the arm is being moved into lateral rotation, clients with a history of dislocation might feel apprehensive. It is critical that you prevent the humeral head from moving anteriorly while you place the arm in lateral rotation.

▨ **Action:** To release the medial rotators, have the client resist as you attempt to press into further lateral rotation for approximately 5 seconds on the distal forearm. Relax and repeat to reduce hypertonicity. To lengthen the muscle and to increase lateral rotation, move the arm into further lateral rotation, and have client resist again for 5 seconds. Repeat three to five times.

4. Contract-Relax and Postisometric Relaxation Muscle Energy Technique of the Lateral Rotators of the Shoulder

▨ **Intention:** The intention is to relax tight lateral rotators, to increase the strength of the lateral rotators if they test weak, to increase the length of these muscles if they were found short by the previous assessment, to stretch the posterior joint capsule, and to increase medial rotation of the shoulder (Fig. 6-24).

▨ **Position:** Client is supine, with the knees flexed and the feet on the table, and with the low back flat on the table. Client then rests the arm at shoulder level (90° abduction) and lowers the forearm into medial rotation as far to the table as comfortable, without lifting the low back off the table.

▨ **Stabilization:** Hold the head of the humerus down to prevent it from moving forward.

▨ **Action:** Have the client resist as you attempt to press into further medial rotation on the distal forearm for approximately 5 seconds. Relax and repeat to reduce hypertonicity. To lengthen the muscle, move the arm into further medial rotation and have the client resist again for 5 seconds. Repeat three to five times.

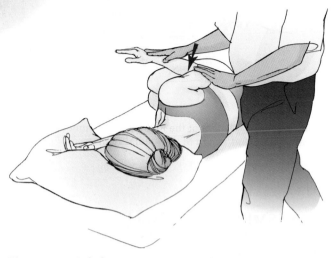

Figure 6-25. Side-lying position CR and RI MET for the lateral rotators.

5. Contract-Relax and Reciprocal Inhibition Muscle Energy Technique in the Side-Lying Position for the Lateral Rotators

▨ **Intention:** The intention is to reduce the hypertonicity of the infraspinatus, teres minor, and teres major with the client in a position that allows for massage of the region after the MET (Fig. 6-25).

▨ **Position:** Client is in the side-lying position. Place the client's arm on the side of the body with the elbow flexed to 90°. Place one hand on the client's elbow to stabilize the arm and the other hand on the distal forearm.

▨ **Action:** Have the client resist as you press down on the distal forearm for 5 seconds. To engage the teres major, which is an internal rotator of the arm, have the client resist as you pull up on the distal forearm for 5 seconds. Repeat these two METs several times and throughout your session as needed.

6. Contract-Relax Muscle Energy Technique for the Pectoralis Major

▨ **Intention:** The intention is to reduce hypertonicity with CR MET if the pectoralis major palpates as tight (Fig. 6-26).

▨ **Position:** Client is supine with knees bent, feet on the table. Place the client's arm in 90° of flexion.

▨ **Action:** Hold the client's distal forearm, and have the client resist as you attempt to pull the arm away from the body (abduction) for approximately 5 seconds. Have the client relax, and then repeat the

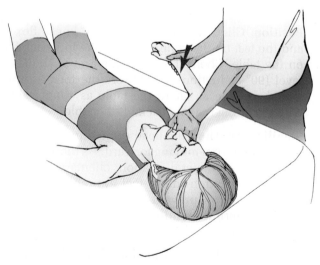

Figure 6-24. CR and PIR MET of the shoulder lateral rotators.

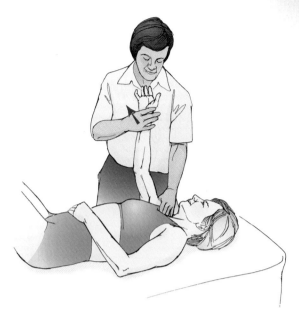

Figure 6-26. CR MET for the pectoralis major.

procedure. To reciprocally inhibit the pectoralis major, have the client resist as you press the arm toward her body.

7. *Postisometric Relaxation Muscle Energy Technique for the Pectoralis Major*

■ **Intention:** The intention is to lengthen the pectoralis major using PIR MET (Fig. 6-27).

■ **Position:** Client is supine with the knees bent, feet on the table. To lengthen the upper fibers, place the

client's arm at 90° of abduction, and to lengthen the lower fibers, place the arm at 135° of abduction.

■ **Stabilization:** Place one hand on the opposite clavicle when working with the upper fibers; place one hand on the glenohumeral joint on the same side when working with the lower fibers.

■ **Action:** To lengthen the upper fibers, hold the client's distal forearm, and slowly move the arm to its tension barrier. Have the client resist as you press the arm toward the floor. Repeat this series until the arm can hang over the side of the table at 90° abduction.

For the lower fibers, move the arm overhead at approximately 135° abduction to its tension barrier, and have the client resist as you press the arm toward the floor. Relax, move the arm to a new length, and repeat.

 CAUTION: If the stretch of this muscle causes numbing and tingling, you are stretching the brachial plexus and need to perform CR technique without the stretch.

8. *Contract-Relax and Postisometric Relaxation Muscle Energy Technique of the Pectoralis Minor*

■ **Intention:** The intention is to relax and lengthen the pectoralis minor (Fig. 6-28).

■ **Position:** Client is supine with the knees bent and feet on the table. Place the palm of one hand over

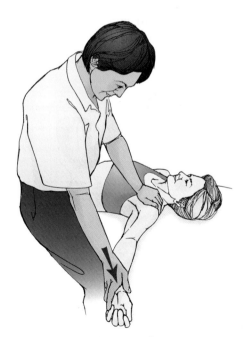

Figure 6-27. PIR MET of the pectoralis major.

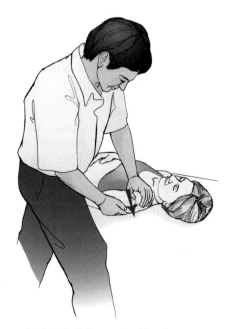

Figure 6-28. CR MET of the pectoralis minor.

the head of the humerus, and place the other hand under the posterior humerus. Lift the shoulder forward and medially, bringing the origin and insertion of the pectoralis minor toward each other.

■ **Action:** Have the client resist as you press on the head of the humerus, attempting to press it back to the table. Press for approximately 5 seconds, relax, and repeat. Move the head of the humerus closer to the table to lengthen the pectoralis minor, and have the client resist as you press toward the table again. Relax, and move the humerus as close to the table as is comfortable and have the client resist again. To reciprocally inhibit the pectoralis minor in its lengthened state, have the client resist as you attempt to lift the scapula off the table.

9. *Contract-Relax Muscle Energy Technique of the Supraspinatus*

■ **Intention:** The intention is to relax the supraspinatus.

■ **Position:** Client is supine, with arms at the sides. Bring one arm away from the client's body approximately 6 inches, to approximately 15° abduction. Place one hand on the client's distal forearm and the other hand on the belly of the supraspinatus in the supraspinous fossa of the scapula.

■ **Action:** Have the client resist as you press toward the client's body. Press for 5 seconds, relax, and repeat. Tap on the belly of the muscle in the supraspinous fossa and say, "Feel this muscle working," to bring sensory awareness to the muscle. The RI is to have the client resist as you attempt to pull the arm away from the body.

10. *Postisometric Relaxation Muscle Energy Technique for the Supraspinatus*

■ **Intention:** The intention is to lengthen the connective tissue of the supraspinatus and the superior portion of the joint capsule. This procedure is for **chronic conditions only** (Fig. 6-29).

■ **Position:** Client is sitting and places one hand on the low back. Hold one hand on the client's distal forearm, and stabilize the client's trunk with the other hand.

■ **Action:** Have the client resist as you attempt to pull the client's arm toward you, across the back. Pull for 5 seconds. Relax for a few seconds, and while the client is completely relaxed, pull the arm slowly into a further stretch across the back. Repeat three to

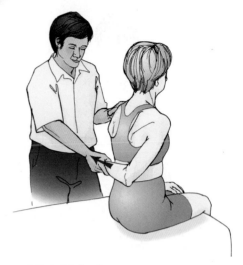

Figure 6-29. PIR MET for the supraspinatus.

five times. This may also be done as a CRAC MET. After the relaxation, have the client actively reach across the back as you gently pull the arm across.

11. *Postisometric Relaxation Muscle Energy Technique to Increase Medial Rotation*

■ **Intention:** The intention is to increase medial (internal) rotation of the glenohumeral joint and to stretch the posterior capsule and subscapularis (Fig. 6-30).

■ **Position:** Client is sitting and places one hand on his or her low back. If this is difficult, the hand is placed on the sacroiliac joint or the greater trochanter area. Hold one hand on the client's elbow and one hand on the distal forearm.

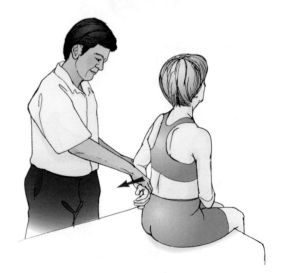

Figure 6-30. PIR MET to increase medial rotation.

Action: Have the client resist as you attempt to pull the distal forearm away from the lower back (i.e., into greater medial rotation). Pull for 5 seconds. Relax for a few seconds, and while the client is completely relaxed, pull the distal forearm slowly away from the lower back into a new resistance barrier or until it begins to be painful for the client. This is usually only approximately 1 inch. If it is painful, release the pull until it is comfortable again. Repeat three to five times. This position may also be used to increase the client's ability to reach up her back. Have the client resist as you attempt to lift the client's hand up the back. Relax. As the client is relaxing, lift the hand up the back to the next comfortable limit.

12. *Muscle Energy Technique to Increase Inferior Glide of the Glenohumeral Joint*

Intention: The intention is to reduce the hypertonicity of the muscles of the shoulder, to relieve pain, and to stretch the joint capsule (Fig. 6-31).

Position: Client is supine, with the involved arm at the side. Stand in the 45° headward position, tuck the client's forearm against your body, and hold it there with your arm. Place one hand in the client's axilla to stabilize the shoulder, and hold the distal humerus with your other hand.

Action: While the client is completely relaxed, press headward slightly with the stabilizing hand while you rotate your trunk away from the table, gently pulling the humerus inferiorly (toward the feet). Hold for 30 to 90 seconds.

Alternate Method: This MET movement is performed with the therapist sitting. Take your shoe off and place your foot in the client's axilla and hold the distal forearm. Lean back to traction the client's arm. Hold for 30 to 90 seconds.

TREATMENT FOR LOSS OF SHOULDER MOTION

13. *Contract-Relax Antagonist Contract to Increase External Rotation in Abduction*

Intention: The intention is to increase the ROM and length of the internal rotators and anterior joint capsule. In chronic shoulder problems, clients lose the ability to abduct and externally rotate the shoulder fully. This technique is a comfortable way to correct these problems (Fig. 6-32).

Position: Client is supine, with the feet on the table and the low back against the table. Place a pillow under the arms if the arms cannot rest comfortably at the end of their tension barrier. Have the client interlace the fingertips and place the hands under the head. Face 45° headward, and place your palms on the client's elbows.

Action: Have the client resist as you attempt to press the elbows toward the pillow or table for about 5 seconds. Relax, then have the client pull her elbows back toward the table to a new resistance barrier. Relax, and repeat the resist, relax, pull toward pillow/table cycle five times.

Home exercise: To increase the ROM of the shoulder, have the client perform the following exercise at home: The client should attempt to pull the

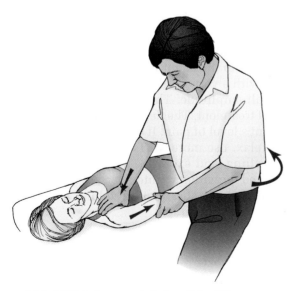

Figure 6-31. MET to increase inferior glide of the glenohumeral joint.

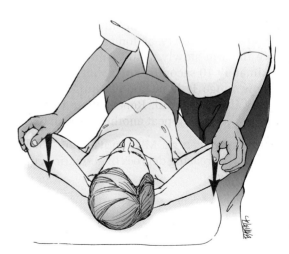

Figure 6-32. PIR MET to increase external rotation in abduction.

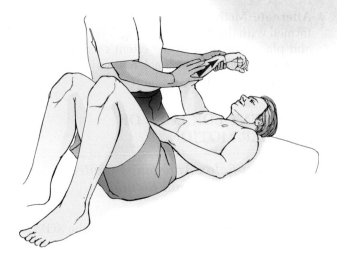

Figure 6-33. Eccentric MET to increase shoulder elevation.

elbows into the pillow for 5 seconds, relax, and repeat five times.

14. Eccentric Muscle Energy Technique to Increase Shoulder Elevation

 CAUTION: This technique is not to be performed on geriatric clients.

▨ **Intention:** The intention is to help dissolve adhesions in the anterior joint capsule, as elevation of the shoulder is one of the primary motions lost in frozen shoulder (Fig. 6-33).

▨ **Position:** Client is supine and elevates the arm to the comfortable limit. Hold the distal humerus, and place one hand on the forearm.

▨ **Action:** Have the client resist as you attempt to move the arm overhead with moderate pressure. Tell the client, "Let me win, and allow me to move your arm very slowly, as long as it is not painful." Move the arm slowly to the pain-free limit for approximately 10 seconds. Relax, but hold the arm in its new range if it is not painful. Bring it back slightly if it is painful. Repeat three to five times, and rest the arm. Repeat another three to five times.

▨ **Variations:** Eccentric MET movement can be performed at increasing degrees of abduction, up to approximately 80°.

SOFT TISSUE MOBILIZATION

BACKGROUND

A thorough discussion of the clinical application of STM can be found on p. 68. In the Hendrickson Method of manual therapy described in this text, the STM movements are called *wave mobilization* and are a combination of joint mobilization and STM performed in rhythmic oscillations with a frequency of 50 to 70 cycles per minute, except in performing brisk transverse friction massage (TFM) strokes, which can be two to four cycles per second. These mobilizations are presented in a specific sequence, which has been found to achieve the most efficient and effective results. This allows the therapist to "scan" the body to determine areas of tenderness, hypertonicity, and decreased mobility. It is important to "follow the recipe" until you have mastered this work. The techniques described below are divided into two sequences: Level 1 and Level II. Level I strokes are designed for every client, from acute injury to chronic degeneration, to enhance health and bring the body to optimum performance. Level II strokes are typically applied after Level I strokes and are designed for chronic conditions. Guidelines for treating acute and chronic conditions are listed below.

GUIDELINES FOR THE THERAPIST

Acute

The primary intention of treatment is to decrease pain and swelling as quickly as possible, maintain as much pain-free joint motion as possible, and induce relaxation. In this method of treatment, the soft tissue is compressed and decompressed in rhythmic cycles. This provides a pumping action that helps to promote fluid exchange, reducing swelling. The strokes that are applied to the client in acute pain need to be performed with a very gentle touch, a very slow rhythm, and small amplitude. There is no uniform "dose" or depth of treatment. The depth of treatment is based on the client's level of pain. If the soft tissue does not begin to relax, use more METs to help reduce discomfort, swelling, and excessive muscle tension. As was mentioned previously, intersperse your STM work with MET. Remember that **stretching is contraindicated** in acute conditions.

Clinical Example: Acute

Subjective: CS is a 64-year-old male health-care administrator who presented to my office complaining of acute left shoulder pain. He reported that the pain began upon awakening a few days previously, after an intense exercise class the previous day. He described the pain as an ache at the mid-arm that could be sharp with certain movements, especially reaching, and that he was unable to elevate the arm overhead.

Objective: Examination revealed active arm elevation limited to 70°, eliciting pain at the anterior portion of the proximal humerus. Active abduction was approximately 20°, at which point pain was elicited in the left mid-humerus region. External rotation was 50% of normal, with pain at the proximal humerus. Speed's test and the empty-can test were both positive, eliciting pain at the superior glenoid. Motion palpation revealed a limitation of posterior glide of the head of the humerus, indicating an anterior fixation of the humeral head. Palpation revealed tight and tender tissue in the area of the anterior humerus.

Assessment: Inflammation of the bicipital tendon (long head), and supraspinatus, with a fixation of the glenohumeral joint.

Treatment (Action): Treatment began with the Level I STM strokes. The subscapularis was tight and tender, which limited external rotation. CR MET was performed to reduce the hypertonicity in the internal rotators and allow more external rotation. In palpating the soft tissue of the second series of Level I strokes, very tight and tender pectoralis major and minor were noted. RI and CR MET were performed on both these muscles (METs #7 and #8). The third series of strokes were then performed to unwind the muscles of the anterior humerus. After unwinding the tissue, I returned to the third stroke of the second series and placed my thumb on the tendon of the long head of the biceps. I palpated that the tendon was riding on the medial rim of the bicipital groove. Next, I mobilized the tendon in an M–L direction to center it in the groove. I performed the fourth series of strokes for the supraspinatus. The tenoperiosteal junction was very tender. I performed CR MET for the supraspinatus (MET #9), to help reduce the inflammation and help increase the nutritional exchange. After the MET, the tissue was much less tender. I then performed gentle STM strokes on the supraspinatus. Next, I perfromed an A–P mobilization on the head of the humerus. After several oscillations, the head of the humerus had normal passive glide. I ended the session with some soft tissue therapy on the cervical spine. I had the client perform active ROM after the session, and elevation was 120°.

Plan: I recommended weekly visits for one month. CS returned to our office in a week and stated that he was feeling significantly less pain and had increased ROM. Elevation was approximately 140°. I repeated the treatment described above. There was much less tension in all of the muscles. CS returned to my office one week later, symptom-free, with full ROM and normal strength. I told him to call as needed for further treatments, and he was discharged from active care.

Chronic

The typical exam findings in clients with chronic shoulder problems are FHP, rounded shoulders, short and tight pectoralis minor and major, and weakness in the external rotators, lower trapezius, and scapular stabilizers. The glenohumeral joint is typically hypomobile, fixated anteriorly, with thick, fibrous ligaments and capsular tissues in the anterior and superior aspects of the joint. Some patients demonstrate the opposite: instability in the joints, weak, deconditioned muscles, and atrophy in the ligaments and capsular tissues. The primary goals of treatment depend on the patient. For patients who are hypomobile, the treatment goals are to reduce the hypertonicity of the muscles; promote mobility and extensibility in the connective tissue by dissolving the adhesions in the muscles, tendons, ligaments, and capsular tissues surrounding the joints; rehydrate the cartilage of the joint; reestablish normal joint play and ROM in the joints; and restore normal neurological function by stimulating the proprioceptors and reestablishing the normal firing patterns in the muscles. Patients who are unstable need exercise rehabilitation. Our treatments can support their stability by reducing tension in the tight muscles with STM and MET and strengthening weak muscles, reestablishing normal firing patterns, and rehabilitating the proprioceptors with MET. With chronic shoulder conditions, it is also important to treat tightness in the cervical and thoracic spine, including the tight upper trapezius, sternocleidomastoid, suboccipitals, and levator scapula. With chronic conditions, we use stronger pressure on the soft tissue and more vigorous mobilizations on the joints. In the Level II sequence, we add deeper soft tissue work as well as work on attachment points, using transverse friction strokes if we find fibrosis (thickening). As was mentioned in the "Acute" section above, intersperse your soft tissue work with METs.

Clinical Example: Chronic

Subjective: RM is a 53-year-old realtor who presented to my office complaining of intense pain and limited motion in the left shoulder. He reported that he was playing basketball with his son a couple of months prior to our visit and jammed his shoulder going for the ball. He immediately felt intense pain at the glenoid area. He went to an orthopedist, and X-rays and MRI were negative for fracture or frank tears of the rotator cuff. He was given anti-inflammatory medication, but his condition did not improve. At the time of our first visit, he described an intense pain at the top of the shoulder that was sharp with certain motions, a deep ache at night, and an inability to lift his arm overhead.

Objective: Examination revealed an elevation of the shoulder on the left side. Active ROM was limited to 90° in flexion, 60° in abduction, and only being able to reach to his back pocket when attempting internal rotation, which elicited pain at the superior glenoid. Passive motion was only slightly better. Isometric testing revealed pain at the superior glenoid with the empty-can test, with only very light pressure. His external rotators were very weak with a light challenge. His pectoralis minor was very tight and tender, and the head of the humerus was fixated anteriorly.

Assessment: Joint and muscle inflammation, especially the supraspinatus, and a fixation of the glenohumeral joint.

Treatment: My first treatment goal was to reduce the pain and swelling. I had the patient lie on his back, and I performed METs #6, #8, and #9 for the pectoralis minor and major and gentle CR MET for the supraspinatus. After the series of METs, I passively oscillated the arm in very small arcs of internal-external rotation to induce relaxation and disperse the fluids in the joint. I next performed MET #3 to reduce the hypertonicity of the internal rotators. The muscles of the anterior chest began to relax and allow greater motion in the arm. I performed the first three series of Level I strokes to unwind the soft tissue of the anterior shoulder, concentrating on both the pectoralis minor and the supraspinatus. Because he had such limited motion, the circumduction mobilization of the glenohumeral joint (MET #2 of the third series of strokes) was performed very slowly and in very small arcs in the beginning. As he became comfortable with the movement and his muscles began to relax, I pressed the head of the humerus more firmly into the joint and performed larger arcs of motion. I ended the session with an A–P mobilization at the head of the humerus. I had him test the ROM at the end of the session, and he was able to elevate the arm to 120° without pain. I showed him simple stretching exercises and one strengthening exercise for the external rotators.

Plan: I recommended a series of weekly visits for one month. I repeated the same basic treatment described above on the second visit. His pain level was reduced so significantly that I was able to begin to stretch the soft tissue of the anterior chest and shoulder and instruct him in exercises to strengthen the external rotators. On the third visit, I began the treatment with him sitting and performed PIR METs to lengthen the supraspinatus and increase internal rotation (METs #10, and #11). Then I had him lie supine and used METs to release and lengthen the pectoralis minor and major (METs #6, #7, and #8), and to increase elevation (MET #14). Because the tissue was much less tender to the touch, I penetrated deeper into the tissue with the STM. I used shorter, more brisk transverse friction strokes on the supraspinatus and anterior joint capsule (Level I STM, fourth series, and Level II, second series). At the fourth visit, he reported that he was completely pain-free, that he was sleeping well, and that his ROM was dramatically better. On examination, his elevation was 160° without pain, and internal rotation was to the T10 vertebrae. I recommended four additional treatments. We performed the same basic protocol described above. At the time of his last visit, he had only slight limitation in his ROM compared with the other side, and isometric testing was strong and pain free. He continued with his strengthening and stretching exercises.

<table>
<tr><td>

Table 6-4 — **Essentials of Treatment**

- Rock the client's body while performing the strokes.
- Shift your weight while performing the strokes.
- Perform the strokes rhythmically.
- Perform the strokes about 50 to 70 cycles per minute.
- Keep your hands and whole body relaxed.

</td></tr>
</table>

Table 6-4 lists some essentials of treatment.

LEVEL I: SHOULDER

1. Release of Serratus Anterior and Subscapularis

- **Anatomy:** Subscapularis (Fig. 6-34), serratus anterior, long thoracic nerve, and median and ulnar nerves (see Fig. 6-7).

- **Dysfunction:** The typical position of dysfunction of the shoulder is a forward and internally rotated position. The subscapularis is typically short and tight. It holds the humerus in an adducted, internally rotated position. The serratus is typically weak in a head-forward, kyphotic posture. The long thoracic nerve lies over the serratus anterior, and the subscapular nerve lies over the subscapularis. These nerves may be entrapped in the overlying fascia.

Position

- **Therapist position (TP):** Standing, facing 45° headward or facing the table.

- **Client position (CP):** Supine, with arm abducted and externally rotated to its comfortable limit. If this position is difficult or painful, keep the arm in the scapular plane without external rotation. As you work toward more external rotation, place a supporting pillow under the client's arm.

Strokes

1. If the shoulder cannot reach 90° of external rotation, perform PIR MET to increase external rotation (see "Muscle Energy Technique" above).

2. With the client's arm abducted and externally rotated, use your fingertips to perform a series of short, scooping strokes on the lateral rib cage to release the serratus anterior and long thoracic nerve (Fig. 6-35). Perform the strokes both posteriorly and toward the axilla. Cover the entire lateral rib cage. The supporting hand rests on the lower rib cage, gently compresses the rib cage, and moves slightly in the same direction with each stroke.

3. Using your superior hand to hold the client's distal forearm, place the fingertips of your inferior hand on the anterior scapula, and perform short, scooping strokes in a headward direction on the subscapularis as you rock the client's arm in a back-stroke-type motion (Fig. 6-36).

4. With the client's arm in the abducted and externally rotated position, place the thumb of your superior hand on the anterior surface of the scapula, and perform short, scooping, headward strokes to release the subscapularis (Fig. 6-37). Grasp the

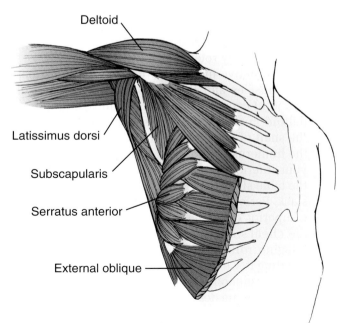

Figure 6-34. Serratus anterior and subscapularis.

Deltoid

Latissimus dorsi

Subscapularis

Serratus anterior

External oblique

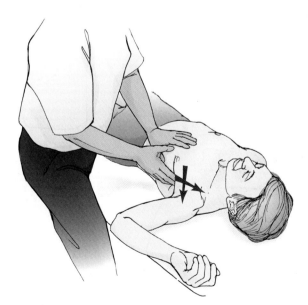

Figure 6-35. Fingertip release of the serratus anterior.

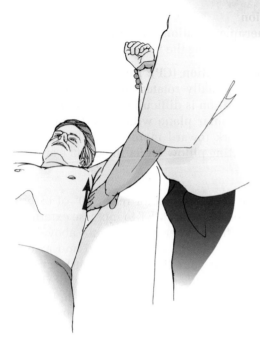

Figure 6-36. Fingertip release of the subscapularis. The fingertips scoop headward as the arm is rocked into a backstroke motion.

entire scapula with your hand. Your fingertips are underneath, and your thumb is on the anterior surface. Gently squeeze with your hand as your thumb performs the stroke.

2. Rolling Soft Tissue of Anterior Shoulder Superiorly

■ **Anatomy:** Pectoralis major and minor, rotator cuff muscles, joint capsule, anterior and middle deltoid, coracobrachialis, and biceps (long and short head) (Fig. 6-38).

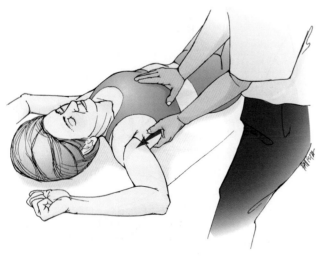

Figure 6-37. Thumb release of the subscapularis.

■ **Dysfunction:** With most dysfunctions, the pectoralis major and minor and the anterior deltoid tend to roll into an anterior, inferior, medial torsion as the humerus is held in an adducted and internally rotated position. This pattern is present with rounded-shoulder FHP; kyphotic thoracic spine; and anterior subluxations of the head of the humerus. The pectoralis minor is typically tight and can entrap the neurovascular bundle that travels under it. The long head of the biceps may become misaligned and rest against the medial rim of the bicipital groove, which can lead to bicipital tendinitis.

Position
■ **TP:** Standing

■ **CP:** Supine

Strokes
1. Hold the client's distal forearm with your superior hand, and move his or her arm into small arcs of external rotation as you perform 1-inch, scooping strokes with the fingertips of your other hand on the upper part of the pectoralis major and minor and the anterior deltoid (Fig. 6-39). Sink into the tissue until you take it into tension, and then scoop the fibers headward in a rhythmic, oscillating fashion, coordinated with the movement of the arm. Change the angle of your strokes so that you are working perpendicular to the line of the fiber.

2. To reset the entire segment into an externally rotated position from the dysfunctional internally rotated position, perform a backstroke-type circular motion with the arm as you perform several additional strokes in this area. The arm is adducted slightly as the backstroke begins and is abducted and externally rotated as it finishes.

3. An alternative method to release both the superficial muscles and the deeper rotator cuff muscles and joint capsule, is to switch hands, and hold the deltoid muscle with your superior hand such that the shaft of your thumb is in line with the shaft of the humerus (Fig. 6-40). Hold the client's arm with your inferior hand at 90° abduction, then lift it off the table slightly to bring the superficial tissue into slack. Perform a series of short, scooping strokes in a superior direction with your thumb as you rock the client's arm in small arcs of external rotation. Imagine rolling the tissue around the bone, unwinding it. Cover the entire area of the anterior and superior glenohumeral joint.

4. The technique described above may also be used to mobilize the long head of the biceps in the bicipital groove. Place your thumb on the medial side of the bicipital tendon, and mobilize the tendon medially

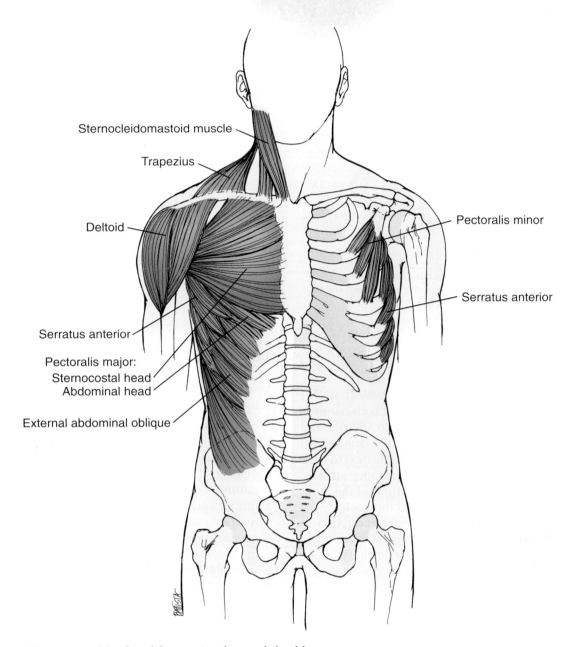

Figure 6-38. Muscles of the anterior chest and shoulder.

to laterally as you rock the client's arm into external rotation. You might need to repeat this many times.

3. *Unwinding the Soft Tissue and Mobilization of the Glenohumeral Joint*

■ **Anatomy:** Superficially—the pectoralis major, anterior and middle deltoid, coracobrachialis, and biceps brachii (Fig. 6-41); deeply—the joint capsule (see Fig. 6-4).

■ **Dysfunction:** The position of dysfunction is for the humerus to sustain an internally rotated position.

The soft tissue winds into an abnormal internal torsion, decreasing the normal lubricant between the fascicles. Eventually, the glenohumeral joint may develop adhesions and begin to dry out, losing full ROM, which leads to calcific deposits.

Position

■ **TP:** Standing. Place the client's arm under your axilla. If the client's shoulder is stiff, it may be more comfortable in your inferior axilla. Otherwise, the arm is better placed on your superior side. If the arm is too heavy, place a pillow under the elbow.

■ **CP:** Supine

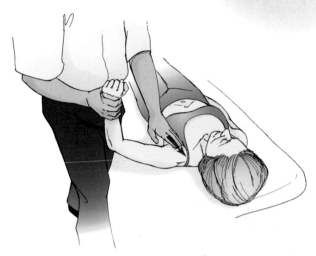

Figure 6-39. Fingertip release of the anterior shoulder muscles. This stroke releases the torsion and unwinds the tissue in a superior and posterior direction.

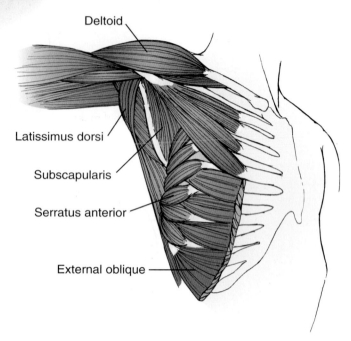

Figure 6-41. Anterior shoulder muscles.

Strokes

1. Hold the proximal humerus with both hands, and compress it slightly into the glenoid cavity to bring the superficial tissues into slack (Fig. 6-42). In this series of strokes, the entire surface of both hands is used to unwind the soft tissue of the anterior and middle humerus. Externally rotate the tissue around the bone. The thumbs of both hands lie next to each other and also perform short, scooping strokes. Cover the anterior and middle portions of the proximal humerus down to the deltoid tuberosity.

2. Mobilize the shoulder. Perform circumduction to help normalize the movement characteristics of the glenohumeral joint and to rehydrate the joint by stimulating the synovial microvilli. Hold the arm as described in the first stroke. Move the entire humerus in a superior direction and then posteriorly, inferiorly, anteriorly, and superiorly again. Repeat this motion either in slow, gentle, small-amplitude circles for acute conditions or in more vigorous, brisk, larger-amplitude circles for chronic conditions. If there is a loss of normal external rotation, you may externally rotate the humerus as you move it superiorly. This stroke is an assessment and a treatment. Perform this movement gently and in small circles if the client is hypermobile or unstable.

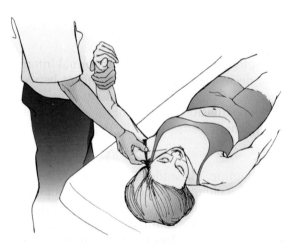

Figure 6-40. Scooping strokes with the thumb for the anterior shoulder muscles.

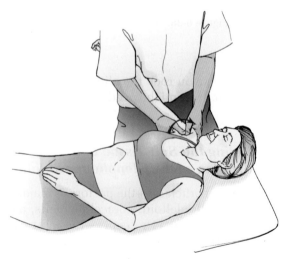

Figure 6-42. Hands used to unwind the torsion that develops in the soft tissue of the glenohumeral joint.

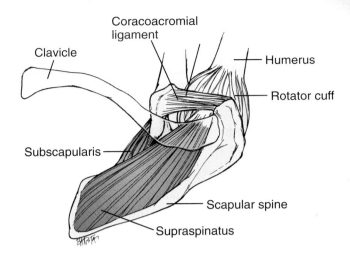

Figure 6-43. Superior view of the supraspinatus and the coracoacromial ligament.

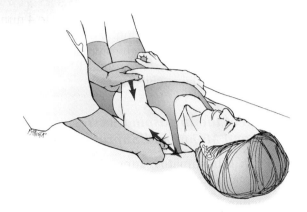

Figure 6-44. Thumb release of the belly and myotendinous junction of the supraspinatus muscle.

4. *Release of the Supraspinatus*

▦ **Anatomy:** Supraspinatus and coracoacromial ligament (Fig. 6-43).

▦ **Dysfunction:** The supraspinatus is the only muscle of the rotator cuff that travels through a tunnel and is therefore susceptible to loss of oxygen when inflamed; the swelling compresses the tissue and can leave a scar on the tendon. The tendon can impinge under the acromion when the arm is abducted or during flexion, especially when combined with internal rotation. The coracohumeral ligament blends with the superior joint capsule and the supraspinatus tendon.

Position
▦ **TP:** Standing

▦ **CP:** Supine

Strokes
1. Release the supraspinatus muscle belly and myotendinous junction using single-thumb or fingertips technique. Place the client's flexed elbow on his or her chest so that the arm rests across the chest. With your inferior hand, grasp just above the client's elbow, and gently impulse the arm headward and posteriorly in the scapular plane. At the same time, the thumb or fingertips of your superior hand perform 1-inch, scooping strokes in the A–P direction in the supraspinous fossa (Fig. 6-44). Reposition the thumb slightly, draw the arm back, and repeat a series of strokes covering the entire supraspinous fossa. If you find thick, fibrotic tissue, stroke back and forth in the A–P direction.

2. To locate the supraspinatus attachment on the greater tuberosity, first have your client rest the hand on the ASIS to internally rotate the humerus. The tendon is located just under the anterolateral aspect of the acromion on the anterior-superior portion of the greater tuberosity.

3. Using the thumb or fingertips of your superior hand, perform TFM strokes on the tenoperiosteal junction of the supraspinatus tendon (Fig. 6-45). The pressure of a TFM stroke is applied in both directions, transverse to the line of the fiber. Hold the client's distal forearm, and rock the arm with each stroke. As the fingertips move forward, the arm moves forward; as the fingertips move back, the arm moves back. This may also be performed as a shearing stroke, with the fingers and arm moving in opposite directions. Palpate for a thickened feel to the tendon, as these strokes are used only as needed. The tendon is usually tender. Perform approximately six to ten strokes on the same spot,

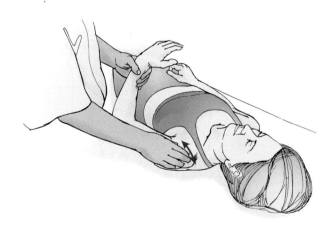

Figure 6-45. Fingertips perform TFM at the tenoperiosteal junction of the supraspinatus. Oscillate the arm with each stroke, which makes the treatment much more comfortable.

and then move to another spot. Work for 3 to 4 minutes per session on the tendon. It often takes six to eight sessions to dissolve the fibrosis. To expose more of the tendon, horizontally adducted the humerus across the client's chest.

5. *Release of the Infraspinatus, Teres Minor and Major, and Supraspinatus*

▨ **Anatomy:** Infraspinatus, supraspinatus, teres minor and major, and suprascapular nerve (Fig. 6-46).

▨ **Dysfunction:** These muscles tend to roll into an inferior torsion as the humeral head migrates superiorly in dysfunction. The external rotators are usually weak, losing their normal function, which is to depress the humerus during arm elevation. This inferior torsion is also created with slumping posture, kyphosis, and weak scapular stabilizers. The suprascapular nerve travels under the infraspinatus on top of the scapula. A site of potential injury to this nerve is under the lateral aspect of the spine of the scapula.

Position

▨ **TP:** Standing

▨ **CP:** Side-lying, with elbows flexed, arms and hands resting on each other. Place a pillow between the client's arms to help support and stabilize the arms.

Strokes

There are three lines of strokes: on the superior aspect of the scapula inferior to the spine of the scapula, in the middle of the scapula, and on the inferior aspect of the scapula. These strokes should be across the bone, not into the bone.

1. To release the hypertonicity or to recruit an inhibited muscle on the posterior scapula, perform CR and RI MET with the client in the side-lying position (see Fig. 6-25, p. 270).
2. Using a double-thumb technique, begin at the superior portion of the scapula inferior to the spine of the scapula, and perform 1-inch, scooping strokes in a superior direction (Fig. 6-47). Begin the series of strokes at the vertebral border, and continue to the posterior humerus.

Note: The suprascapular nerve travels under the infraspinatus and lies on top of the scapula. It is most exposed inferior to the most lateral aspect of the spine of the scapula. A sharp radiating pain is elicited if the nerve is compressed. It can be released with gentle scooping strokes.

3. Begin a second and third line of strokes on the middle and inferior aspects of the scapula, continuing to the posterior humerus.

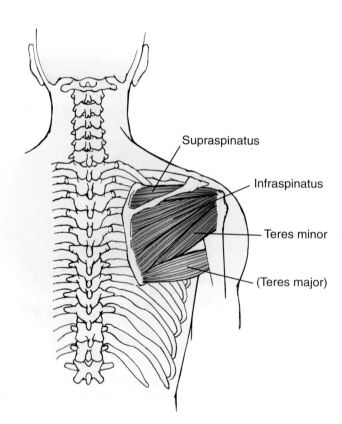

Figure 6-46. Teres minor, infraspinatus, and supraspinatus.

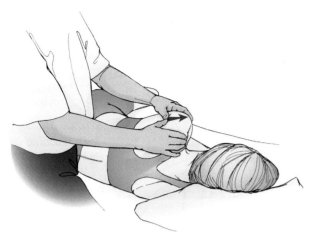

Figure 6-47. Double-thumb technique to release the infraspinatus and the teres minor.

4. As an alternative method to release the supraspinatus, face 45° headward. Tuck your arm under the client's arm, and place both hands on the supraspinous fossa of the scapula (Fig. 6-48). Using your fingertips, perform back and forth strokes in an A–P direction on the supraspinatus muscle. Move your arms and the client's arm with each stroke. Cover the entire area of the supraspinous fossa.

6. *Prone Release of the Posterior Rotator Cuff and Posterior Deltoid*

▨ **Anatomy:** Supraspinatus, infraspinatus, teres minor, and posterior deltoid (Fig. 6-49).

▨ **Dysfunction:** As has been mentioned, the muscles of the posterior shoulder tend to roll into an inferior torsion and need to be moved superiorly.

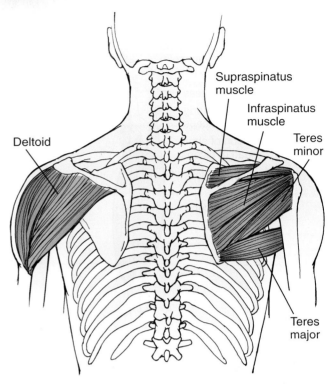

Figure 6-49. Posterior rotator cuff muscles, the posterior deltoid, and teres major.

With a loss of the normal thoracic curve and a retracted scapula, the posterior cuff muscles shorten.

Position
▨ **TP:** Standing
▨ **CP:** Prone

Strokes
1. Place both thumbs on the posterior aspect of the proximal humerus, and perform a series of gentle, scooping strokes, rolling the soft tissue fibers superiorly (Fig. 6-50). The intention is to unwind the

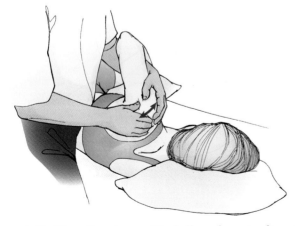

Figure 6-48. Fingertip release of the belly and myotendinous junction of the supraspinatus.

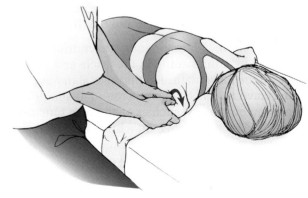

Figure 6-50. Release of the posterior shoulder muscles. Both hands wrap around the soft tissue of the posterior shoulder and roll the tissue in a headward direction.

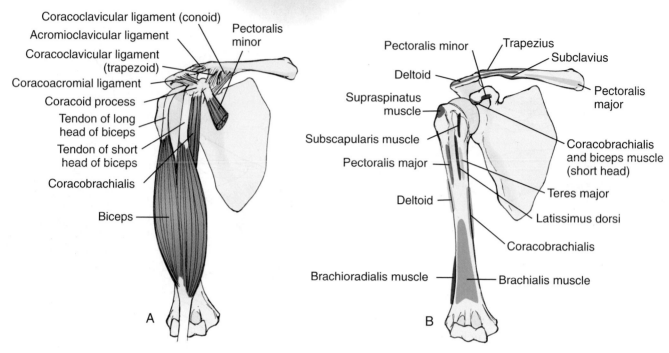

Figure 6-51. **A.** Attachments to the coracoid process. **B.** Attachments to the anterior shoulder complex.

tissue around the bone. This releases the adhesions that develop from sustained contraction and inferior torsion. Grasp the entire arm with your hands, and move all the soft tissue that wraps around the humerus with each stroke. Release the pressure at the end of each stroke, place your hands in a slightly new location, and perform another stroke. Cover the entire posterior humerus.

LEVEL II: SHOULDER

1. Release of the Clavicle and the Coracoid Process Attachments

▨ **Anatomy:** Pectoralis major and minor, anterior deltoid, subclavius, and coracobrachialis; and coracoacromial, coracohumeral, coracoclavicular, and AC ligaments (Figs. 6-51**A** and 6-51**B**).

▨ **Dysfunction:** Thoracic outlet syndrome can be caused by a thickening in the fascia and a shortening of the musculature in the areas above and below the clavicle. Causes include rounded-shoulder FHP or previous injury, such as a fall on an outstretched hand. The ligaments attaching to the coracoid process are often fibrotic because of FHP, rounded shoulders, or impingement syndrome.

Position

▨ **TP:** Standing, facing the direction of your stroke

▨ **CP:** Supine

Strokes

1. Press the base of your superior hand under the clavicle as you wrap your fingertips over the sternum or clavicle (Fig. 6-52). Perform a series of short, back-and-forth strokes in the medial to lateral plane. Rock your body with your strokes. This technique cleans the superior and posterior portions of the medial clavicle and sternum for the sternocleidomastoid and superficial and deep cervical and pectoral fascia. Place your other hand on the lower rib cage. Press posteriorly and superiorly on the lower rib cage with your strokes to give some slack to the area being worked. Alternatively,

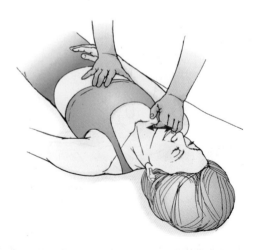

Figure 6-52. Fingertip release of the clavicle attachments.

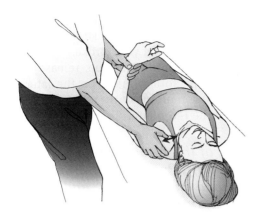

Figure 6-53. Thumb release of the inferior border of the coracoid process.

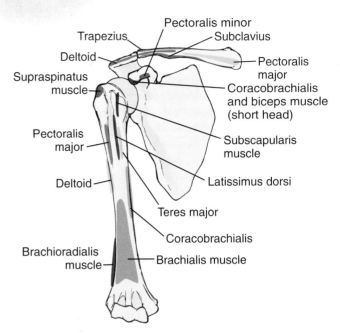

Figure 6-54. Attachments to the anterior shoulder complex.

you can hold the client's distal forearm and move the arm into small arcs of abduction and adduction with your strokes to help mobilize the clavicle.

2. Perform short, back-and-forth strokes in the medial-to-lateral plane with your thumb on the anterior and inferior clavicle. This technique releases the clavicular portion of the pectoralis major, the anterior deltoid, and the subclavius on the inferior portion of the clavicle.

3. Using the thumb of your superior hand, perform back-and-forth strokes on the inferior border of the coracoid process to release the pectoralis minor, coracobrachialis, and short head of the biceps (Fig. 6-53). Hold the client's distal forearm to abduct the arm, and elevate it slightly to bring the tissue into slack.

4. Holding the client's arm as in the previous stroke, perform transverse strokes with the thumb or fingertips beginning on the superior portion of the coracoid process for the coracoclavicular and coracoacromial ligaments and continuing your strokes to the clavicle and acromion. Move your fingertips to the AC joint and perform back-and-forth strokes in the A–P plane for the AC ligament. Rock the client's arm in the direction of your stroke, and coordinate the movement of the arm with the stroke.

2. *Release of the Joint Capsule and Muscle Attachments on the Anterior Humerus*

▓ **Anatomy:** Subscapularis, long head of the biceps in the bicipital groove, pectoralis major, teres major, latissimus dorsi, transverse humeral ligament, coracohumeral ligament, and joint capsule (Fig. 6-54).

▓ **Dysfunction:** The muscles attaching to the anterior humerus are usually short and tight, pulling

the arm into an adducted and internally rotated position. The tenoperiosteal and myotendinous junctions become fibrotic from the cumulative stress of poor posture, previous inflammation caused by overuse, or injury. The long head of the biceps is irritated with an internally rotated humerus because it forces the tendon to rub against the medial aspect of the groove. The anterior joint capsule is often thick and fibrotic after injury or cumulative stress and may develop adhesive capsulitis.

Position

▓ **TP:** Standing

▓ **CP:** Supine

Strokes

1. Facing 45° headward, use a single-thumb technique to release the transverse humeral ligament by moving in the inferior-to-superior (I–S) plane on both sides of the bicipital groove (Fig. 6-55). Rock the client's arm as you rock your entire body with each stroke. Let your hand and thumb stay relaxed, and let the thumb move with the arm motion. Next, release any adhesions to the bicipital tendon by keeping your thumb on the bicipital tendon and moving the client's arm into small arcs of medial and lateral rotation, letting the tendon roll under your thumb.

2. With the client's arm at his or her side and the elbow flexed to 90°, place your thumb or fingertips to the most medial part of the lesser tuberosity. You can palpate the subscapularis by having your client

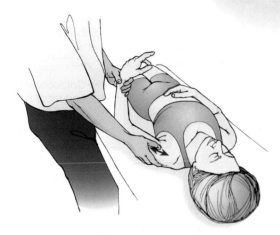

Figure 6-55. Release of the muscle attachments to the anterior humerus.

resist as you attempt to pull laterally on the distal forearm. Perform a series of back-and-forth strokes approximately 30° headward on the broad, tendinous attachment of the subscapularis. To expose the tendon more fully, move the arm into more external rotation.

3. From the lesser tuberosity, slide your thumb distally along the humerus to find the attachments of the teres major, latissimus, and coracobrachialis. Lift the arm off the table slightly to bring the tissue into slack. Perform back-and-forth strokes in the I–S plane on the medial side of the humerus to release these muscles.

In this technique, the strokes are along the bone and not into the bone. With each stroke, rock the entire arm in the direction of your stroke.

4. Using single-thumb technique, release the attachment of the pectoralis major on the lateral side of the bicipital tendon with short back-and-forth strokes in the I–S plane.

3. *Release of the Attachments of the Rotator Cuff, Posterior Joint Capsule, Long Head of the Triceps, and the Radial Nerve*

▨ **Anatomy:** Attachments of the posterior rotator cuff, posterior joint capsule, triceps, and radial nerve (Figs. 6-56A and 6-56B).

▨ **Dysfunction:** With an irritation or inflammation of the infraspinatus or teres minor, the tenoperiosteal attachment points thicken and become fibrotic. As these muscles interweave with the posterior joint capsule, the capsule also thickens. Thickening of the posterior joint capsule draws the head of the humerus anteriorly and superiorly, contributing to impingement syndrome and limiting medial rotation.

Position

▨ **TP:** Standing

▨ **CP:** Prone, with forearm over edge of table, in 90° of abduction

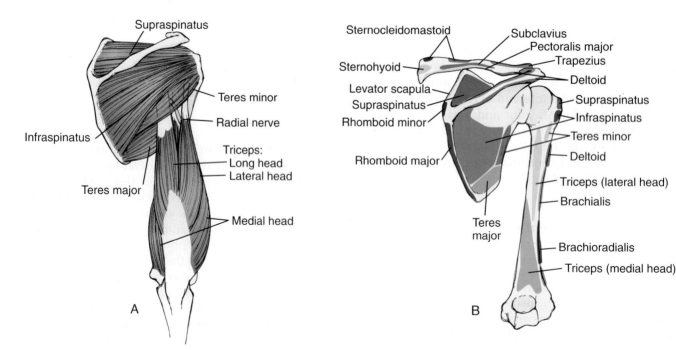

Figure 6-56. A. Posterior rotator cuff muscles, the triceps, and radial nerve. **B.** Muscle attachments to the posterior shoulder complex.

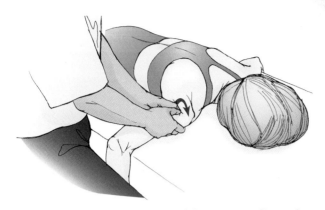

Figure 6-57. Double-thumb release of the rotator cuff muscles, posterior joint capsule, the triceps, and the radial nerve.

Strokes

1. Place both thumbs next to each other, and wrap your hands around the proximal portion of the humerus (Fig. 6-57). Use the thumbs to penetrate through the muscle to perform short, back-and-forth strokes transverse to the shaft of the humerus to release the attachments of the infraspinatus, teres minor, and joint capsule on the posterior glenoid fossa and proximal humerus. For a hypermobile shoulder, it is important to stabilize the anterior humerus with your fingertips and not allow excessive forward translation of the head of the humerus.

2. To palpate the attachment of the long head of the triceps at the infraglenoid tubercle of the scapula, place the fingertips of one hand on the inferior aspect of the glenoid fossa, and have the client resist as you attempt to press his or her elbow into flexion. Using a double-thumb technique, perform a series of back-and-forth, transverse strokes on the attachment site.

3. Release the radial nerve, triceps, posterior deltoid, and the posterior brachialis attachments on the posterior humerus. Use the same double-thumb technique described in the first stroke (see Fig. 6-56). Beginning at the proximal humerus, perform a series of short, scooping strokes transverse to the shaft of the humerus. To release the posterior deltoid with CR MET, have your client lift his or her arm slightly off the table and resist as you press the arm lightly toward the table.

4. *Repositioning of the Rotator Cuff Muscles and Deltoid in the Seated Position*

- **Anatomy:** Deltoid, supraspinatus, infraspinatus, teres minor, and subscapularis (Figs. 6-58**A** and 6-58**B**).

- **Dysfunction:** The most common dysfunction of the glenohumeral joint is for the humeral head to sit high in the glenoid fossa. The rotator cuff muscles tend to part at the top of the joint and roll inferiorly as the humeral head is held in this sustained superior position. The technique is performed in the sitting position with the arm at 90° abduction, as this is a position of function for eating, reaching, and so on.

Position

- **TP:** Standing, facing the table at 45° angle. For treatment, place your front foot on the table. If you have a tall client, have the client sit in a chair.

- **CP:** Sitting on the table or a chair, a few inches from the edge

Strokes

These strokes often follow the passive circumduction assessment (p. 264). Your assessment findings help you to determine which of the following strokes to use.

1. Place your foot on the edge of the table or chair, and rest the client's forearm on your thigh, with the humerus in the scapular plane. To help reestablish normal function and position, perform CR MET with special attention to areas of restriction.
   a. Abduction—Lift the client's arm off your thigh, and have the client resist as you press down on the elbow.
   b. Adduction—Tuck your fingers under the client's elbow, and have the client resist as you attempt to lift the arm off your leg.
   c. Internal rotation—Tuck your hand under the client's distal forearm. Have the client resist as you attempt to lift the arm.
   d. External rotation—First, lift the wrist a few inches off your leg. Have the client resist as you attempt to press down on the distal forearm (Fig. 6-59).
   e. Horizontal flexion or extension—Have the client resist as you pull the humerus posteriorly or press anteriorly into the client's elbow.

2. After each MET is performed, use either your fingertips on the anterior muscles or your thumbs on the posterior muscles to scoop the soft tissue superiorly and toward the midline of the superior glenohumeral joint (see Fig. 6-59B). The intention is to lift the soft tissue toward the highest point of the shoulder. You may perform more brisk, back-and-forth strokes if you find areas of fibrosis.

3. Stand next to your client, and perform passive circumduction again. The movement should be smooth and pain free. If not, perform this series of METs and STMs again.

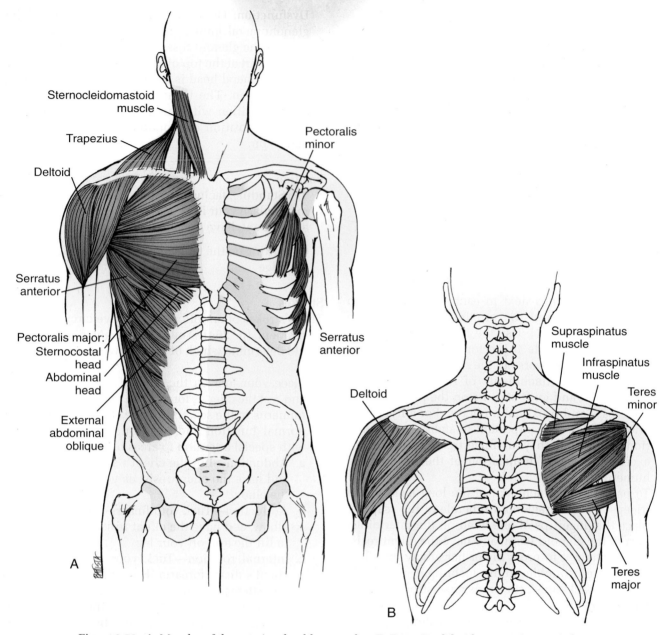

Figure 6-58. A. Muscles of the anterior shoulder complex. **B.** Posterior deltoid, supraspinatus, infraspinatus, and teres minor, and teres major.

5. *Treatment of the Subdeltoid Bursa*

▨ **Anatomy:** The subdeltoid bursa is located deep under the deltoid and inferior to the acromial arch. It acts as a lubricant during shoulder motion, particularly abduction, and secretes synovium into the joint space (Fig. 6-60).

▨ **Dysfunction:** Bursae swell when they are inflamed, whether as a result of acute trauma or of cumulative stress, such as repetitive overhead activities. With an acute bursitis, the client experiences severe pain in the shoulder region and loses all ability to elevate the arm. Chronic shoulder dysfunction may

lead to a drying out of the bursa, eventually leading to adhesions, and an inferior migration of the bursa.

Position
▨ **TP:** Standing

▨ **CP:** Sitting

Strokes
Apply some oil or lotion to the client's upper arm so that you can easily slide on the skin. Hold the client's distal forearm with one hand, and pull the arm into a gentle traction (Fig. 6-61). Place the shaft of your thumb a few inches distal to the acromion on the

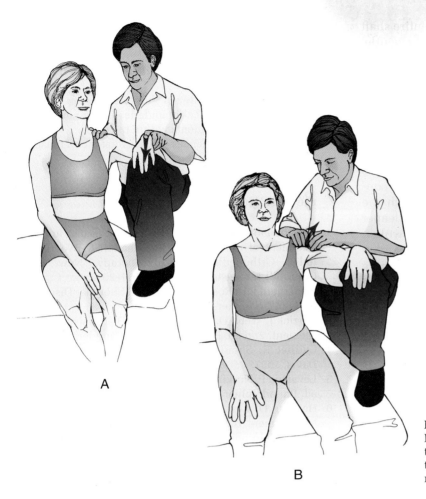

A

B

Figure 6-59. A. Sitting MET and OM. Perform METs to release hypertonicity in the muscles of the glenohumeral joint. **B.** Next, use fingertips or thumbs to reposition the soft tissue toward the most superior part of the joint.

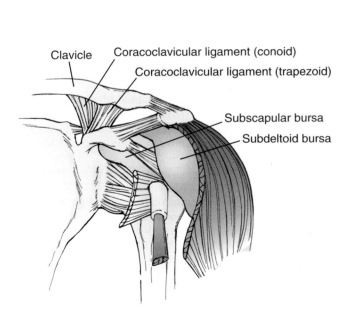

Clavicle
Coracoclavicular ligament (conoid)
Coracoclavicular ligament (trapezoid)
Subscapular bursa
Subdeltoid bursa

Figure 6-60. Subdeltoid (subacromial) bursa.

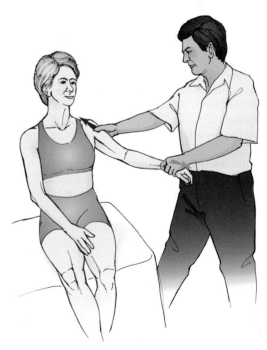

Figure 6-61. Using the web space of the hand, perform slow, gentle strokes on the subdeltoid bursa.

lateral arm. Using the fleshy portion of the entire shaft of your thumb and webspace, perform a slow, gentle, continuous stroke toward the acromion. When you reach the acromion, traction the arm and lift it slightly into abduction as you use your thumb to gently press into the arm. Coordinate the movements of the arm and the stroke so that the arm is lifting as the thumb is pumping the excess fluid from the bursa under the acromion. Repeat this pumping a few times. Then begin the stroke again, placing your hand a few inches below the acromion, and perform another long, continuous stroke. In chronic conditions in which the area has a dry and gristly feel, you may use deeper pressure to rehydrate the bursa. For an acute, swollen bursa, begin your stroke close to the acromion, moving superficially. Your next stroke begins a little more distally, milking the excess fluid headward a little bit at a time. Repeat the stroke about ten times.

 CAUTION: *In acute bursitis, use gentle pressure, and do not repeat this stroke more than ten times.*

■ *Study Guide*

Level I

1. List the four muscles of the rotator cuff. Describe their origins, insertions, and actions.
2. List which muscles are tight and which are weak in the shoulder.
3. Describe the MET for the pectoralis minor and the supraspinatus.
4. Describe the common positional dysfunction of the anterior deltoid. Describe the direction of the massage strokes to correct it.
5. Describe the signs and symptoms of a supraspinatus, infraspinatus, and subscapularis tendinitis.
6. Describe the stroke direction for the teres minor and infraspinatus.
7. Describe the MET for the internal and the external rotators.
8. List the scapular stabilizing muscles.
9. List some common causes of thoracic outlet syndrome.
10. When treating tightness or weakness imbalances, which muscles must be treated first?

Level II

1. Describe how to differentiate rotator cuff symptoms from a nerve root irritation in the neck.
2. Describe the signs and symptoms of bicipital tendinitis, subacromial bursitis, impingement syndrome, and adhesive capsulitis.
3. Describe the empty-can test and Speed's test, and describe the significance of a positive test.
4. List the muscles and ligaments that attach to the coracoid process.

5. Describe the scapular stabilization test.
6. List the muscle attachments to the anterior humerus and their relation to the bicipital groove.
7. Describe what is indicated when the shoulder hikes upward in active abduction.
8. Describe the MET for frozen shoulder.
9. Describe the anatomical boundaries of the coracoacromial arch and the contents within the arch.
10. Describe the consequences of weak rotator cuff muscles.

■ *References*

1. Boissonnault W, Janos S. Dysfunction, evaluation, and treatment of the shoulder. In Donatelli R, Wooden M (eds): Orthopedic Physical Therapy. New York: Churchill Livingstone, 1994, pp 169–201.
2. Porterfield J, DeRosa C. Mechanical Shoulder Disorders. St. Louis: Saunders, 2004.
3. Garrick J, Webb D. Sports Injuries: Diagnosis and Management, 2nd ed. Philadelphia: WB Saunders, 1999.
4. Cailliet R. Shoulder Pain, 3rd ed. Philadelphia: FA Davis, 1991.
5. Levangie P, Norkin C. Joint Structure and Function, 3rd ed. Philadelphia: FA Davis, 2001.
6. Hertling D, Kessler R. Shoulder and Shoulder Girdle. Management of Common Musculoskeletal Disorders, 4th ed. Baltimore: Lippincott Williams & Wilkins, 2006, pp 281–355.
7. Hammer W. The Shoulder. In Hammer W (ed): Functional Soft Tissue Examination and Treatment by Manual Methods. Gaithersburg, MD: Aspen, 1999, pp 36–135.
8. Corrigan B, Maitland GD. Practical Orthopaedic Medicine. London: Butterworths, 1983.
9. Kendall F, McCreary E, Provance P, Rodgers, M, Romani, W. Muscles: Testing and Function, 5th ed. Baltimore: Lippincott Williams & Wilkins, 2005.
10. Janda V. Evaluation of muscular imbalance. In Liebenson C. Rehabilitation of the Spine, 2nd ed. Baltimore: Lippincott Williams & Wilkins, 2007, pp 203–225.
11. Halbach J, Tank R. The shoulder. In Gould J (ed): Orthopedic and Sports Physical Therapy. St. Louis: CV Mosby, 1990, pp 483–521.
12. Greenman PE. Principles of Manual Medicine, 2nd ed. Baltimore: Williams & Wilkins, 1996.
13. Faber K, Singleton S, Hawkins R. Rotator cuff disease: Diagnosing a common cause of shoulder pain. J Musculoskeletal Med 1998;15:15–25.
14. Neer OS. Impingement lesions. Clin Orthop 1983;173:70–77.
15. Wilk K. The Shoulder. In Malone T, McPoil T, Nitz A (eds): Orthopedic and Sports Physical Therapy, 3rd ed. St. Louis: Mosby, 1997, pp 410–458.
16. Brukner P, Khan K, Kibler WB, Murrel G. Shoulder pain. Clinical Sports Medicine, 3rd ed. Sydney: McGraw-Hill, 2006, pp 243–288.
17. Oatis CA. Kinesiology: The Mechanics and Pathomechanics of Human Movement. Philadelphia: Lippincott Williams & Wilkins, 2004.

▌ *Suggested Readings*

Chaitow L. Muscle Energy Techniques, 3rd ed. New York: Churchill Livingstone, 2006.

Corrigan B, Maitland GD. Practical Orthopaedic Medicine. London: Butterworths, 1983.

Cyriax J, Cyriax P. Illustrated Manual of Orthopedic Medicine. London: Butterworths, 1983.

Garrick J, Webb D. Sports Injuries, 2nd ed. Philadelphia: WB Saunders, 1999.

Greenman PE. Principles of Manual Medicine, 2nd ed. Baltimore: Williams & Wilkins, 1996.

Hoppenfeld S. Physical Examination of the Spine and Extremities. New York: Appleton-Century-Crofts, 1976.

Kendall F, McCreary E, Provance P, M Rogers, W Romani. Muscles: Testing and Function, 5th ed. Baltimore: Williams & Wilkins, 2005.

Magee D. Orthopedic Physical Assessment, 3rd ed. Philadelphia: WB Saunders, 1997.

Levangie P, Norkin C. Joint Structure and Function, 3rd ed. Philadelphia: FA Davis, 2001.

Platzer W. Locomotor System, vol. 1, 5th ed. New York: Thieme Medical, 2004.

Reid DC. Sports Injury and Assessment. New York: Churchill Livingstone, 1992.

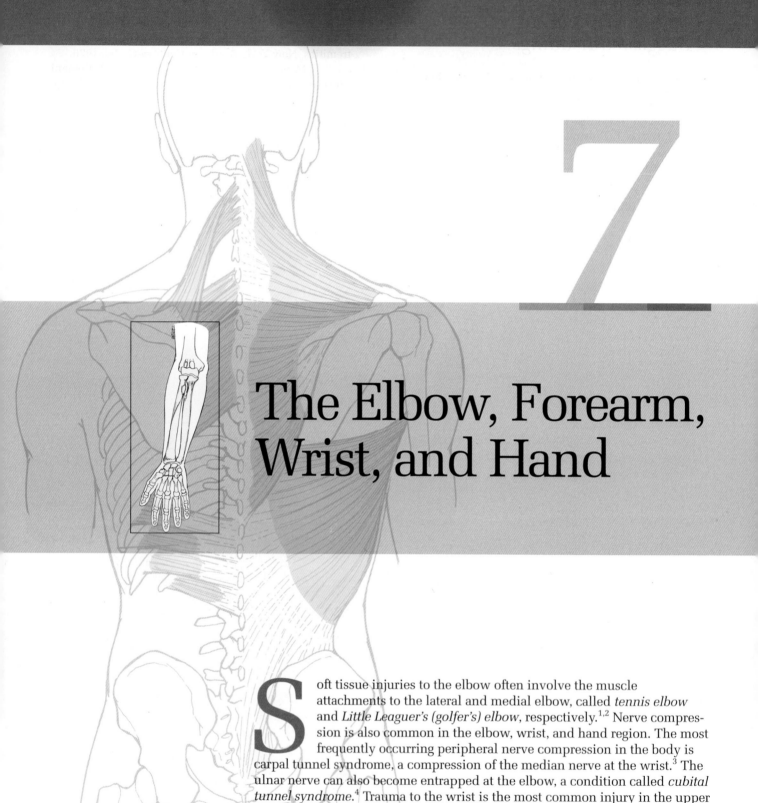

7

The Elbow, Forearm, Wrist, and Hand

Soft tissue injuries to the elbow often involve the muscle attachments to the lateral and medial elbow, called *tennis elbow* and *Little Leaguer's (golfer's) elbow*, respectively.[1,2] Nerve compression is also common in the elbow, wrist, and hand region. The most frequently occurring peripheral nerve compression in the body is carpal tunnel syndrome, a compression of the median nerve at the wrist.[3] The ulnar nerve can also become entrapped at the elbow, a condition called *cubital tunnel syndrome*.[4] Trauma to the wrist is the most common injury in the upper extremity, followed by injuries to the interphalangeal (IP) joints of the hand.[5] Fracture of the distal radius is the most common fracture in adults over age 50.

Anatomy, Function, and Dysfunction of the Elbow and Forearm

OVERVIEW OF THE ELBOW, FOREARM, WRIST, AND HAND

The bones of the upper limb are the **humerus** (the arm), the **radius** and **ulna** (the forearm), the **carpals** (the wrist), and the **metacarpals** and **phalanges** (the hand). The elbow is the articulation of the distal humerus with the proximal radius and ulna. Flexion and extension occur between the humerus and the ulna, and pronation and supination occur between the radius and the ulna. The wrist consists of 8 bones in two rows, and 15 muscles cross the wrist: 9 on the extensor surface (dorsum) and 6 on the anterior (palmar) surface. The hand consists of 19 bones and 19 joints.

BONES AND JOINTS OF THE ELBOW AND FOREARM

See Figure 7-1.

HUMERUS

■ **Structure:** The distal end of the humerus expands into the medial and lateral epicondyles. The trochlea and the capitulum of the humerus form condyles that articulate with the ulna and radius, respectively. On the posterior surface is a large indentation, the olecranon fossa, that accepts the olecranon process of the ulna during extension. On the medial side of the trochlea is a groove (sulcus) for the ulnar nerve. The radial nerve travels in a groove on the posterior surface of the humerus.

ULNA

■ **Structure:** The ulna has a large hook-shaped proximal end called the olecranon process, to which the triceps attaches. The anterior surface is the cartilage-lined trochlear notch, which articulates with the humerus to form the humeroulnar joint. The proximal portion of the ulna has a small curved surface, the radial notch, for articulation with the radius, forming the proximal radioulnar joint.

RADIUS

■ **Structure:** The proximal end of the radius is called the *head* and articulates with the capitulum of the humerus on its superior side and with the ulna on its medial side. The radius carries most of the load from the arm to the hand and therefore widens at its distal end and articulates with the first row of carpal bones. On the medial aspect of the proximal shaft is the radial tuberosity, which serves as the attachment site for the biceps brachii.

JOINTS OF THE ELBOW AND FOREARM

■ **Structure:** The three bones of the arm and forearm form three joints at the elbow and one joint at the

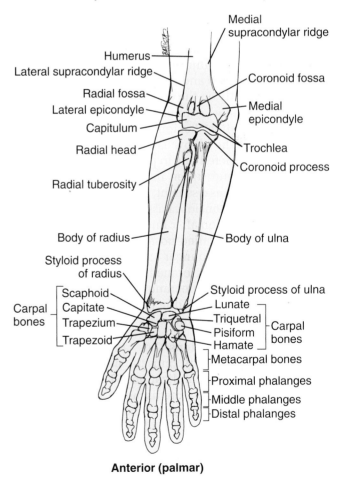

Anterior (palmar)

Figure 7-1. Bones of the elbow, forearm, wrist, and hand.

distal forearm. The three joints of the elbow are the humeroulnar, humeroradial, and proximal radioulnar joints. The joint of the distal forearm is the distal radioulnar joint, located proximal to the wrist.

- ☐ The **humeroulnar joint** is the articulation between the trochlea of the humerus and the trochlear notch of the ulna.
- ☐ The **humeroradial joint** is the articulation between the capitulum of the humerus and the head of the radius.
- ☐ The **proximal radioulnar joint** is the articulation between the head of the radius, the radial notch of the ulna, and the annular ligament.
- ☐ The **distal radioulnar joint** is the articulation between the head of the ulna and the ulnar notch of the radius.

- ▪ **Function:** Flexion and extension occur at the humeroulnar and humeroradial joints. Pronation and supination involves the rotation of the radius around the ulna. This motion occurs at the proximal and distal radioulnar joints. The resting, open position of the elbow joint is about 70° of flexion, and the closed position is extension.

- ▪ **Dysfunction and injury:** Dysfunctions and injuries of the bones of the elbow are not nearly as common as are soft tissue injuries. The elbow can develop traumatic arthritis and consequent degeneration after a fall directly on the elbow or on an outstretched hand. If the elbow is injured and swells, it assumes a position of slight flexion to accommodate the excess fluid. If the elbow is immobilized or if joint motion is restricted due to pain, it can develop capsular fibrosis and stiffen in this flexed position. In passive motion assessment, flexion will be more restricted than extension. Passive extension can have a painful limitation after injury or as a consequence of degeneration, called *posterior impingement syndrome*.[6] In the younger client, impingement is caused by the posterior medial corner of the olecranon abutting the olecranon fossa. In the older client, impingment is due to osteoarthritis (OA) at the radiocapitellar joint.

- ▪ **Treatment implications:** Loss of joint motion is treated initially with muscle energy technique (MET). Soft tissue mobilization (STM) is performed on the periarticular soft tissue to dissolve adhesions and to allow for greater extensibility. Postisometric relaxation (PIR) MET is performed on the short and tight muscles that could be inhibiting the joint's normal range of motion (ROM). Finally, joint mobilization is performed to stimulate nutritional exchange in the cartilage and to help dissolve calcium deposits on the articular surfaces.

SOFT TISSUE STRUCTURES OF THE ELBOW AND FOREARM

JOINT CAPSULE AND LIGAMENTS OF THE ELBOW AND FOREARM

- ▪ **Structure:** The joint capsule of the elbow is thin and lax. It encloses the three joints of the elbow, but it does not enclose the medial and lateral epicondyles. Strong **ulnar** and **radial collateral ligaments** blend with the capsule, reinforcing it.
  - ☐ The **ulnar (medial) collateral ligament** usually has two portions: the anterior portion, which travels from the medial epicondyle to the coronoid portion of the ulna, and the posterior portion, which travels from the medial epicondyle to the olecranon. The ulnar nerve travels under the fibers to the olecranon.
  - ☐ The **radial (lateral) collateral ligament** travels from the lateral epicondyle of the humerus to the annular ligament, which encloses the radial head. The radial collateral ligament is interwoven with the superficial extensor muscles.
  - ☐ The **annular ligament of the radius** attaches to the ulna and encircles the radial head. It is lined with cartilage on its inner surface to reduce friction as the head of the radius turns in pronation and supination.
  - ☐ As in the leg, an **interosseous membrane** connects the radius and ulna, strengthening the two bones.

- ▪ **Function:** As in the other joints of the body, the ligaments and joint capsule provide passive stability to the joints of the elbow. These structures also play a neurosensory role and have reflex connections with the surrounding muscles. The joint capsule interweaves with the fascia of the brachialis, triceps, and anconeus muscles.[7] To prevent pinching of the joint capsule between the articular surfaces during extension, these muscles contract and pull the capsule out of the joint space. The interosseous membrane provides a site for muscle attachments and helps to distribute the forces applied to the distal radius, as in a pressing action.

- ▪ **Dysfunction and injury:** A thickening of the ligaments of the elbow typically follows cumulative stress or an acute injury. Acute injury typically results in swelling and sustained flexion of the elbow (the open position) to mimimize tension on the capsule and allow more fluid, which reduces pain.[7] Passive supination is restricted with fibrosis of the annular ligament, and passive medial and lateral glide are reduced with fibrosis of the lateral and medial collateral ligaments. Weakness or sustained contraction of the triceps and brachialis potentially causes an impingement of the joint capsule. A loss of full passive extension can be due to adhesions in the anterior joint capsule, collateral ligaments, or tight and short flexors of the elbow.

■ **Treatment implications:** Acute injuries are first treated with MET in flexion and extension to pump out the excess fluid, reduce hypertonicity, and decrease pain. Passive movement of the elbow in flexion and extension also assists in reducing swelling and maintaining motion in the joint. In chronic conditions, the ligaments typically become fibrotic and thickened because of the deposit of excessive collagen after an injury or cumulative stress. Perform contract-relax (CR) MET to the muscles that attach to the capsule and ligaments, including the triceps, brachialis, and superficial extensors or the wrist and hand. Next, perform STM, including transverse friction massage, to the body (midportion) and attachment points of the ligaments. This process helps to dissolve the adhesions and restores normal extensibility to the soft tissue. If the ligaments have become too slack and the elbow is unstable, exercise rehabilitation is recommended to restore stability.

FASCIA

■ **Structure:** The fascia of the arm is called the *brachial fascia* and forms two compartments: the **anterior compartment,** which contains the flexors of the elbow, and the **posterior compartment,** which contains the extensors of the elbow.

The fascia of the forearm is called the antebrachial fascia and forms three compartments: the **anterior,** which contains the flexors; the **posterior,** which contains the extensors; and the **radial,** which contains a muscle of elbow flexion, the brachioradialis, and two extensors of the wrist, the extensor carpi radialis longus (ECRL) and the extensor carpi radialis brevis (ECRB).

NERVES

■ **Structure:** The nerves that exit from the neck and travel into the arm are called the **brachial plexus.** After they travel under the clavicle, they form seven long nerves into the arm, forearm, and hand. We consider the three main nerves—the **ulnar, median,** and **radial nerves**—because they are commonly involved clinically. The ulnar and median nerves travel along the medial side of the arm between the two heads of the biceps muscle in a groove called the *median bicipital sulcus.* The radial nerve travels on the posterior side of the humerus in the groove under the lateral head of the triceps. At the elbow, each of the nerves can become entrapped at the following sites:

☐ The **ulnar nerve** travels through a fibro-osseous tunnel behind the medial epicondyle called the **cubital tunnel.** The tunnel is formed by a fibrous arch called the *arcuate ligament,* which is a fascial expansion of the origins of the humeral and ulnar heads of the flexor carpi ulnaris. It then travels through the two heads of the flexor carpi ulnaris (Fig. 7-2).

☐ The **median nerve** travels through a fibro-osseous tunnel on the anterior-medial surface of the distal end of the humerus, beneath the edge of the aponeurosis of the biceps called the lacertus fibrosis, and then between the two heads of origin of the pronator teres (Fig. 7-3).

☐ The **radial nerve** travels from the extensor compartment to the flexor compartment between the brachialis and the brachioradialis. It passes under the fibrous origin of the ECRB and then enters the supinator canal between the two heads of the supinator muscle, which are connected by a fibrous arch called the *arcade of Frohse,* approximately 2 inches distal to the lateral epicondyle (Fig. 7-4).

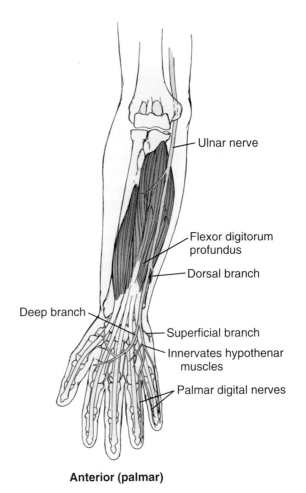

Anterior (palmar)

Figure 7-2. Course of the ulnar nerve through the elbow, forearm, wrist, and hand.

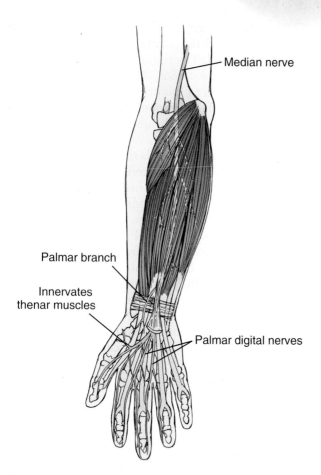

Figure 7-3. Course of the median nerve through the elbow, forearm, wrist, and hand.

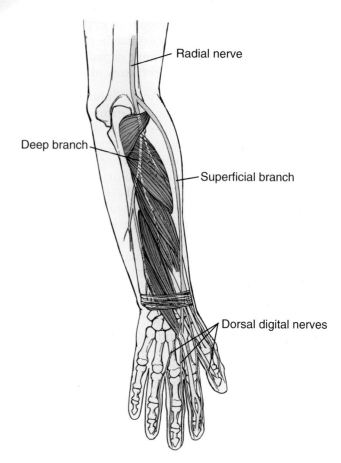

Figure 7-4. Course of the radial nerve through the elbow, forearm, wrist, and hand.

■ **Function:** The three main nerves—the ulnar, median, and radial nerves—function as follows:
- ☐ The **ulnar nerve** supplies the flexors in the forearm and hand and the skin on the ulnar side of the hand and fourth and fifth fingers.
- ☐ The **median nerve** innervates most of the flexors of the arm, forearm, and hand as well as the skin of the wrist, thenar eminence, palm, flexor side of the thumb, and index and middle fingers.
- ☐ The **radial nerve** innervates all the extensors of the arm and forearm and the skin on the extensor side of the arm and hand.

■ **Dysfunction and injury:** The nerves of the elbow can be injured as a result of any trauma to the elbow or cumulative stress. The **ulnar nerve** is often irritated with repetitive elbow flexion or from sustained elbow flexion, which commonly occurs with sleeping. This is called *cubital tunnel syndrome.* The fibrous arch (arcuate ligament) through which the ulnar nerve travels is slack in extension and becomes more taut in flexion, which narrows the cubital tunnel.[8] The **median nerve** is often irritated or entrapped as it travels underneath the edge of the lacertus fibrosis, the fascial expansion of the biceps, or as it passes between the two heads of the

pronator teres, due to repetitive pronation or pronation and flexion of the elbow.[4] This is called *pronator syndrome.* The **radial nerve** can be irritated by a repeated pronation, elbow extension, and wrist flexion (wringing motion) or by overuse of the extensor muscles. The nerves can also become entrapped in the sustained contraction of overused muscles, which creates a thickening in the fascia at its attachment sites, or in the fibro-osseous tunnel through which the nerve travels. This is called *radial tunnel syndrome.* The specific anatomy of the entrapment sites is described above in "Structure."

■ **Treatment implications:** The treatment protocol for nerve entrapment is for the therapist first to perform MET to the muscles that interweave with the particular tunnel to reduce the hypertonicity in the muscles and to increase the length and extensibility of the connective tissue that forms the tunnel. For example, to release the cubital tunnel, perform MET to the flexor carpi ulnaris, as its fascial expansion interweaves with the cubital tunnel. Next, perform manual release of the nerve by gentle, scooping strokes transverse to the line of the nerve. This dissolves the adhesions surrounding the nerve and releases the tension in the fascia suspending the nerve. Deep STM strokes, including transverse friction massage, are often needed to release the fibrosis in the fascia that forms the tunnels. The specific treatment protocol for the common entrapment sites is listed in the "Technique" section.

MUSCLES

▨ **Structure:** The muscles that move the elbow are three flexors and two extensors. The flexors are the brachialis, biceps brachii, and brachioradialis. The two extensors are the triceps and the anconeus.

The forearm has 19 muscles, 11 in the extensor and radial compartments and 8 in the flexor compartment. Of these 19, 6 forearm muscles move only the wrist, and 9 additional muscles move the thumb and fingers and act secondarily at the wrist.

☐ The **superficial anterior compartment** includes the pronator teres, flexor digitorum superficialis, flexor carpi radialis, flexor carpi ulnaris, and palmaris longus, which is frequently absent (Fig. 7-5**A**).

☐ The **deep anterior compartment** includes the pronator quadratus, flexor digitorum profundus, and flexor pollicis longus (Fig. 7-5**B**).

☐ The **radial compartment** includes the brachioradialis, ECRL, and ECRB (Fig. 7-6**A**).

☐ The **superficial posterior compartment** includes the extensor digitorum, extensor digiti minimi, and extensor carpi ulnaris (Fig. 7-6**B**).

☐ The **deep posterior group** includes the supinator, abductor pollicis longus, extensor pollicis brevis, extensor pollicis longus, and extensor indicis (Fig. 7-6**C**).

☐ Two muscles are involved in pronation: the pronator teres and pronator quadratus; and two muscles are involved in supination: the biceps brachii and supinator.

☐ Forearm muscles can also be categorized by the location of their attachments. The medial and lateral epicondyles of the distal end of the humerus are attachment points for many of the muscles that move the wrist and hand.

☐ Muscles attach to the medial epicondyle of the humerus by the common flexor tendon. These

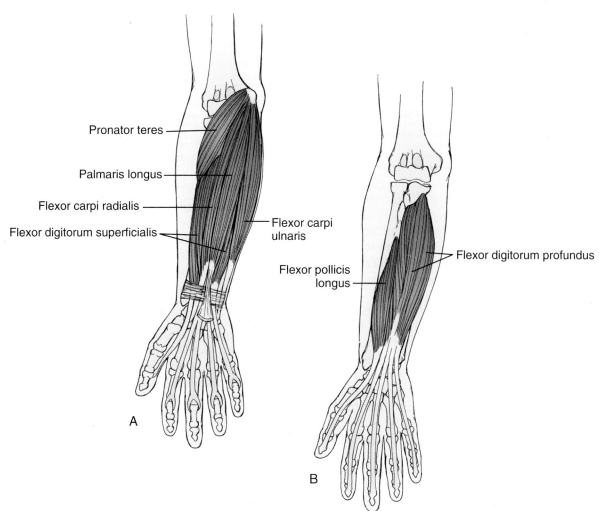

Figure 7-5. Forearm muscle compartments. **A.** Superficial anterior. **B.** Deep anterior.

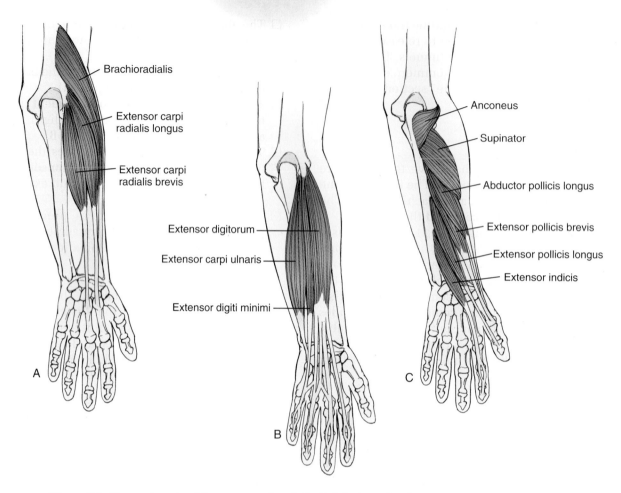

Figure 7-6. Compartments of forearm muscles. **A.** Radial. **B.** Superficial posterior. **C.** Deep posterior.

muscles include the flexor carpi radialis, flexor carpi ulnaris, palmaris longus, flexor digitorum superficialis, and flexor digitorum profundus.

☐ Muscles attaching to the lateral epicondyle of the humerus are the extensors of the wrist and hand, including the ECRL, ECRB, extensor carpi ulnaris, and extensor digitorum.

▨ **Function:** The muscles that cross the elbow and forearm are essential to movement of the hand in all activities of daily living and for recreation and sport. The hand and wrist muscles also help to reinforce the joint capsule of the elbow and produce a compressive force to the elbow during muscle contraction; therefore, these muscles contribute to joint stability.[9] Many of the muscles that move the wrist and hand attach to the humerus because it provides a much more stable base than the forearm. Co-contraction of the flexor and extensor muscles of the elbow, wrist, and hand provides stability to the elbow and forearm for movements of the wrist and hand and keeps the flexors in their optimum length-tension relationship for maximum grip strength.

▨ **Dysfunction and injury:** Dysfunction and injuries to the muscles and associated fascia attaching in the elbow region are common. **Tennis elbow,** or lateral epicondylitis, is considered an acute manifestation of a chronic condition. The acute episode is a tenoperiosteal tear of the wrist extensors, most commonly the ECRB. The chronic problem is a degenerative disorder caused by tissue fatigue from repetitive gripping. Tennis players, musicians, massage therapists, and carpenters are all susceptible to overuse of gripping motions. **Golfer's elbow (Little Leaguer's elbow),** or medial epicondylitis, is considered a tenoperiosteal tear of the wrist flexors and the pronator teres. It is caused by repetitive wrist flexion and pronation (e.g. golf, throwing, gripping).

▨ **Treatment implications:** Perform CR MET to reduce the hypertonicity in the involved muscles. Lengthen the myofascia with PIR MET. Perform STM to the involved muscles, including transverse friction massage at the attachment sites.

ANATOMY OF THE MUSCLES OF THE ELBOW, FOREARM, WRIST, AND HAND

See Table 7-1.

Table 7-1	Anatomy of the Muscles of the Elbow, Forearm, Wrist, and Hand

Muscle	Origin	Insertion	Action
Anterior Compartment Muscles of the Arm			
Biceps brachii	Two heads—short head from the coracoid process, long head from the upper lip of the glenoid fossa (supraglenoid tubercle)	Tuberosity of the radius; bicipital aponeurosis inserts into the fascia of the forearm	Flexion and supination of the elbow; flexion and abduction of the arm; stabilization of the glenohumeral joint
Brachialis	Distal half of the anterior portion of the humerus	Coronoid process of the ulna and the joint capsule	Flexion of the elbow
Posterior Compartment Muscles of the Arm			
Triceps brachii	Long head—lower edge of the glenoid cavity (infraglenoid tubercle); lateral head—upper one-third of the posterior surface of the humerus; medial head—lower two-thirds of the posterior surface of the humerus	Olecranon process of the ulna and the posterior joint capsule	Extension of the elbow and assistance in extension of the shoulder joint
Anconeus	Posterior surface of the lateral condyle of the humerus	Posterior surface of the proximal ulna and lateral aspect of olecranon	Extension of the forearm and tension of the posterior joint capsule of the elbow
Anterior Group of the Forearm: Superficial Layer			
Pronator teres	Two heads—humeral head from the medial epicondyle of the humerus, ulnar head from the coronoid process of the ulna	On the pronator tuberosity on the middle one-third of the radius	Pronation of forearm and flexion of the elbow
Flexor digitorum superficialis	Humeral head—medial epicondyle of the humerus; ulnar head—medial coronoid process; radial head—radial tuberosity area	Split tendons attach to the sides of the middle phalanx of the four fingers (palmar surface); at the MCP joint the tendon splits in two, through which the tendon of the flexor digitorum profundus travels	Flexion of the PIP joints of the fingers; assists in flexion of MCP joints and the wrist
Flexor carpi radialis	Medial epicondyle of the humerus	Base of the second and the third metacarpals (palmar surface)	Flexion and radial deviation of the wrist; weak flexion of the elbow
Palmaris longus (may be absent)	Medial epicondyle of the humerus	Palmar surface of the hand into the palmar aponeurosis	Wrist flexion; cupping of the hand
Flexor carpi ulnaris	Humeral head—medial epicondyle of the humerus; ulnar head—olecranon and posterior margin of the ulna	Pisiform bone and the base of the fifth metacarpal; extends to the pisohamate ligament and the hamate bone	Flexion and ulnar deviation of the wrist; weak flexion of the elbow

(continued)

| Table 7-1 | Anatomy of the Muscles of the Elbow, Forearm, Wrist, and Hand (*Continued*) |

Muscle	Origin	Insertion	Action
Anterior Group of the Forearm: Deep Layer			
Pronator quadratus	Distal one-fourth of the anterior surface of the ulna	Distal one-fourth of the anterior surface of the radius	Pronation of the forearm
Flexor digitorum profundus	Proximal three-fourths of the ulna and interosseous membrane	Base of the palmar surface of the distal phalanges of each finger	Flexion of DIP joints of the fingers and assists in flexion of PIP, MCP, and wrist
Flexor pollicis longus	Middle anterior surface of the radius	Base of the distal phalanx of the thumb (palmar surface)	Flexion of the IP joint of the thumb; assists in flexion of the wrist
Radial Group of Forearm Muscles			
Extensor carpi radialis brevis	Lateral epicondyle of the humerus, the radial collateral ligament, and the annular ligament	Base of the third metacarpal (dorsal surface)	Extension and radial deviation of the wrist
Extensor carpi radialis longus	Distal one-third of the lateral supracondylar ridge of the humerus	Base of the second metacarpal	Extension of the wrist; radial deviation of the wrist
Brachioradialis	Proximal two-thirds of the lateral supracondylar ridge of the humerus	Lateral surface of the styloid process of the radius	Brings forearm into neutral and flexes elbow from this position
Posterior Group of the Forearm: Superficial Layer			
Extensor digitorum	Posterior surface of the lateral epicondyle of the humerus, the radial collateral ligament, and the annular ligament	Four tendons to the bases of the second and the third phalanges of the four fingers on the dorsal surfaces; tendon broadens into the dorsal aponeurosis (hood) of fingers 2 to 5	Extension and spreading of the fingers, wrist, and forearm
Extensor digiti minimi	Arises together with the extensor digitorum at lateral epicondyle	Dorsal aponeurosis of the fifth digit	Extends the fifth digit and assists ulnar deviation of hand
Extensor carpi ulnaris	Posterior surface of the lateral epicondyle of the humerus	Base of the fifth metacarpal (dorsal surface)	Extension of the wrist; ulnar deviation of the wrist together with the flexor carpi ulnaris; and extension of the forearm
Posterior Group of the Forearm: Deep Layer			
Supinator	Lateral epicondyle of the humerus and supinator crest of the ulna and joint capsule	Outer surface of the proximal one-third of the radius	Supination of the forearm
Abductor pollicis longus	Posterior surface of the ulna	Trapezium and base of the first metacarpal, radial side	Extension and abduction of the CMC joint of the thumb

Table 7-1	Anatomy of the Muscles of the Elbow, Forearm, Wrist, and Hand (*Continued*)		
Muscle	**Origin**	**Insertion**	**Action**
Posterior Group of the Forearm: Deep Layer			
Extensor pollicis brevis	Posterior surface of the radius and ulna, distal to abductor pollicis longus	Dorsal surface of base of the proximal thumb	Extension of the MCP joint of the thumb; extension and abduction of the CMC joint of the thumb
Extensor pollicis longus	Posterior surface of the middle one-third of the ulna	Base of the distal phalanx of the thumb (dorsal surface)	Extension of the IP and MCP joints of the thumb; extension of the wrist
Extensor indicis	Distal one-third of the dorsal surface of the ulna	Extensor aponeurosis of the index finger	Extension of the index finger

MUSCULAR ACTIONS OF THE ELBOW AND FOREARM

See Table 7-2.

Table 7-2	Muscular Actions of the Elbow and Forearm

Flexion

- Biceps brachii—flexes and supinates the forearm
- Brachialis
- Brachioradialis—pronates forearm if supinated; supinates if pronated
- Pronator teres—pronates forearm and flexes the elbow
- Palmaris longus—weak flexor of elbow and wrist
- Flexor carpi ulnaris—flexes elbow; flexes and adducts wrist
- Flexor carpi radialis—flexes wrist and elbow; abducts wrist and pronates forearm
- Flexor digitorum superficialis—flexes forearm; flexes middle phalanges of four middle fingers

Extension

- Triceps brachii—also extends and adducts arm
- Anconeus—also responsible for pulling the synovial membrane out of the way of the olecranon process during extension

Supination

- Supinator
- Biceps brachii

Pronation

- Pronator teres—also flexes elbow
- Pronator quadratus

Anatomy, Function, and Dysfunction of the Wrist

BONES AND JOINTS OF THE WRIST

▨ **Structure:** The distal ends of the radius and ulna form the **distal radioulnar joint**. The wrist is composed of eight carpal bones in two rows (see Fig. 7-1). This distal radius articulates with the scaphoid and lunate bones of the wrist, forming the **distal radiocarpal joint**. The distal ulna articulates with an articular disc (meniscus) called the *triangular fibrocartilage complex* and with the proximal row of carpal bones. The **midcarpal joint** is the articulation of the proximal and distal rows of the carpal bones.

☐ The proximal row of carpal bones, from lateral to medial, are the navicular (scaphoid), lunate, triquetrum, and pisiform, which sits on the triquetrum.

☐ The distal row, from lateral to medial, are the trapezium, trapezoid, capitate, and hamate.

▨ **Function:** The radius carries approximately 80% of the load from the arm to the hand. The radius of the forearm is analogous to the tibia in the leg, which carries approximately 80% of the load to the foot. The main function of the wrist is precise control of the hand position for fine motor control and optimum strength. Achieving optimum strength is possible by maintaining control of the length–tension relationship of the extrinsic muscles of the hand.[9]

The distal radioulnar joint allows pronation and supination. The wrist has four basic movements: radial abduction, ulnar abduction, flexion, and extension. These movements can be combined to perform circumduction. The pisiform bone functions as a sesamoid for the flexor carpi ulnaris. The close-packed position of the wrist is full extension, and the open position is neutral to slight extension.

▨ **Dysfunction and injury:** A fall on an outstretched hand (FOOSH) injury typically involves a position of extension of the wrist and the elbow. Because the radius carries the majority of the load, its distal end is a common site of fracture, called a *Colles' fracture*. A FOOSH injury is also a common cause of ligamentous sprains. Injuries or chronic overuse can lead to fixation of the bones of the wrist, most commonly the lunate and scaphoid. **Impaction syndromes** of the scaphoid, capitate, and lunate refer to microtrauma and resulting pain, typically the result of repetitive hyperextension from gymnastics, yoga, or racquet sports.

▨ **Treatment implications:** A posttraumatic injury to the wrist, especially one that has been immobilized because of fracture, typically has a significant loss of motion. To treat this type of injury, perform MET to increase the joint ROM. Then perform PIR MET to lengthen the shortened myofascia and interweaving ligaments. Perform STM, including transverse friction massage, to help dissolve adhesions. Next, perform joint mobilization to help normalize the accessory motion between the bones of the wrist, reduce calcium deposits, and rehydrate the cartilage.

SOFT TISSUE STRUCTURES OF THE WRIST

JOINT CAPSULE AND LIGAMENTS

▨ **Structure:** The distal radioulnar joint has a strong capsule and is strengthened by ligaments. The midcarpal joint depends primarily on ligaments for support. The ligaments also provide significant passive control of wrist motion. As in the foot, the carpal bones of the wrist form a transverse and longitudinal arch that is concave anteriorly. This bony arch is covered with the dense **flexor retinaculum (transverse carpal ligament)** and forms the **carpal tunnel** through which the **median nerve** travels, along with nine tendons of the fingers and thumb: the flexor pollicis longus and four tendons each of the flexor digitorum superficialis and flexor digitorum profundus (see "Muscles").

The joint capsule of the wrist is reinforced by the flexor and extensor retinaculum, which is a thickening of the fascia of the forearm, and an extensive system of ligaments, including the radial and ulnar collateral ligaments, the palmar and dorsal radiocarpal ligaments, and the pisohamate ligament.

▨ **Function:** The wrist ligaments help to transmit the forces that move through the wrist and hand, stabilize the carpal bones, and perform a neurosensory role. The arches in the hand are created by the bones, which are suspended and reinforced by the flexor retinaculum and the intercarpal ligaments.

Increase in the arch can occur through the action of the palmaris longus, flexor carpi ulnaris, and intrinsic muscles of the hand. Contraction of the flexor carpi ulnaris tightens the proximal portion of the flexor retinaculum.

- **Dysfunction and injury:** Injuries to the ligaments of the wrist are common and are usually the result of an acute injury rather than a cumulative stress. A FOOSH is a common injury that sprains the wrist, either the dorsal or palmar ligaments. The joint capsule of the distal radioulnar joint can develop adhesions after injury, which would limit pronation and supination.[10] The flexor retinaculum can thicken in response to cumulative use of the finger flexors (such as keyboard work), contributing to a narrowing of the carpal tunnel and compression of the median nerve, called **carpal tunnel syndrome** (see "Nerves").

- **Treatment implications:** To treat the wrist ligaments, first perform CR MET to the muscles that interweave with the involved ligaments. On the anterior wrist, these muscles are the flexors of the wrist, fingers, and thumb; and on the posterior wrist, these muscles are the extensors of the wrist, fingers, and thumb. This treatment creates a contracting and relaxing force, which helps to realign the healing fibers and acts as a pump to promote nutritional exchange. Next, perform STM, including gentle scooping strokes in the more acute phase and transverse friction massage in the chronic phase, to dissolve thick and fibrotic tissue. To lengthen the joint capsule of the distal radioulnar joint, perform MET to increase pronation and supination.

LIGAMENTS OF THE WRIST

See Table 7-3.

NERVES

See Figures 7-2 to 7-4.

- **Structure:** After traveling through the tunnels at the elbow, the **ulnar, median,** and **radial nerves** travel through the forearm to the wrist area and hand.
  - □ The **ulnar nerve** travels with the flexor carpi ulnaris to the wrist, where it travels on top of (anterior) the flexor retinaculum on the radial side of the pisiform. It divides into superficial and deep branches that then travel under the pisohamate ligament, which is a fibro-osseous space between the pisiform and the hook of the hamate called the **tunnel of Guyon.**[11] It contributes

Table 7-3		Wrist Ligaments
Ligament	**Origin**	**Insertion**
Transverse carpal ligament (distal flexor retinaculum)	Navicular (scaphoid) and tubercle of the trapezium	Pisiform and hook of the hamate
Pisohamate ligament	Pisiform bone	Hook of the hamate
Ulnar collateral ligament	From the distal end of the styloid process of the ulna	Medial side of the triquetral and pisiform bones
Radial collateral ligament	Distal end of the styloid process of the radius	Radial side of the scaphoid bone

branches called the *interdigital nerves* to the fingers (see "Nerves of the Hand").

- □ The **median nerve** exits the elbow region between the two humeral heads of the pronator teres and then travels between the superficial and the deep flexors. It continues in the midline of the palmar aspect of the wrist through the **carpal tunnel** formed by the carpal bones and the flexor retinaculum.
- □ The **radial nerve** divides into superficial and deep (interosseous) branches distal to the elbow. The deep branch travels between the superficial and deep layers of the extensors and under the extensor pollicis longus. The superficial radial nerve travels under the skin on the distal aspect of the radius to the dorsum of the thumb and index finger.

- **Function:** The ulnar, median, and radial nerves provide sensory and motor functions to the hand.
  - □ The **ulnar nerve** has muscular branches to the flexor carpi ulnaris and the ulnar portion of the deep flexors of the fingers, the hypothenar muscles, the interossei, the adductor pollicis, and the deep head of the flexor pollicis brevis. It is sensory to the ulnar side of the hand, most specifically at the tip of the little finger.
  - □ The **median nerve** supplies most of the flexors of the forearm and the thenar muscles. It is sensory to the lateral portion of the palm and thenar eminence. Its innervation is most specific at the tip of the index finger.
  - □ The **radial nerve** has muscular branches that innervate all the extensors and has a sensory branch to the dorsum of the hand, most specifically the webspace between the thumb and the index fingers.

▨ **Dysfunction and injury:**
  ☐ Compression of the **median nerve** at the wrist is called **carpal tunnel syndrome.** A common cause is overuse of the finger flexors, which can create inflammation and swelling. Chronic irritation leads to fibrosis or thickening of the sheath and thickening of the transverse carpal ligament, which narrows the tunnel. Other causes include previous injury, subluxation of the lunate, edema from pregnancy, and OA.
  ☐ The **ulnar nerve** can be trapped as it passes through the **tunnel of Guyon,** which is formed by the pisohamate ligament between the pisiform and the hook of the hamate. Or it can be irritated from swelling of the flexor carpi ulnaris at the insertion into the pisiform.

▨ **Treatment implications:** To treat carpal tunnel syndrome, perform CR MET to the wrist and finger flexors to reduce hypertonicity and increase the extensibility of the fascia of the wrist and hand attaching to these muscles. Next, perform CR MET to the palmaris longus, flexor carpi ulnaris, flexor carpi ulnaris, and intrinsic muscles of the hand that attach to the transverse carpal ligament (flexor retinaculum) to increase the extensibility of the ligament and to help decompress the tunnel. Then perform a gentle distraction of the flexor retinaculum. For chronic conditions, perform STM to the attachment points of the flexor retinaculum.
  ☐ For the ulnar nerve, perform CR MET to the flexor carpi ulnaris to release the tension in the pisohamate ligament. Next perform STM transverse to the line of the ligament. Then perform gentle scooping strokes transverse to the line of the nerve in the tunnel of Guyon.

MUSCLES

▨ **Structure:** Six muscles have tendons crossing the anterior wrist. Three of these act only on the wrist: the palmaris longus, flexor carpi radialis, and flexor carpi ulnaris. The other three flex the fingers and thumb and act secondarily on the wrist: the flexor digitorum superficialis, flexor digitorum profundus, and flexor pollicis longus. In addition to the median nerve, nine tendons pass through the carpal tunnel: the flexor pollicis longus and the four tendons each of the flexor digitorum superficialis and profundus.

Nine muscles cross the dorsum of the wrist. Three of these muscles are wrist muscles: the ECRB, ECRL, and extensor carpi ulnaris. The other six are finger and thumb muscles that act secondarily on the wrist: the extensor digitorum, extensor indicis, extensor digiti minimi, extensor pollicis longus, extensor pollicis brevis, and abductor pollicis longus.

The tendons that cross the wrist are stabilized and lubricated to ensure precise control of movement and smooth gliding. The structures that stabilize the tendons are the retinaculum of the wrist and the fibrous connective tissue holding the flexor tendons to the fingers and thumb called *annular ligaments.* The flexor tendons are lubricated by synovial sheaths in the palm and fingers.

▨ **Function:** The primary roles of the muscles that cross the wrist are to provide strength and stability for the hand and to allow fine positional movements. Achieving this strength and stability is possible by maintaining the optimal length–tension relationship of the extrinsic muscles of the fingers and thumb (see "Muscles of the Hand" below).[9]

▨ **Dysfunction and injury:** Tendinitis at the attachment points of the wrist, called **insertional tendinitis**, is common from injury and overuse. These include the ECRB, ECRL, extensor carpi ulnaris, flexor carpi radialis, and flexor carpi ulnaris. Another common dysfunction is **stenosing tenosynovitis (De Quervain's tenovaginitis)** of the extensor pollicis brevis and the abductor pollicis longus. These two muscles travel together through a fibroosseous tunnel formed by the extensor retinaculum over the radial styloid. Repetitive gripping motions cause the tendons to rub against each other, creating irritation and inflammation. This inflammation creates swelling in the acute stage and fibrosis in the chronic stage. Both conditions narrow the tunnel and create pain with movement using the muscles. **Intersection syndrome** is described as either a bursitis or a tenosynovitis, which occurs at the site where the abductor pollicis longus and extensor pollicis brevis cross over the extensor carpi radialis tendons. Clients report a tenderness on the dorsal side of the radius just proximal to the wrist.

▨ **Treatment implications:** For De Quervain's tenovaginitis, perform CR MET to the involved tendons, and perform STM, using gentle scooping strokes transverse to the line of the tendons. Deeper friction strokes are indicated if thickened, fibrotic tissue is palpated in the chronic condition. For insertional tendinitis, perform MET for the involved tendon to reduce the hypertonicity, to lengthen the myofascia, and to increase the resilience of the fascia at the tenoperiosteal junctions. Perform STM for the entire length of the muscle and transverse friction massage at the insertion points.

MUSCULAR ACTIONS AT THE WRIST

See Table 7-4.

Table 7-4	Muscular Actions at the Wrist

Two compound joints compose the wrist: the radiocarpal and the midcarpal joints. There are four basic motions: flexion, extension, radial deviation (abduction), and ulnar deviation (adduction). Six muscles of the forearm move only the wrist. Nine additional muscles that move the thumb and fingers also move the wrist.

Wrist

Flexion

- Flexor carpi ulnaris
- Flexor carpi radialis
- Palmaris longus

Extension

- Extensor carpi ulnaris
- Extensor carpi radialis longus
- Extensor carpi radialis brevis

Radial Deviation (Abduction)

- Extensor carpi radialis longus
- Extensor carpi radialis brevis
- Flexor carpi radialis
- Palmaris longus

Ulnar Deviation (Adduction)

- Flexor carpi ulnaris
- Extensor carpi ulnaris

Anatomy, Function, and Dysfunction of the Hand

BONES AND JOINTS OF THE HAND

The hand has 19 bones and 19 joints (see Fig. 7-1). There are five metacarpals and three phalanges for each of the four fingers and two phalanges for the thumb.

CARPOMETACARPAL JOINTS

 Structure: The articulations between the distal row of carpal bones and the base of the metacarpals are called the carpometacarpal (CMC) joints. The thumb is the first CMC joint and is the articulation of the first metacarpal and the trapezium.

 Function: The CMC joints of the second, third, and fourth fingers are synovial joints with simple flexion and extension movements. The second and third CMC joints are nearly immobile, providing a stable base for the cupping and holding motions of the palm. The fifth CMC (the little finger) has the capability of a slight amount of abduction and adduction in addition to flexion and extension.

The first CMC joint (the thumb) is also called the metacarpal triquetral joint. It is described as a saddle joint and has a wide variety of movements, including flexion, extension, abduction, adduction, and circumduction. This joint is the key to mobility of the thumb. The thumb faces the palm instead of anteriorly like the other fingers, which allows it to touch the other fingers (called *opposition*), an essential motion in holding, gripping, and pinching.

 Dysfunction and injury: The hand is a common site for arthritis, both the degenerative and systemic types, such as rheumatoid arthritis (RA). Hereditary factors can be related to arthritis of the fingers and thumb. OA typically manifests as joint swelling at the distal IP (DIP) joints, called *Heberden's nodes*, or at the proximal IP (PIP) joints, called *Bouchard's nodes*. The CMC joint of the thumb is one of the most commonly arthritic joints in the body. OA is common in the DIP joints, less common in the PIP joints, and fairly rare in the metacarpophalangeal (MCP) joints.[3]

Degenerative arthritis is related to overuse and inflammation leading to capsular fibrosis, loss of the normal synovial fluid, and cartilage degeneration. Often, predisposing factors such as subluxation or fixation of the normal gliding characteristics of the joint are present. The most common cause of swelling at the PIP is collateral ligament tears.[12] The thumb is also a common site of sesamoiditis, an inflammation of the ligaments and joint capsule surrounding the sesamoid bones.

■ **Treatment implications:** The treatment protocol for OA of the hand is MET for the finger flexors and extensors to help stimulate the normal joint lubrication by tensing the joint capsule through its attachment to the muscles. Perform STM to release adhesions in the annular ligaments of the flexor tendons and at the tenoperiosteal attachments of the flexors to the thumb and fingers. Perform transverse friction massage to the ligament system of the fingers and thumb, concentrating on transverse strokes to the collateral ligaments and transverse metacarpal ligaments. Then perform joint mobilization to the involved joint.

METACARPOPHALANGEAL JOINTS

■ **Structure:** MCP joints are the articulations of the convex heads of the metacarpals and the concave bases of the phalanges (fingers). They are synovial joints with a joint capsule and three ligaments: the palmar, transverse metatarsal, and collateral. The MCP joint of the thumb has two **sesamoid bones** embedded within the adductor pollicis and the flexor pollicis brevis tendons.

■ **Function:** The MCP joint has four possible motions: flexion, extension, adduction, and abduction. The sesamoids improve the mechanics of the MCP joint by increasing the angle of insertion to improve leverage and to help distribute the force of contraction.

■ **Dysfunction and injury:** The MCP joints are also prone to acute injury and OA. The sesamoids of the thumb can become inflamed after injury or repetitive stress, called **sesamoiditis**, and also can misalign (sublux) toward the palm.

■ **Treatment implications:** Treatment for MCP injuries is the same as that for the CMC joint.

INTERPHALANGEAL JOINTS

■ **Structure:** The IP joints are the articulations between the proximal and distal phalanges. Each of these joints has a joint capsule, two collateral ligaments, and a fibrocartilage palmar plate (see "Joint Capsules and Ligaments of the Interphalangeal Joints").

■ **Function:** IP joints are synovial hinge joints with two possible motions: flexion and extension. The flexion of these joints toward the palm allows the holding and gripping action of the hand.

■ **Dysfunction and injury:** IP joint dysfunction and injury are the same as those of the CMC joint.

■ **Treatment implications:** Treatment for IP dysfunction is the same as that for the CMC joint.

SOFT TISSUE STRUCTURES OF THE HAND

JOINT CAPSULES AND LIGAMENTS

The clinically important ligaments of the hand can be described by location (Figs. 7-7**A** and 7-7**B**).

JOINT CAPSULES AND LIGAMENTS OF THE CARPOMETACARPAL JOINTS

■ All CMC joints of the hand have transverse and longitudinal ligaments. The CMC joint of the thumb has a loose joint capsule, reinforced by

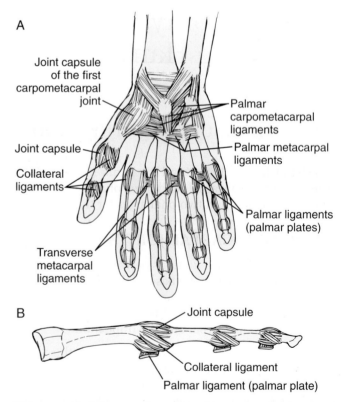

Figure 7-7. A. Joint capsule, collateral ligaments, deep transverse metacarpal ligaments, and palmar ligaments of the MCP and IP joints. **B.** Lateral view of the joint capsule and collateral ligaments of the MCP and IP joints.

radial, ulnar, palmar, and dorsal ligaments. An intermetacarpal ligament exists between the first and second metacarpals.

JOINT CAPSULES AND LIGAMENTS OF THE METACARPOPHALANGEAL JOINTS

- The **joint capsules** of the MCP joints are interwoven with medial and lateral collateral ligaments; accessory collateral ligaments; transverse metacarpal ligaments; the palmar ligament (palmar plate), a thick, dense fibrocartilage structure; and the extensor hood (see below).

- The **collateral ligaments** of the MCP joints are thick, rounded cords on the sides of the joints, which suspend the palmar plate.

- The **transverse metacarpal ligaments** interweave with the joint capsules of the MCP joints and the palmar plates. They have a deep and superficial portion, through which the palmar digital nerve travels.

- The **palmar ligaments (palmar or volar plates)** are embedded in the walls of the joint capsules on the palmar side of the MCP joints. They are attached to the heads of the metacarpals and the proximal phalanges of the MCP joints. The distal portion of these ligaments has a cartilage lining, and the proximal portion is membranous. They have a groove in them for the flexor tendons of the fingers and are interwoven with the transverse metacarpal and collateral ligaments of the MCP joints. They move with the finger, proximally with flexion, and distally with extension.

- At the level of the MCP joints is the **extensor hood (expansion)**, a broad, flat fibrous sheet composed of lateral bands of the extensor tendons, and fibrous extensions of the interosseous and lumbrical muscles.[10]

JOINT CAPSULE AND LIGAMENTS OF THE INTERPHALANGEAL JOINTS

- The **joint capsule** of the IP joints is reinforced with two collateral ligaments, two accessory collateral ligaments, and a palmar ligament. The flexor tendons of the fingers interweave with the joint capsules of the IP joints.

- The **collateral ligaments** of the IP joints connect the IP joints. The fibers are oriented in a proximal-to-distal direction following the shaft of the bone. They help to guide the flexion and extension movement of the IP joints.

- The **palmar ligaments (palmar or volar plates)** are embedded in the walls of the joint capsules on the palmar side of the IP joints of the fingers and the thumb. They are attached from the proximal to the distal portion of the IP joints. They are interwoven to

the joint capsule and collateral ligaments and have a groove in them for the flexor tendons of the fingers.

- The flexor tendons are held in place by a fibrous sheath called the **annular ligament,** which functions as a retinaculum to stabilize and guide the tendons. They attach to the palmar plate and underlying bone, creating a fibro-osseous tunnel with the bone.

- **Function:**
  - ☐ The **joint capsule** has a fibrous and synovial layer. The joint capsule provides passive stability to the joint, guides joint motion, provides lubrication to the joint through stimulation of the synovial layer, and plays a neurosensory role. The joint capsule also contains mechanoreceptors and pain receptors that provide information about movement, position, pressure, and pain as well as reflex connections to the surrounding muscles.
  - ☐ The **collateral ligaments** of the IP joints stabilize the articulating bones and suspend the palmar plate and flexor sheath.[13]
  - ☐ The **transverse metacarpal ligament** holds the heads of the metacarpals together.
  - ☐ The **palmar plate** functions to expand the articular surface for the metacarpal head and prevents the long flexor tendons from impinging into the joint.[9]

- **Dysfunction and injury:**
  - ☐ Fibrosis of the collateral ligaments and joint capsule of the fingers is common as a consequence of acute trauma; after cumulative stresses, such as repetitive gripping motions; or in degenerative conditions of the joints.
  - ☐ The PIP joint is the most commonly injured joint of the hand.[11] The incident typically involves jamming a finger, which hyperextends the joint, spraining the joint capsule and collateral ligaments. A chronic microtearing of the IP collateral ligament is also common, especially at the PIP joint. This tearing creates swelling in the acute stage and can cause joint degeneration by preventing the normal gliding of the joint surfaces.[12]
  - ☐ Injury to the collateral ligaments of the MCP joints can lead to adhesions that result in decreased flexion of that joint. Injury to the medial (ulnar) collateral ligament of the thumb is a common ski injury caused by forceful hyperextension or abduction of the thumb, called **skier's thumb**.
  - ☐ A thickening of the deep transverse metacarpal ligaments is common with acute or degenerative conditions. Shortening, which is subsequent to the ligament thickening, compresses the metacarpal heads together, leading to dysfunction and pain at the MCP joints. With thickening also comes decreased space for the palmar digital nerve, and this can lead to pain, numbing, and tingling in the fingers.

☐ The annular ligament can thicken and shorten from excessive use of the flexor tendons, such as keyboard work, or from repetitive gripping motions. Increased friction of the flexor tendons develops at the tunnel formed by these ligaments, especially at the MCP joints. This increased friction creates irritation, inflammation, and potential fibrosis of the ligament, which narrows the tunnel and leads to **trigger finger**.

☐ The palmar ligament can thicken as a result of degenerative arthritis, or can be injured from a FOOSH. When the hand is immobilized after an injury, the membranous portion of the ligament can retract and develop adhesions, leading to flexion contracture of the joint.[14]

■ **Treatment implications:** Treat the ligaments of the hand by first performing MET to the muscles that interweave with the ligaments. As the most involved ligaments are usually on the palmar side, concentrate the MET on the flexors of the fingers and thumb. Next, perform STM to the involved ligaments, transverse to the line of the fiber. If the ligament is thickened, use transverse friction strokes. If the finger is held in sustained flexion, release the torsion in the collateral ligaments by performing a palmar to dorsal scooping motion on the ligaments. Finally, mobilize the joints in the area of the involved ligament to help normalize neurologic function and hydrate the area of the ligament. To treat the palmar ligaments, use a scooping stroke in a proximal to distal direction to reduce adhesions and tethering in the membranous portion of the ligament.

FASCIA

■ **Structure:** The antebrachial fascia of the forearm is strengthened on the extensor surface of the wrist by the extensor retinaculum, which continues as the dorsal fascia of the hand. On the palmar surface, the antebrachial fascia thickens into the **palmar fascia,** which is interwoven into the aponeurosis of the palmaris longus muscle. The fascia continues as the fascia covering the thenar and hypothenar eminences, and interweaves with the flexor retinaculum at the wrist. The palmar fascia has deep and superficial layers connected by fascia, separating the palm into compartments containing the tendons. It continues distally and interweaves with the transverse metacarpal ligament and the flexor tendon sheaths.

■ **Function:** The palmar fascia provides a surface to prevent slipping while grasping an object, stabilizes the tendons and neurovascular stuctures, and provides protection to the nerves and blood vessels.[10]

■ **Dysfunction:** Thickening and nodular formation of the palmar fascia can occur spontaneously for unknown reasons, a condition called **Dupuytren's**

contracture. It can create a severe disability of the hand, owing to flexion contracture of the tendons of the fourth and fifth fingers.

■ **Treatment implications:** Symptoms from Dupuytren's disease can be relieved somewhat through deep longitudinal and transverse work on the palmar fascia. This condition typically requires surgical intervention.

NERVES OF THE HAND

■ **Structure:** The median and ulnar nerves have terminal branches called the **palmar digital nerves (interdigital nerves).** Palmar digital nerves travel between the superficial and deep layers of the transverse metacarpal ligament between the heads of the metacarpals. In the fingers and thumb, they travel on the radial and ulnar side of each digit rather than on the palmar side, where they might be compressed with gripping (see Figs. 7-2 to 7-4).

■ **Function:** Each palmar digital nerve gives off sensory branches to the skin on the front and sides of the fingers as well as articular branches to the MCP and IP joints.

■ **Dysfunction and injury:** Interdigital nerves can become entrapped in between the superficial and deep layers of the transverse metacarpal ligament. The ligaments thicken because of injury, overuse, or disease. In dysfunction, the hand is typically held in sustained flexion, compressing the metacarpal heads and the interdigital nerves.

■ **Treatment implications:** To treat the interdigital nerves, perform STM to first release the transverse metacarpal ligament. Then perform gentle scooping strokes perpendicular to the line of the nerve in between the heads of the metacarpals.

MUSCLES OF THE HAND

■ **Structure**: The hand has 18 intrinsic muscles and 9 extrinsic muscles (Figs. 7-8 to 7-10). The fingers have two extrinsic flexors and three extensors. The thumb has four extrinsic muscles: one on the palmar side and three on the dorsal side. Most of the intrinsic muscles of the hand are contained in two distinct pads: the thenar eminence at the base of the thumb and the hypothenar eminence at the base of the fifth finger. In addition to these pads, the intrinsic muscles include the lumbricals and the dorsal and palmar interossei.

As the flexor tendons travel over the MCP and IP joints, they are enclosed within a lubricated tendon sheath, sometimes called a *digital sheath*, with a synovial inner layer and a fibrous outer layer, allowing

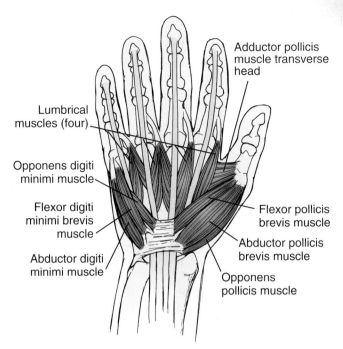

Figure 7-8. Muscles and flexor tendons of the hand.

the tendons to slide freely within them. The flexor tendons are connected to the extensor hood by oblique and transverse retinacular ligaments. The annular ligaments form a fibro-osseous tunnel that encloses the flexor tendons and their sheaths to the heads of the metacarpals in the fingers and thumb. These ligaments act like a retinaculum, stabilizing and guiding the movement of the tendons.

The extensors pass under the extensor retinaculum, are enclosed within their own tendon sheaths, and form an extensor hood on the dorsal surface of each digit that replaces the posterior portion of the joint capsule. This hood wraps around the joint and attaches to the transverse metacarpal ligament.

The lumbricals and interossei are the intrinsic muscles of the fingers. They expand into a fibrous sheet, which forms part of the extensor hood.

▨ **Function:** The main function of the hand is to grasp and manipulate objects, requiring fine motor control. A strong grip is performed mainly by the extrinsic flexors, and delicate movement, such as a pinch, will use more of the intrinsics. Extension of the fingers is caused by the combined action of the extensors and the intrinsics. The lumbrical muscles have been described as functioning as the primary organ of sensory feedback in the hand. These muscles have more muscle spindles than any other muscle in the body.[5]

The wrist and hand have an optimum position in which all the extrinsic muscles of the hand are under equal tension, which provides the finger flexors and thumb optimum power. This is called the **position of function** of the wrist and hand. In this position, the wrist is held in neutral, and the fingers are moderately flexed at the MCP joints and slightly flexed at the PIP and DIP joints.

▨ **Dysfunction and injury:** The hand is susceptible to acute and chronic dysfunctions and injuries. Tearing of the extensor tendon away from the bone (avulsion)

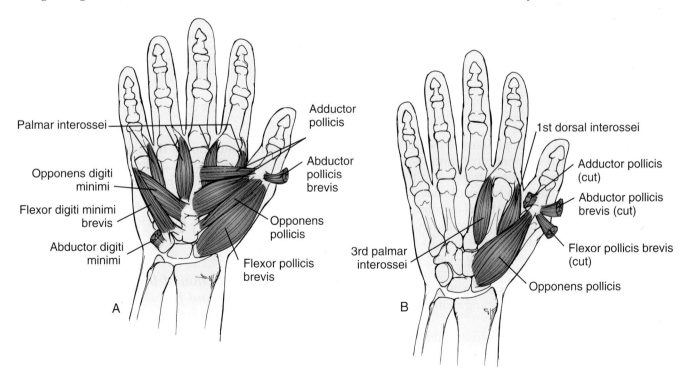

Figure 7-9. A. Deep layer of hand muscles. **B.** Deep layers of the hand muscles with both heads of the adductor pollicis sectioned to reveal the interossei underneath.

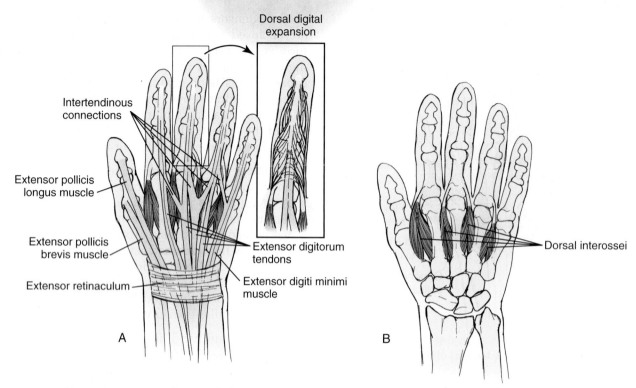

Figure 7-10. A. Muscles and tendons of the dorsum of the hand. **B.** Dorsal interossei muscles.

at the end of the finger is the most common closed-tendon (does not cut the skin) injury to athletes.[5] The incident usually involves a forceful impact on the tip of the finger and is called **mallet finger.**[7]

☐ Chronic dysfunctions are often due to fatigue. Through overuse, the muscles are held in a sustained contraction and build up metabolic waste products, creating an acidic environment and decreased oxygen. This manifests as ischemic pain that leaves the muscles sensitive to modest pressures.

☐ Weakness of the intrinsic muscles and sustained contraction of the finger extensors produce a **clawing** of the fingers.

☐ The tendons of the finger flexors can develop a thickening of their tendon sheath, forming a nodule that can become entrapped in the annular ligament, creating a **trigger finger.** The other cause of trigger finger that was mentioned previously is a thickening of the annular ligament. Trigger finger develops at the base of the proximal phalanx. The client feels a "snap" as the tendon moves between flexion and extension.

☐ The flexor pollicis longus can become irritated because of repetitive gripping motions or acute trauma, such as a FOOSH.

☐ The dorsal and palmar interossei and lumbricals can become irritated because of repetitive fine motor movements of the fingers, such as those done by musicians.

▨ **Treatment implications:** The basic protocol is to first perform CR or PIR MET to the involved muscles and fascia to increase their extensibility and help restore normal neurologic function. Next, perform STM with scooping strokes, transverse to the line of the fiber. Transverse friction strokes may be used if fibrosis is palpated. Mobilization of the associated joint is performed to help increase lubrication, restore joint play, and normalize the articular and periarticular nerves that communicate with the muscle.

Muscle Imbalances of the Elbow, Wrist, and Hand

▨ **Muscles that tend to be tight and short:** Pronator teres, flexor carpi ulnaris and radialis, flexors of the fingers, and muscles of the thenar eminence

▨ **Muscles that tend to be weak and inhibited:** Finger and wrist extensors, lumbricals, interossei, and supinator

Positional Dysfunction of the Muscles of the Elbow, Wrist, and Hand

▨ The muscles of the forearm tend to develop a torsion toward pronation. The muscles of the hand develop a torsion that folds the thenar and hypothenar muscles toward the midline of the palm, and the fingers into a sustained flexed position.

INTRINSIC MUSCLES OF THE HAND

See Table 7-5.

Table 7-5	Intrinsic Muscles of the Hand		
Muscle	**Origin**	**Insertion**	**Action**
Thenar Eminence			
Abductor pollicis brevis	From the flexor retinaculum and the tubercles of the scaphoid and trapezium.	Radial side of the proximal phalanx and radial sesamoid of the MP joint; lies superficial to opponens pollicis and partly superficial and lateral (radial) to the flexor pollicis brevis	Draws the thumb at right angles to the palm, rotates it medially, and extends it
Opponens pollicis	Deep to the abductor pollicis brevis, arises from the tubercle of the trapezium and the flexor retinaculum	Attaches the entire length of the lateral border and palmar surface of the first metacarpal	Bends it medially across the palm and rotates it medially (i.e., in opposition); abducts, flexes, and rotates first metacarpal
Flexor pollicis brevis	Superficial part arises from the flexor retinaculum and tubercle of the trapezium; deep part arises from the capitate and trapezoid	Radial sesamoid bone of the MCP joint of the thumb and proximal phalanx	Flexes the proximal phalanx of the thumb; flexes the MCP joint and rotates it medially in cooperation with opponens
Adductor pollicis	Arises by transverse and oblique heads: Oblique head—capitate, bases of the second and the third metacarpals; transverse head—entire length of the shaft of the third metacarpal bone	Ulnar sesamoid bone of the MCP joint of the thumb and proximal phalanx	Produces adduction and assists in opposition and flexion of the thumb on the first phalanx
Hypothenar Eminence			
Abductor digiti minimi	Arises from the pisiform bone, the tendon of the flexor carpi ulnaris, and the pisohamate ligament	Into the base of the proximal phalanx (ulnar side) of the fifth digit	Abducts the little finger
Flexor digiti minimi	From the hook of the hamate and the flexor retinaculum	On the ulnar side of the base of the proximal phalanx; separated at its origin from abductor digiti minimi by the deep branches of ulnar artery and nerve	Flexes the little finger at its MCP joint
Opponens digiti minimi	Deep to the abductor and flexor digiti minimi, arising from the hook of the hamate and flexor retinaculum	Into the entire length of the ulnar margin of the fifth metacarpal	Draws the fifth metacarpal forward and laterally (radially) at the same time, rotating it about its axis so that its anterior surface comes to face the thumb in opposition
Lumbricals (I through IV)	Arise from the radial side of the tendons of the flexor digitorum profundus	To the radial side of the extensor hood of each finger and to the joint capsules of the MCP joint	Act in association with the interossei to flex the digits at the MCP joints, and extend at the IP joints

(continued)

Table 7-5	Intrinsic Muscles of the Hand (*Continued*)		
Muscle	**Origin**	**Insertion**	**Action**
Hypothenar Eminence			
Dorsal interossei	Four double-headed muscles, each arising from adjacent sides of the five metacarpal bones	Attach to the bases of the proximal phalanges and the dorsal aponeurosis; first attaches to the radial side of the proximal phalanx of the index finger; the second and the third attach to the sides of the proximal phalanx of the middle finger; and the fourth attaches to the ulnar side of the ring finger	Abduct the finger from the axis of the middle finger, flex at the MCP joint, and extend at the IP joint
Palmar interossei	Three single-headed muscles that arise from the palmar surfaces of the second, fourth, and fifth metacarpals	Attach to the extensor hood of corresponding phalanges	Adduct the fingers to the midline, flex at the MCP and extend at the IP joints

MUSCULAR ACTIONS OF THE HAND

See Table 7-6.

Table 7-6	Muscular Actions at the Hand

The hand consists of 19 bones and 19 joints. Nine muscles from the forearm move the fingers or thumb, and the hand has 18 intrinsic muscles. For clarity, the actions of the fingers and thumb are differentiated.

Fingers

Flexion
- Flexor digitorum superficialis
- Flexor digitorum profundus
- Flexor digiti minimi
- Lumbricals and interossei assist flexion

Extension
- Extensor digitorum
- Extensor indices
- Extensor digiti minimi

Adductors
- Long finger flexors are principal adductors, assisted by palmar interossei

Abductors
- Dorsal interossei, assisted by long extensors
- Abductor digiti minimi

Thumb

Flexion
- Flexor digitorum longus (extrinsic)
- Flexor pollicis brevis (intrinsic)

Extension
- Extensor pollicis longus
- Extensor pollicis brevis

Abduction
- Abductor pollicis longus (extrinsic)
- Abductor pollicis brevis (intrinsic)

Adduction
- Adductor pollicis, oblique and transverse heads

Opposition
- Opponens pollicis
- Opponens digiti minimi

Dysfunction and Injury of the Elbow, Forearm, Wrist, and Hand

FACTORS THAT PREDISPOSE TO ELBOW, FOREARM, WRIST, AND HAND PAIN

▨ Repetitive gripping, such as playing tennis or hammering, can fatigue and weaken the wrist and finger flexors and extensors, predisposing them to an acute tear at their tenoperiosteal attachments at the elbow and wrist.

▨ Repetitive or prolonged use of finger flexors, such as keyboard work, can cause a tendinitis, leading to localized pain, swelling, or both at the wrist, leading to carpal tunnel syndrome.

▨ Repetitive elbow flexion and extension, such as carpentry work or playing instruments such as the violin, can cause elbow pain.

▨ Repetitive elbow extension, such as throwing a ball, irritates the muscle attachments at the elbow.

▨ Repetitive pronation or supination (twisting) motions.

▨ Previous injury to the joints can cause a thickening of the joint capsule and collateral ligaments, limiting joint motion, leading to degeneration of the cartilage and OA.

▨ A subluxation of the lunate in the wrist can cause carpal tunnel syndrome. A fixation of the MCP or IP joint can lead to degeneration and OA.

▨ Immobility

▨ Fatigue

DIFFERENTIATION OF ELBOW, FOREARM, WRIST, AND HAND PAIN

It is important to realize that pain in the elbow, wrist, and hand can come from disease processes rather than from injuries and dysfunctions to the neuromusculoskeletal system. See "Contraindications to Massage Therapy: Red Flags" in Chapter 2, "Assessments and Technique" for guidelines on when massage is contraindicated and when to refer the client to a doctor.

▨ The elbow, wrist, and hand are common areas where a combination of pain, numbing, and tingling can be referred from the cervical spine and shoulder. As was mentioned in Chapter 5, "Cervical Spine," one type of referred pain is caused by muscle, ligament, joint capsule, disc, or dura mater. These tissues elicit what is called **sclerotomal** pain when they are injured. Usually, the sclerotomal pain is described as deep, aching, and diffuse. A second type of referred pain, called **radicular** pain, is caused by an irritation of the spinal nerve root. If the sensory (dorsal) root is irritated, there is sharp pain, numbing, or tingling that is well localized in what are called dermatomes. A dermatome is an area of the skin supplied by the sensory root of a single spinal nerve (see Chapter 3, "Lumbosacral Spine" for a figure of the dermatomes). If there is compression of the motor (ventral) nerve root, in addition to the pain, numbing, and tingling, there might be weakness in the muscles supplied by that nerve root, called the **myotome.** The relevant myotomes of the elbow, wrist, and hand are C6 wrist extension, C7 wrist flexion, and C8 thumb extension.

▨ The entrapment of a peripheral nerve in the area of the elbow, wrist, and hand can also lead to some combination of pain, numbing, or weakness. In peripheral entrapment, manual pressure over the entrapped nerve typically increases the intensity of the symptoms temporarily. This increased intensity of symptoms is an indication for treatment. The STM techniques that release peripheral nerve entrapment are highly effective. If symptoms do not resolve after several treatments, refer the client to a chiropractor or osteopath for spinal evaluation.

▨ Differentiation of other conditions can be categorized according to the region involved.

▨ An ache at the medial and lateral epicondyles that is increased with gripping or isometric challenge of the wrist flexors, pronators, or extensors is typically a tenoperiosteal tear of the muscle attachments.

▨ Pain in the same region might also be a nerve entrapment. Lateral epicondylitis, radial tunnel syndrome, flexor tendinopathy, and cubital tunnel syndrome have similar symptoms. Unlike tendinitis or a tenoperiosteal tear, an entrapment is not typically aggravated by isometric challenge.

▨ Pain in the anterior forearm can be a bicipital or pronator teres tendinitis. Both conditions are often painful with isometric challenge.

▨ Pain at the wrist can be a tendinitis at the insertion points of the wrist flexors and extensors. With tendinitis, flexors and extensors are tender to palpation and painful with isometric challenge. Pain at the wrist can also be a ligament sprain. Sprains are often associated with an acute injury. They are not painful to isometric challenge, but they are painful to passive stretch.

▨ Numbing and tingling in the thumb, index, and middle fingers can be carpal tunnel syndrome. Phalen's test (pressing the dorsum of the hands together in front of the chest for 1 minute) is usually positive.

▨ Aching and stiffness in the thumb or fingers can be OA. With OA, there is a loss of normal joint play, and thickened and tender joint capsule and collateral ligaments.

COMMON DYSFUNCTIONS AND INJURIES OF THE ELBOW, FOREARM, WRIST, AND HAND

LATERAL EPICONDYLITIS (TENNIS ELBOW)/EXTENSOR TENDINOPATHY

▨ **Causes:** Lateral epicondylitis, or tennis elbow, is considered an acute manifestation of a chronic condition. The acute episode is a tenoperiosteal tear of the wrist extensors, most commonly the ECRB. The chronic problem is a degenerative disorder caused by tissue fatigue from repetitive gripping. Tennis players, musicians, massage therapists, and carpenters are susceptible to overuse of gripping motions.

▨ **Symptoms:** A gradual or intermittent mild ache often develops insidiously. Usually, the most tender area is at the anterior portion of the lateral epicondyle at the tenoperiosteal junction of the wrist extensors, particularly the ECRB. The client might also feel pain in the body of the tendon over the radial head or at the musculotendinous junction of the extensors several inches distal to the radial head. The ache can increase to severe pain and progress down the back of the forearm to the wrist and hand.

▨ **Signs:** Clients experience increased pain with gripping motions and resisted wrist extension. They also experience pain on resisted extension of the middle finger, with their elbow extended. Pain

could occur with passive flexion of the wrist and with pronation of the forearm as the ECRB is stretched over the proximal radial head, making the muscle susceptible to injury.

▨ **Treatment:** For **acute** extensor tendinitis (tennis elbow), perform METs #4 and #5 to help reduce the swelling and pain and decrease muscle tension and tenderness. Next, perform Level I, third series, of gentle STM strokes, with emphasis on the ECRB. Palpate the area to assess for hypertonicity and tenderness and perform MET and STM as indicated. For **chronic** extensor tendinopathy, perform PIR MET #5 to lengthen the ECRB and ECRL. Perform Level I, second series, and Level II, first series, at the myotendinous and tenoperiosteal junctions of the extensor muscles to dissolve adhesions. Finally, mobilize the elbow, Level II, sixth series, to help normalize joint play and induce normal neurological function.

MEDIAL EPICONDYLITIS (GOLFER'S ELBOW)/FLEXOR TENDINOPATHY

▨ **Causes:** Repetitive wrist flexion and pronation (e.g. golfing, throwing, and gripping) can lead to medial epicondylitis. This condition is common to computer workers, massage therapists, carpenters, golfers, and tennis players.

▨ **Symptoms:** Medial epicondylitis symptoms are pain at the medial side of the elbow at the tenoperiosteal junction of the pronator teres, pain at the flexor carpi radialis on the anterior medial epicondyle of the humerus, and possible pain at the musculotendinous junction of flexors just distal to the medial epicondyle. Usually, this condition has little radiation, but it can involve an ulnar nerve entrapment.

▨ **Signs:** Clients experience painful resisted wrist flexion with the elbow in extension and supination. Pain might be elicited on resisted pronation, implicating pronator teres.

▨ **Treatment:** For **acute** flexor tendinitis, perform METs for the flexors of the wrist and fingers and for the pronators (METs #7, #8, and #9) to help reduce the swelling and pain and to decrease muscle tension and tenderness. Next, perform Level I, third series, of gentle STM strokes, with emphasis on the flexors and pronators. Palpate the area to assess for hypertonicity and tenderness, and perform MET and STM as indicated. For **chronic** flexor tendinopathy, perform PIR MET for the flexors of the wrist and fingers and for the pronators (METs #7, #8 and #9). Perform Level I, first series, and Level II, second series, at the myotendinous and tenoperiosteal junctions of the flexor muscles to dissolve adhesions. Finally, mobilize the elbow, Level II, sixth series, to help normalize joint play and induce normal neurological function.

CUBITAL TUNNEL SYNDROME (ENTRAPMENT OF ULNAR NERVE AT ELBOW)

▦ **Causes:** Repetitive elbow flexion, which narrows the cubital tunnel, or sustained elbow flexion, which commonly occurs with sleeping, can cause cubital tunnel syndrome. The ulnar nerve can be entrapped at several locations: at the fascia of the subscapularis (see Chapter 6, "The Shoulder"), at the distal third of the medial arm, and at the cubital tunnel. The ulnar nerve can also be entrapped between the two heads of the flexor carpi ulnaris or at the tunnel of Guyon (see "Wrist").

▦ **Symptoms:** Clients experience pain, tingling, and numbing to the fourth and fifth fingers. They might also experience medial elbow ache, which can extend to the forearm.

▦ **Signs:** Cubital tunnel syndrome signs include weakness of the intrinsic muscles of the hand and wasting of the hypothenar eminence, which is innervated by the ulnar nerve. Digital pressure over the ulnar nerve behind the medial epicondyle, sustained passive flexion of the elbow for 1 minute, or resisted wrist flexion with ulnar deviation reproduces ulnar nerve entrapment symptoms.

▦ **Treatment:** Perform the treatment described above for the flexors of the wrist and fingers and the pronators. Perform CR MET to the flexor carpi ulnaris (MET #8) to reduce swelling, pain, and muscle hypertonicity. In chronic conditions, perform PIR MET (MET #8) to increase the length and extensibility of the fascia forming the cubital tunnel. Then perform Level II, second series of STM strokes, for the fibrous arch (arcuate ligament) of the cubital tunnel. Release the ulnar nerve with gentle, scooping strokes transverse to the line of the nerve.

CARPAL TUNNEL SYNDROME

▦ **Causes:** Carpal tunnel syndrome symptoms are elicited by median nerve compression, which leads to decreased circulation and therefore decreased oxygen. Causes of this condition include overuse of finger flexors (e.g., keyboard work, building trades, and massage therapy), which can cause inflammation and swelling of the tendon sheaths, which can

develop into fibrosis or thickening of the flexor tendon and fibrosis of the transverse carpal ligament. Carpal tunnel syndrome can also occur because of previous injury or other chronic microtrauma, subluxation of the lunate, edema from pregnancy, and OA.

▦ **Symptoms:** Clients experience insidious onset of numbing and tingling in the first three fingers. Symptoms are worse at night or upon rising in the morning and are usually relieved by moving the hand ("shaking it out"). There might be pain at the wrist that can radiate to the elbow.

▦ **Signs:** Pressing the dorsum of the hands together in front of the chest for 1 minute (Phalen's test) reproduces carpal tunnel syndrome symptoms. If flexor tendinitis is an underlying factor, resistive testing of the finger flexors increases symptoms.

▦ **Treatment:** Repeat the protocol described above for flexor tendinitis. To increase the extensibility of the transverse carpal ligament (flexor retinaculum), perform CR MET to the muscles that attach to it: the palmaris longus, the muscles of the thenar and hypothenar eminence, and the flexor carpi ulnaris. Next, perform Level II, fourth series of strokes, which describes treatment for both acute and chronic carpal tunnel syndrome.

LIGAMENTOUS WRIST SPRAINS

▦ **Cause:** A common cause of a wrist sprain is a FOOSH.

▦ **Symptoms:** Pain is usually well localized to the site of injury. The most commonly involved ligaments are the lunocapitate on the dorsal side and the radiolunate on the palmar side.[3]

▦ **Signs:** Passive wrist flexion yielding pain on the dorsum of the wrist typically indicates the lunocapitate ligament. Leaning on an extended wrist is painful for the dorsal lunocapitate and the palmar radiolunate ligaments as well as fixations of the carpal bones.

▦ **Treatment:** The first goal in treating **acute** ligament injuries is to reduce pain, swelling, and muscle guarding as quickly as possible. Perform CR and reciprocal inhibition (RI) METs #8 and #9 for the wrist and finger flexors for the palmar ligaments and METs #5 and #6 for the wrist extensors for the dorsal ligaments. Since the muscles interweave with the ligaments, MET provides a gentle pumping action, which reduces swelling as well as muscle spasms. Perform gentle STM strokes, including the Level I, fourth and fifth series, and Level II, third and fourth series, to provide gentle movement to the ligaments, promoting repair and preventing adhesions. Finally, induce gentle joint mobilization to the wrist (Level II, sixth series). The goals for **chronic** injures are to reduce the adhesions in the ligaments, to reduce protective muscle spasms, and to promote normal joint motion. Perform Level I strokes to scan for areas of restriction and hypertonicity. Use CR MET to reduce excess tightness, and use PIR MET to lengthen shortened muscles. Perform Level II strokes, especially the third and fourth series. Identify areas of fibrosis, and perform back-and-forth and friction strokes on areas of fibrosis. Ligaments often take six weeks to one year to heal.

ABDUCTOR POLLICIS LONGUS AND EXTENSOR POLLICIS BREVIS TENOVAGINITIS (DE QUERVAIN'S TENOVAGINITIS)

- **Causes:** These two tendons are enclosed within the same sheath, and repetitive gripping motions cause the tendons to rub against each other, creating irritation of the synovial lining and leading to inflammation and swelling. The irritation and inflammation create swelling in the acute stage and fibrosis in the chronic stage. Both conditions narrow the tunnel and create pain with movement using the muscles.

- **Symptoms:** A tenovaginitis symptom is the insidious onset of pain at the anatomic "snuffbox," the area over the scaphoid bounded by the tendons of the abductor pollicis longus and the extensor pollicis brevis and the extensor pollicis longus on the other side. Another possible symptom is pain in the distal lateral forearm, especially with gripping activities.

- **Signs:** There are two common tests. In the first test, resisted thumb extension and resisted thumb abduction increase pain. In the second test, have the client flex his or her thumb, wrap his or her fingers around the thumb, and ulnar deviate the wrist (**Finkelstein's test**). A positive test elicits pain at the snuffbox.

- **Treatment:** Perform MET for the brachioradialis (MET #4), abductor pollicis logus, and extensor pollicis brevis. (See Kendall and colleagues[15] for descriptions on how to "muscle test" and perform MET to these muscles.) Perform STM, transverse to the line of the tendons (Level II, third series, third stroke). For acute conditions, the METs and STM are very gentle. For chronic conditions, deeper friction strokes are indicated if you palpate thickened fibrotic tissue.

OSTEOARTHRITIS OF THE THUMB AND FINGERS

- **Causes:** Hereditary factors related to arthritis of the fingers can be a cause of thumb and finger OA. Degenerative arthritis is related to overuse and inflammation leading to capsular fibrosis, loss of the normal synovial fluid, and cartilage degeneration. Often, predisposing factors, such as subluxation or fixation of the normal gliding characteristics of the joint, are present.

- **Symptoms:** OA of the thumb causes pain at the base of the thumb that increases with thumb movements, especially gripping. There is often crepitation and weakness. With degenerative changes, the thumb assumes an adduction deformity. With OA of the fingers, there is pain and loss of ROM at the involved joint.

- **Signs:** With OA of the thumb, clients experience pain on passive abduction of the thumb and painful crepitation in mobilization of the first CMC joint. With OA of the fingers, clients experience pain and limited flexion of the MCP, PIP, and DIP joints, with a thickened feel to the joint capsule and ligaments.

- **Treatment:** The treatment protocol for arthritis of the hand is twofold: First, we take a global approach that includes treatment for the neck and shoulder to enhance vascular and neurological function to the hand, as well as the entire MET protocol, and Level I and Level II wrist and hand series; second, we focus our treatment on the involved joints and perform MET on the flexors and extensors of the that joint; STM of the muscular attachments, ligaments, and joint capsule of the involved joints; and mobilization of the joints. MET for the finger flexors and extensors helps to stimulate normal joint lubrication by tensing the joint capsule through its attachment to the muscles. STM of the collateral ligaments and joint capsule is important to release adhesions and stimulate the synovial membrane to induce the normal lubrication into the joint (Level I, sixth series, and Level II, fifth series). Joint mobilization induces normal glide of the joint surfaces and stimulates the normal lubrication of the joint.

LESS COMMON DYSFUNCTION AND INJURIES

BICIPITAL TENDINITIS AT THE ELBOW

- **Causes:** Repetitive throwing and repetitive pronation or supination are causes of bicipital tendinitis at the elbow.

▨ **Symptom:** Pain, usually well localized to either the lower myotendinitis junction in the middle of the cubital fossa, just proximal to the elbow crease, or the lower tenoperiosteal junction between the radial tuberosity and ulna, is a bicipital tendinitis symptom.

▨ **Signs:** Clients experience painful resisted elbow flexion with their forearm supinated or resisted supination.

▨ **Treatment:** Perform MET for the biceps (MET #1) and Level II, second series STM strokes, at the above-named sites.

TRICEPS TENDINITIS AT THE ELBOW

▨ **Causes:** Repetitive elbow extension, as in tennis backhand, or repetitive or excessive arm pressing, as in the handstands of gymnastics, causes triceps tendinitis at the elbow.

▨ **Symptom:** Pain at the tenoperiosteal insertion of the olecranon of the elbow is a symptom of triceps tendinitis at the elbow.

▨ **Sign:** Clients experience pain with resisted elbow extension.

▨ **Treatment:** Perform MET for the triceps (MET #1) and STM for the tenoperiosteal attachment on the olecranon.

ENTRAPMENT OF THE MEDIAN NERVE AT THE ELBOW

▨ **Causes:** Repetitive pronation or pronation and flexion of the elbow cause median nerve entrapment at the elbow. The nerve can be entrapped in a fibro-osseous tunnel on the anterior-medial surface of the distal end of the humerus, beneath the edge of the aponeurosis of the biceps (lacertus fibrosis), or between the two heads of the origin of the pronator teres (pronator syndrome).

▨ **Symptoms:** Similar to those of carpal tunnel, symptoms of median nerve entrapment at the elbow are numbing and tingling of the first three fingers.

▨ **Signs:** Symptoms can be aggravated by full passive pronation of the elbow or by digital pressure at the anterior-medial surface of the distal humerus. If entrapment is severe, clients experience a loss of strength when pinching the tip of the thumb to the index finger, called *Froment's sign*.

▨ **Treatment:** Perform MET to the biceps and pronator (METs #1, and #7) to reduce the hypertonicity and to increase the length and extensibility of the connective tissue. Perform manual release of the

nerve with gentle, scooping strokes transverse to the line of the nerve (Level II, second series).

RADIAL TUNNEL SYNDROME (ENTRAPMENT OF RADIAL NERVE AT THE ELBOW)

▨ **Causes:** Repeated pronation, elbow extension, and wrist flexion (wringing motion) or overuse of the extensor muscles can cause radial tunnel syndrome. This condition is found in musicians, tennis and golf players, and massage therapists. The nerve can be entrapped at the anterolateral aspect of the distal humerus as the nerve travels between the brachialis and the brachioradialis, as it passes under the fibrous origin of the ECRB, and as it enters the supinator canal approximately 2 inches distal to the lateral epicondyle under a fibrous arch called the *arcade of Frohse*.[16]

▨ **Symptoms:** Deep, dull ache and paresthesia at the lateral epicondyle and posterior aspect of the proximal forearm are symptoms of radial nerve entrapment. Extensor muscle weakness might also occur.

▨ **Signs:** Clients experience increased pain with resisted supination of the forearm or passive extension and pronation of the elbow and flexion of the wrist. Grip weakness can also occur.

▨ **Treatment:** Perform METs for the extensors of the wrist and fingers (METs #5 and #6), supinator (MET #7), and brachioradialis (MET #4). Perform manual release of the nerve with gentle, scooping strokes transverse to the line of the nerve (Level II, first series).

EXTENSOR CARPI RADIALIS BREVIS AND LONGUS TENDINITIS

▨ **Cause:** Repetitive wrist extension causes ECRB and ECRL tendinitis.

▨ **Symptoms:** Localized pain or a vague deep ache on the dorsum of the hand are symptoms of this condition. The usual sites are the tenoperiosteal junction at the base of the second metacarpal (for ECRL) or the base of the third metacarpal (for ECRB).

▨ **Signs:** Clients experience pain with resisted wrist extension with radial deviation.

▨ **Treatment:** For **acute** conditions, perform CR and RI MET for the ECRB and ECRL (MET #5) to reduce the swelling and pain, and provide gentle stimulation to help realign the fibers. Perform gentle STM along the entire length of the muscle (Level I, second and third series). For **chronic** conditions, perform PIR MET for the extensors of the wrist (MET #5) to lengthen the myofascia and dissolve adhesions. Perform STM for the tenoperiosteal junctions (Level II, third series). Mobilize the wrist to prevent fixations and to help rehydrate the joint (Level II, sixth series).

EXTENSOR CARPI ULNARIS TENDINITIS

- **Causes:** Playing tennis and racquet sports and excessive keyboard work are common causes of extensor carpi ulnaris tendinitis.

- **Symptoms:** Localized pain or a vague deep ache at the ulnar styloid, between the ulna and the triquetral, or at the base of the fifth metacarpal are symptoms of this condition.

- **Signs:** Clients experience pain with resisted ulnar deviation of the wrist and with wrist extension.

- **Treatment:** For **acute** conditions, perform gentle CR or RI MET for the extensor carpi ulnaris, which is the same as described in MET #5, except the wrist is ulnar deviated. Perform STM along the entire length of the muscle to reduce hypertonicity and promote nutritional exchange. For **chronic** conditions, perform PIR MET to lengthen the myofascia (MET #5) and deep back-and-forth strokes across the attachment points (Level II, third series).

FLEXOR CARPI ULNARIS TENDINITIS

- **Cause:** Repetitive wrist flexion, such as excessive keyboard work or massage therapy, causes flexor carpi ulnaris tendinitis.

- **Symptoms:** Localized pain or a vague ache at the tenoperiosteal junction on the pisiform (palmar surface) or at the base of the fifth metacarpal are symptoms of this condition.

- **Sign:** Clients might experience increased pain with resisted wrist flexion with ulnar deviation.

- **Treatment:** For **acute** conditions, perform CR and RI MET for the flexor carpi ulnaris (MET #8) and STM (Level I, first and third series). For **chronic** conditions, perform PIR MET #8 to help lengthen the myofascia and STM at the attachment sites at the elbow and wrist (Level I first series, and Level II second series).

FLEXOR CARPI RADIALIS TENDINITIS

- **Cause:** Repetitive wrist flexion causes flexor carpi radialis tendinitis.

- **Symptoms:** Localized pain or ache at the tenoperiosteal insertion of the palmar surface at the base of the second metacarpal that can radiate to the elbow is a symptom of this condition.

- **Signs:** Clients might experience increased pain with resisted wrist flexion with radial deviation.

- **Treatment:** For **acute** conditions, perform CR and RI MET for the flexor carpi radialis (MET #8) and STM (Level I, first and third series). For **chronic** conditions, perform PIR MET #8 to help lengthen the myofascia and STM at the attachment sites at the elbow and wrist (Level I, first series, and Level II, second series).

ULNAR NERVE COMPRESSION AT THE WRIST (HANDLEBAR PALSY)

- **Causes:** Prolonged pressure on the hypothenar eminence and a FOOSH injury cause ulnar nerve compression at the wrist. The ulnar nerve passes through the tunnel of Guyon, which is formed by the pisohamate ligament between the pisiform and the hook of hamate and can be compressed in the tunnel or be irritated from swelling of the flexor carpi ulnaris at its insertion into the pisiform.

- **Symptoms:** Symptoms include numbing and tingling to the ring and little fingers if the superficial branch is affected or deep, aching pain in the palm of hand if the deep branch is affected.

- **Signs:** Digital pressure over the nerve near the pisiform increases the intensity of symptoms.

- **Treatment:** Perform MET to the flexor carpi ulnaris to release the tension in the pisohamate ligament (MET #8). Perform STM strokes transverse to the ligament, and then perform gentle, scooping strokes perpendicular to the line of the nerve at the tunnel (Level II, fourth series, fifth stroke).

FLEXOR POLLICIS LONGUS TENDINITIS

- **Cause:** Repetitive gripping, such as that done in racquet sports, causes flexor pollicis longus tendinitis.

- **Symptoms:** The symptoms of this condition are a deep ache, most commonly at the thenar eminence as the tendon runs along the extent of the first metacarpal or at the tenoperiosteal insertion on the palmar surface at the base of the distal phalanx.

- **Sign:** Clients experience pain that increases with resisted thumb flexion at the IP joint.

- **Treatment:** Perform MET for the flexor pollicis longus (MET #3), and perform STM at the muscle belly, the myotendinous junctions, and the attachment points in the thenar eminence (Level I, fifth series, Level II, fifth series).

DORSAL AND PALMAR INTEROSSEOUS TENDINITIS

▨ **Cause:** Repetitive fine motor movements of the fingers, such as those done by musicians, cause dorsal and palmar interosseous tendinitis.

▨ **Symptom:** Pain between the metacarpal shafts is a symptom of this condition.

▨ **Signs:** Clients experience pain on resisted abduction (dorsal) or adduction (palmar).

▨ **Treatment:** Perform MET for the interossei, which is resisted abduction and adduction. Perform STM in between the shafts of the metacarpals (Level I, fourth and sixth series).

STENOSING TENOSYNOVITIS OF THE FINGER AND THUMB (TRIGGER FINGER)

▨ **Causes:** Repetitive forceful gripping causes a thickening of the flexor tendon sheath (annular ligament) and/or a nodule to form on the tendons. Hereditary factors can also be a cause.

▨ **Symptom:** The fingers locking in flexion and needing to be passively extended or extended with a snap that can be painful are typical symptoms.

▨ **Sign:** Observation of this above-mentioned snapping is a sign of this type of tenosynovitis.

▨ **Treatment:** This condition can be unresponsive to manual therapies, but treatment can reduce intensity and frequency of symptoms. Perform MET for the flexor tendons of the thumb and fingers (METs #1 and #9). Perform transverse strokes on the tendon, the involved tendon sheath, and the annular ligament that suspends the tendon to the bone (Level I, sixth series, and Level II, fifth series).

ENTRAPMENT NEUROPATHY OF PALMAR DIGITAL NERVE

▨ **Causes:** The interdigital nerves can become entrapped in between the superficial and deep layers of the transverse carpal ligament. The ligaments thicken because of injury or repetitive gripping motions. The hand is typically held in sustained flexion, compressing the metacarpal heads and the nerves.

▨ **Symptoms:** Burning pain in one or more fingers, with either increased or decreased sensation, and cold fingers are symptoms of this condition.

▨ **Signs:** Clients might experience acute tenderness of the palmar surface of the webspace between the metacarpal heads. Hyperextension of the finger can increase pain at this site.

▨ **Treatment:** Perform METs #8 and #9 to release the flexors of the wrist and fingers, as the fascia interweaves with the transverse metacarpal ligament. Then perform gentle, scooping strokes perpendicular to the nerve, in between the heads of the metacarpals (Level I, sixth series).

Assessment of the Elbow, Wrist, and Hand

BACKGROUND

Pain at the elbow is often localized to the lateral and medial epicondyles and usually represents a tendinitis of the muscle attachments at those sites. Examination reveals pain with isometric testing and with passive stretching of the involved muscles. The elbow is also the site of neurologic symptoms referred from C6–C7 nerve root irritation. This pain is deep and gripping and often is present even at rest. Examination findings typically include painless weakness of the wrist extensors and flexors, which would require a referral to a chiropractor or an osteopath.

Pain at the wrist has traumatic and cumulative origins. A FOOSH can sprain the ligaments, as can fracture the distal end of the radius, a common injury. Pain at the wrist is also commonly associated with chronic overuse, such as tendinitis associated with retail clerks, carpenters, and massage therapists. Either of these histories can lead to neurologic symptoms or conditions such as carpal tunnel syndrome. Conditions of traumatic and cumulative origin are fairly easy to assess.

Pain and disability in the hand is one of the most common complaints presented to the therapist. The thumb is one of the most common sites for OA and can lead to great disability. The fingers are also common sites for arthritis of the degenerative and rheumatoid types. The hand is a common site for referral of numbing and tingling from the C6–C8 nerves. Such referral leads to painless weakness, unlike the pain with isometric contraction of an involved musculotendinous unit.

HISTORY QUESTIONS FOR THE CLIENT WHO HAS ELBOW, FOREARM, WRIST, AND HAND PAIN

▨ When does it hurt?
  ☐ Local problems in the elbow, wrist, and hand usually involve pain with use, with some notable exceptions. For example, carpal tunnel and cubital tunnel syndromes cause numbing and tingling at night. Referral of pain from the cervical spine exists independent of movement of the extremity. It is important to realize that a client could have both a local and a referred problem overlapping.

ELBOW

INSPECTION AND OBSERVATION

▨ **Position:** Client must be suitably undressed so that you can observe the skin. Have the client stand in front of you, in the anatomical position (i.e., arms at sides, palms facing forward).

▨ **Observation:** Note the position of the neck and shoulders as well as the elbows, and compare sides. A sustained deviation of the neck could indicate a cervical problem. Note any redness, heat, swelling, scars, or other abnormalities about the elbow. Normally, the forearms have approximately a 10° to 15° lateral deviation relative to the arm; this deviation is called the **carrying angle.** A deviation from the normal side might indicate a previous trauma.

ACTIVE MOVEMENTS

Flexion and Extension

▨ **Position:** Client stands facing you.

▨ **Action:** Instruct the client to follow your movements. First, abduct the arms to 90° with the palms

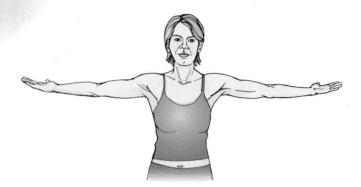

Figure 7-11. Active elbow extension is best observed with the client's arms abducted to 90°.

up to compare elbow extension (Fig. 7-11). Next, place your fingertips on your shoulders to compare elbow flexion (Fig. 7-12).

▨ **Observation:** The normal range for extension is 0° (i.e., fully straight), although you might observe some hyperextension in women and children. Inability to fully extend the elbow often indicates a joint problem. The typical ROM for elbow flexion is 140° to 160°.

Pronation and Supination (Figs. 7-13A and 7-13B)

▨ **Position:** Client stands facing you, with elbows against the body and flexed 90° and with thumb facing up (i.e., with the forearm in neutral).

▨ **Action:** Ask the client to turn his or her palms down fully and then turn both palms up fully.

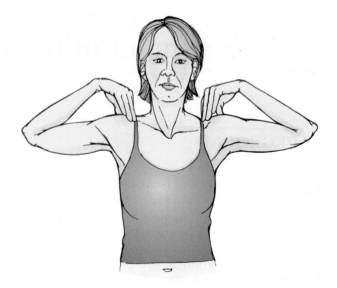

Figure 7-12. Active elbow flexion is done by having the client attempt to touch the shoulders with the fingertips.

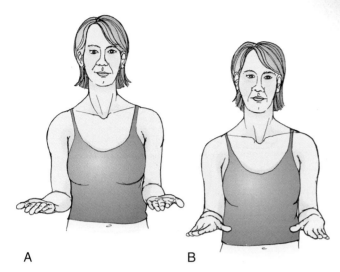

Figure 7-13. A. Active supination. **B.** Active pronation, with the thumbs abducted, which allows for an easy measure of the ROM.

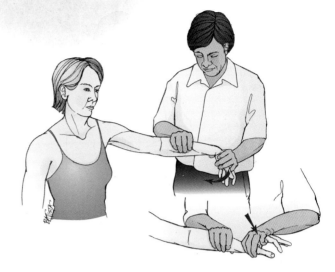

Figure 7-14. *Left and upper right.* One test for lateral epicondylitis is to extend the elbow and then press the wrist into flexion. *Lower right.* A second test for lateral epicondylitis is to have the client resist as you attempt to flex the wrist.

▨ **Observation:** Inability to supinate fully can indicate fixation of the proximal or distal radioulnar joints, shortened forearm flexors, or OA.

PASSIVE AND RESISTED MOVEMENTS

Flexion, Extension, Pronation, and Supination

▨ **Position:** Client is sitting.

▨ **Action:** Place one hand on the elbow and the other hand on the distal forearm. Take the joint to the limit of pain, tissue tension, or both. If it is not painful, move the joint with some overpressure to assess the end feel.

▨ **Observation:** Flexion range is approximately 160°. Normally, there is a soft tissue end feel. If there is decreased motion and a thick, leathery end feel, they indicate fibrosis of the capsule. Decreased flexion is the capsular pattern of the elbow and is an early sign of arthritis. If there is a decreased ROM and a bony end feel, they indicate arthritis. Loss of extension is a common outcome of immobilization after injury, usually due to adaptive shortening of the anterior joint capsule. A mushy end feel during extension indicates swelling in the joint. Inability to supinate fully can indicate a fixation of the proximal or distal radioulnar joints, shortened forearm flexors, or OA.

Tests for Lateral Epicondylitis

▨ **Position:** Client is sitting.

▨ **Action:** Two tests are common for lateral epicondylitis. In the first test, the client's elbow is in

extension, and the forearm is pronated. Press the wrist into flexion and ulnar deviation (Fig. 7-14**A**). In the second test, the client's elbow and wrist are extended, and the forearm is pronated. Have the client resist as you attempt to press the wrist into flexion (Fig. 7-14**B**).

▨ **Observation:** The first test places maximum stretch on the common extensor tendon. The second test isometrically challenges the wrist extensors. These tests are typically painful with lateral epicondylitis. The first position is also used as a PIR MET to lengthen the extensors in a chronically shortened condition.

Tests for Medial Epicondylitis

▨ **Position:** Client is sitting.

▨ **Action:** Two tests are common for medial epicondylitis. In the first test, the client's elbow is extended, and the forearm is supinated. Press the wrist into extension (Fig. 7-15**A**). In the second test, the client's elbow and wrist are extended, and the forearm is supinated. Have the client resist as you attempt to press the wrist into further extension (Fig. 7-15**B**).

▨ **Observation:** The first test places maximum stretch on the common flexor-pronator tendon. The second test isometrically challenges the wrist flexors. These tests are typically painful with medial epicondylitis. The first position is also used as a PIR MET to lengthen the flexors in a chronically shortened condition.

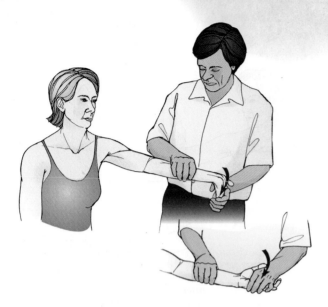

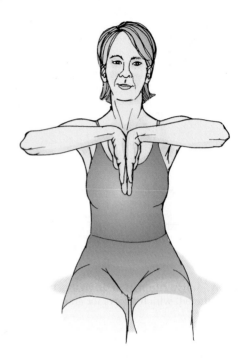

Figure 7-15. *Left and upper right.* One test for medial epicondylitis is to extend the elbow and then passively stretch the wrist into extension. *Lower right.* A second test is to have the client resist as you attempt to press the wrist into extension.

Figure 7-16. Active flexion of the wrist is performed by having the client place the backs of the hands together. This allows easy comparison of both sides. If this position is held for 1 minute, it is called Phalen's test, a test for carpal tunnel syndrome.

WRIST

ACTIVE MOVEMENTS

Flexion

■ **Position:** Client is sitting and is asked to follow your movements.

■ **Action:** Have the client bring the backs of the hands together in front of the chest with the forearms parallel to the floor (Fig. 7-16).

■ **Observation:** Note whether the backs of the hands can touch each other equally and whether the forearms are at the same level. Loss of flexion manifests either as the inability to touch the back of the other hand or as the elbow being higher on the involved side.

Carpal Tunnel Syndrome Test (Phalen's Test)

■ **Position:** The position described above is held for 1 minute or until numbing or tingling arises in the thumb, index finger, and middle fingers. This is called **Phalen's test**; it tests whether there is a compression of the median nerve in the carpal tunnel.

■ **Observation:** The client reports a numbing and tingling in the thumb and the index and middle

fingers that is elicited or worsened if he or she began the test with these symptoms.

Extension

■ **Position:** Client is sitting and asked to follow your movements.

■ **Action:** Have the client bring the palms together in a "prayer position" in front of the chest with the forearms parallel to the floor (Fig. 7-17).

■ **Observation:** Note whether the forearms are at the same level. Loss of extension manifests as the elbow being lower on the involved side. The normal range is 60° to 70°. This tests the joint capsule and ligaments on the palmar surface and is most limited in joint injuries or dysfunction, as extension is the close-packed position for the wrist.

Functional Screening Test for the Wrist

■ **Position:** Client is sitting.

■ **Action:** Have the client rest the hand on the table and attempt to lean his or her weight to that side on the extended wrist.

■ **Observation:** A sharp, localized pain at the dorsum of the wrist usually indicates a joint problem, whether a fixation or subluxation of one of the

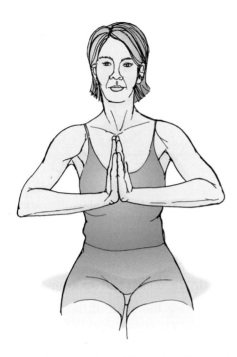

Figure 7-17. Active extension of the wrists. Comparison of both sides.

carpals or an arthritic joint. A positive finding can also indicate a sprain. Inability to perform this motion can indicate a fracture.

PASSIVE MOVEMENTS: NOTE THE RANGE OF MOTION AND THE END FEEL

Flexion, Extension, and Radial or Ulnar Deviation

▨ **Position:** Client is sitting.

▨ **Action:** Stabilize the forearm with one hand, hold the client's hand with the other hand, and move the wrist into the four motions. Note that radial and ulnar deviations are done with the wrist in 0° of flexion and extension.

▨ **Observation:**
  ☐ Flexion tests ligaments on the dorsum of the hand and the joint capsule.
  ☐ Extension tests the joint capsule and ligaments on the palmar surface and is most limited in joint injuries or dysfunction, as extension is the close-packed position for the wrist.
  ☐ Radial deviation tests the ulnar collateral ligament.
  ☐ Ulnar deviation tests the radial collateral ligament and compresses the triangular fibrocartilage complex.

HAND

HAND INSPECTION

▨ **Position:** If the wrist or hand is the area of complaint, have the client sit and place both hands on the thighs. Inspect these areas for swelling and scars, and feel the hands for temperature differences from one side to the other.

▨ **Observation:** Note any nodular swellings on the MCP, PIP, or DIP joints, which can indicate OA. If there is a single or a few joints involved, it is usually a result of OA. If there are multiple swollen joints, primarily at the MCP joints and they are fairly uniform bilaterally, it usually indicates RA. Note if the fingers have an ulnar deviation, which is typical of RA.

THUMB MOVEMENTS

▨ In anatomical position, abduction of the thumb occurs by moving the thumb perpendicular to the palm, and adduction moves it toward the palm. Extension moves the thumb laterally, and flexion moves the thumb across the palm. Opposition is considered full when the tip of the thumb can touch the base of the little finger.

ACTIVE MOVEMENTS

Flexion, Extension, Adduction, Abduction, and Opposition

▨ **Position:** Client is sitting with hands resting on the thighs and is asked to follow your movements.

▨ **Action:** For easy comparison, have the client perform the following movements with both hands: flexion, extension, adduction, abduction, and opposition.

▨ **Observation:** Abduction and extension are painful in capsulitis and OA of the first CMC joint.

Abduction

▨ **Position:** Client is sitting. Have the client reach his or her arms out in front, with forearms supinated and hands together, and have the client place the palms up.

▨ **Action:** Have the client abduct both thumbs to their full range. Compare sides.

▨ **Observation:** A clinically significant motion of the thumb to assess is abduction. An injured or arthritic thumb has decreased abduction, extension, and opposition.

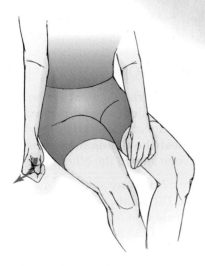

Figure 7-18. Finkelstein's test, to rule out stenosing tenosynovitis of the extensor pollicis brevis and abductor pollicis longus.

Test for Tenovaginitis of the Thumb (Finkelstein's Test)

▨ **Position:** Client is sitting. Have the client flex his or her thumb to the palm and wrap the fingers around the thumb.

▨ **Action:** Have the client cock the wrist into ulnar deviation (Fig. 7-18).

▨ **Observation:** Pain at the radial styloid, anatomical snuffbox, or both indicates the presence of a tenovaginitis of the extensor pollicis brevis and abductor pollicis longus tendons.

PASSIVE MOVEMENTS

Abduction and Extension

▨ **Position:** Client is sitting. Sit next to the client.

▨ **Action:** Stabilize the hand, and gently pull the thumb into abduction and then into extension. Always do the painful side last.

▨ **Observation:** Abduction and extension stretch the anterior capsule and are painful in capsulitis, arthritis, or arthrosis of the first CMC joint. Painful, crepitant limitation of motion indicates OA. The range of passive abduction can be increased with an injury and consequent insufficiency of the ulnar collateral ligament, a common injury in skiers.

Test to Assess Whether a Client Has Osteoarthritis of the Thumb

▨ **Position:** Client is sitting. Sit next to the client. Hold the client's thumb below the CMC joint with your

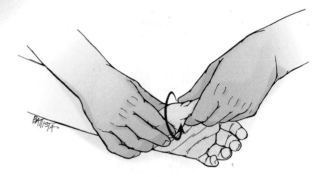

Figure 7-19. To assess the function of the first carpometacarpal joint, hold the joint between your thumb and index finger, and gently circumduct the thumb.

thumb in the distal part of the snuffbox and your index finger in the thenar pad opposite the thumb.

▨ **Action:** Holding the shaft of the thumb with your other hand, gently circumduct the thumb (Fig. 7-19).

▨ **Observation:** Pain and crepitation indicate OA of the first CMC joint. As in the patellar grinding test, this test is also used as a treatment. Gently mobilize the CMC articulation to "clean" the surfaces of calcium spicules that have deposited. Perform this for only a few minutes per session and only within the client's comfortable limits.

FINGERS

Active Movements

Flexion and Extension
▨ **Position:** Client is sitting.

▨ **Action:** First, have the client make a fist and attempt to touch the tips of the fingers to the distal palmar crease (Fig. 7-20). Second, have the client fully extend the fingers.

▨ **Observation:** If the client cannot touch the fingertips to the palm, note the distance from the fingertip to the palm, and reevaluate after your treatment to see whether the client can get closer. Inability to flex fully is caused by joint capsule fibrosis, lumbricals,

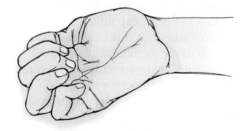

Figure 7-20. Active finger flexion. Notice the ring finger's inability to touch the palm.

or OA of the joint. In the second movement, note whether the fingers can extend past neutral, which is the normal range.

PASSIVE MOVEMENTS

FLEXION OF THE METACARPOPHALANGEAL, PROXIMAL INTERPHALANGEAL, AND DISTAL INTERPHALANGEAL JOINTS

▨ **Position:** Client is sitting.

▨ **Action:** Passively flex the MCP, PIP, and DIP joints, one at a time.

▨ **Observation:** In capsular fibrosis and degenerative joint disease, passive flexion is limited.[13] If passive flexion is limited in the MCP joint, perform the **Bunnel-Littler test** to differentiate whether the restriction is from tight lumbricals and interossei or from a tight joint capsule. The MCP joint is held in slight extension as you attempt to move the PIP into flexion. If the PIP joint is difficult to flex, next move the MCP joint into slight flexion, as this relaxes the intrinsic muscles. If the PIP joint is still tight, the capsule is restricting the movement.

Techniques

GUIDELINES TO APPLYING TECHNIQUES

A thorough discussion of treatment guidelines can be found on p. 86 in Chapter 2. In the method of treatment described in this text, we make two underlying assumptions. The first is that an injury or dysfunction in one structure causes compensations in the entire region of the injury as well as in other areas of the body. Carpal tunnel syndrome, for example, is not an isolated condition but is influenced by forward-head posture, rounded shoulders, and arm and forearm tension. It is important for the therapist to refer to other chapters to learn the protocol for assessment and treatment in each area involved.

The second assumption is that an injury or dysfunction that localizes in one tissue affects many other tissues in the area. A tendinitis in the thumb, for example, involves not only the irritated tendon, but also the muscle belly, thumb joint, ligaments, and joint capsule. It is important for the therapist to assess and treat the surrounding muscles, tendons, ligaments, and joints of the elbow, wrist, and hand in addition to treating the tendinitis of the thumb.

The treatment protocols listed under "Common Dysfunctions and Injuries" typically limit the recommendations to a few specific guidelines regarding that particular condition. It is important to remember that in the clinical setting, it is necessary to take a more global approach and treat the entire person rather than just a local area. The treatments described in this text address all the structures of the region through three techniques: muscle energy technique (MET), soft tissue mobilization (STM), and joint mobilization. These techniques can be applied to every type of elbow, wrist, and hand pain, but the "dose" of the technique varies greatly from slow movements and light pressures for acute conditions to stronger pressures and deeper-amplitude mobilizations for chronic problems. Each aspect of the treatment is also an assessment to determine pain, tenderness, hypertonicity, weakness, and hypomobility or hypermobility. We use the philosophy of treating what we find when we find it. Remember that the goal of treatment is to heal the body, mind, and emotions. Keep your hands soft, keep your touch nurturing, and work only within the comfortable limits of your client so that he or she can completely relax into the treatment.

THE INTENTIONS OF TREATMENT FOR ACUTE CONDITIONS ARE AS FOLLOWS

▨ To stimulate the movement of fluids to reduce edema, increase oxygenation and nutrition, and eliminate waste products.

▨ To maintain as much pain-free joint motion as possible to prevent adhesions and maintain the health of the cartilage, which is dependent on movement for its nutrition.

■ To provide mechanical stimulation to help align healing fibers and stimulate cellular synthesis.

■ To provide neurological input to minimize muscular inhibition and help maintain proprioceptive function.

 *CAUTION: Stretching is **contraindicated** in acute conditions.*

THE INTENTIONS OF TREATMENT FOR CHRONIC CONDITIONS ARE AS FOLLOWS

■ To dissolve adhesions and restore flexibility, length and alignment to the myofascia.

■ To dissolve fibrosis in the ligaments and capsular tissues surrounding the joints.

■ To rehydrate the cartilage and restore mobility and ROM to the joints.

■ To eliminate hypertonicity in short and tight muscles, strengthen weakened muscles, and reestablish the normal firing pattern in dysfunctioning muscles.

■ To restore neurological function by increasing sensory awareness and proprioception.

Clinical examples are described below under "Soft Tissue Mobilization."

MUSCLE ENERGY TECHNIQUE

THERAPEUTIC GOALS OF MUSCLE ENERGY TECHNIQUE (MET)

A thorough discussion of the clinical application of MET can be found on p. 76. The MET techniques described below are organized into one section for teaching purposes. In the clinical setting, the METs and STM techniques are interspersed throughout the session. METs are used for assessment and treatment. A healthy muscle or group of muscles is strong and pain free when isometrically challenged. MET will be painful if there is ischemia or inflammation in the muscles or their associated joints. The muscle will be weak and painless if the muscle is inhibited or the nerve is compromised. During treatment, MET is used as needed. For example, when you find a tight and tender flexor carpi ulnaris, use CR MET to reduce the hypertonicity and tenderness. If the flexor carpi ul-

naris is painful while contracting, perform an RI MET, inducing a neurological relaxation. If the finger extensors are weak and inhibited, first release the tight finger flexors, and then use CR MET to recruit and strengthen the finger extensors.

MET is very effective for an acute, painful elbow, wrist, and hand, but the pressure that is applied must be very light so as not to induce pain. Gentle, pain-free contraction and relaxation of the elbow, wrist, and finger flexors and extensors and related muscles provide a pumping action to reduce swelling, promote the flow of oxygen and nutrition, and eliminate waste products.

THE BASIC THERAPEUTIC INTENTIONS OF MET FOR ACUTE CONDITIONS ARE AS FOLLOWS

■ Provide a gentle pumping action to reduce pain and swelling, promote oxygenation of the tissue, and remove waste products.

■ Reduce muscle spasms.

■ Provide neurological input to mimimize muscular inhibition.

THE BASIC THERAPEUTIC INTENTIONS OF MET FOR CHRONIC CONDITONS ARE AS FOLLOWS

■ Decrease excessive muscle tension.

■ Strengthen muscles.

■ Lengthen connective tissue.

■ Increase joint movement and increase lubrication to the joints.

■ Restore neurological function.

The MET section below shows techniques that are used for most clients. In acute conditions, use METs #1, #2, and #3. For chronic conditions, our goal is to treat the tight muscles before trying to strengthen weak muscles. Remember that the flexors and pronators are typically short and tight, and the extensors and supinators are typically weak. It is important to realize that the muscles in the elbow, wrist, and hand are often weak because of an irritation, injury, or dysfunction of the nerves in the cervical spine. PIR MET, which lengthens muscles and fascia, is used in chronic conditions only and is **contraindicated** for acute conditions. Remember that MET should not be painful. Mild discomfort as the client resists the pressure is normal if the area is irritated or inflamed. Refer to Chapters 5 and 6 for METs for the cervical spine and shoulder.

MUSCLE ENERGY TECHNIQUE FOR ACUTE ELBOW, WRIST, AND HAND PAIN

1. *Contract-Relax Muscle Energy Technique for Acute Elbow Pain*

 Intention: The intention is to contract and relax the muscles of flexion and extension of the elbow. This pumps the waste products and swelling out of the injured area, increases the nutritional exchange, and helps to realign the healing fibers.

> ! *CAUTION: This technique is performed only within pain-free limits. There are beneficial effects with only grams of pressure.*

 Position: Client is supine with the elbow in 90° of flexion and the forearm supinated. Hold the distal forearm in one hand, and place the other hand on the anterior arm to stabilize it (Fig. 7-21).

 Action: Have the client resist as you slowly and gently press the elbow toward flexion for approximately 5 seconds. Relax for a few seconds. Have the client resist as you slowly and gently pull the forearm, attempting to extend the elbow. Relax, and repeat the cycle several times.

2. *Contract-Relax Muscle Energy Technique for Acute Wrist Pain*

 Intention: The intention is to contract and relax the muscles of flexion and extension of the wrist. This pumps the waste products and swelling out of an injured area, increases the nutritional exchange, and helps to realign the healing fibers.

> ! *CAUTION: This technique is performed only within pain-free limits. There are beneficial effects with only grams of pressure.*

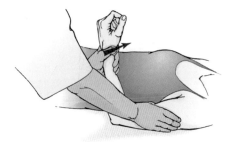

Figure 7-21. CR MET for acute elbow pain.

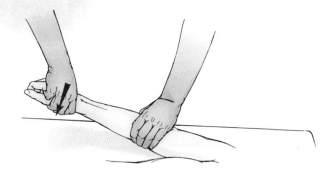

Figure 7-22. CR MET for acute wrist pain.

 Position: Client is supine with the arm resting on the table; the forearm is pronated and slightly elevated. The elbow is slightly flexed, and the wrist and hand are in the position of function (i.e., with the wrist in slight extension and the MCP and IP joints in slight flexion). Place a stabilizing hand on the proximal forearm and the other hand on the dorsum (top) of the wrist (Fig. 7-22).

 Action: Have the client resist as you slowly and gently press the dorsum of the wrist toward flexion for approximately 5 seconds. Relax for a few seconds. Place the fingertips of your working hand on the client's palm, and have the client resist as you slowly and gently pull up on the palm toward wrist extension. Relax, and repeat the cycle several times.

3. *Contract-Relax Muscle Energy Technique for Acute Finger and Thumb Pain*

 Intention: The intention is to contract and relax the fingers and thumb muscles of flexion and extension. This pumps the waste products and swelling out of an injured area, increases the nutritional exchange, and helps to realign the healing fibers.

> ! *CAUTION: This technique is performed only within pain-free limits. There are beneficial effects with only grams of pressure.*

 Position: Client is supine with the arm resting on the table; the forearm is pronated and slightly elevated. The elbow is slightly flexed, and the wrist and hand are in the position of function (i.e., with the wrist in slight extension and the MCP and IP joints in slight flexion). Place a stabilizing hand on the proximal forearm. For the fingers, place the other hand on the dorsum of the fingers. For the thumb, turn the client's hand to face the body, and place your working hand on the dorsum of the client's thumb.

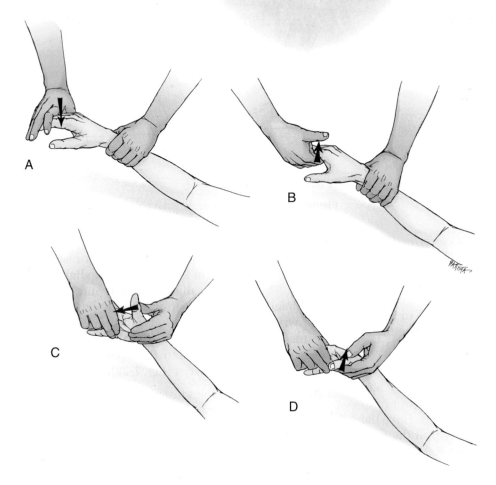

Figure 7-23. **A.** CR MET for finger extension. **B.** CR MET for finger flexion. **C.** CR MET for thumb extension. **D.** CR MET for thumb flexion.

■ **Action:** *For the fingers,* have the client resist as you slowly and gently press the top of the fingers toward flexion for approximately 5 seconds (Fig. 7-23**A**). Relax for a few seconds. Place the fingertips of the working hand on the palmar aspect of the client's fingers, and have the client resist as you slowly and gently pull the fingers up toward finger extension (Fig. 7-23**B**). Relax, and repeat the cycle several times. *For the thumb,* have the client resist as you slowly and gently press the dorsum of the thumb toward flexion (toward the palm) for approximately 5 seconds (Fig. 7-23**C**). Relax for a few seconds. Place the fingertips of the working hand on the palmar aspect of the client's thumb, and have the client resist as you slowly and gently pull the thumb up, toward extension (Fig. 7-23**D**). Relax, and repeat the cycle several times.

MUSCLE ENERGY TECHNIQUE FOR ELBOW, FOREARM, WRIST, AND HAND MUSCLES

4. Contract-Relax Muscle Energy Technique for the Brachioradialis

■ **Intention:** The intention is to reduce the hypertonicity or to facilitate (strengthen) and bring sensory awareness to this muscle. This muscle is often short and tight and contributes to entrapment of the radial nerve.

■ **Position:** Client is supine with the elbow in slight flexion and the forearm in neutral (i.e., with the palm facing the client's body). Place the working hand on the distal forearm (Fig. 7-24).

■ **Action:** Have the client resist as you attempt to extend the elbow for approximately 5 seconds. Relax

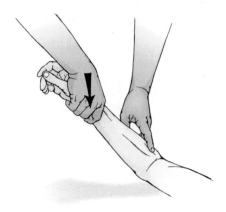

Figure 7-24. CR MET for the brachioradialis.

and repeat several times. For sensory awareness, tap lightly on the muscle belly.

5. Contract-Relax and Postisometric Relaxation Muscle Energy Technique for the Extensor Carpi Radialis Brevis and Longus

▥ **Intention:** The intention is to reduce the hypertonicity, to facilitate (strengthen) and bring sensory awareness, or to lengthen the myofascia of these muscles. These muscles are commonly involved in lateral epicondylitis (tennis elbow) and are part of the myotome of the C6 nerve root.

▥ **Position:** Client is supine with the elbow extended, the forearm pronated and slightly elevated off the table, the wrist in slight extension, and the hand in the position of function. Place the palm of the working hand on the dorsum of the hand.

▥ **Action:** For acute lateral epicondylitis, begin with the elbow in flexion and with light resistance. As symptoms resolve, move the elbow toward greater extension and increase the amount of pressure. For CR MET, have the client resist as you press on the dorsum of the hand toward wrist flexion for approximately 5 seconds (Fig. 7-25**A**). Relax and repeat several times. For PIR MET, move wrist into greater flexion, and have the client resist as you press toward flexion (Fig. 7-25**B**). Relax and repeat the CR–lengthen cycle several times.

▥ **Observation:** Painless weakness can implicate a problem with the C6 nerve root. Pain at the lateral elbow implicates lateral epicondylitis.

6. Contract-Relax Muscle Energy Technique for the Extensor Digitorum, Extensor Indicis, and Extensor Digiti Minimi

▥ **Intention:** The intention is to reduce the hypertonicity, to facilitate (strengthen) and bring sensory awareness, or to lengthen the myofascia of these muscles. The extensor digitorum is also commonly involved in lateral epicondylitis (tennis elbow) and with OA of the fingers, as the extensor hood interweaves with the joint capsule.

▥ **Position:** Client is supine with the elbow extended, the forearm pronated and slightly elevated off the table, the wrist in slight extension, and the fingers extended. Place the palm of the working hand on the dorsum of the fingers (Fig. 7-26).

▥ **Action:** Have the client resist as you press on the dorsum of the fingers toward finger flexion for approximately 5 seconds. Relax and repeat several times.

▥ **Observation:** Painless weakness might implicate a problem with the C7 nerve root.

7. Contract-Relax and Postisometric Relaxation Muscle Energy Technique for the Pronator Teres and Supinator, and to Increase Pronation and Supination

▥ **Intention:** The intention is to reduce the hypertonicity, to facilitate (strengthen), and to lengthen the myofascia of the pronator teres and supinator muscles. These muscles are often short and tight and contribute to entrapment of the median and radial nerves.

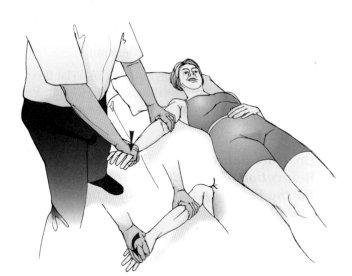

Figure 7-25. A. *Left and upper right.* CR MET for the ECRB and ECRL. **B.** *Bottom and center.* PIR MET for the ECRB and ECRL.

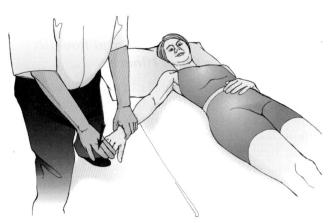

Figure 7-26. CR MET for the extensor digitorum, extensor indicis, and extensor digiti minimi.

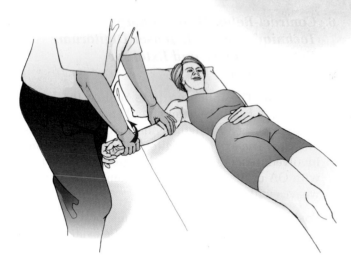

Figure 7-27. CR and PIR MET for the pronator teres.

■ **Position:** Client is supine with the elbow extended and the forearm in neutral (i.e., with the palm facing the client's body). Instruct the client to avoid using the finger flexors (e.g., the client should not make a fist). Place the palm of the working hand on the flexor surface of the distal forearm for the pronator and on the extensor surface for the supinator (Fig. 7-27).

■ **Action:** For CR MET for the pronator, have the client resist as you attempt to turn the forearm into supination for approximately 5 seconds. Relax and repeat several times. For PIR MET, move the forearm into greater supination, and have the client resist as you attempt to turn the forearm into greater supination. Relax, and repeat the CR–lengthen cycle several times. For the supinator, have the client resist as you attempt to turn the forearm into pronation for approximately 5 seconds. For PIR MET, move the forearm into greater pronation, and have the client resist as you attempt to turn the forearm into greater pronation. Relax, and repeat the CR–lengthen cycle several times.

8. Contract-Relax Muscle Energy Technique for the Flexor Carpi Radialis and the Flexor Carpi Ulnaris

■ **Intention:** The intention is to reduce the hypertonicity, to facilitate (strengthen) and bring sensory awareness, or to lengthen the myofascia of these muscles. The flexor carpi ulnaris is typically short and tight, especially in people who overuse the computer, and is commonly involved in compression of the ulnar nerve (cubital tunnel syndrome).

■ **Position:** Client is supine with the elbow flexed, the forearm supinated, the wrist slightly flexed, and the fingers relaxed (to prevent substitution of the finger flexors). For the flexor carpi radialis, place your

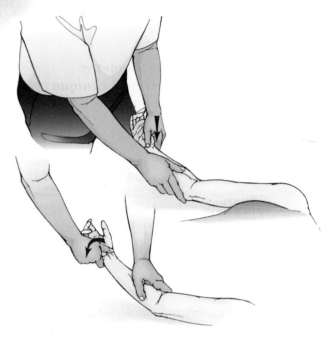

Figure 7-28. A. *Upper.* CR MET for the flexor carpi radialis. **B.** *Lower.* CR MET for the flexor carpi ulnaris.

hand on the thenar eminence. For the flexor carpi ulnaris, place your hand on the hypothenar eminence.

■ **Action:** For the flexor carpi radialis, flex the wrist toward the radial (thumb) side, and have the client resist as you press the wrist toward wrist extension toward the ulnar (pinkie) side (Fig. 7-28**A**). Relax and repeat several times. For the flexor carpi ulnaris, flex the wrist toward the ulnar side, and have the client resist as you press the wrist toward wrist extension toward the radial (thumb) side (Fig. 7-28**B**). The flexor carpi ulnaris MET is also commonly performed with the therapist sitting next to the table with the client's elbow flexed. Have the client bend the pinkie toward the medial elbow and resist as you attempt to pull the hand into extension.

■ **Observation:** Painless weakness of the wrist flexors implicates a problem with the C7 nerve root. Pain at the medial elbow implicates medial epicondylitis.

9. Contract-Relax and Postisometric Relaxation Muscle Energy Technique for the Flexor Digitorum Superficialis and Flexor Digitorum Profundus

■ **Intention:** The intention is to reduce the hypertonicity, to facilitate (strengthen) and bring sensory awareness, or to lengthen the myofascia of these muscles. These flexors are typically short and tight. This MET is used for trigger fingers and OA, as the flexors interweave with the joint capsule.

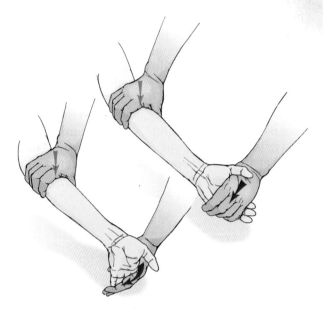

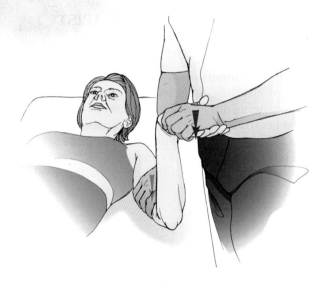

Figure 7-30. MET to increase the wrist extension ROM.

Figure 7-29. A. *Upper and right.* CR MET for the flexor digitorum superficialis and profundus. **B.** *Lower and left.* PIR MET for the flexor digitorum superficialis and profundus.

Position: Client is supine with the elbow extended, the forearm supinated, and the wrist over the edge of the table. Place your fingers on the palmar surface of the fingers, and place your stabilizing hand on the distal forearm.

Action: For CR MET, have the client resist as you press the fingers toward finger extension (Fig. 7-29**A**). Relax, and repeat several times. For PIR MET, after the relaxation phase, press fingers toward greater extension, and have the client resist as you press toward greater finger extension (Fig. 7-29**B**).

MUSCLE ENERGY TECHNIQUE FOR CHRONIC LOSS OF WRIST MOTION

10. *Muscle Energy Technique for Loss of Range of Motion in the Wrist*

Intention: The wrist is typically limited in its ROM after a traumatic injury, such as a Colles' fracture to the distal radius. This MET is focused on increasing joint motion rather than muscle length.

Position: Client is supine with the elbow flexed to 90°. To increase extension, place one hand on the palm of the hand, and bend the wrist into the comfortable limit of extension. To increase flexion, place your hand on the dorsum of the client's hand, and flex the wrist to its comfortable limit.

Action: To increase extension, move the wrist into its comfortable limit of extension. Have the client resist as you press toward greater extension (Fig. 7-30).

Relax, and as the client relaxes, press the wrist into greater extension. Repeat the CR–lengthen cycle several times. To increase flexion, have the client resist as you press toward wrist flexion for approximately 5 seconds. Relax, and as the client relaxes, press the wrist into greater flexion. Repeat the CR–lengthen cycle several times.

SOFT TISSUE MOBILIZATION

BACKGROUND

A thorough discussion of the clinical application of STM can be found on p. 68. In the Hendrickson Method of manual therapy described in this text, the STM movements are called *wave mobilization* and are a combination of joint mobilization and STM performed in rhythmic oscillations with a frequency of 50 to 70 cycles per minute, except in performing brisk transverse friction massage strokes, which can be two to four cycles per second. These mobilizations are presented in a specific sequence, which has been found to achieve the most efficient and effective results. This allows the therapist to "scan" the body to determine areas of tenderness, hypertonicity, and decreased mobility. It is important to "follow the recipe" until you have mastered this work. The techniques described below are divided into two sequences: Level I and Level II. Level I strokes are designed for every client, from acute injury to chronic degeneration, to enhance health and bring the body to optimum performance. Level II strokes are typically applied after Level I strokes and are designed for chronic conditions. Guidelines for treating acute and chronic conditions are listed below.

GUIDELINES FOR THE THERAPIST

Acute

The primary intentions of treatment are to decrease pain and swelling as quickly as possible, maintain as much pain-free joint motion as possible, and induce relaxation. In this method of treatment, the soft tissue is compressed and decompressed in rhythmic cycles. This provides a pumping action, which helps to promote fluid exchange, reducing swelling.

The strokes that are applied to the client who is in acute pain need to be performed with a very gentle touch, a very slow rhythm, and small amplitude. There is no uniform "dose" or depth of treatment. The depth of treatment is based on the client's level of pain. If the soft tissue does not begin to relax, use more METs to help reduce discomfort, swelling, and excessive muscle tension. As was mentioned previously, intersperse your STM work with MET. Remember that **stretching is contraindicated** in acute conditions.

Clinical Example: Acute

Subjective: KK is a 48-year-old, mother of two children who presented to my office complaining of acute left wrist and hand pain. She reported that she fell on her outstretched hand while playing tennis on the morning of her visit. When she entered the treatment room, she was holding her hand because she was in so much pain. She described the pain as an ache in the wrist and distal forearm and a severe pain at the base of the thumb when she tried to move the thumb in any direction.

Objective: Observation revealed normal skin tone without any redness. Palpation revealed a diffuse warmth without any hot spots. Active wrist flexion was limited and elicited a pain at the thenar pad. Active wrist extension was 50% of normal and elicited a pain at the dorsal wrist crease. She was able to move the thumb actively only a few degrees in each direction. Passive motion was limited and painful. Isometric testing was very painful in thumb abduction, eliciting a pain at the base of the thumb. Palpation revealed very spastic and tender thenar muscles.

Assessment: Spastic and tender thenar muscles, with a loss of passive glide at the thumb.

Treatment (Action): Treatment began with RI and CR MET for the wrist and thumb (METs #2 and #3). In the beginning of the treatment, only a few grams of pressure could be applied to the thumb in abduction and extension without eliciting pain. METs for the other directions were used to reduce the swelling, pain, and spasticity of the thenar muscles. Eventually, she was able to resist with moderate pressure in both abduction and extension. Level I STM was performed, especially the third and fourth series of strokes to disperse the inflammation and to promote adequate circulation of oxygen to the area. In performing the strokes, I found that the posterior joint capsule of the thumb and the lateral collateral ligament were extremely tender to the touch. I performed the third, fourth and fifth series of Level II strokes very slowly and gently to mobilize the soft tissue. As I was performing the strokes, I slowly and gently mobilized the thumb to induce normal joint play. I ended the session with gentle mobilizations of the elbow and wrist (Level II, sixth series). At the end of the session, she was able to move her wrist and thumb without pain to about 75% of normal ROM. I discussed natural anti-inflammatories with her and instructed her in active and passive movement for the wrist and thumb.

Plan: I recommended a follow-up visit in a few days. KK returned to our office in five days and stated that she was completely pain free except at the limits of thumb motion or if she attempted a strong grip. Upon examination, she had slight discomfort at the end ranges of both active and passive motion of the thumb. Isometric testing was mildly tender to thumb abduction and extension, eliciting a pain at the base of the thumb. I repeated the treatment described above, concentrating on the snuffbox area for the posterior joint capsule of the thumb and the lateral collateral ligament. The thenar muscles were much less tender and spastic. KK returned to my office one week later, symptom free, with full ROM and normal strength. I told her to call as needed for further treatments, and she was discharged from active care.

Chronic

The typical exam findings in clients with chronic elbow, wrist, and hand problems are short and tight flexors and pronators and weak extensors and supinators. The elbow, wrist, and fingers tend to assume a flexed position. Chronic soft tissue problems often have degenerated soft tissue rather than inflammatory tissue and often have loss of joint play in the involved joints, degenerated joints (osteoarthritis), or both. The pariarticular soft tissue (joint capsule and ligaments) are typically thick and fibrous but can be atrophied, leading to instability in the joint. Degenerated joints lose neurological function, leading to problems with fine motor control. Chronic pain clients often have forward-head posture and rounded shoulders, with the upper crossed syndrome of muscular imbalances. The thumb joint is typically hypomobile, fixated toward the palm, with thick, fibrous ligaments and capsular tissues. The primary goals of treatment depend on the patient. For patients who are hypomobile, with thick fibrous tissue and tight muscles, the treatment goals are to reduce the hypertonicity of the muscles; promote mobility and extensibility in the connective tissue by dissolving the adhesions in the muscles, tendons, ligaments and capsular tissues surrounding the joints; rehydrate the cartilage of the joint; establish normal joint play and ROM in the joints; and restore normal neurological function by stimulating the proprioceptors and reestablishing the normal firing patterns in the muscles. Patients who are unstable need exercise rehabilitation. Our treatments can support their stability by reducing tension in the tight muscles and performing MET to the weak muscles to help reestablish normal firing patterns and rehabilitate the proprioceptors. With chronic conditions in the elbow, wrist, and hand, it is also important to treat the cervical and thoracic spine. Irritation, injury, or dysfunction of the nerves from the cervical spine can cause pain and altered sensations in the elbow, wrist, and hand, as well as tightness or weakness in the muscles of the upper extremity. With chronic conditions, we use stronger pressure on the soft tissue and more vigorous mobilizations on the joints. In the Level II sequence, we add deeper soft tissue work and work on attachment points, using transverse friction strokes if we find fibrosis (thickening). As was mentioned in the "Acute" section above, intersperse your soft tissue work with METs.

Clinical Example: Chronic

Subjective: RK is a 65-year-old, 5'2", 115-pound female administrative assistant who presented to my office with a chief complaint of pain at the left wrist. She stated that she had fractured the wrist when she fell on her outstretched hand approximately 10 weeks prior to her visit. She was diagnosed with a Colles' fracture, a fracture to the distal radius, and surgery was performed to fixate the displaced bone. After surgery, she was referred to physical therapy, but she stated that it was difficult for her to continue because the treatments seemed to make the pain worse. At the time of her visit, she described the pain as aching and burning with any movement of the wrist and said that the pain was sharp with certain motions.

Objective: Upon examination, active ROM was approximately 2°of motion in flexion, extension, supination, pronation, and radial and ulnar deviation. Passive motion was minimally greater than active motion and had a capsular end feel initially, with a bony end feel at the end range. Joint play of the wrist was severely restricted in anterior-to-posterior (A–P) glide. Isometric testing was weak and painful in wrist and finger extension, radial and ulnar deviation, and pronation and supination. Grip strength was 35 pounds on the left and 70 pounds on the right. The patient is right-handed. To palpation, there was a thickened, fibrous feel to the tissue on the dorsum of the wrist. Touching the area of the fracture was emotionally distressing for the patient.

Assessment: Loss of ROM in the wrist, loss of joint play (accessory motion), weakness in the muscles of the left hand, and fibrosis of the soft tissues of the left wrist.

Treatment: My first treatment goal was to reduce the pain and increase the ROM of the wrist. Treatment began with the patient supine, with her elbow at 90° of flexion. CR MET was performed for the wrist flexors and extensors and to increase radial and ulnar deviation, as well as pronation and supination (METs #7 through #10). Light pressures were used. The patient was instructed in how to perform these techniques at home. STM was performed with light scooping strokes at the radiocarpal, midcarpal, and CMC joints (Level II, third and fourth series). There was extreme tenderness over the fracture site, but the patient tolerated light pressure very well. Joint mobilization was performed to help rehydrate the cartilage and increase joint play (Level II, sixth series).

Plan: Recommendations were made for four treatments, with a reevaluation after the fourth visit. RK returned to the office one week later and reported that she did not flare up after our session. Upon examination, there was a slight increase in wrist extension. The same treatment described above was performed. Slight increases in the pressure were applied in the MET and in the STM. On her next visit, she stated that she was feeling a slight decrease in pain. Active ROM was approximately 10°in all ranges. MET, STM, including transverse friction massage, and joint mobilization were performed. The STM concentrated on the soft tissue over the fracture site. After her sixth visit, she stated that the pain was reduced 50% and that she was using the hand more in daily activities. She was seen for 12 visits over a six-month period. At the time of our last visit, she was pain free, and she stated that her hand and wrist were functioning normally. Her ROM was normal except in flexion and supination, which were reduced 25%. Grip strength was 60 pounds on the left and 70 pounds on the right. The patient was discharged from ongoing care and was encouraged to continue with her home exercise program.

Table 7-7 lists some essentials of treatment.

LEVEL I: ELBOW, FOREARM, WRIST, AND HAND

1. Release of the Flexor-Pronator Muscles of the Forearm

- **Anatomy:** The flexors and extensors of the wrist and fingers and the pronator of the forearm (Figs. 7-31**A** and 7-31**B**).

- **Dysfunction:** The flexors of the wrist and fingers are susceptible to both acute injury and chronic dysfunction. Repetitive wrist or finger flexion from sports, such as golf or tennis; gripping such as gardening, massage therapy, or carpentry; and computer work can cause pain at their attachments at the medial epicondyle or at the musculotendinous junction a few inches distally. Chronic overuse fatigues the soft tissue, leading to microfailure. The flexors are typically tight and short. The fascia surrounding the muscles (epimysium) and fascicles (perimysium) develop fibrosis (thickening), creating a restriction of the normal movement in the soft tissue.

Position
- **Therapist Position (TP):** standing

- **Client Position (CP):** supine

Table 7-7	Essentials of Treatment

- Rock the client's body while performing the strokes.
- Shift your weight while performing the strokes.
- Perform the strokes rhythmically.
- Perform the strokes about 50 to 70 cycles per minute.
- Keep your hands and whole body relaxed.

MET
To reduce hypertonicity and discomfort in the soft tissue, perform METs for the pronators (METs #7) and flexors of the wrist and fingers (METs #8 and #9).

Strokes

CAUTION: *These first two strokes are contraindicated for acute conditions in which there is swelling and heat, and for atrophied tissue.*

1. Our first intention is to lengthen the superficial fascia. Using a soft fist, perform a series of long, continuous strokes starting at the wrist and continuing to the elbow (Fig. 7-32). Use a small amount of lotion to avoid skin burn. Keep your wrist in neutral, and let your hand mold gently to the client's arm. Begin with the client's forearm supinated. Repeat over the entire flexor surface of the forearm, and continue the strokes on the flexor surface of the humerus, including the biceps, brachialis, and brachioradialis. Repeat the stroke several times until you feel a relaxation in the soft tissue.

2. Using either a single- or double-thumb technique, perform short, scooping strokes from the midforearm to the elbow, covering the entire flexor surface (Fig. 7-33). Flex your thumb slightly by gently squeezing the client's forearm as you stroke. This allows the thumb joint to stay open and disperses the force through your entire hand. Be careful not to push the arm into the glenoid fossa, which would compress the shoulder. This stroke releases the fascial coverings of the individual muscles and helps to separate the muscles from one another to allow them to slide freely.

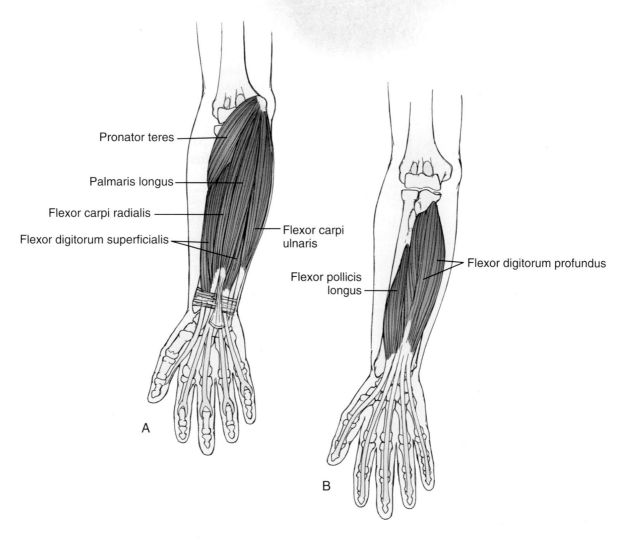

Figure 7-31. Forearm muscle compartments. **A.** Superficial anterior. **B.** Deep anterior.

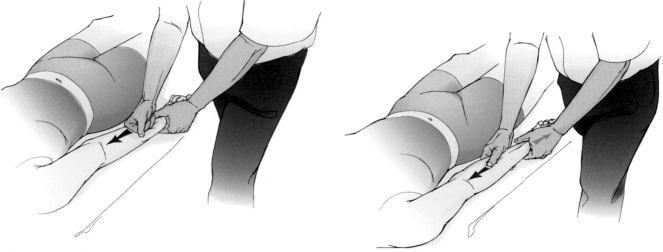

Figure 7-32. Soft fist technique to stretch the antebrachial fascia.

Figure 7-33. Thumb release of the forearm muscles.

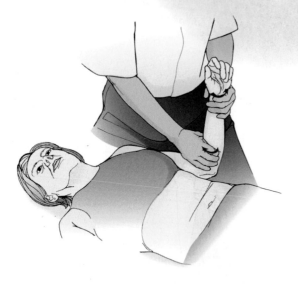

Figure 7-34. Gentle fingertip release of forearm muscles for acute conditions.

3. For acute conditions, flex the elbow to relax the muscles of the forearm, and perform gentle, transverse, scooping strokes with fingertips in the medial-to-lateral (M–L) plane (Fig. 7-34). Cover the entire flexor, radial, and extensor surface scanning for hypertonic and tender tissue.

2. *Release of Sustained Contraction in the Extensor Muscles of the Wrist and Fingers*

▪ **Anatomy:** Extensors of the wrist and fingers, and brachioradialis (Figs. 7-35**A** and 7-35**B**).

▪ **Dysfunction:** Extensors of the wrist and fingers are involved in "tennis elbow," especially the ECRB and ECRL. All of the extensors can become involved in extensor tendinopathy, a chronic degenerative condition of the tendon. If muscles remain

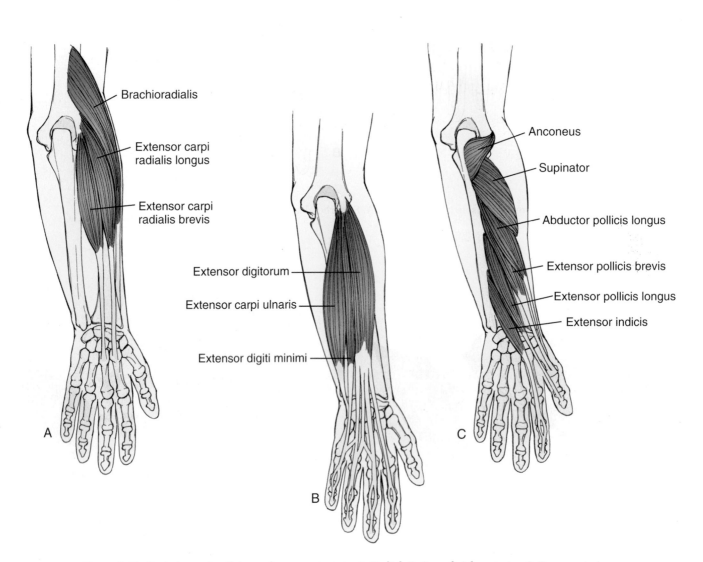

Figure 7-35. Posterior and radial muscle compartments. **A.** Radial. **B.** Superficial posterior. **C.** Deep posterior.

in a sustained contraction, the fascia that covers the muscle, fascicles, and fibers themselves can develop adhesions. The extensors tend to be weak. A tight muscle is often a weak muscle, and it fatigues easily. Sustained contraction also causes acidic buildup from metabolic wastes and decreases oxygen, leading to ischemic pain.

Position
▧ **TP:** Standing

▧ **CP:** Supine

MET
To reduce hypertonicity and discomfort in the soft tissue in this region, perform METs for the brachioradialis and the wrist and finger extensors (METs #4 , #5, and #6).

Strokes
1. We repeat the same two strokes from the first series on the extensor and radial surfaces. First place the client's forearm in pronation. Using a soft fist, perform a series of long, continuous strokes starting at the wrist and continuing to the elbow.
2. Using either a single- or double-thumb technique, perform short, scooping strokes from the midforearm to the elbow, covering the entire extensor surface. Use the same hand position that is shown in Fig. 7-33, and apply it to the extensor and radial surfaces. This releases the fascial coverings of the extensors of the wrist and hand and helps to separate the individual muscles.
3. To release the brachioradialis, place the forearm in neutral (i.e., with the client's thumb pointed toward the ceiling). Using either a single- or double-thumb technique, begin at the radial styloid, and perform longitudinal scooping strokes, continuing to the supracondylar ridge above the elbow (Fig. 7-36). Perform longitudinal and transverse strokes on the ridge. If you are using a single-thumb technique, you may start this series of strokes with the client's elbow in flexion, and as you stroke, move the client's elbow into extension, as this increases the stretch of the fascia.
4. For acute conditions, flex the elbow to relax the muscles and perform gentle, transverse, scooping strokes using the same positions that are illustrated in Fig. 7-34.

3. *Release of the Torsion in the Flexor and the Extensor Muscles*

▧ **Anatomy:** Flexors and extensors of the wrist, fingers, and thumb (Figs. 7-35**A** and 7-35**B** and Figs. 7-37**A** and 7-37**B**), and superficial radial nerve (see Fig. 7-4).

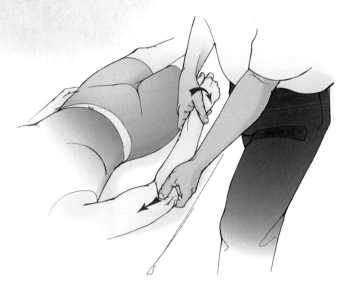

Figure 7-36. Thumb release of the brachioradialis. Extend the client's elbow as you stroke the brachioradialis.

▧ **Dysfunction:** Muscles that undergo sustained contraction develop torsion. Sustained tension on the ventral (anterior) surface pronates the wrist; excessive tension on the dorsal surface tends to supinate the wrist. Typically, the flexors and pronators are tight and short, and the extensors are weak. The superficial radial nerve can become entrapped in the fascia in the distal forearm. The extensor pollicis brevis and abductor pollicis longus cross over the ECRL and ECRB in the distal forearm, a site of potential irritation (called **intersection syndrome**). Transverse strokes dissolve adhesions between the fascicles and fibers. One of the intentions is to broaden the fibers, rehydrate the tissue, and induce mobility deep within the soft tissue.

Position
▧ **TP:** Standing for the first three strokes and sitting for the fourth stroke

▧ **CP:** Supine, with the client's elbow in slight flexion, or sitting

MET
To reduce the hypertonicity and tenderness of the pronators and supinators and to increase the ROM of pronation and supination, perform MET #7.

Strokes
1. The intention of these strokes is to release the torsion in the forearm muscles. If you are on the client's right side, hold the distal forearm with your right hand. Your left thumb should rest on the lateral epicondyle (Fig. 7-38). Perform short, scooping strokes by flexing your left thumb toward your palm. Pronate the forearm with each stroke in

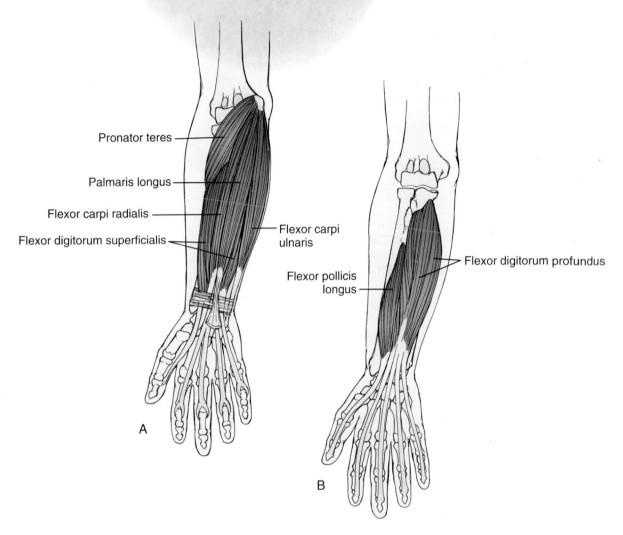

Pronator teres

Palmaris longus

Flexor carpi radialis

Flexor digitorum superficialis

Flexor carpi ulnaris

Flexor pollicis longus

Flexor digitorum profundus

A

B

Figure 7-37. Forearm muscle compartments. **A.** Superficial anterior. **B.** Deep anterior.

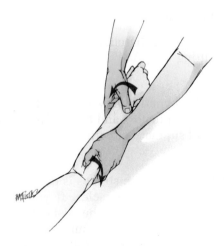

Figure 7-38. Roll the extensors laterally as you pronate the forearm.

an oscillating rhythm of approximately one to two cycles per second. Repeat this motion to cover the entire surface of the dorsal and radial aspects of the forearm. These are gentle strokes and should be comfortable for the client.

As you stroke on the distal third of the dorsum and lateral aspects of the radius, you are releasing the superficial radial nerve and the site of intersection syndrome.

2. Switch hand positions so that your right hand is on the origin of the flexor-pronator group at the medial epicondyle. Your left hand is on the distal aspect of the lateral forearm (Fig. 7-39). Perform a series of short, scooping strokes beginning on the medial epicondyle with the thumb of one hand as you supinate the forearm with the other hand. Continue this series of strokes on the entire flexor

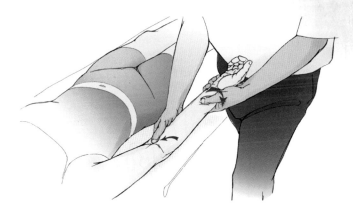

Figure 7-39. Roll the flexors medially as you supinate the forearm.

compartment. Follow the pronator teres to its insertion on the middle of the radius.

3. An alternative method for patients who have bulky forearms is for you to sit on the table and place the patient's forearm on your thigh (Fig. 7-40). Using a double- or braced-thumb technique, roll the flexor muscles laterally. For the extensors, place the client's forearm on the table in pronation. The therapist faces the table and, using double- or braced-thumb technique, performs oscillating scooping strokes to roll the extensors and radial muscles medially.

4. Release of the Dorsum of the Wrist and Fingers and the Webspace of the Thumb

▥ **Anatomy:** The extensor retinaculum; dorsal interossei; adductor pollicis; transverse metacarpal ligament; and extensor aponeurosis (hood), which includes the fascial expansion of the extensor ten-

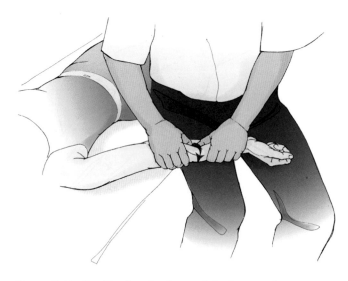

Figure 7-40. Double-thumb release of the forearm flexors.

dons and the lumbricals and interossei on the lateral sides of the MCP and IP joints (Fig. 7-41).

▥ **Dysfunction:** The dorsum of the wrist is the site of thick adhesions after a FOOSH, due to adhesions in the ligaments and capsular tissue. The extensor aponeurosis can become thickened and adhered to the bone at the MCP joints from inflammation due to injury, overuse, or degeneration. The thumb tends to be held is an adducted and flexed position, which shortens the adductor pollicis, the first dorsal interossei, and the intermetacarpal ligament.

Position
▥ **TP:** Standing, or sitting on the table or in a chair

▥ **CP:** Supine

MET
Perform METs for the extensors of the wrist and hand (METs #5 and #6). Use very light CR MET for acute conditions and PIR MET for chronic conditions. You may perform MET for the adductor pollicis by having the client hold the thumb and index fingers together and resist as you attempt to pull them apart.

Strokes
1. Use a soft thumb to perform 1-inch scooping strokes between the metacarpals to release the dorsal interossei (Fig. 7-42). Support the hand from the palmar surface with your fingertips resting between the metacarpals you are working on to wedge the bones apart as you work. Continue these scooping strokes in between the MCP joints.

2. Using thumbs or fingertips, perform back-and-forth strokes in the dorsal-palmar direction on either side of the MCP joint and the sides of each finger and thumb to release the extensor aponeurosis, lumbricals, and interossei. Continue your strokes in the M–L plane on the dorsal surface of each finger to release the extensor aponeurosis (Fig. 7-43).

3. Sit on the table, and place the client's hand on your flexed thigh. Perform a series of short, scooping strokes in the proximal to distal direction in three areas: along the shaft of the thumb; in midbelly, midway between the thumb and index finger; and finally next to the shaft of the index finger (Fig. 7-44). You are releasing the first dorsal interossei, the adductor pollicis, and the intermetacarpal ligament. Place your index finger under the muscle you are working on to add a counterforce. This stroke can also be done as a shearing stroke, with the working finger moving in one direction and the finger underneath moving in the opposite direction as you stroke.

4. Next, release the same area described above with transverse strokes. Begin a series of short, scooping strokes on the dorsal-medial surface of the thumb

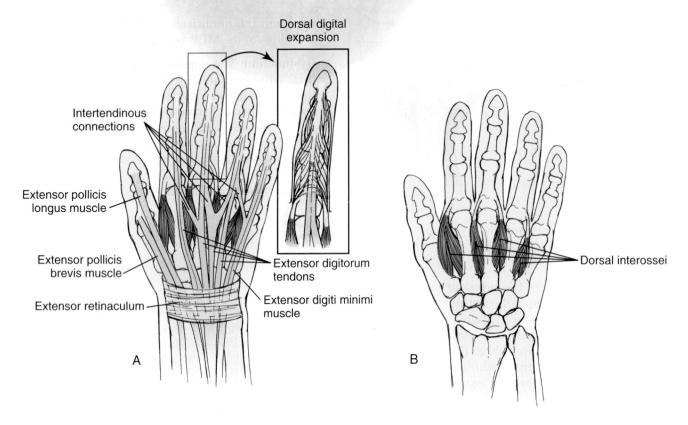

Figure 7-41. **A.** Muscles and tendons of the dorsum of the hand. **B.** Dorsal interossei muscles.

transverse to the shaft, taking the tissue "off the bone."

5. Now stand facing the table, and place a flexed knee on the table. With the client's hand resting on your thigh, perform a series of short, scooping strokes along the dorsal-lateral surface of the index finger. Take the tissue off the bone, toward the thumb (Fig. 7-45).

5. *Release of the Thenar and the Hypothenar Eminences*

■ **Anatomy:** *Thenar muscles*—abductor pollicis brevis; flexor pollicis brevis (superficial and deep heads); adductor pollicis (transverse and oblique heads); opponens pollicis; *hypothenar muscles*—abductor digiti minimi, flexor digiti minimi brevis,

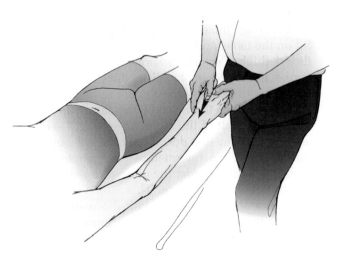

Figure 7-42. Single-thumb release of the dorsal interossei between the metacarpals.

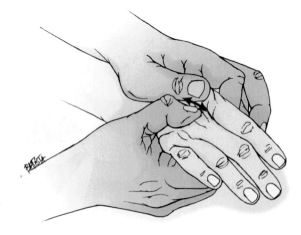

Figure 7-43. Thumbs or fingertip back-and-forth strokes in the dorsal-palmar direction on either side of the MCP joint and sides of each finger and thumb to release the extensor aponeurosis, lumbricals and interossei.

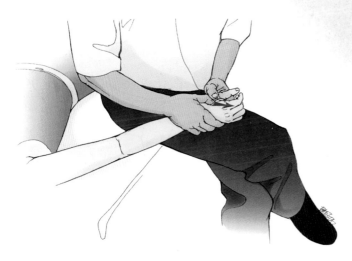

Figure 7-44. Single-thumb technique of longitudinal strokes on the first dorsal interossei, the adductor pollicis, and the intermetacarpal ligament.

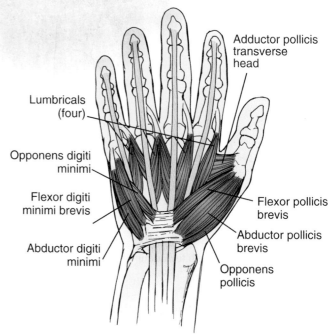

Figure 7-46. Muscles and flexor tendons of the hand.

opponens digiti minimi; palmar aponeurosis; and sesamoids of the thumb (Fig. 7-46).

Dysfunction: The hand tends to move into sustained flexion in chronic dysfunction, after injury or because of degeneraton or arthritis. This rolls the thenar muscles into medial torsion and the hypothenar muscles into a lateral torsion, which folds these muscular pads toward the center of the palm. Sesamoiditis of the thumb can develop after a fall or repetitive gripping motions. The sesamoids tend to misalign toward the palm and need to be mobilized laterally.

Position

TP: Either standing or sitting on the table or in a chair, resting the client's hand on your thigh

CP: Supine

MET

You may perform METs for the thenar eminence, which is described in the section on MET for acute thumb pain (MET #3). The hypothenar is released by having the client resist flexion and opposition of the little finger.

Strokes

1. To release the palmar aponeurosis, place your thumbs on the midline of the palm and your fingers on the dorsum of the hand. Perform a series of slow, spreading strokes with your thumbs to part the midline of the palm. Repeat many times, and cover the entire palm (Fig. 7-47).

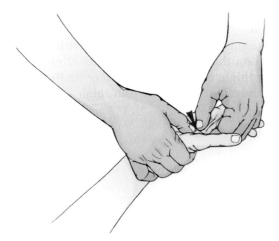

Figure 7-45. Double-thumb release of the first dorsal interossei.

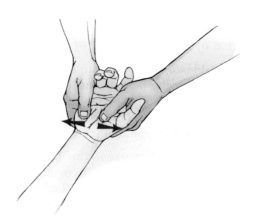

Figure 7-47. Double-thumb release of the palmar interossei.

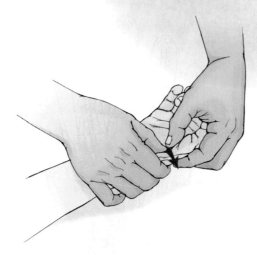

Figure 7-48. Double-thumb technique with scooping strokes on the thenar eminence.

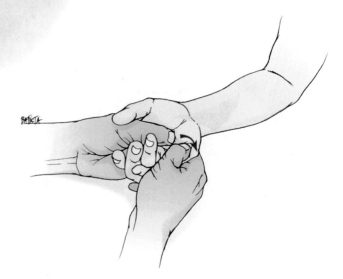

Figure 7-49. Double-thumb technique with scooping strokes on the hypothenar eminence.

2. Sit on the table, and rest your client's hand on your thigh, palm up. Using a double-thumb technique, perform short, scooping strokes in the M–L direction on the thenar eminence (Fig. 7-48). Begin at the proximal portion of the most lateral aspect of the thenar for the opponens pollicis and the abductor pollicis brevis. Continue to the MCP joint. Begin a second line of M–L scooping strokes closer to the palm for some of the fibers of the abductor pollicis brevis and for the superficial head of the flexor pollicis. Again, continue to the MCP joint. Support your strokes by placing your fingertips on the dorsum of the thumb. Rock your body into each stroke, and externally rotate the thumb with each stroke.

3. To release the hypothenar eminence, sit on a chair facing 45° headward. Place the client's hand on your thigh, palm up. Using a double-thumb technique, perform short, scooping strokes to roll the muscles from lateral to medial (Fig. 7-49). Begin at the pisiform, and perform short, scooping strokes with the thumbs for the abductor digiti minimi, flexor digiti minimi, and opponens digiti minimi. Continue to the fifth MCP joint.

6. *Release of Palmar Aspect of Fingers*

- **Anatomy:** Flexor digitorum superficialis and profundus, lumbricals, palmar and dorsal interossei, joint capsule, medial and lateral collateral ligaments, annular ligament, transverse metacarpal ligament, and palmar ligament (Fig. 7-50A–C).

- **Dysfunction:** The flexors of the fingers tend to shorten and become fibrotic with overuse or injury, keeping the fingers in a sustained flexion. The digital synovial sheaths are surrounded by a fibrous sheath and are stabilized to the bone by annular and cruciate ligaments. After injury or overuse, the tendon sheaths can develop adhesions, drying out the synovial membrane. The flexor tendons can also become inhibited in their normal glide through the annular ligament, known as *trigger finger*. The joint capsule and collateral ligaments become fibrotic and shorten as a result of inflammation from overuse, injury, or arthritis, and they hold the joint in a sustained flexion. The collateral ligament's position of dysfunction is to "fall" into an anterior torsion (toward the palm) with the MCP or IP joints becoming fixed toward a sustained flexed position. The membranous portion of the palmar ligament can develop adhesions if the joint is held in a sustained flexion. The palmar digital nerve can misalign to the palmar aspect of each finger (under the finger) from their normal position at the sides of the fingers or can become entrapped between the superficial and deep portions of the metacarpal ligament.

Position
- **TP:** Standing, facing headward with your flexed knee on the table, supporting the client's hand on your thigh, or sitting in a chair or on the table, resting the client's hand on your thigh

- **CP:** Supine

MET
Perform MET for the finger flexors (MET #9).

Strokes
1. Release the tendons of the flexor digitorum superficialis and profundus with strokes in two directions. First, using a single- or double-thumb technique,

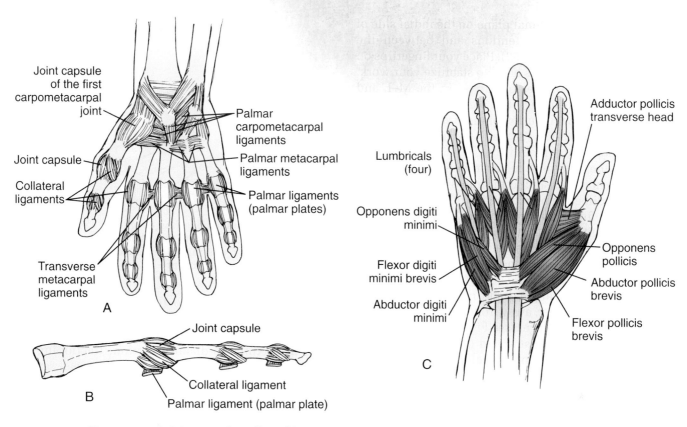

Figure 7-50. A. Joint capsule, collateral ligaments, deep transverse metacarpal ligaments, and palmar ligaments of the MCP and IP joints. **B.** Lateral view of the joint capsule and collateral ligaments of the MCP and IP joints. **C.** Muscles and flexor tendons of the hand.

perform short back-and-forth strokes in the M–L plane transverse to the line of the tendons. Begin at the base of the hand, and continue to the tip of each finger and thumb (Fig. 7-51). Next, perform a series of back-and-forth strokes in the proximal-to-distal plane along the sides of the flexor tendons to re-lease the flexor sheath and the annular ligaments. Concentrate you attention in the areas of the MCP and IP joints (Fig. 7-52).

2. Release the lumbricals and interossei with strokes in two directions. First, perform a series of short back-and-forth strokes with the tip of your thumb

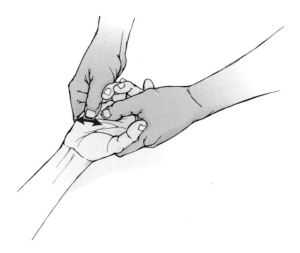

Figure 7-51. Single-thumb technique with transverse strokes on the flexor tendons.

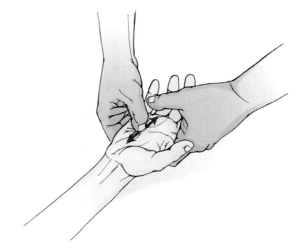

Figure 7-52. Single-thumb release of the lumbricals and palmar interossei.

in the distal to proximal plane on the radial side of the flexor digitorum tendons and between the metacarpals (see Fig. 7-52). Place your fingertips on the back of the client's hand to stabilize your work. Next, perform a series of strokes in the M–L and A–P planes "cleaning" the palmar surface of the MCP joints. The intention of these strokes is to dissolve fibrosis and to "spread" the metacarpals, allowing for greater mobility.

3. Release the transverse metacarpal ligament by performing short back-and-forth strokes in the proximal-to-distal direction on either side of the heads of the second to fifth metacarpals (Fig. 7-53). Release the palmar digital nerve by gently scooping back and forth in the M–L plane between the heads of the metacarpals and scooping away from the midline on each finger. The palmar digital nerve occasionally becomes misaligned and migrates toward the midline of the finger, away from its normal position on the side of the finger (see Fig. 7-53).

4. Release the joint capsule and collateral ligaments of the IP joints by using a single- or double-thumb technique and performing short back-and-forth strokes transverse to the shaft on the medial and lateral sides of the IP joint of each finger and thumb (Fig. 7-54).

5. To help normalize the position of the medial and lateral collateral ligaments, turn the client's hand so that it is resting palm down on your thigh. Place your index finger on the medial or lateral side of the IP joint. Begin with the IP joint in flexion, and lift the ligaments in a palmar-to-dorsal direction as you extend the finger (see Fig. 7-54).

6. To release adhesions in the membranous portion of the palmar plate, first place the lateral portion of

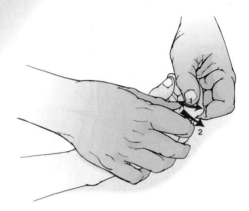

Figure 7-54. Single-thumb technique with (1) a series of back-and-forth strokes transverse to the collateral ligaments and joint capsule and (2) a lifting of the collateral ligaments dorsally as you extend the client's finger.

your index finger into the flexor surface of the client's finger, proximal to the IP or the MCP joint while the joint is flexed. Perform a scooping stroke in a proximal-to-distal direction, tractioning the tissue as you extend the finger. Repeat several times (Fig. 7-55).

LEVEL II: ELBOW, WRIST, AND HAND

1. Release of the Attachments at the Lateral Epicondyle and the Radial Nerve

■ **Anatomy:** Extensor muscles of the wrist and hand, brachioradialis, supinator, and radial nerve (Fig. 7-56).

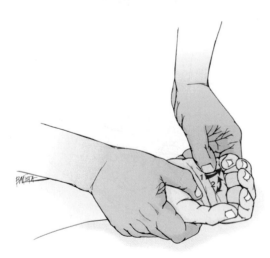

Figure 7-53. Single-thumb technique with (1) short back-and-forth strokes in the proximal to distal plane for the transverse metacarpal ligament and (2) gentle scooping strokes in the M–L place to release the palmar digital nerve.

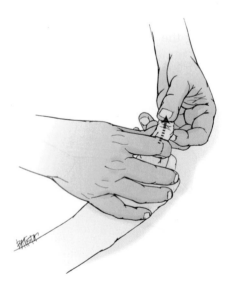

Figure 7-55. To release any adhesions in the membranous portion of the palmar ligament, the lateral portion of the index finger presses into the flexor surface proximal to the IP joint while it is flexed. As you extend the finger, the index finger scoops distally, tractioning the tissue.

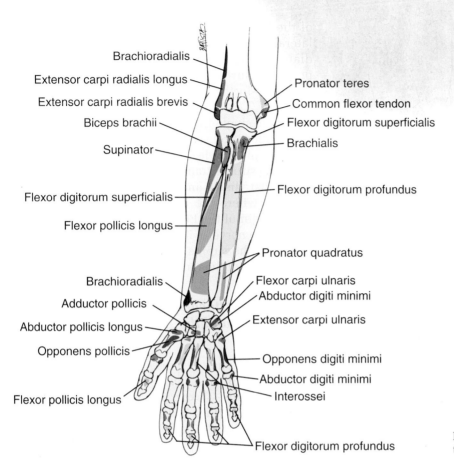

Figure 7-56. Muscle attachments on the anterior forearm, wrist, and hand.

Dysfunction: The lateral epicondyle is the site of tennis elbow, an overuse or acute strain of the origins of the extensor tendons of the wrist and hand, especially the ECRB. Radial tunnel syndrome is an entrapment of the radial nerve at the elbow.

Position
 TP: Standing

 CP: Supine

MET
Perform METs for the extensors of the wrist and fingers (METs #5 and #6), supinator (MET #7), and brachioradialis (MET #4).

Strokes
1. Tuck the client's right arm into your right axilla, and hold the arm with both hands. Your thumbs will be together at the distal third of the lateral arm. Using a double-thumb technique, perform a series of short posterolateral scooping strokes on the distal humerus (Fig. 7-57). You have two intentions: One intention is to release the radial nerve as it

passes between the brachialis and the brachioradialis. The second intention is to release the attachments of the brachioradialis and ECRL from the supracondylar ridge. Begin your strokes just

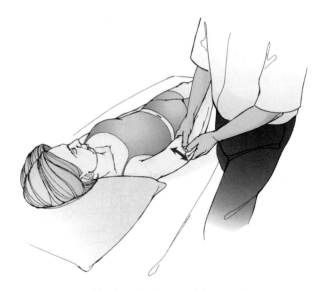

Figure 7-57. Double-thumb release of the attachments on the lateral epicondyle and release of the radial nerve.

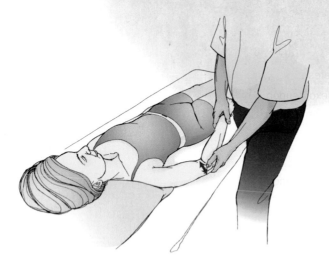

Figure 7-58. Single-thumb release of the attachments on the lateral epicondyle and release of the radial nerve.

lateral to the biceps, and push the biceps medially slightly to make your tissue contact. Have the client's elbow in midflexion, and flex it more as you stroke. Add a slight external rotation of the humerus with each stroke.

2. Holding the distal forearm in one hand, use a single-thumb technique to release the attachments

of the ECRB and common extensor tendon at the lateral epicondyle (Fig. 7-58). Next, release the radial collateral ligament and joint capsule from the posterior surface of the lateral epicondyle with back-and-forth strokes using your flexed index finger.

3. Using the single-thumb technique described in the stroke above, release the radial nerve distal to the lateral epicondyle. Perform a series of gentle, scooping strokes transverse to the nerve in the M–L plane just distal and medial to the lateral epicondyle where the nerve travels through the fibrous origin of the ECRB. Using your index finger, release the nerve as it enters the supinator canal as it pierces the supinator muscle on the posterolateral portion of the radial head.

2. *Release of Attachments at the Medial Epicondyle and the Ulnar and Median Nerves*

▨ **Anatomy:** Pronator teres, flexor carpi radialis, flexor carpi ulnaris, flexor digitorum superficialis and profundus, flexor pollicis longus, palmaris longus, biceps (Fig. 7-59), and ulnar and median nerves (see Figs. 7-2 and 7-3).

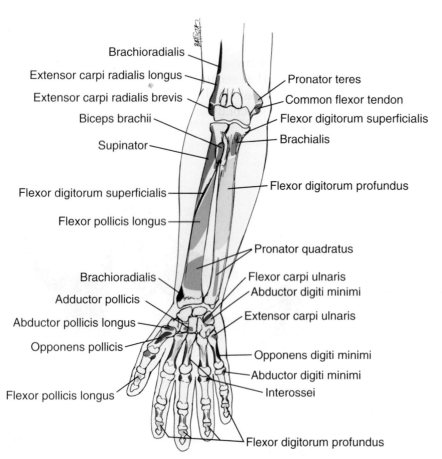

Figure 7-59. Muscle attachments on the anterior forearm, wrist, and hand.

▨ **Dysfunction:** The medial epicondyle is the site of golfer's elbow, which is a strain of the tenoperiosteal junction of the pronator teres and common flexor tendon, and the myotendinous junctions of the wrist and fingers flexors. The flexors and pronator teres are typically short and tight. The ulnar and median nerves can be entrapped in the elbow region.

Position

▨ **TP:** Standing

▨ **CP:** Supine or sitting

MET

Perform METs for the pronators, flexors of the wrist and fingers (METs #7, #8, and #9) and biceps (MET #1).

Strokes

1. Release the biceps attachment to the radial tuberosity by placing your thumb on the biceps tendon at that site. Hold your thumb on the tendon as you oscillate the forearm/arm into small arcs of pronation/medial rotation and supination/lateral rotation to provide transverse friction to the tendon (Fig. 7-60). Keep moving the thumb onto different sites after a few oscillations.
2. To release the flexor pollicis longus, flexor digitorum superficialis, and flexor digitorum profundus attachments, flex the client's elbow to 90°, and have the client's wrist and fingers relaxed to bring the muscles into slack. Facing the table and with the client's forearm in neutral, use your fingertips to perform deep back-and-forth strokes in the M–L plane on the radius and ulna as your supporting hand pronates the forearm (Fig. 7-61).

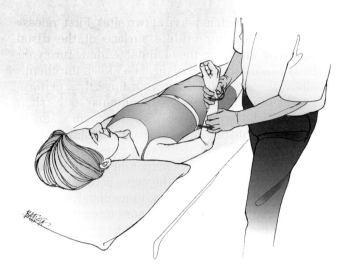

Figure 7-61. Fingertip release of the flexor surface of the forearm. The support hand pronates and supinates the forearm as the fingertips scoop back-and-forth on the soft tissue.

3. Release the ulnar nerve at two sites. At the first site, tuck the client's arm into your axilla, as shown previously. First, use fingertips to scoop in the posterior-to-anterior and the M–L planes at the medial aspect of the distal humerus where the nerve travels through the fibrous expansion of the common flexor tendon (called the *cubital tunnel*). Next, to release the ulnar nerve as it travels through the ulnar and humeral heads of the flexor carpi ulnaris, turn to face the foot of the table, and flex the client's elbow to 90° (Fig. 7-62). Hold the distal forearm with one hand, and use the fingertips of your superior hand to scoop in a posterior-to-anterior, M–L direction two finger widths distal to the medial epicondyle as you pronate the forearm.

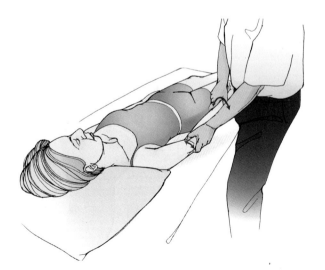

Figure 7-60. Release of the bicipital attachments on the proximal radius.

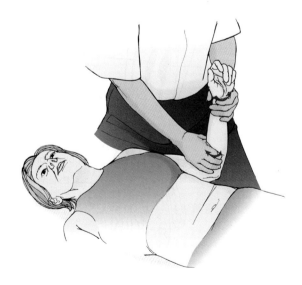

Figure 7-62. Fingertip release of the ulnar nerve at the proximal forearm.

4. Release the median nerve at two sites. First, release it at the anterior middle surface of the distal humerus, medial to the bicipital tendon. Turn your body toward the head of the table. Keep the client's elbow flexed to 90°. Using your fingertips, perform gentle, scooping strokes perpendicular to the shaft of the distal arm as you rock the client's arm in short arcs of internal and external rotation with each stroke. Second, using your fingertips, perform gentle, scooping strokes perpendicular to the shaft of the forearm to release the nerve between the two heads of the pronator teres, immediately distal to the medial epicondyle and more toward the midbody of the muscle (see Fig. 7-61).

3. *Release of the Extensor Attachment Points and the Ligaments on the Dorsum of the Wrist*

■ **Anatomy:** ECRL and ECRB, extensor pollicis longus and brevis, abductor pollicis longus, extensor carpi ulnaris, ulnar and radial collateral ligaments, dorsal ligaments of the wrist, and brachioradialis (Fig. 7-63).

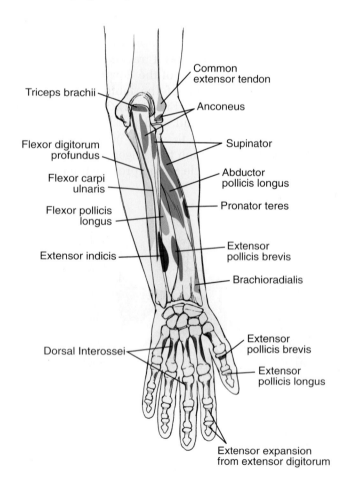

Triceps brachii

Flexor digitorum profundus

Flexor carpi ulnaris

Flexor pollicis longus

Extensor indicis

Dorsal Interossei

Common extensor tendon

Anconeus

Supinator

Abductor pollicis longus

Pronator teres

Extensor pollicis brevis

Brachioradialis

Extensor pollicis brevis

Extensor pollicis longus

Extensor expansion from extensor digitorum

Figure 7-63. Attachments on the posterior surface of the forearm, wrist, and hand.

■ **Dysfunction:** Tenoperiosteal junctions tend to become fibrotic with overuse or injury. The ligaments on the dorsum of the wrist shorten and become fibrotic after a FOOSH injury, predisposing the wrist to arthritis. The lateral side of the distal radius and base of the thumb are sites of a potentially disabling condition called De Quervain's tenosynovitis.

Position
■ **TP:** Either standing, facing headward for strokes on the hand and wrist, or sitting

■ **CP:** Supine

MET
Perform METs for the extensors of the wrist and hand (METs #5 and #6) and the abductor pollicis and extensor pollicis brevis by placing the thumb in a comfortable abducted or extended position and having the client resist while you press on the back of the thumb toward adduction and flexion.

Strokes
1. Use a double- or single-thumb technique and perform back-and-forth strokes in the M–L plane, from the bases of the second and third metacarpals, to release the ECRL and ECRB, and the dorsal ligaments of the wrist underneath (Fig. 7-64). Oscillate the forearm in a radioulnar glide as you perform these strokes.
2. Release the extensor carpi ulnaris and the ulnar collateral ligament by performing short back-and-forth strokes in the M–L plane, from the ulnar styloid to the base of the fifth metacarpal. Cover the dorsum and medial aspect of the wrist. Oscillate the wrist in short arcs of a radioulnar glide as you

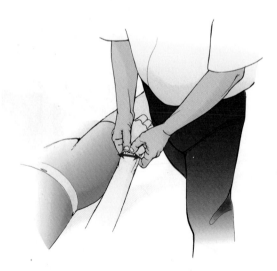

Figure 7-64. Double-thumb release of the extensor attachments at the wrist.

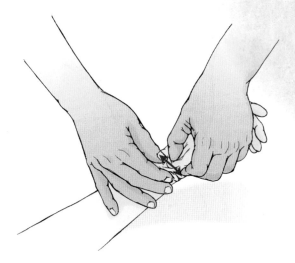

Figure 7-65. Double-thumb release of the extensor pollicis brevis and abductor pollicis longus.

perform these strokes. Using your index finger, perform back-and-forth strokes in the A–P plane between the ulnar styloid and the pisiform to release the ulnar collateral ligament.

3. Perform gentle back-and-forth strokes transverse to the shaft of the radius with a single- or double-

thumb technique or a fingertips technique in the area of the anatomical snuffbox. Turn the client's wrist so that it is in neutral, and perform a series of strokes from the lateral aspect of the radial styloid process to the base of the first metacarpal (Fig. 7-65). You are releasing the extensor pollicis brevis and the abductor pollicis longus—the potential site of tenovaginitis; the brachioradialis attachment; and the radial collateral ligament. Begin another series of strokes at Lister's tubercle, a bony prominence on the dorsum of the radius, to release the extensor pollicis longus, which bends around this bony prominence, and continue to the distal aspect of the dorsum of the thumb.

4. Release of Wrist Flexor Insertion Points and the Median and Ulnar Nerves at the Wrist

▣ **Anatomy:** Flexor carpi radialis, flexor carpi ulnaris, median and ulnar nerves, flexor retinaculum, ulnar collateral ligament, and pisohamate ligament (Fig. 7-66).

▣ **Dysfunction:** The wrist flexors tend to thicken at their insertion points at the wrist as a result of the

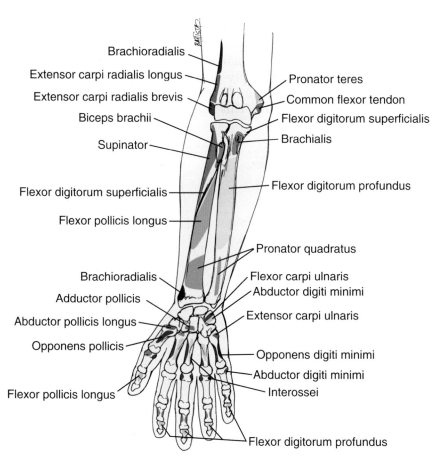

Figure 7-66. Muscle attachments on the anterior forearm, wrist, and hand.

muscles being overworked in gripping, holding, and keyboard work. This can lead to carpal tunnel syndrome, a compression of the median nerve at the wrist. The flexor retinaculum which forms the "roof" over the carpal tunnel, can thicken due to irritation or inflammation of the finger flexors. The ulnar nerve can become entrapped within the tunnel of Guyon. The pisohamate ligament, which forms the roof over the tunnel of Guyon, can thicken because of injury or overuse of the flexor carpi ulnaris.

Position

■ **TP:** Standing

■ **CP:** Supine

MET

You can perform METs for the wrist flexors (MET #8) and for the thenar and hypothenar muscles, which attach to the flexor retinaculum, by folding them toward the center of the palm and having the client resist as you attempt to draw them apart.

Strokes

1. Using a double-thumb technique, perform a series of back-and-forth strokes in the M–L plane from the palmar aspect of the distal radius to the base of the second and the third metacarpals (Fig. 7-67). You are releasing the flexor carpi radialis, the lateral side of the flexor retinaculum, and the base of the thenar pad. Oscillate the wrist in gentle arcs of radial and ulnar glide as you perform these strokes.

2. Using a double-thumb technique, perform a series of back-and-forth strokes in the M–L plane from the ulnar styloid to the pisiform and the fifth

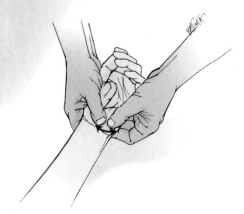

Figure 7-68. Double-thumb release of the flexor carpi ulnaris and the medial aspect of the flexor retinaculum.

metacarpal. You are releasing the flexor carpi ulnaris and the medial aspect of the flexor retinaculum (Fig. 7-68). Oscillate the wrist in gentle arcs of radial and ulnar deviation as you perform these strokes. To release the ulnar collateral ligament, place your index finger just distal to the medial aspect of the ulnar styloid process, and perform back-and-forth strokes in the A–P plane as you rock the wrist in pronation and supination to shear the tissue.

3. To release the carpal tunnel in acute conditions, stretch the flexor retinaculum with a myofascial-holding technique. Place your thumbs at the bases of the thenar and hypothenar eminences (Fig. 7-69). Apply a gentle spreading pressure away from the midline, and hold this for approximately 1 minute. This lengthens the flexor retinaculum.

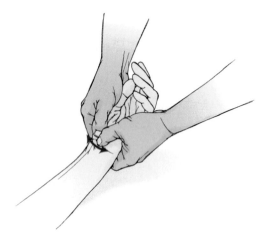

Figure 7-67. Double-thumb release of the attachments of the flexor carpi radialis, the lateral side of the flexor retinaculum, and the muscle attachments on the base of the thenar pad.

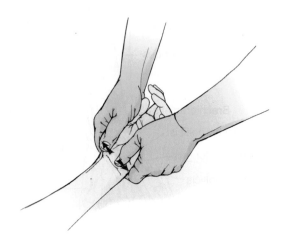

Figure 7-69. Myofascial-holding technique to stretch the flexor retinaculum for acute conditions of carpal tunnel syndrome.

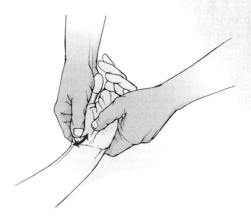

Figure 7-70. Single-thumb release of the attachment points of the flexor retinaculum on the tubercles of the navicular and the trapezium.

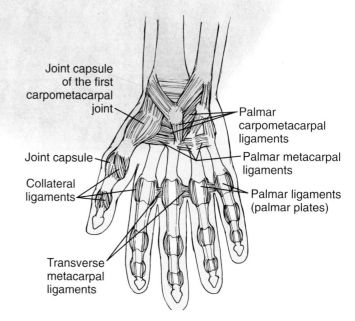

Figure 7-72. Joint capsule, collateral ligaments, deep transverse metacarpal ligaments, and palmar ligaments of the MCP and IP joints.

4. In subacute and chronic carpal tunnel syndrome, perform back-and-forth strokes in an inferior-to-superior plane on the attachments of the transverse carpal ligament at two sites: on the lateral side of the pisiform and hook of the hamate and on the medial side of the tubercles of the navicular and trapezium (Fig. 7-70).
5. Using a single-thumb technique, perform gentle back-and-forth strokes in the inferior-to-superior plane in between the pisiform and the hook of the hamate to release the pisohamate ligament (Fig. 7-71). Next, release the ulnar nerve as it travels under this ligament through the tunnel of Guyon with gentle back-and-forth strokes in the M–L plane between these two bony landmarks.

5. Release of the Joint Capsule and Ligaments of the Thumb and Mobilization of the Thumb

▨ **Anatomy:** Flexor pollicis brevis; flexor pollicis longus; joint capsule of the thumb; flexor pollicis longus; deep head of flexor pollicis brevis; first CMC joint; palmar and dorsal CMC ligaments, which strengthen the joint capsule; and sesamoids of the thumb (Fig. 7-72).

▨ **Dysfunction:** The CMC joint of the thumb is one of the most commonly arthritic joints of the body. The joint capsule thickens, decreasing the normal glide of the articulating surfaces. Aching in the thenar pad can be caused by these degenerative changes.

Position
▨ **TP:** Sitting or standing

▨ **CP:** Supine, with palm up

MET
Perform METs for the muscles of the thumb (MET #3) to help increase the extensibility of the capsular tissues.

Strokes
1. Sit on the table, and place the client's hand on your thigh, palm up. Using a single- or double-thumb

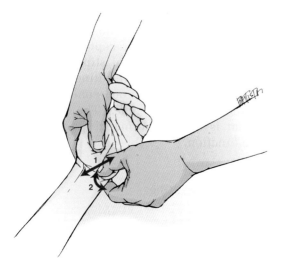

Figure 7-71. (1) Release of the pisohamate ligament. (2) Release the ulnar nerve traveling through the tunnel of Guyon.

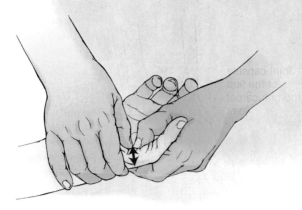

Figure 7-73. Double-thumb release of the deepest layers of the thenar muscles and the anterior joint capsule.

technique, perform scooping strokes in the M–L direction and then back-and-forth strokes in the M–L plane on the thenar pad. You are releasing the deep head of the flexor pollicis brevis, the flexor pollicis longus tendon, and the palmar joint capsule and ligaments (Fig. 7-73). Cover the entire thenar pad, and work until you can penetrate through the muscles to the bone without pain. This can take many sessions.

2. Stand, and place your flexed knee on the table. Rest the client's hand on your thigh, with the forearm in neutral, that is, with the client's thumb toward the ceiling. Using a single- or double-thumb technique, perform back-and-forth strokes in the M–L plane on the dorsal aspect of the joint capsule of the first CMC joint (Fig. 7-74). Oscillate the forearm in pronation and supination while performing these strokes.

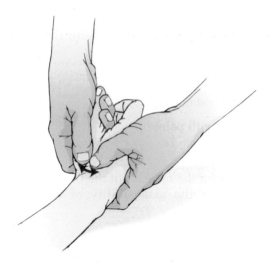

Figure 7-74. Release of the joint capsule of the dorsal surface of the thumb (the first CMC joint).

3. To mobilize the first CMC joint, place your flexed knee on the table, and rest the client's hand on your thigh. Hold the client's thumb at the CMC joint with your thumb in the distal part of the snuffbox, and place your index finger on the thenar pad opposite the thumb. Holding the shaft of the client's thumb with your other hand, gently circumduct the thumb (see Fig. 7-19). Always work within your client's comfortable limit. The client should be able to relax completely into this mobilization. It is normal to hear and feel some grinding (crepitation) if the joint is arthritic. Perform this for only a few minutes each session. This mobilization can help to dissolve calcium spicules on the joint surfaces and can dissolve small deposits on larger spurs on the rims of the joint.

4. To help normalize the position of the sesamoids, place the flexed index finger of your superior hand on the medial side of the palmar aspect of the MCP joint. Circumduct the thumb as in the previous stroke, and as the thumb is moving toward the palm, gently press your finger into the medial side of the client's thumb. As you bring the thumb away from the palm, pull your index finger laterally, mobilizing the sesamoids.

6. *Mobilization of the Elbow, Carpals, Metacarpals, and Phalanges*

▨ **Anatomy:** Joints of the elbow, wrist, and hand (see Fig. 7-1).

▨ **Dysfunction:** Loss of joint play (accessory motion) between the bones can be caused by chronic muscular tension, overuse, or injury. This limitation of the normal gliding of the joint can profoundly affect active ROM. Because of this loss of motion, the joint capsule and ligaments thicken, leading to degeneration of the joint. As the joint loses motion, sensory nerves (mechanoreceptors) from the soft tissue surrounding the joint stimulate reflexes to the surrounding muscles, resulting in either weakness (inhibition) or sustained contraction. This is called the *arthrokinetic reflex*. The intention of the treatment is to help normalize joint motion and muscle function.

Position
▨ **TP:** Standing or sitting

▨ **CP:** Sitting

MET
MET can be used to increase the extensibility of the soft tissue surrounding the joint you want to mobilize. As the myofascia interweaves with the capsular tissues, MET is an effective therapy to warm up the joint,

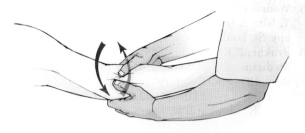

Figure 7-75. Mobilization of the elbow.

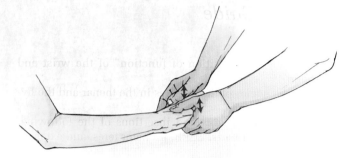

Figure 7-77. A–P glide of the metacarpals. Move the adjacent metacarpals in opposite directions.

stimulate lubrication, and release fascial restrictions that prevent normal glide.

Strokes

1. To mobilize the elbow, grasp the client's elbow by placing your flexed index fingers between the medial and lateral epicondyles and the olecranon while resting your thumbs on the anterior cubital fossa (Fig. 7-75). Tuck the client's distal arm into your axilla. Mobilize the elbow by first flexing the client's elbow slightly as you rock it up and laterally while increasing the pressure of your lateral and medial index fingers in the joint space. Bring the elbow down and in toward the client's body, and repeat these movements several times to normalize the joint capsule function and the articular surfaces. Then have the client lean back to add some traction, and gently bring the elbow into full extension.
2. To release potential calcium deposits from the joint space, bring the client's elbow to full extension, squeeze the joint with your hands, and rock it back-and-forth in an M–L glide.
3. To mobilize the wrist, place the client's forearm in pronation. Wrap your hands around the wrist such that one hand is holding the distal forearm and

your index finger and webspace of the other hand is wrapped around the wrist. Gently oscillate your hands in opposite directions to perform an A–P glide (Fig. 7-76).
4. To perform an A–P glide of the metacarpals, grasp adjacent metacarpals with your thumbs on the dorsal surface and your fingertips underneath. Shear the metacarpals in opposite directions in short, oscillating strokes (Fig. 7-77).
5. To perform an A–P glide of the MCP, PIP, and DIP joints, stabilize the proximal portion of the joint. Grasp the distal portion with your thumb and forefinger, performing the glide to the distal portion of the joint in short, oscillating strokes (Fig. 7-78).
6. To have the client perform self-care for the fingers, instruct the client to wrap his or her entire hand around one finger, place the hand in the pronated position, then move the hand in an M–L, back-and-forth motion to mobilize the IP joints into lateral bending. This helps to clean the lateral rim of the joint, the first site of calcium deposits.

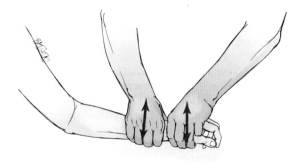

Figure 7-76. Mobilization of the wrist. Hands move in opposite directions.

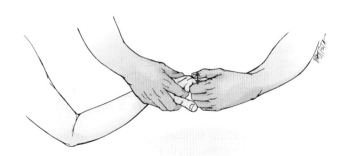

Figure 7-78. A–P glide of the MCP, PIP, and DIP joints.

Study Guide

Level I

1. Describe the "position of function" of the wrist and hand.
2. List the names of the muscles in the thenar and the hypothenar groups.
3. Describe the origins and insertions of the following: flexor carpi ulnaris, ECRB, pronator teres, and extensor carpi ulnaris.
4. Describe the signs and symptoms for the seven common dysfunctions and injuries in the elbow, wrist, and hand.
5. Describe the MET for acute elbow, wrist, and hand pain.
6. Describe the treatment protocol for injured ligaments.
7. Describe the stroke direction to release the thenar and the hypothenar eminences.
8. List the muscles in the five fascial compartments of the forearm.
9. Describe the stroke direction to release the collateral ligaments of the fingers.
10. Describe the implication if your client has painless weakness while attempting to perform MET.

Level II

1. Describe the direction of mobilization in self-care for the fingers.
2. List the origins and insertions of the muscles of the thenar and the hypothenar eminence.
3. Describe the signs and symptoms of the less common injuries and dysfunctions of the elbow, wrist, and hand.
4. Describe the common entrapment sites of the median, radial, and ulnar nerves at the elbow.
5. Describe the two muscles that are involved in De Quervain's tenovaginitis at the wrist, and describe the treatment protocol.
6. Describe the attachment sites for the transverse carpal ligament and the treatment protocol for acute and chronic carpal tunnel syndrome.
7. Describe the common entrapment sites of the median and ulnar nerves at the wrist.
8. Describe the MET for the muscles of the elbow, wrist, and hand.
9. Describe the mobilizations of the elbow, wrist, and hand.
10. Describe the treatment protocol for degenerative arthritis of the hand.

References

1. Parkes J. Common injuries about the elbow in sports. In Scott WN, Nisonson B, Nicholas J (eds): Principles of Sports Medicine. Baltimore: Williams & Wilkins, 1984, pp 140–155.
2. Garrick J, Webb D. Sports Injuries, 2nd ed. Philadelphia: WB Saunders, 1999.
3. Szabo R, Madison M. Carpal tunnel syndrome. Orthop Clin North Am 1992;23:103–109.
4. Hertling D, Kessler R. Management of Common Musculoskeletal Disorders, 4th ed. Baltimore: Lippincott Williams & Wilkins, 2006.
5. Wadsworth C. The wrist and hand. In Malone T, McPoil T, Nitz A (eds): Orthopedic and Sports Physical Therapy. St. Louis: Mosby, 1997, pp 327–378.
6. Brukner P, Khan K, Kibler WB, Murrel G. Clinical Sports Medicine, 3rd ed. Sydney: McGraw-Hill, 2006.
7. Reid DC. Sports Injury and Assessment. New York: Churchill Livingstone, 1992.
8. Frick H, Leonhardt H, Starck D. Human Anatomy, vol. 1. New York: Thieme Medical, 1991.
9. Levangie P, Norkin C. Joint Structure and Function, 3rd ed. Philadelphia: FA Davis, 2001, pp 226–250.
10. Oatis CA. Kinesiology: The Mechanics and Pathomechanics of Human Movement. Philadelphia: Lippincott Williams & Wilkins, 2004.
11. Pecina M, Krmpotic-Nemainic J, Markiewitz A. Tunnel Syndromes. Boca Raton, FL: CRC Press, 1991.
12. McRae R. Clinical Orthopedic Examination, 2nd ed. Edinburgh: Churchill Livingstone, 1983.
13. Posner M. Wrist injuries. In Scott WN, Nisonson B, Nicholas J (eds): Principles of Sports Medicine. Baltimore: Williams & Wilkins, 1984, pp 156–177.
14. Cailliet R. Hand Pain and Impairment, 4th ed. Philadelphia: FA Davis, 1994.
15. Kendall F, McCreary E, Provance P, Rodgers, M, Romani, W. Muscles: Testing and Function, 5th ed. Baltimore: Lippincott Williams & Wilkins, 2005.
16. Hammer W. Functional Soft Tissue Examination and Treatment by Manual Methods, 2nd ed. Gaithersburg, MD: Aspen, 1999.

Suggested Readings

Cailliet R. Hand Pain and Impairment, 4th ed. Philadelphia: FA Davis, 1994.

Corrigan B, Maitland GD. Practical Orthopaedic Medicine. London: Butterworths, 1983.

Cyriax J, Cyriax P. Illustrated Manual of Orthopedic Medicine. London: Butterworths, 1983.

Garrick J, Webb D. Sports Injuries, 2nd ed. Philadelphia: WB Saunders, 1999.

Greenman PE. Principles of Manual Medicine, 3rd ed. Baltimore: Lippincott Williams & Wilkins, 2003.

Hammer W. Functional Soft Tissue Examination and Treatment by Manual Methods, 2nd ed. Gaithersburg: Aspen, 1999.

Hertling D, Kessler R. Management of Common Musculoskeletal Disorders, 4th ed. Baltimore: Lippincott Williams & Wilkins, 2006.

Hoppenfeld S. Physical Examination of the Spine and Extremities. New York: Appleton-Century-Crofts, 1976.

Levangie P, Norkin C. Joint Structure and Function, 3rd ed. Philadelphia: FA Davis, 2001

Magee D. Orthopedic Physical Assessment, 3rd ed. Philadelphia: WB Saunders, 1997.

Platzer W. Locomotor System, vol 1, 5th ed. New York: Thieme Medical, 2004.

Wadsworth C. The wrist and hand. In Malone T, McPoil T, Nitz A (eds): Orthopedic and Sports Physical Therapy. St. Louis: Mosby, 1997, pp 327–378.

8

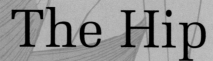

The Hip

D ysfunction, injury, and degeneration of the hip joint are common complaints in all age groups.[1] Hip pain is one of the primary causes of gait impairment in children and in the elderly. Restoration of normal gait is one of the primary goals of therapy, as walking is the most essential activity to maintain health. The hip joint is much more susceptible to degenerative conditions than to traumatic conditions. Degeneration is more common in the elderly, but it is not uncommon in young athletes or performers. Osteoarthritis of the hip results in more significant disability than does osteoarthritis of any other joint.[2]

Anatomy, Function, and Dysfunction of the Hip

GENERAL OVERVIEW

The hip joint is the articulation between the head of the femur and a deep socket in the hip bone called the *acetabulum* (Fig. 8-1). The hip bone is also called the *innominate bone* and is the fusion of three bones: the ilium, ischium, and pubis (see Fig. 8-1). The pelvis includes the two hip bones: the sacrum and coccyx. Twenty-two muscles surround the hip joint, as well as a dense joint capsule, numerous ligaments, and bursae.

BONES AND JOINTS OF THE HIP

HIP BONE AND ACETABULUM

◼ The acetabulum is a cuplike socket in the lateral aspect of the innominate bone of the pelvis for articula-

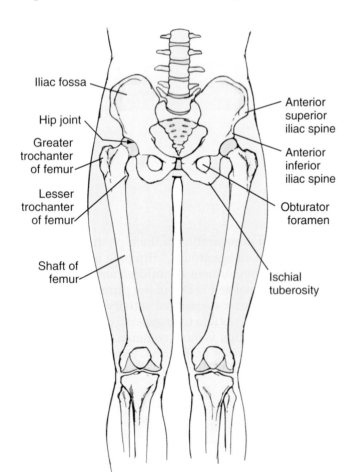

Figure 8-1. Bony landmarks of the hip.

tion with the head of the femur. The socket forms a hemisphere, but the outer lip of the acetabulum is discontinuous, as it has a deep notch on the inferior portion called the *acetabular notch*. The transverse acetabular ligament attaches across the gap, completing the acetabular rim. As in the shoulder, a ring of fibrocartilage called a **labrum** deepens the socket. The acetabulum faces laterally, anteriorly, and inferiorly.

FEMORAL HEAD

◼ **Structure:** The femur is the longest and strongest bone in the body (see Fig. 8-1). The femoral head is its proximal expansion that sits in the acetabulum. It forms approximately two-thirds of a sphere and is completely covered by articular cartilage except for a central portion called the fovea. The primary blood supply to the femoral head is intracapsular (i.e., between the capsule and the bone). There are nerve fibers, including pain receptors in the bone under the cartilage (subchondral bone), that potentially communicate with the mechanoreceptors in the joint capsule and ligaments.[3]

◼ **Function:** The femoral head supports the weight of the trunk and transmits all of the reactive force from the ground up through the leg. While a person stands on one leg and during the support phase of walking, the femoral head sustains as much as 300% of body weight. These forces can increase to 600% of body weight with jumping and carrying weight.

◼ **Dysfunction and injury:** If intracapsular pressure increases because of acute swelling or chronic tightening, it can lead to loss of blood to the femoral head, called *avascular necrosis*, and predisposes the joint to degeneration.[2]

FEMORAL NECK AND SHAFT

◼ **Structure:** The femoral neck is a short piece of bone that connects the femoral head to the shaft. There are also two important bony protuberances on the femur: the greater and lesser trochanters, which serve as attachment sites for muscles.

◼ **Function:** In the standing posture, the acetabulum and the femoral neck are directed anteriorly. The femoral neck dictates the angle at which the head fits into the pelvis. There are two important angles that determine the function of the hip:

□ **Angle of inclination:** The angle of the femoral neck to the femoral shaft. In the adult, it is normally approximately 125°.

□ **Angle of torsion:** The angle of torsion describes the amount of spiral twist between the femoral neck and the condyles. A line through the femoral neck and a line through the condyles form the angle. The angle is normally approximately 15° anterior.

▥ **Dysfunction and injury:** Developmental changes can create variations in the angles of how the neck and shaft fit together. These variations alter the range of motion (ROM) and function of the hip.

□ An increased angle of inclination is called **coxa valga,** and a decreased angle is called **coxa vara.**

□ An increased angle of torsion is called an **anteverted** hip, and the client tends to walk with a toe-in gait. When the client is lying supine on the treatment table, the foot on the side of the anteverted hip may point straight up or toe in slightly, instead of the normal 15° of external rotation. The client has increased internal hip rotation and decreased external hip rotation.

□ A decreased angle of torsion is called a **retroverted** hip, and the client walks with a toe-out gait. When the client is lying supine on the treatment table, the foot on the side of the retroverted hip is turned out excessively. The client has increased external rotation and decreased internal rotation.

□ Loss of bone cells in the femoral neck is called **osteopenia** and is common in the elderly. This condition predisposes the region to fracture.[1]

▥ **Treatment implications:** It is important during the assessment of the hip to determine whether a client has lost medial (internal) rotation. This loss of motion is associated with adhesions in the capsule and predisposes the hip joint to degeneration. During the assessment, always compare both sides because the client might have a normal retroversion in the hip and not a loss of medial rotation. With retroverted hips, both sides have a painless, resilient decrease in medial rotation. Painful hips in the elderly are treated with special precautions. Never vigorously mobilize a geriatric hip because of the potential weakening of the femoral neck owing to osteopenia.

GREATER TROCHANTER OF THE FEMUR

▥ **Structure:** The greater trochanter is a bony projection on the lateral side of the femur where the neck and shaft of the femur meet.

▥ **Function:** It is the site of attachments of muscles that abduct and externally rotate the hip.

LESSER TROCHANTER OF THE FEMUR

▥ **Structure:** The lesser trochanter is a bony projection on the posteromedial side of the junction of the neck and the shaft of the femur.

▥ **Function:** It is the site of the attachment of the iliacus and psoas muscles that are blended into one tendon at their insertion.

HIP JOINT

▥ **Structure:** The hip joint is a synovial, ball-and-socket joint formed by the articulation of the acetabulum of the hip bone and the femoral head. The head of the femur and acetabulum are lined with articular cartilage. The joint is located approximately 1 inch inferior to the inguinal ligament, approximately midway between the anterior superior iliac spine (ASIS) and the pubic symphysis (Fig. 8-2).

▥ **Function:** The primary functions of the hip joint are weight bearing, walking, and stabilizing the trunk to the lower extremity. It has six possible motions: flexion, extension, abduction, adduction, and medial and lateral rotation. The closed-packed position of the joint is extension and medial rotation, and the open-packed position is flexion, lateral rotation, and abduction. The hip joint is stable because two-thirds of the femoral head fits within the acetabulum. This is different from the glenohumeral joint of the shoulder, in which the bones have little contact. This stability sacrifices mobility, and the hip has limited ROM compared with the shoulder.

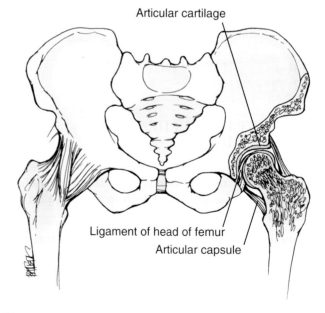

Figure 8-2. Hip joint. Two-thirds of the femur head sits within the acetabulum (socket) of the hip bone.

■ **Dysfunction and injury:** Acute injuries to the hip can result from sports, motor vehicle accidents, or falls from bikes, skis, or horses or in daily life. In an elderly person, a fall can result in fracture of the femoral neck due to senile osteoporosis, resulting in surgical repair. If acute injuries are not treated properly, the hip joint is susceptible to developing degenerative arthritis years after the original injury. Dysfunction and injury usually manifests as pain, limited motion, and gait disturbances. The pain is described as an ache, typically felt deep inside the hip and in the inguinal region, at the midpoint between the ASIS and the pubis. The pain can refer to the greater trochanter, anterior thigh, and knee. The typical position of dysfunction of the hip is for the head of the femur to be fixed in an anterior position, with a loss of posterior glide. This is often due to sustained tension in the flexors and weak extensors.

■ **Treatment implications:** Acute injuries are treated with muscle energy technique (MET), joint mobilization, and soft tissue mobilization (STM). The treatment goals are to reduce the swelling, pain, and muscle guarding and to maintain as much pain-free ROM as possible. In an arthritic or prearthritic hip, assessment typically reveals loss of passive medial rotation, flexion, and adduction with a hard end feel in degeneration of the cartilage and a capsular end feel with fibrosis of the joint capsule. The primary treatment for degeneration is to increase the joint ROM, especially medial rotation. This increase in ROM is accomplished with MET. It is also important to balance the length and strength of the muscles crossing the pelvic region, as minor imbalances in joint alignment repeated over a lifetime of use induce wear and tear on the joint. Loss of posterior glide of the hip is treated with anterior-to-posterior (A–P) joint mobilization.

SOFT TISSUE STRUCTURES OF THE HIP

LIGAMENT OF THE HEAD OF THE FEMUR

■ **Structure:** The ligament of the head of the femur (ligamentum teres) extends from the nonarticular portion of the acetabular notch to the fovea on the femoral head (see Fig. 8-2).

■ **Function:** The ligament forms a sleeve for the ligamentum teres artery that provides nutrition to the femoral head. The ligament is also surrounded by a synovial membrane, so it spreads a layer of synovium to the joint with hip movement. Lauren Berry, RPT, describes this structure as a "wick" that

weeps fluid out of the synovial membrane when the ligament brushes against the acetabulum.

■ **Dysfunction and injury:** The ligament of the head of the femur is one mechanism that provides lubrication and nutrition to the hip joint. Decreased motion in the hip or any joint eventually causes the joint to dry out. The synovial membrane needs to be stimulated by movement to generate and release the synovial fluid. Because most clients do not move their hips in full ROM, the periphery of the cartilage tends to dry out.

■ **Treatment implications:** One goal of treatment is to mobilize the hip to sweep the ligament of the head of the femur across the acetabulum. The rhythmic oscillations of wave mobilization stimulates the secretion of synovial fluid and distributes that lubrication into the cartilage surfaces of the femoral head and the acetabulum.

JOINT CAPSULE AND CAPSULAR LIGAMENTS

■ **Structure:** The joint capsule is a connective tissue sleeve that attaches proximally around the entire circumference of the labrum and distally around the femoral neck. It is thick and strong and has a spiral orientation as it winds around the femur. It tightens in extension, as in standing upright and in internal rotation, and it becomes slack in flexion and external rotation, as in a cross-legged position. In addition to the capsular sleeve that coils around the hip joint, three capsular ligaments—named according to their bony attachments—spiral around the joint (Figs. 8-3 and 8-4).

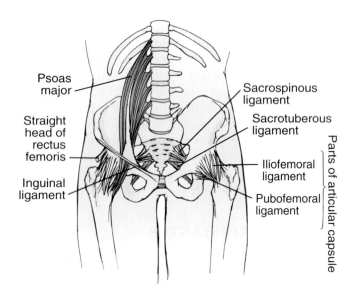

Figure 8-3. Anterior view of the hip joint, showing the joint (articular) capsule that includes the iliofemoral and pubofemoral ligaments and the straight head of the rectus femoris.

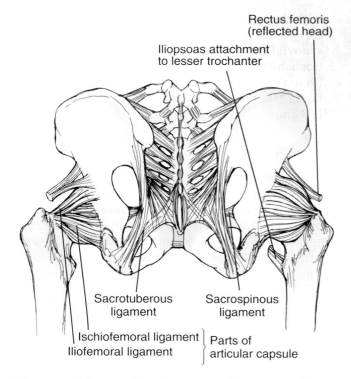

Rectus femoris (reflected head)

Iliopsoas attachment to lesser trochanter

Sacrotuberous ligament

Sacrospinous ligament

Ischiofemoral ligament
Iliofemoral ligament

Parts of articular capsule

Figure 8-4. Joint capsule and ligaments of the posterior hip. The reflected head of the rectus femoris interweaves with the posterior joint capsule.

☐ **Iliofemoral ligament:** It forms an inverted "V," spirals anteriorly and medially, and attaches to the inferior portion of the anterior inferior iliac spine (AIIS) proximally and to the intertrochanteric line inferiorly. It reinforces the capsule anteriorly. It becomes taut in extension, as in standing upright. It is the strongest ligament in the body.[3]

☐ **Pubofemoral ligament:** It attaches to the pubic ramus and the intertrochanteric line. It reinforces the capsule medially. It becomes taut in hip abduction and extension.

☐ **Ischiofemoral ligament:** It forms a spiral weave from the acetabular rim to the inner surface of the greater trochanter. It reinforces the capsule posteriorly. It becomes taut in hip flexion and medial rotation, and it limits adduction when the hip is flexed.[4]

▌ **Function:** The joint capsule and capsular ligaments add passive stability to the joint in standing and moving. The inner layer of the capsule is lined with a synovial membrane that secretes lubricant into the joint with joint movement. The capsule and ligaments provide mechanoreceptor information regarding position, movement, balance, and coordination of the hip. As in all synovial joints, there are reflexive connections between the capsule and the ligaments to the surrounding muscles.

▌ **Dysfunction and injury:** Injuries to the joint capsule and ligaments are common after a traumatic incident or repetitive microtrauma. Inflammation and capsular swelling result, leading to painful limitation of motion. The hip assumes a more flexed, open position, but sustained flexion can lead to contractures of the hip flexors, especially the iliopsoas, and adhesions in the joint capsule and ligaments. Eventually, this shortening leads to degeneration of the joint. One of the first manifestations of degeneration is capsular thickening, assessed by painful loss of passive medial (internal) rotation. The posterior capsule and ischiofemoral ligament thicken and shorten, pulling the joint into external rotation. The joint assumes its more open position (i.e., flexion, abduction, and lateral rotation) and loses its ability to move into medial rotation. Arthrokinetic (regarding movement) and arthrostatic (regarding posture) reflexes are abnormal in degenerating joints.[3] This disturbs normal movement, coordination, balance, and posture, making the joint more vulnerable to further injury.

▌ **Treatment implications:** Therapy for acute capsular swelling is through contract-relax (CR) MET. The muscle contraction causes a tightening or winding of the capsule and ligaments, and the relaxation causes an unwinding of the capsule and ligaments. This winding (tightening) and unwinding (loosening) of the capsule theoretically pumps fluid out of the joint if it is swollen and stimulates the normal secretion of the synovial fluids if the joint has dried out. Therapy for capsular and ligamentous thickening is focused on MET to increase medial rotation. This is followed by MET to increase flexion and adduction. Release of the pectineus, rectus femoris, and gluteus minimus is also critical because they interweave with the capsule.

LABRUM

▌ **Structure and function:** The labrum is a ring of fibrocartilage that surrounds the acetabulum. It functions to deepen the acetabulum and stabilize the hip.[4]

▌ **Dysfunction and injury:** The labrum may be bruised, abraded, or torn from both traumatic events and repetitive microtrauma. A fall on the side of the hip; repetitive flexion during cycling, dance, or martial arts; or weight-bearing stresses due to pelvic imbalances can injure the labrum. Instability of the hip, manifested as excessive ROM, is another source of irritation to the labrum. The instability might be due to prior injury or deconditioning.

▌ **Treatment implications:** The goal of treatment is to help normalize ROM and help to stabilize the joint with balanced muscle function. Passive motion assessment is used to determine ROM. MET is used to

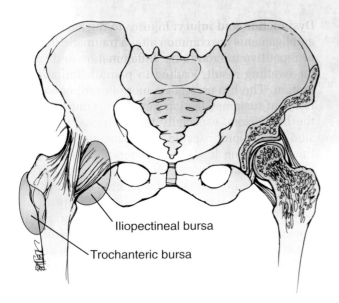

Figure 8-5. Iliopectineal and trochanteric bursae.

assess muscle strength and correct imbalances in muscle function by reducing tension in hypertonic muscles and strengthening inhibited muscles.

BURSAE

- **Structure and function:** A bursa is a synovial-lined sac filled with synovial fluid that functions to decrease friction. Of the many bursae around the hip, only two are commonly involved clinically (Fig. 8-5).
  - ☐ **Iliopectineal:** The iliopectineal bursa is located between the iliopsoas muscle and the joint capsule over the hip joint. The synovial cavity of the hip joint often connects anteriorly with the iliopectineal bursa.
  - ☐ **Trochanteric:** The trochanteric bursa lies between the gluteus maximus and greater trochanter.

- **Dysfunction and injury:** As with all bursae, there are two possibilities of dysfunction and injury. First, the bursa can become inflamed and swell, owing to either a traumatic event or cumulative or repetitive stresses. Second, the bursa can develop adhesions and dry out, decreasing its synovial lubricant. The iliopectineal bursa can become irritated with excessive hip flexion or because of shortened capsular tissue due to degeneration of the hip joint. The trochanteric bursa can become irritated from a fall on the side of the hip or with repetitive stresses, such as running, tennis, or cycling. Lauren Berry, RPT, taught that the positional dysfunction of the bursae of the hip is that they migrate inferiorly.

- **Treatment implications:** The bursae need to be stroked superiorly, either with slow, gentle strokes to milk the excess fluid out for an acute bursitis or

with deeper strokes in a superior direction to dissolve adhesions and stimulate the secretion of the synovial membrane to rehydrate the bursae. The trochanteric bursa is typically irritated by friction from a short iliotibial band (ITB) and tight tensor fascia lata (TFL). The treatment is to lengthen the ITB and strengthen the gluteus medius.

NERVES

- The **femoral nerve** is a branch of the lumbar plexus that travels through the psoas muscle and enters the anterior thigh through the **femoral triangle,** medial to the iliopsoas. The femoral triangle is defined as the space between the sartorius, adductor longus, and inguinal ligament. The **femoral nerve** innervates the muscles of the anterior thigh (Fig. 8-6).

- The **lateral femoral cutaneous nerve** enters the thigh under the inguinal ligament, approximately one-half inch medial to the ASIS. It supplies innervation to the skin on the lateral thigh (see Fig. 8-6).

- The **genitofemoral nerve** is a branch of the lumbar plexus that travels through the belly of the psoas major and along the medial border of the psoas. It supplies the scrotum in the male, the labia in the female, and the skin over the femoral triangle (see Fig. 8-6).

- The **obturator nerve** is a branch of the lumbar plexus that travels into the medial thigh under the pectineus and then between the adductor muscles. It supplies innervation to the skin on the medial thigh to the knee (Fig. 8-7).

- The **sciatic nerve** travels just posterior to the hip joint and innervates the muscles of the posterior thigh and the muscles of the leg and foot through the posterior tibial and peroneal nerves (Fig. 8-8).

- **Dysfunction and injury:** These nerves can be compressed with sustained muscle contraction, can be entrapped in adhesions resulting from previous inflammation or injury, or can become excessively stretched because of pelvic imbalance. See Chapter 3, "Lumbosacral Spine," for information on nerve root irritation and injury where these nerves originate at the spine.

- **Treatment implications:** STM can effectively release peripheral compression and entrapment of the nerves. These techniques are fully described in the technique section.

MUSCLES

- **Structure:** Twenty-two muscles surround the hip. These muscles can be divided into five groups:
  - ☐ **Flexors:** Iliacus, psoas, rectus femoris, TFL, and sartorius

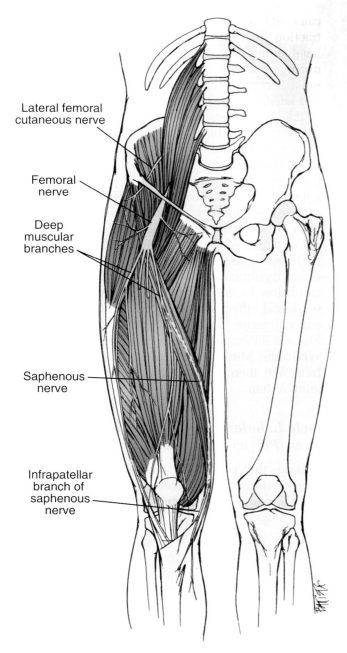

Figure 8-6. Femoral and lateral femoral cutaneous nerves.

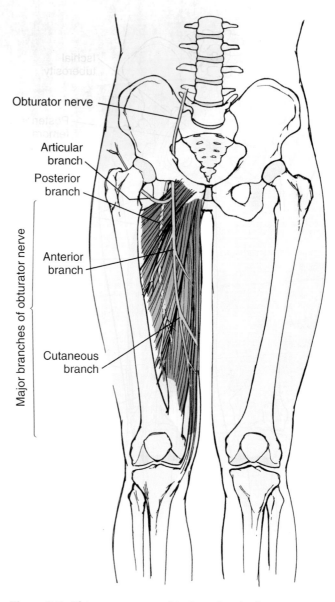

Figure 8-7. Obturator nerve and its branches in the anterior thigh.

□ **Extensors:** Gluteus maximus, semimembranosus, semitendinosus, and biceps femoris
□ **Abductors:** TFL and gluteus medius and minimus
□ **Adductors:** Gracilis; pectineus; and adductor magnus, longus, and brevis
□ **Lateral rotators:** Piriformis, obturator internus and externus, superior and inferior gemelli, and quadratus femoris
□ **Medial rotators:** Gluteus medius (anterior fibers) and minimus and TFL

▓ **Function:** The primary functions of the muscles of the hip are to provide tension to control joint movement, to stabilize the hip, and to provide movement and stability to the knee and lumbosacral region.
□ **Flexors:** The iliopsoas is an important stabilizer of the lumbosacral spine. However, sustained contraction adds a compressive load to the spine and discs and can irritate these structures.
□ **Extensors:** The hip extensors not only are important in normal walking, but also are active in getting into and out of a chair and in ascending and descending stairs.
□ **Abductors:** The abductors are essential to normal gait because they prevent excessive downward displacement of the pelvis during weight bearing. The gluteus minimus attaches to the joint capsule and protects the capsule from impingement by pulling it up during abduction.[4]

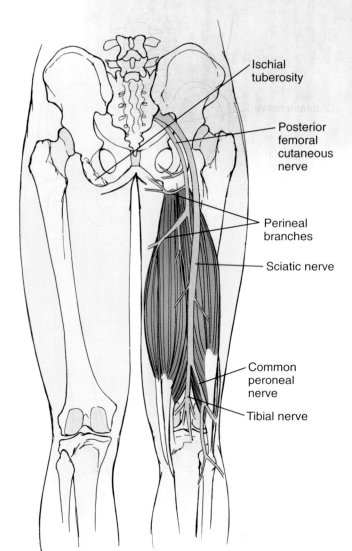

Figure 8-8. Sciatic nerve innervates the posterior thigh, leg, and foot.

□ **Adductors:** Working synergistically with the abductors, the adductors stabilize the pelvis during the weight shift from one limb to the other.

□ **Lateral rotators:** These muscles stabilize the hip by drawing the head of the femur into the acetabulum during the stance phase of gait. They also act like a rotator cuff for fine postural control.[1]

□ **Medial rotators:** The medial rotators are active during the stance phase of gait when the pelvis rotates over a fixed femur.

▪ **Dysfunction and injury:** The most commonly injured muscles of the hip region are the two-joint muscles, especially the rectus femoris and biceps femoris. Two-joint muscles incur these injuries be-

cause one of their main functions is eccentric contraction, that is, to contract while the muscle is lengthening. Muscles are much more prone to injury during eccentric contraction. The rectus femoris must eccentrically contract to decelerate the hip and knee, and the hamstrings eccentrically contract as the knee comes to full extension at heel strike.[5] Contractures of the hip flexors are very common for clients who spend most of their day sitting, such as office workers, people who drive as a large part of their day, and sedentary seniors.[4] For a person with a flexible lumbar spine, a short iliopsoas will lead to increased lumbar curve (lordosis). For a client with a stiff spine, a short iliopsoas will produce a forward lean of the trunk. Muscle dysfunction has two basic categories: muscle imbalance and positional dysfunction. Muscle imbalance describes a condition in which certain muscles are usually weak and others are usually short and tight. Janda and colleagues[6] call this muscle imbalance in the hip and lumbopelvic region **lower (pelvic) crossed syndrome.** Muscle imbalances alter movement patterns and therefore add a continuing stress to the joint system.

Muscle Imbalances of the Hip Region (Lower [Pelvic] Crossed Syndrome)

▪ **Muscles that tend to be tight and short:** the iliopsoas, piriformis, rectus femoris, TFL, adductors, external rotators, quadratus lumborum, ITB, and hamstrings

▪ **Muscles that tend to be weak and inhibited:** the quadriceps (except the rectus femoris), especially the vastus medialis obliquus; abdominals; and gluteus maximus, medius, and minimus.

Positional Dysfunction of the Hip Region Muscles

▪ The psoas tends to wind into a medial torsion along with the adductors.

▪ The pectineus, rectus, sartorius, and TFL all tend to wind into a medial torsion.

▪ The gluteus maximus and medius, piriformis, and other external rotators tend to roll into an inferior torsion.

ANATOMY OF THE HIP MUSCLES

See Table 8-1.

(Labels on figure: Ischial tuberosity; Posterior femoral cutaneous nerve; Perineal branches; Sciatic nerve; Common peroneal nerve; Tibial nerve)

Table 8-1   Anatomy of the Hip Muscles

Flexors (see Fig. 8-9)

Muscle	Origin	Insertion	Action	Dysfunction
Psoas major	Transverse processes of the lumbar vertebrae, vertebral bodies and intervening discs; the psoas interweaves with the diaphragm; the lumbar plexus runs between the superficial and deep parts of the psoas major	Passes behind the inguinal ligament and in front of the joint capsule, ending in a tendon that receives almost all the fibers of the iliacus on its lateral side and attaches to the lesser trochanter of femur and joint capsule	Flexion of the hip; flexes the trunk against the thigh; side-bends the lumbar spine; stabilization of the lumbar spine; assists in lateral rotation and abduction of the hip.	If the psoas is contracted or short unilaterally, the trunk is flexed and side-bent to the same side. Bilateral contraction increases the lumbar curve if the spine is flexible and can flatten the lumbar curve and pull the trunk forward if the lumbar spine is inflexible. Psoas contraction can increase low back pain and aggravate a herniated disc, because the psoas attaches to the disc. Hip flexion contractures are common in people who sit a great deal, such as office workers and sedentary elders.[4]
Psoas minor	Lies in front of the psoas major from the sides of the T12–L1 bodies and discs	Attached to the iliopubic eminence and to the iliopectineal arch, a fascial expansion of the inguinal ligament; the psoas minor is absent in approximately 50% of the population		
Iliacus	A triangular sheet of muscle arising from the upper two-thirds of the iliac fossa; from the inner lip of the iliac crest, anterior sacroiliac, and iliolumbar ligaments; and from the lateral surface of the sacrum	Most fibers converge into the lateral side of the tendon of the psoas major and insert on the lesser trochanter of the femur and anterior joint capsule.	Hip flexion; flexes the trunk against the leg; performs lateral rotation of the hip.	The iliacus has the same dysfunction patterns as the psoas. Tightness in the iliopsoas can create weakness and decreased hip flexor strength, such as in climbing stairs. The iliopsoas tends to roll into a medial torsion
Tensor fascia lata (TFL)	Anterior aspect of the external lip of the iliac crest, lateral surface of the ASIS	Attached to the two layers of the iliotibial band, which attaches to the lateral tubercle of the tibia	Hip flexion, abduction and medial rotation; knee extension and lateral rotation; serves as a stabilizer of the pelvis	Weakness contributes to a bow-legged position; shortness contributes to knock-knees and anterior pelvic tilt. Tightness of the TFL is associated with both anterior and lateral knee pain, called *iliotibial band friction syndrome*. Excessive tightness of the TFL/ITB causes rubbing and friction against the lateral condyle of the femur. Tightness also causes excessive lateral pull of the patella, creating patellar tracking dysfunction.

(continued)

363

Table 8-1 Anatomy of the Hip Muscles (Continued)

Flexors (see Fig. 8-9)

Muscle	Origin	Insertion	Action	Dysfunction
Rectus femoris (for other quadriceps, see Chapter 9, "The Knee")	Arises by two tendinous heads: a straight head from the AIIS and a reflected head from a groove above the acetabulum and from the fibrous capsule of the hip	Ends in a broad, thick aponeurosis and flattened tendon attached to the upper surface of the patella; superficial, central part of the quadriceps tendon	Assists in flexing the hip and extends the knee; efficiency as a hip flexor increases the more the knee is flexed because flexion lengthens this muscle	For dysfunction of the rectus femoris and other quadriceps, see Chapter 9, "The Knee."
Sartorius	A narrow, strap muscle, the longest muscle in the body, arises from the medial side of the ASIS	Ends in a thin, flat tendon that curves forward into a broad aponeurosis attached in front of the gracilis and semitendinosus to the medial surface of tibia	Hip flexion, lateral rotation and abduction of the hip; knee flexion	A weak sartorius decreases dynamic stabilization of the knee. Tightness and overuse contributes to pes anserinus bursitis.

Adductors of the Hip (see Fig. 8-10)

Muscle	Origin	Insertion	Action	Dysfunction
Pectineus	A flat, quadrangular muscle arising from the pectineal line on the superior pubic ramus between the iliopubic eminence and the pubic tubercle	Attach on the pectineal line on posterior surface of femur; can also interweave with the joint capsule	Flexion and adduction of the hip.	Pectineus tends to be short and tight. Thickens with hip flexion contractures and degeneration of the hip.
Adductor longus	Most anterior of the three adductors; arises by a flat tendon from the front of the pubis in the angle between the crest and the symphysis	Expands in a broad, fleshy belly that is inserted into the linea aspera in the middle third of the posterior femur between the vastus medialis and the adductor brevis and magnus	Adduction and flexion of the hip. Functional role of adductors is to stabilize the pelvis during transfer of weight from one side to another.	Adductor longus tends to roll into a medial torsion. Commonly injured in sports with kicking and quick pivoting activities.
Adductor brevis	Posterior to the pectineus and adductor longus, arises along the body and inferior ramus of the pubis	Attached to the posterior femur along a line from the lesser trochanter to the linea aspera between the pectineus and the adductor magnus	Adducts hip; aids in flexion and medial rotation of hip.	Adductor brevis tends to be short and tight.

Muscle			
Adductor magnus	A massive triangular muscle arising from the lower lateral aspect of the ischial tuberosity, the ischial ramus, and the adjacent pubic ramus	Pubic fibers attach to the medial margin of the gluteal tuberosity; fibers from the ischial ramus attach to the linea aspera; from the ischial tuberosity attaches to the adductor tubercle	Powerful adductor of the hip; lower portion of the muscle extends the hip and rotates it medially; also acts as a dynamic stabilizer of the medial patella, as the vastus medialis obliquus inserts into the adductor magnus tendon.[7]	With sustained contraction, the hip adductors cause a lateral pelvic tilt, with the pelvis high on the side of contraction[8]
Gracilis	Most superficial of the adductor group; arises by a thin aponeurosis from the medial margins of the lower pubic bone, the inferior pubic ramus, and the adjoining ischial tuberosity.	Attaching to the medial surface of the proximal tibia below the condyle, immediately anterior to the semitendinosus	With the knee extended, adducts the hip; also flexes and medially rotates the knee	The gracilis, sartorius, and semitendinosus form a common tendinous insertion called the *pes anserinus*, which provides dynamic stabilization of the knee against rotary and valgus stresses.[4] Weakness contributes to instability of the knee.

Gluteal Region *(see Fig. 8-11)*

Gluteus maximus	Largest and most powerful muscle, it is the most characteristic feature of the human, associated with bringing the trunk upright; arises from the posterior line of the ilium, the posterior aspect of the sacrum, coccyx, and sacrotuberous ligament	Ends in a thick, tendinous lamina attached to the iliotibial tract of the fascia lata; deeper fibers of the lower part attach to the gluteal tuberosity of the femur	Extensor and powerful lateral rotator of the hip; inferior fibers assist in adduction, and upper fibers are abductors; balances the trunk on the femur; balances the knee joint via the ITB	Tends to be weak, inhibited by sustained contraction of the hip flexors, especially the iliopsoas, causing overuse of the hamstrings.
Gluteus medius	Broad, thick muscle arises from the outer surface of the ilium, between the anterior and posterior gluteal lines	Fibers converge to a strong, flat tendon that is attached to the superior aspect of the lateral surface of greater trochanter	Principal muscle of hip abduction; anterior fibers medially rotate and can assist in flexion; posterior fibers laterally rotate and can assist in extension of the hip	If weak, leads to lateral pelvic tilt and elevated pelvis on the side of weakness; if contracted, pelvis is low on side of contracture. Short and tight abductors are associated with degeneration of the hip, as joint seeks open position, which is flexion and abduction, shorting the abductors.

(continued)

Table 8-1   Anatomy of the Hip Muscles (Continued)

Muscle	Origin	Insertion	Action	Dysfunction
Gluteal Region (see Fig. 8-11)				
Gluteus minimus	Deep to the gluteus medius, arises from outer surface of the ilium between the ASIS and greater sciatic notch	Attached to the anterior and superior portion of the greater trochanter and the hip joint capsule.	Acting with the gluteus medius, abducts the hip; the anterior fibers of the minimus rotate the hip medially; both can also act as hip flexors	Tightness causes abduction and medial rotation of the hip; in standing, there is a lateral pelvic tilt, low on the side of shortness, accompanied by medial rotation of the femur.
Deep Lateral Rotators of Hip (see Fig. 8-11)				
Piriformis	Anterior surface of sacrum between the margin of the greater sciatic notch and the pelvic surface of the sacrotuberous ligament	Passes out of the pelvis through the greater sciatic foramen and attaches by a rounded tendon to the superior-posterior border of the greater trochanter; often blended with the common tendon of obturator internus and gemelli	Laterally rotates the extended hip; abducts the hip when the hip is flexed	Piriformis is typically short and tight as a result of excessive sitting and because it substitutes for a weak gluteus medius.[1] Sustained contraction can compress the sciatic nerve, leading to pain, numbing, and tingling into the thigh.
Quadratus femoris	Proximal part of the lateral border of tuberosity of the ischium	Attaches to the posterior femur, extending down the intertrochanteric crest	All of these muscles not only are lateral rotators of the hip, but also act like a rotator cuff for fine postural control and serve as dynamic stabilizers of the hip by drawing the head of the femur into the acetabulum during stance phase of gait.[1]	Tends to be short and tight, contributing to toe-out stance in standing.
Obturator internus	Internal or pelvic surface of the obturator membrane and margin of the obturator foramen, the inferior ramus of the pubis and ischium; exits the pelvis through the lesser sciatic notch	Fibers make a right-angled bend over the grooved surface of the ischium between the spine and the tuberosity, passing horizontally across the hip joint capsule, and interweave with the insertions of the gemelli, inserting on medial superior surface of the posterior greater trochanter.		Lauren Berry, RPT, taught that the obturator internus rolls into an abnormal inferior torsion in dysfunction and injury to the lumbopelvic region. This torsion puts a tethering or pulling force on the fascia suspending the sciatic nerve, which can irritate the nerve, causing diffuse sciatic pain into the thigh and leg.

Muscle	Origin	Insertion	Action	Notes
Gemellus superior	Superior aspect of the spine of the ischium	Lies on the superior surface of the obturator internus and attaches to the medial surface of greater trochanter.		Lateral rotators are nearly three times stronger than medial rotators; if there is lateral rotator weakness, there is a medial rotation of the femur, and a tendency for knock-knees; if there is lateral rotator shortness, there is lateral rotation of the femur and an out-toeing of the foot in standing.[8]
Gemellus inferior	Inferior aspect of the ischial tuberosity.	Lies on the inferior surface of the obturator internus and attaches to the medial surface of the greater trochanter		
Obturator externus	Flat, triangular muscle covering the external surface of the anterior pelvic wall, arising from the bone around the obturator foramen	Trochanteric fossa of femur		

Hamstrings (see Fig. 8-12)

Muscle	Origin	Insertion	Action	Notes
Biceps femoris (long head)	Ischial tuberosity (blending with the sacrotuberous ligament)	The long and short heads blend together and attach to the head of the fibula and lateral condyle of the tibia and lateral collateral ligament	Flexion of the knee, extension of the hip (except short head); the only lateral rotator of the knee	Weakness of hamstrings contributes to an anterior pelvic tilt and to increased lordosis; bilateral contraction causes a posterior pelvic tilt and a decreased lumbar curve; weakness of the medial hamstrings contributes to knock-knees, and a lateral rotation of the femur.

Hamstring weakness also increases instability of the knee, especially after injury to the ACL, because hamstrings provide active resistance to anterior glide of the tibia on the femur.[4] Hamstring tightness can prevent the knee from achieving full extension. |
Biceps femoris (short head)	Middle third of the lateral lip of the linea aspera.			
Semitendinosus	From the ischial tuberosity, blended with the long head of the biceps	Medial margin of the tuberosity of the tibia; together with the sartorius and gracilis, they form the pes anserinus tendons	Extension of the hip, flexion of the knee, and medial rotation of the flexed knee	
Semimembranosus	Ischial tuberosity	Tendon attaches to three places: to the posteromedial corner of the tibia; to the fascia of the popliteus; and into the posterior wall of the joint capsule as the oblique popliteal ligament, attaching to the medial meniscus	Extension of the hip; flexion and medial rotation of the knee; during knee flexion, it pulls the meniscus backward.	

Quadriceps (refer to the Chapter 9, "The Knee")

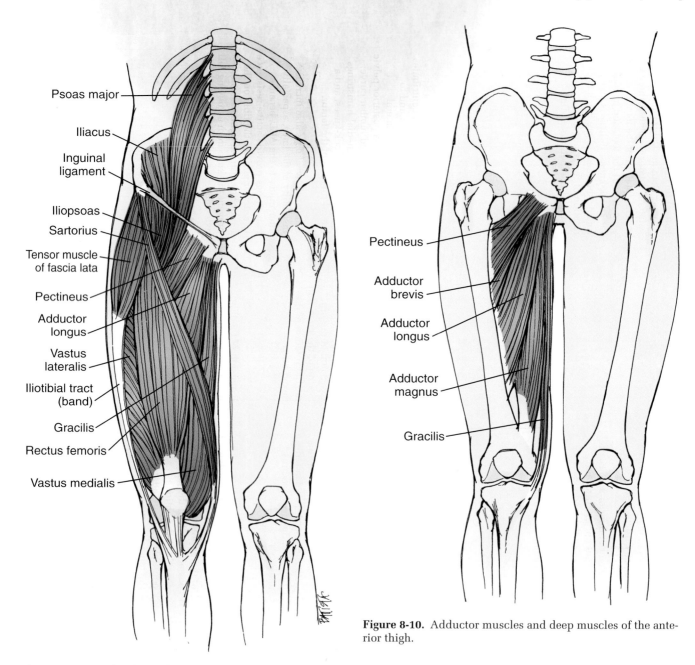

Psoas major
Iliacus
Inguinal ligament
Iliopsoas
Sartorius
Tensor muscle of fascia lata
Pectineus
Adductor longus
Vastus lateralis
Iliotibial tract (band)
Gracilis
Rectus femoris
Vastus medialis

Figure 8-9. Superficial muscles of the anterior thigh.

Pectineus
Adductor brevis
Adductor longus
Adductor magnus
Gracilis

Figure 8-10. Adductor muscles and deep muscles of the anterior thigh.

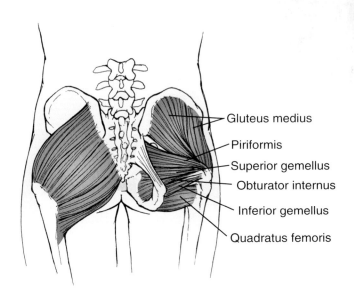

Figure 8-11. Gluteal muscles and deep rotators of the hip.

Gluteus medius

Piriformis

Superior gemellus

Obturator internus

Inferior gemellus

Quadratus femoris

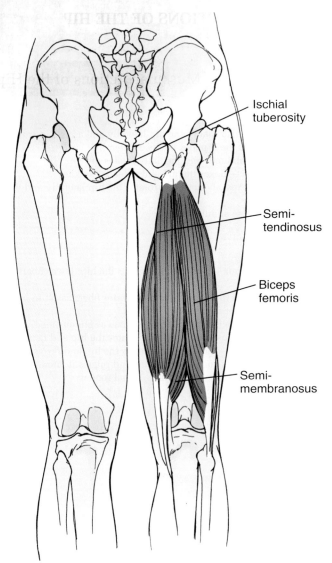

Figure 8-12. Posterior hip and thigh muscles.

Ischial tuberosity

Semi-tendinosus

Biceps femoris

Semi-membranosus

MUSCULAR ACTIONS OF THE HIP

See Table 8-2.

Table 8-2	Muscular Actions of the Hip

Flexion

- Psoas major—also rotates the hip laterally and assists in trunk flexion
- Iliacus—flexes the hip and rotates it laterally
- TFL—flexes, abducts, and medially rotates the hip
- Rectus femoris—flexes the hip and extends the knee
- Sartorius—flexes, abducts, and rotates the hip laterally and flexes and rotates the knee medially
- Pectineus—also adducts the hip

Extension

- Gluteus maximus—also laterally rotates the hip; lower fibers adduct and upper fibers abduct the hip
- Gluteus medius (posterior fibers)—anterior fibers assist in hip flexion and medial rotation; a strong abductor of the hip
- Gluteus minimus (posterior fibers)—same as gluteus medius
- Semimembranosus—also medially rotates the hip and flexes and medially rotates the knee
- Semitendinosus—also medially rotates the hip and flexes and medially rotates the knee
- Biceps femoris—also flexes the knee and rotates it laterally
- Piriformis—acts primarily as an external rotator

Abduction

- Gluteus medius
- Piriformis
- TFL
- Obturator internus
- Gluteus maximus
- Gluteus minimus

Adduction

- Adductor magnus—also flexes the hip; lower fibers cause medial rotation
- Adductor longus—also flexes the hip and rotates it laterally
- Adductor brevis—also flexes the hip and rotates it laterally
- Gluteus maximus—also extends the hip
- Gracilis—also medially rotates the hip and flexes the knee
- Pectineus—also flexes the hip

Lateral Rotation (acts like shoulder rotator cuff for fine postural control)

- Gluteus maximus
- Quadratus femoris—also adducts the hip
- Obturator internus
- Gluteus medius and minimus—posterior fibers
- Iliopsoas
- Obturator externus
- All adductors
- Biceps femoris—also extends the hip
- Piriformis—also abducts the hip

Medial Rotation

- Gluteus minimus—anterior fibers
- Gluteus medius—anterior fibers
- TFL
- Gracilis—also adducts and flexes the hip and flexes the knee
- Adductor magnus (which is inserted into adductor tubercle)
- Semimembranosus and semitendinosus—also extend the hip

Hip Dysfunction and Injury

FACTORS THAT PREDISPOSE TO HIP PAIN

▨ Predisposing factors to hip pain include capsular thickening caused by previous trauma, leg-length inequality, pelvic unleveling (pelvic obliquity), chronic lower back dysfunction or pain, chronic sacroiliac joint (SIJ) dysfunction or pain, muscle imbalances, anteverted hip, muscle fatigue, obesity, and sedentary lifestyle.

▨ Leg-length inequality creates pelvic unleveling and a high ilium relative to the other side. The ilium rolls anteriorly slightly as it elevates, compressing the hip joint on that side. This compression predisposes the joint on the side of the long leg to arthrosis.[9] This unleveling also creates gait disturbances, which create uneven stress through the joint, predisposing it to degeneration.

▨ Chronic lower back dysfunction or pain or chronic SIJ dysfunction or pain creates compensations throughout the hip region, causing uneven distribution of the weight through the cartilage.

▨ Anteversion in the hip causes the hip to assume its closed-packed position, creating increased compression in the joint and winding the joint capsule into its tightened position.

▨ Muscle imbalance creates abnormal movement through the joint, which means that an imbalanced stress on the cartilage will occur. Tight muscles add a compressive load to the joint, and hypertonic muscles are more easily fatigued and therefore more easily strained.

DIFFERENTIATION OF HIP PAIN

▨ It is important to realize that on rare occasions, hip pain can represent a pathologic condition. See "Contraindications to Massage Therapy: Red Flags" in Chapter 2, "Assessment and Technique," for guidelines on when massage is contraindicated and when to refer. Hip pain can also come from structures other than the hip, most commonly the lumbar spine. Chronic hip pain also requires a thorough examination of the lumbar spine. Assuming that pain in the

hip is not pathologic, differentiation can be categorized according to the structures that are involved.

▨ Myofascial pain of acute onset is described as a sharp, localized pain that is often associated with swelling, heat, and redness. The pain is increased with isometric contraction, performed during CR MET, and is better with rest. It is typically localized to the attachment sites or the myotendinous junctions. Gluteus medius tendinitis is well localized to the greater trochanter; adductor strains are localized to the groin; rectus femoris to the AIIS, midbelly, or patellar attachments; hamstrings to the ischial tuberosity, midthigh, or patellar attachments; and iliopsoas to the groin.

▨ Bursitis is manifested as a diffuse ache, a burning sensation, or both. It is worse with movement or, in the case of the trochanteric bursa, worse with lying on it. A swollen bursa elicits an empty end feel on passive motion (i.e., the client feels pain before the tissue is in tension).

▨ A capsulitis manifests as a deep, diffuse, aching pain and stiffness in the groin. The pain is worse with sitting and climbing stairs and is stiffer in the morning. The first sign of capsulitis of the hip is a painful decrease in passive medial rotation. Remember that capsulitis is the precursor of osteoarthritis (hip degeneration).

▨ Arthritis is an inflammation of the hip joint, and arthrosis is a degeneration of the joint. Arthritis or arthrosis elicits a deep ache in the groin, greater trochanter, buttock, anterior thigh, and eventually the knee. In the early stages, it is painful with excessive movement, but as it progresses, it manifests as a toothache-like pain even at rest. Passive medial rotation and flexion are limited and have a hard end feel, unlike a chronic capsular shortening which has a thick, leathery end feel.

▨ The hip region is a common area for peripheral nerve entrapment. The pain is described as burning, as numbing or tingling, or as a combination of the two. Peripheral entrapment is typically in a larger area, and the pain is more diffuse.

▨ The anterior, lateral, and posterior thigh are also common sites of dermatomal pain from nerve root irritation. Nerve root pain is a sharp pain in a well-described patch of skin.

COMMON DYSFUNCTIONS AND INJURIES OF THE HIP

GLUTEUS MEDIUS TENDINITIS

- **Causes:** Pelvic unleveling stresses the hip abductors on the side of the high ilium; running, dancing, and racquet sports all stress the gluteus medius.

- **Symptoms:** Pain is well localized over the greater trochanter and superior iliac fossa and can radiate down the lateral or posterior thigh. Pain is brought on by hip movements, especially climbing stairs or prolonged walking or running.

- **Signs:** Pain is reproduced by resisted hip abduction. Pain occurs on tendon stretch with full passive adduction. The gluteus medius usually tests weak, and the TFL becomes hypertonic, substituting for the weak gluteus medius.

- **Sites:** Gluteus medius tendinitis occurs at the tenoperiosteal junction at the lateral aspect of the greater trochanter and the myotendinous junction. The fasciculi in the belly of the muscle tend to roll into an inferior torsion.

- **Treatment:** For **acute** conditions, perform CR and reciprocal inhibition (RI) MET for the gluteus medius (MET #8) with light pressure. If the position shown in that MET is still painful, place a pillow under a straightened leg, and have the client just begin to attempt to lift the leg off the pillow to engage the abductors. Have the client then pull the leg back into the table to engage adductors. Repeat MET with increasing pressure to engage more of the muscle if the technique remains within client's comfort level. Perform Level I, first series, with gentle pressure and a slow rhythm. As you perform the strokes, palpate the tissues to assess for hypertonicity and perform more MET if the area remains tender and hypertonic. For **chronic** conditions, first reduce the hypertonicity with MET #8. The gluteus medius is typically weak, but it may also be tight—a tightness-weakness pattern. Perform MET #9 to relax and lengthen the adductors, as tight adductors inhibit the abductors. Next, perform STM, especially Level II, first series, to dissolve fibrosis in the muscle, especially at the attachment points. Because joint dysfunction can inhibit normal muscle function, assess the passive ROM of the hip, especially medial and lateral rotation, and A–P glide. Perform MET and joint mobilization as indicated if you find a loss of normal hip motion.

ADDUCTOR TENDINITIS OR GROIN STRAIN

- **Causes:** A typical pattern of dysfunction is for the adductors to be tight and short and for the abductors to be weak. This pattern is associated with anteverted hips, genu valgus, and unleveling of the pelvis. Sustained contraction fatigues the muscle and makes it more susceptible to injury; the adductor longus is most commonly involved. Adductor strain is a common injury in sports, usually of acute onset, with well-localized pain.[10]

- **Symptoms:** Pain is usually well localized to the groin and inner thigh.

- **Signs:** Adductor tendinitis or groin strain signs are pain with resisted hip adduction, possible pain with full passive abduction, and pain to palpation.

- **Sites:** Groin strain or adductor tendinitis occurs at the tenoperiosteal junction at the anterior pubis and at the musculotendinous junction a few centimeters distally. Adductor fasciculi develop a medial and posterior torsion.

- **Treatment:** For **acute** conditions, perform CR and RI MET for the adductors (MET #2) with light pressure. Perform Level I, second and fourth series, with gentle pressure and a slow rhythm. As you perform the strokes, palpate the tissues to assess for hypertonicity, and perform more MET if the area remains tender and hypertonic. If it is comfortable for the client, perform MET #7 to release the adductors in the side-lying position. For **chronic** conditions, first perform the STM and METs described for acute conditions to reduce the hypertonicity. Because the adductors are typically short and tight, perform MET #9 to lengthen the adductors. Next, perform STM, Level II, second series, to dissolve fibrosis at the attachment points of the adductors on the posterior femur. It is important to remember to treat the entire area of complaint as well as the other side of the body to release compensations to the injury. Perform Level II, fourth and fifth series, to release the attachment points in the region.

QUADRICEPS TENDINITIS (MOST COMMONLY RECTUS FEMORIS)

- **Causes:** The rectus femoris is most commonly involved. Soccer, running, and jumping all stress the rectus femoris. It is particularly susceptible to injury because it is a two-joint muscle and acts eccentrically to decelerate the hip and knee.[11] It is typically tight and short.

- **Symptoms:** Pain is usually well localized to the AIIS, approximately 3 inches inferior to the ASIS, in the midbelly of the muscle, or at the patellar attachments either above or below the patella.

- **Signs:** Pain with resisted knee extension with hip extended (i.e., with the client supine and attempting to lift the straight leg) and pain with passive flexion of the knee more than 120° (i.e., with the client prone) are typical signs of rectus femoris tendinitis.

- **Sites:** Rectus femoris tendinitis occurs at the tenoperiosteal junction at the AIIS, at the insertion of reflected head into the superior aspect of the acetabulum, in the midbelly, or at the patella.

- **Treatment:** For **acute** conditions, perform CR and RI MET for the quadriceps (MET #3) with light pressure. Perform Level I, fourth and fifth series, with gentle pressure and a slow rhythm. As you perform the strokes, palpate the tissues to assess for hypertonicity and perform more MET if the area remains tender and hypertonic. If it is comfortable for the client, perform MET #5 to release the hamstrings. For **chronic** conditions, first perform the STM and MET described for acute conditions to reduce the hypertonicity. Because the rectus femoris is typically short and tight, perform PIR MET #6 in Chapter 9 to lengthen the quadriceps, specifically the rectus femoris. Next, perform STM, Level II, fifth series, to dissolve fibrosis at the attachment points. It is important to treat the entire area of complaint as well as the other side of the body to release compensations to the injury.

HAMSTRING TENDINITIS

- **Causes:** The hamstrings are short and tight in most people for two reasons. First, we live in a sedentary culture, and sitting shortens the hamstrings and the iliopsoas. The shortened iliopsoas inhibits the gluteus maximus and thus overloads the hamstrings. This overload predisposes the muscle to fatigue. Second, the hamstrings eccentrically contract as the knee comes to full extension at heel strike, making it vulnerable; thus overexertion, such as can occur in running, jumping, and racquet sports, leads to injury. The biceps femoris is most commonly involved.[7]

- **Symptoms:** Pain may be present at three common sites: at the ischial tuberosity, in the midbelly, and less commonly behind the knee.

- **Signs:** Pain that can be reproduced with resisted knee flexion, possible pain with resisted hip extension, and pain in the muscle with a straight-leg-raising (SLR) test are signs of hamstring tendinitis.

- **Sites:** Hamstring tendinitis occurs at the tenoperiosteal insertions at the ischial tuberosity, at the myotendinous junction at various sites on the posterior thigh, and at tenoperiosteal insertions behind the knee.

- **Treatment:** For **acute** conditions, perform CR and RI MET for the hamstrings (MET #5) with light pressure. Perform Level I, second and third series, with gentle pressure and a slow rhythm. As you perform the strokes, palpate the tissues to assess for hypertonicity, and perform more MET if the area remains tender and hypertonic. For **chronic** conditions, first perform the STM and MET described for acute conditions to reduce the hypertonicity. Because the hamstrings are typically short and tight, perform CRAC MET #10 to lengthen the hamstrings and MET #9 to lengthen the adductors. Next, perform STM, Level I, second and third series, and Level II, second series, to dissolve fibrosis at the attachment points of the adductors and hamstrings.

ILIOPSOAS TENDINITIS

- **Causes:** As with the hamstrings, the iliopsoas tends to be short and tight. Repetitive hip flexion, such as occurs in stair climbing, soccer, dancing, and kicking, can fatigue and strain this muscle. Excessive sitting shortens the muscle.

- **Symptoms:** Pain in the groin, often poorly localized, especially with hip flexion, is a symptom of iliopsoas tendinitis.

- **Signs:** Pain on resisted hip flexion and pain under the inguinal ligament with passive hip flexion and adduction of the hip perpendicular to the inguinal ligament are signs of iliopsoas tendinitis.

- **Sites:** Iliopsoas tendinitis occurs at the tenoperiosteal junction of the lesser trochanter and within the belly of the muscle, especially in the area of the inguinal ligament.

- **Treatment:** The primary intention in treating **acute** injuries is to reduce pain, swelling, and muscle spasms. Perform CR and RI MET for the iliopsoas with light pressure (METs #6 and #7 in Chapter 3). Perform Level I, seventh series (see Chapter 3) STM, with gentle pressure and a slow rhythm. As you perform the strokes, palpate the tissues to assess for hypertonicity, and perform more MET if the area remains tender and hypertonic. For **chronic** conditions, first perform the STM and MET described for acute conditions to reduce the hypertonicity. Because the iliopsoas is typically short and tight, perform PIR MET #8 in Chapter 3 to lengthen the iliopsoas. Next, perform STM, Level I, seventh series from Chapter 3, and Level II, fourth series, to dissolve adhesions in the belly of the muscle and to release fibrosis at the attachment points of the iliopsoas at the lesser trochanter. Assess the ROM of the hip joint, including A–P glide. Perform MET to normalize ROM, and perform A–P mobilization of the hip to help normalize joint play at the hip.

TROCHANTERIC BURSITIS

- **Causes:** Trochanteric bursitis occurs as a result of a fall on the side of the hip; a repetitive circular motion of the hip, as in riding a bicycle; or a sustained contraction of the TFL, ITB, and gluteus maximus caused by hip joint pathology or lumbosacral injury or dysfunction.

- **Symptoms:** Clients usually experience an acute onset of a diffuse, deep ache and burning sensation over the greater trochanter; this pain can ache and throb down the lateral thigh and can worsen when the client climbs stairs or lies on it at night.

- **Signs:** Resisted abduction and extension can cause pain that is achy and diffuse; passive adduction with hip flexion causes pain. An inflamed bursa is tender to palpation.

- **Sites:** Trochanteric bursitis occurs at the posterolateral aspect of the greater trochanter and down the lateral thigh.

- **Treatment:** For **acute** conditions, perform very gentle manual therapy to drain the excess fluid from the bursa, Level I, sixth series. Once the swelling in the area goes down, perform CR and RI MET for the TFL (MET #7) and gluteus maximus (MET #6) with light pressure. Repeat Level I, sixth series, to drain out the bursa as needed. It can take six weeks to resolve an acute bursitis. For **chronic** conditions, first perform METs #6 and #7 for the TFL and gluteus maximus, and perform PIR MET for the ITB (MET #12). Perform manual therapy for the bursa, Level I, sixth series, at an increased depth. If the area feels fibrotic, use greater depth to dissolve adhesions and help rehydrate the bursa.

ILIOPECTINEAL BURSITIS

- **Causes:** Repetitive hip flexion, as in stair climbing, dancing, or martial arts, or sustained hip flexion, as in a sedentary lifestyle, compresses the iliopsoas over the bursa.

- **Symptoms:** Clients experience a diffuse, deep ache in the groin and anterior thigh.

- **Signs:** Passive adduction in flexion compresses the bursa and elicits an empty end feel or an ache in the groin before the tension barrier; full passive extension reproduces the pain.

- **Sites:** The iliopectineal bursa is located between the psoas muscle and the hip joint capsule.

- **Treatment:** For **acute** conditions, perform very gentle MET for the iliopsoas (MET #6 and #7, Chapter 3) to help pump the excess fluid from the area. Perform manual therapy, Level II, third series, to drain the excess fluid from the bursa. For **chronic** conditions, repeat the treatment for acute conditions, but with greater depth.

HIP CAPSULITIS (SYNOVITIS)

- **Causes:** Trauma, repetitive hip flexion, such as occurs in stair climbing or hiking, or an overuse of the hip flexors through dance or racquet sports can inflame the joint capsule and lead to acute capsulitis (synovitis). If the acute condition is not properly rehabilitated, it will lead to fibrosis of the capsule, limited hip motion, and eventual degeneration.

- **Symptoms:** Clients experience a sometimes rapid onset of pain and stiffness, made worse with activity, usually localized in the groin, but sometimes in the anterior thigh and knee.

- **Signs:** Medial rotation of the hip is most limited, accompanied by limited flexion and adduction. With acute capsulitis, there is an empty end feel; chronic capsulitis elicits a leathery end feel with a decreased ROM.

- **Sites:** Hip capsulitis occurs at the capsule between the trochanter and the acetabulum.

- **Treatment:** The first treatment goal for an **acute** synovitis is to reduce the swelling, which will reduce the pain and muscle spasms. Perform MET #1 very gently, followed by METs for the flexion-extension planes at 90° of hip flexion (METs #6 and #7 from Chapter 3). Next, perform MET #14 to contract and release the joint capsule in both medial and lateral rotation. This MET is performed to increase the ROM by pumping the excess fluid out of the joint. Follow the MET with gentle passive motion in flexion-extension and medial-lateral rotation planes. This helps to pump the swelling out of the joint.

DEGENERATION OF THE HIP (OSTEOARTHRITIS)

- **Causes:** A degenerated or osteoarthritic hip means that the cartilage has worn down. Fibrosis, dyhydration, and shortening of the joint capsule typically precede degeneration. Dehydration and fibrosis diminish the blood supply to the femoral head as the artery to the head of the femur is intracapsular. Clients are usually middle-aged or older, often with a history of prior trauma, usually a fall. Osteoarthritis is typically associated with cumulative stress, such as pelvic unleveling, often due to leg-length disparity. The side of the high ilium rolls forward slightly, compressing the hip joint on that side. The long limb also assumes a position of relative adduction, causing excessive pressures on the hip joint. Chronic low back pain often leads to gait disturbances and secondary problems in the hips caused by altered weight distribution. Anteverted hip and a sedentary lifestyle are also predisposing factors. A sedentary lifestyle shortens the anterior capsule of the hip, decreasing its mobility. Degeneration of the hip is not associated with aging,[2] and healthy geriatric patients should have full ROM in the hips.

▨ **Symptoms:** Insidious onset of an ache that begins in the groin and extends to the greater trochanter, medial buttock, and anterior thigh and that can refer to the knee is a typical symptom of osteoarthritis of the hip. Patients describe being stiff in the morning or after sitting for long periods and having pain after extended walking.

▨ **Signs:** Medial rotation of the hip is most limited, accompanied by limited flexion. Painful limitation of medial rotation with a capsular end feel is typical. A hard (bony) end feel with passive flexion and medial rotation is noted if there is a significant loss of cartilage. The gluteus medius and maximus are weak, and there is a late-onset recruitment of the gluteus maximus (see MET #6). The piriformis, adductors, and iliopsoas are typically short and tight.

▨ **Treatment:** It is critical to maintain or restore the normal length to the capsule, because a shortened capsule can diminish the blood supply to the femoral head and predisposes the joint to degeneration. Perform MET #14 and passive extension to increase the length of the capsule by increasing medial rotation and extension. If the client has **acute** hip pain, follow the protocol described above for capsulitis (synovitis). For **chronic** conditions, the intention is to identify short and tight muscles, fibrous tissue, weak muscles, the ROM of the hip, and joint play. Typically, the iliopsoas, rectus femoris, TFL, adductors, and hamstrings are short and tight and need to be treated first. The gluteus medius and gluteus maximus are typically weak and need to be recruited. The hip is typically fixed in an anterior position and needs to be mobilized in the A–P direction to restore normal joint play. In addition to releasing the hypertonicity and

strengthening the inhibited muscles around the hip, it is critical to stretch the joint capsule and to increase medial rotation, flexion, and adduction of the hip with MET.

SNAPPING HIP SYNDROME

▨ **Causes:** There are three common explanations: (1) The ITB snaps over the greater trochanter as the hip moves from flexion to extension; (2) the iliopsoas tendon snaps over the iliopectineal eminence; and (3) the iliofemoral ligament snaps over the femoral head.[11]

▨ **Symptoms:** Clients experience a snapping or pain at the anterior or lateral aspect of the hip.

▨ **Signs:** When the leg is lowered to the table with the knee extended, the "snap" occurs.

▨ **Treatment:** All three typical causes of snapping hip are typically chronic. The treatment consists of PIR MET to reduce the hypertonicity of the involved muscles and stretch the fascia of the ITB (METs #11 and #12), the iliopsoas (METs #6–8 from Chapter 3), and the anterior joint capsule (MET to increase extension, under "Passive Extension"). Perform STM for the TFL and ITB, Level I, sixth series; the iliopsoas, Level I, seventh series (see Chapter 3); and the anterior joint capsule, Level II, fifth series.

ENTRAPMENT OF THE LATERAL FEMORAL CUTANEOUS NERVE

▨ **Causes:** Pregnancy, obesity, or repetitive hip flexion such as occurs in stair climbing or hiking can entrap the lateral femoral cutaneous nerve of the thigh.

▨ **Symptoms:** Clients experience burning pain with numbness and tingling over the anterolateral aspect of the thigh to just above the knee.

▨ **Signs:** Increased symptoms brought on by passive hip extension are a sign of entrapment.

▨ **Sites:** The nerve is usually entrapped under the inguinal ligament approximately one-half inch medial to the ASIS in the fibro-osseous tunnel formed by the iliac fascia and the inguinal ligament.

▨ **Treatment:** Release the nerve by working transverse to it, medially to laterally, superior and deep to the inguinal ligament (Level II, third series).

ENTRAPMENT OF THE OBTURATOR NERVE

▨ **Causes:** Overuse of the hip adductors, such as riding a horse, or direct pressure on the adductor attachments, such as riding a bicycle, can irritate the area, leading to fibrosis and peripheral entrapment.

▨ **Symptoms:** Clients experience burning pain or numbing and tingling in the medial thigh.

▨ **Signs:** Pain elicited by passive hip adduction can be a sign of obturator nerve entrapment.

▨ **Sites:** Obturator nerve entrapment occurs medial to the psoas above the inguinal ligament and between the adductor longus and the pectineus immediately distal to the pubis.

▨ **Treatment:** Perform Level II, third and fourth series STM, to release the nerve by working transverse to the nerve at the sites mentioned above.

ENTRAPMENT OF THE FEMORAL NERVE

▨ **Symptoms:** Sustained hypertonicity of the psoas is a common source of nerve entrapment. Unlike most nerves, the lumbar plexus, which is the root of the femoral nerve, travels through the body of the psoas rather than alongside the muscle.

▨ **Symptoms:** Clients experience pain, numbing, and tingling in the anterior thigh.

▨ **Signs:** Increased symptoms elicited with passive hip extension is a sign of femoral nerve entrapment.

▨ **Sites:** Entrapment is usually superior to the inguinal ligament within a psoas contracture.

▨ **Treatment:** Perform Level I, seventh series (see Chapter 3), to release the iliopsoas, and perform Level II, third and fourth series STM, to release the nerve by working transverse to its line in a medial-to-lateral (M–L) direction at the sites mentioned above. These are the same strokes as those used for the psoas muscle release, with a different intention.

ENTRAPMENT OF SCIATIC NERVE

▨ **Causes:** The most common causes are contracture of the piriformis, obturator internus, or biceps femoris. Any inflammation in the gluteal region can create a fibrosis that tethers (pulls) on the loose irregular connective tissue that suspends the sciatic nerve as it travels through the gluteal region.

▨ **Symptoms:** Clients experience a diffuse ache in the buttock and diffuse pain, numbing, or tingling down the posterior thigh. Symptoms rarely extend to the calf and foot.

▨ **Signs:** The SLR test can be mildly positive, with diffuse pain, numbing, or tingling in the leg at approximately 70°. If a lumbar disc herniation creates nerve root pressure, it usually creates a sharp, well-localized pain during the SLR test well below 70°.

▨ **Sites:** Sciatic nerve entrapment can occur at the following sites:
☐ Piriformis muscle
☐ Greater sciatic notch
☐ Lateral-superior aspect of the ischial tuberosity tethered by inferior torsion of the obturator internus
☐ Between the greater trochanter and the ischial tuberosity entrapped under the biceps femoris attachment
☐ Adhesions between the adductor magnus and the short head of the biceps femoris

▨ **Treatment:** Sciatic neuritis can be caused by many lesions not listed above, including a herniated disc and serious pathology. Refer to Chapter 3 for guidelines in the treatment of disc herniation and to Chapter 2 for contraindications to massage therapy (red flags). The list above represents common entrapment sites that can be addressed safely by the massage therapist. Perform CR and PIR METs for the piriformis (METs #4 and #5 from Chapter 3) external rotators of the hip (MET #4), adductors (MET #9), and hamstrings (MET #10). Perform STM at the common entrapment sites, including Level I, first, second, and third series, from Chapter 3, and Level II, first series, in this chapter.

Hip Assessment

BACKGROUND

One of the primary intentions of the assessment for the massage therapist is to differentiate a shortened joint capsule and degeneration of the joint from muscle dysfunction and injury. This objective is accomplished primarily through passive ROM assessment, which is addressed in this section. The second goal is to assess the length, strength, and proper firing sequence of the muscles that affect the hip. The third goal is to assess soft tissue accurately after an acute injury. The second and third goals are primarily addressed in the "Muscle Energy Technique" section.

HISTORY QUESTIONS FOR THE CLIENT WHO HAS HIP PAIN

- Where does it hurt? (Ask the client to place his or her hand over the area.)
  - ☐ The primary goal of taking a history in a person with hip and groin pain is to localize the anatomical region.[10] Clients can usually touch a tendinitis, bursitis, or muscle strain. If the pain is hard to locate, it is usually from the joint or a referral from the lumbosacral spine. Problems in the hip joint itself will be felt in the inguinal region, midway between the ASIS and the pubic symphysis. With worsening conditions, the pain can radiate to the anterior thigh and knee. Because the nerves to the knee and hip have the same embryologic origin, dysfunction in one joint can refer pain to the other. Pain over the greater trochanter and lateral thigh can be a referral from the hip joint or lumbar spine, a tendinitis of the gluteus medius, or a trochanter bursitis. Pain in the buttock can be caused by piriformis or gluteus medius tendinitis or dysfunctions of the SIJ or lumbar spine. Clients often point to the SIJ when asked to locate their hip problem. Pain localized to the SIJ implicates that joint.
- Do you have a history of back problems?
  - ☐ Pain in the hip region is often referred from the lumbosacral spine. Asymmetry in the pelvis can create lower back and hip joint problems due to the abnormal stresses on those joints. These two conditions are differentiated through active and passive ROM studies. Typically, if a client has full and pain-free active and passive ROM in the lumbosacral spine and a full and painless SLR test (see Chapter 3), that region is eliminated as the source of referral.

OBSERVATION

GAIT

Observe as the client walks around your treatment room. Indications that there could be a hip problem include a limp; guarded weight bearing, in which the knee is bent to help absorb the shock of weight bearing, shorter stride length, a stiff hip during gait, or shifting of the trunk from side to side in transferring the weight from one leg to the other.

POSTURE

- **Position:** The client is standing, facing away from the therapist.
- **Action:** Place your hands on the iliac crests to determine whether they are level.
- **Observation:** A pelvis that is not level is called a pelvic obliquity. Pelvic obliquity can be caused by leg-length difference, muscle imbalance, SIJ or lumbar spine dysfunction or degeneration, or scoliosis. (See Chapter 3 for further discussion of postural assessment.)

TRENDELENBURG'S TEST

- **Intention:** To assess the balance, stability, and strength of the gluteus medius.
- **Position:** Have the client stand with the back to you and next to a wall, in case he or she needs to reach out a hand for support.
- **Action:** Ask the client to stand on one leg (the uninvolved leg first).
- **Observation:** Normally, the pelvis on the side of the lifted leg should rise because the gluteus medius pulls the hip down on the standing leg. If the gluteus medius on the standing leg is weak, the pelvis

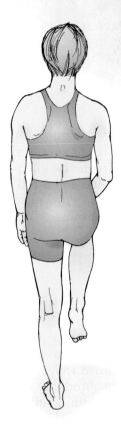

Figure 8-13. Trendelenburg's test. The hip on the standing leg should lower as the opposite leg is lifted. An elevation of the hip on the standing leg side indicates weakness of the gluteus medius on that side.

rises on the standing leg side, lowering the pelvis on the side of the lifted leg. This is called Trendelenburg's sign (Fig. 8-13). If the test is negative, have the client repeat the test with eyes closed. This tests balance and the integrity of the proprioceptors. If the client's balance is impaired, standing on one leg for 10 to 30 seconds several times a day is an excellent exercise to help reeducate the proprioceptors.

ACTIVE MOVEMENTS

Observe the ROM. Ask whether movement hurts.

EXTENSION

See MET #6 for the hip extension test.

FLEXION

▨ **Position:** Ask the client to stand facing you.

▨ **Action:** Ask the client to march in place slowly, bringing the thigh as close to the chest as possible. Ask the client not to lean back to perform this action.

▨ **Observation:** This is a good screening test for hip joint problems and for iliopsoas tendinitis. The normal range is approximately 110° to 120°. With joint involvement, the ROM is limited in flexion. With tendinitis, this movement can elicit pain in the groin.

ABDUCTION

▨ **Position:** Ask the client to stand facing you.

▨ **Action:** Have the client bring one leg out to the side to his or her comfortable limit, abducting the hip. Instruct the client to keep the trunk upright and the foot facing forward and not externally rotated as the movement is performed.

▨ **Observation:** Abduction assessment when the client is standing is more accurate than when the client is supine. If there is a dysfunction in the hip, then there is a tendency to bend the trunk to the opposite side as the client attempts to lift the hip, giving a false reading. The normal range is from 30° to 50°. Painless inability to perform this movement might indicate gluteus medius weakness or degenerative joint disease of the hip. Usually, joint degeneration elicits groin ache with this motion. Pain at the greater trochanter could be a trochanteric bursitis, and pain in the buttock could be a gluteus medius tendinitis.

LATERAL ROTATION

▨ **Position:** The client is prone, with one knee bent to 90°.

▨ **Action:** Place your hand on the sacrum to ensure that it does not move, and ask the client to move the bent leg toward the midline.

▨ **Observation:** The normal range is from 40° to 60°. Always compare both sides. A person who has retroverted hips has an increased range on both sides of lateral rotation and equal limitation of medial rotation on both sides.

MEDIAL ROTATION

▨ **Position:** The client is prone, with one knee bent to 90°.

▨ **Action:** Place your hand on the sacrum to ensure that it does not move, and ask the client to move the bent leg away from the midline.

▨ **Observation:** The ROM is normally approximately 30° to 40°. As with all active and passive tests, compare both sides. A person who has anteverted hips has an increased range of medial rotation on both sides and equal limitation of lateral rotation on both sides. Loss of medial rotation is one of the key assessment findings in hip degeneration.

PASSIVE MOVEMENTS

Always begin with the "good side," that is, the non-involved side. Ask the client to tell you if the movement begins to elicit pain. If there is pain, ask where the pain is felt (location) and what kind of pain or discomfort is felt (quality). Note the ROM and the end feel when you put overpressure on the movement.

EXTENSION

- **Position:** The client is prone, with the knee fully flexed. Place your hand over the client's sacrum to stabilize it, and tuck your other hand under the client's distal thigh.

- **Action:** Slowly lift the client's hip into extension until there is pain or until tissue tension. Keep the leg in neutral; do not abduct it as it is extended (Fig. 8-14).

- **Observation:** The normal ROM is approximately 10° to 15°. This movement places a stretch on the iliopsoas and anterior capsule. A tight iliopsoas has a muscle tension end feel; a tight capsule has a thick, leathery end feel. This motion is typically limited with degenerative joint disease of the hip. This is also a *femoral nerve stretch test.* If there is pain, numbing, or tingling in the anterior thigh,

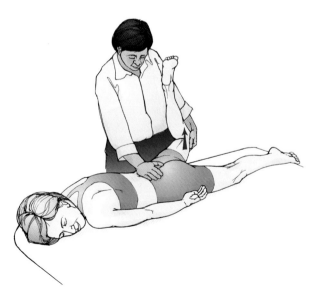

Figure 8-14. Passive extension.

there could be a peripheral entrapment within the iliopsoas or a more central lesion at the L2, L3, or L4 nerve root. If the nerve test is positive, perform MET and manual release of the iliopsoas and femoral nerve for several sessions. If there is no significant improvement, refer the client to a chiropractor or osteopath.

- **MET to Increase Extension:** This position is also used as a PIR MET to increase extension of the hip and to stretch the iliopsoas and anterior joint capsule. Have the client resist as you attempt to pull the hip into greater extension. Relax for a few seconds. Slowly pull the hip into greater extension to a new resistance barrier. Have the client resist as you attempt to pull the hip into further extension. Relax, and move the hip again into further extension. Repeat this cycle three to five times.

FLEXION

- **Position:** The client is supine. Bring the client's hip and knee into flexion, and place the foot on the table. Place your hand on the client's knee and your other hand on the lateral side of the crest of the ilium.

- **Action:** With your inferior hand, bring the hip into flexion by moving the thigh toward the client's chest until you feel the pelvis move. As soon as you feel the pelvis move, you are at the end range of hip flexion.

- **Observation:** The normal pattern of movement for the thigh is in a straight line toward the chest, independent of movement of the pelvis. The normal range is approximately 140°. A dysfunctional movement pattern for the thigh is to move toward abduction and external rotation as you bring it toward the chest (i.e., toward the open position of the joint) and for the pelvis to move with the thigh. This dysfunctional pattern combined with a limited ROM typically indicates a shortness and fibrosis of the ischiofemoral ligament and hip joint degeneration. Pain in the groin at the end of the range indicates psoas tendinitis, and pain in the groin with an empty end feel indicates iliopectineal bursitis. If the range is normal, note whether the opposite leg rises off the table. This indicates a short and tight iliopsoas of the extended leg. Passive hip flexion on one leg to determine psoas tightness on the extended leg is called the **Thomas test.**

ABDUCTION

- **Position:** For easy comparison, both hips are tested together. The client is supine, with hips in a flexed and abducted position and the soles of the feet together in the center of the table.

▨ **Action:** If this position is comfortable, permit the client to rest the legs in this position. If the hips cannot rest in this position comfortably, ask the client to locate the pain and describe its quality. If the client can rest in this position comfortably, place your hands on the client's knees, and slowly press the knees toward the table, pressing the hips into abduction.

▨ **Observation:** Compare the height of the knees to determine the ROM of hip abduction. This is a quick screening test that allows you to easily compare the two sides. Discomfort or pain in the groin might indicate a strain of the adductor longus. Pain in the posterior hip might indicate posterior capsule impingement. Loss of motion on one side with a capsular end feel indicates capsular fibrosis and possible hip joint degeneration. Loss of passive internal rotation would confirm degenerative joint disease of the hip.

 CAUTION: Clients who have had total hip replacements should not be pushed past 90° of hip flexion or to the end range of adduction or internal and external rotation.

ADDUCTION

▨ **Position:** The client is supine. Have the client flex the knee and place the foot on the table. Stabilize the pelvis by placing one hand on the client's ASIS closest to you. Place your other hand on the client's knee.

▨ **Action:** Flex the hip fully, and then move the hip into adduction by pressing the thigh toward the opposite shoulder, 90° to the inguinal ligament (Fig. 8-15).

▨ **Observation:** This flexion compresses the iliopsoas muscle, the iliofemoral ligament, and the iliopectineal bursa and stretches the piriformis muscle. Groin pain with tissue stretch indicates iliopsoas muscle tension; groin pain with limited motion and capsular end feel indicates iliofemoral ligament fibrosis; and groin pain with an empty end feel indicates iliopectineal bursitis. Buttock pain might indicate piriformis shortness.

MEDIAL OR LATERAL ROTATION

▨ **Position:** The client is supine. Bring the hip and knee to 90° of flexion, with no abduction or adduction of the hip. Hold the ankle in one hand, and place the other hand on the outside of the knee.

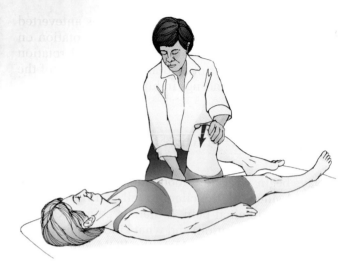

Figure 8-15. Passive hip adduction. The best clinical information is gathered if the hip is pressed into adduction perpendicular to the inguinal ligament.

▨ **Action:** Stabilize the knee, and slowly pull the ankle toward you to medially rotate the hip joint, and then move the leg away from you to laterally rotate the hip joint (Fig. 8-16).

▨ **Observation:** Lateral rotation should be 10° to 20° greater than medial rotation. Compare both sides. If the client has retroverted hips, there is excessive lateral rotation bilaterally. If the hips are anteverted, there is excessive medial rotation bilaterally. Decreased medial rotation on one side, eliciting

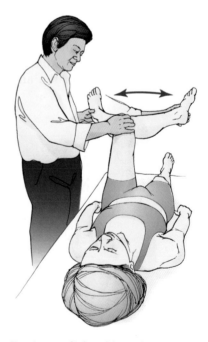

Figure 8-16. Passive medial and lateral rotation. This is one of the most important tests in hip assessment. Medial rotation is the first motion that is decreased in capsulitis, fibrosis of the joint capsule, and degeneration of the articular surfaces. These three conditions are differentiated by the end feel.

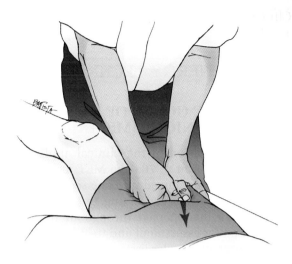

Figure 8-17. Anterior-to-posterior mobilization of the hip joint.

groin pain at the end range, is usually indicative of hip joint degeneration or of ligamentous or capsular fibrosis. Joint degeneration has a hard end feel or a capsular end feel with decreased ROM. Shortness of the ligaments or capsule has a capsular, leathery end feel. The capsular pattern of the hip is decreased medial rotation and abduction.

MOBILIZATION OF THE HIP JOINT

▓ **Intention:** This mobilization is performed to assess motion restrictions of the femoral head in the acetabulum and to induce an A-P glide (Fig. 8-17).

Typically, the femur is fixed anteriorly due to sustained tightness in the hip flexors and weakness in the extensors. This mobilization is shown here for teaching purposes, but in the context of the treatment, it is typically performed after METs for the iliopsoas, rectus femoris, and TFL and Level I strokes.

▓ **Position:** The client is supine. Place your hands next to each other below the inguinal ligament, midway between the ASIS and the pubic symphysis (midline of the body).

▓ **Action:** Gently push the proximal femur posteriorly, in brisk, oscillating pulses. Repeat several times.

▓ **Observation:** The typical motion restriction and positional dysfunction of the head of the femur is an anterior fixation. Mobilizing the head of the femur posteriorly helps to reestablish its normal position and movement. Compare to the non-involved side and to other healthy hips to get a feeling for what is normal.

PALPATION

▓ Most of the soft tissue palpation is done while performing the strokes. As you perform each stroke, feel for temperature, texture, tenderness, and tone. Be aware that in addition to groin tenderness caused by irritation of the muscle or bursa, the groin is also an emotionally vulnerable area. Approach this area with sensitivity.

Techniques

GUIDELINES TO APPLYING TECHNIQUES

A thorough discussion of treatment guidelines can be found on p. 86 in Chapter 2. In the method of treatment described in this text, we make two underlying assumptions. The first is that pain or dysfunction in one localized area affects the entire region, so we assess and treat an entire region rather than localized

pain. A degenerated hip, for example, is not an isolated condition but typically affects the knee and low back as well as the muscles of the hip and lumbosacral region. The second assumption is that pain and dysfunction that localize in one tissue affect many other tissues in the area. Iliopsoas tendinitis, for example, typically involves not only the iliopsoas muscle and tendon, but also the ligaments and joint capsule of the hip as well as the alignment and motion of the hip joint. The treatments described in this text address all the structures of the region through three techniques: muscle energy technique (MET), soft tissue mobilization (STM), and joint mobilization. These techniques can be applied to every type of hip pain, but the "dose" of the technique varies greatly from slow movements and light pressures for acute conditions, to stronger pressures and deeper amplitude mobilizations for chronic problems. Each aspect of the treatment is also an assessment to determine pain, tenderness, hypertonicity, weakness, and hypomobility or hypermobility. We use the philosophy of treating what we find when we find it. Remember that the goal of treatment is to heal the body, mind, and emotions. Keep your hands soft, keep your touch nurturing, and work only within the comfortable limits of your client so that he or she can completely relax into the treatment.

THE INTENTIONS OF TREATMENT FOR ACUTE CONDITIONS ARE AS FOLLOWS

▨ To stimulate the movement of fluids to reduce edema, increase oxygenation and nutrition, and eliminate waste products.

▨ To maintain as much pain-free joint motion as possible to prevent adhesions and maintain the health of the cartilage, which depends on movement for its nutrition.

▨ To provide mechanical stimulation to help align healing fibers and stimulate cellular synthesis.

▨ To provide neurological input to minimize muscular inhibition and help maintain proprioceptive function.

 CAUTION: Stretching is ***contraindicated*** in acute conditions

THE INTENTIONS OF TREATMENT FOR CHRONIC CONDITIONS ARE AS FOLLOWS

▨ To dissolve adhesions and restore flexibility, length and alignment to the myofascia.

▨ To dissolve fibrosis in the ligaments and capsular tissues surrounding the joints.

▨ To rehydrate the cartilage and restore mobility and ROM to the joints.

▨ To eliminate hypertonicity in short and tight muscles, strengthen weakened muscles, and reestablish the normal firing pattern in dysfunctioning muscles.

▨ To restore neurological function by increasing sensory awareness and proprioception.

Clinical examples are described below under "Soft Tissue Mobilization."

MUSCLE ENERGY TECHNIQUE

THERAPEUTIC GOALS OF MUSCLE ENERGY TECHNIQUE (MET)

A thorough discussion of the clinical application of MET can be found on p. 76. The MET techniques described below are organized into one section for teaching purposes. In the clinical setting, the METs and STM techniques are interspersed throughout the session. METs are used for assessment and treatment. A healthy muscle or group of muscles is strong and pain free when isometrically challenged. MET will be painful if there is ischemia or inflammation in the muscles or their associated joints. The muscle will be weak and painless if the muscle is inhibited or the nerve is compromised. During treatment, MET is used as needed. For example, when you find a tight and tender piriformis, use CR MET to reduce the hypertonicity and tenderness. If the piriformis is painful while contracting, perform RI MET, inducing a neurological relaxation. If the hip extensors are weak and inhibited, first release the tight hip flexors, then use CR MET to recruit and strengthen the hip extensors. A primary goal in performing MET for the hip is to lengthen a shortened joint capsule (MET #14), as this helps to prevent joint degeneration.

MET is very effective for an acute, painful hip, but the pressure that is applied must be very light so as not to induce pain. Gentle, pain-free contraction and relaxation of the hip flexors and extensors and related muscles provide a pumping action to reduce swelling, promote the flow of oxygen and nutrition, and eliminate waste products.

THE BASIC THERAPEUTIC INTENTIONS OF MET FOR ACUTE CONDITIONS ARE AS FOLLOWS

▨ Provide a gentle pumping action to reduce pain and swelling, promote oxygenation of the tissue, and remove waste products.

▨ Reduce muscle spasms.

▨ Provide neurological input to mimimize muscular inhibition.

THE BASIC THERAPEUTIC INTENTIONS OF MET FOR CHRONIC CONDITIONS ARE AS FOLLOWS

▨ Decrease excessive muscle tension.

▨ Strengthen muscles.

▨ Lengthen connective tissue.

▨ Increase joint movement and increase lubrication to the joints.

▨ Restore neurological function.

The hip flexors and adductors are typically short and tight, and the extensors and abductors are typically weak. First assess and treat the muscles that tend to be tight. In the muscles of the hip, the iliopsoas (see Chapter 3), adductors, rectus femoris, pectineus, TFL, and hamstrings are usually found to be short and tight. Next, functionally test the firing pattern of the gluteus medius, and facilitate the muscle if it tests weak. The MET section ends with a remarkably effective treatment for degeneration of the hip: MET #14, "Muscle Energy Technique to Increase Medial Rotation."

The MET section below shows techniques that are used for most clients. In acute conditions, use MET #1 to reduce swelling and pain in the joint. METs #9, #12, and #13 are for chronic conditions only, as they involve increasing the length of the myofascia. Remember that stretching is **contraindicated** in acute conditions.

MET should not be painful. Mild discomfort as the client resists the pressure is normal if the area is irritated or inflamed. Refer to Chapters 3 and 9 for METs for the lumbar spine and the knee, which directly influence the hip.

MUSCLE ENERGY TECHNIQUE FOR ACUTE HIP PAIN

1. Contract-Relax Muscle Energy Technique and Traction for Acute Hip Pain

▨ **Intention:** The flexors of the hip are most commonly involved in acute hip pain. Use CR MET to help reduce the hypertonicity in the flexors and to help decompress the joint.

▨ **Position:** The client is supine, with the hip flexed and the foot on the table. Hold the distal thigh with both your hands.

▨ **Action:** Have the client resist as you pull inferiorly on the thigh to provide traction on the hip joint for approximately 5 seconds. Relax, and repeat three to five times. After a few cycles, as the client is relaxing, pull the thigh footward for approximately 30 to 90 seconds. Repeat several times (Fig. 8-18).

MUSCLE ENERGY TECHNIQUE FOR HYPERTONIC MUSCLES

2. Contract-Relax and Postisometric Relaxation Muscle Energy Technique for the Pectineus and Adductors

▨ **Intention:** The intention is to perform CR and PIR MET to reduce the hypertonicity and lengthen the

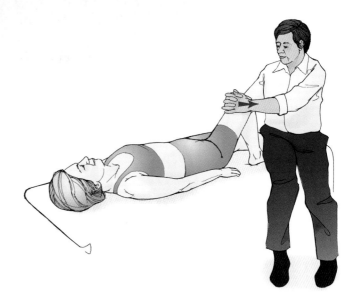

Figure 8-18. CR MET and hip traction for acute hip pain.

short adductors and the pectineus. These muscles are often strained, causing a painful limitation of abduction.

▨ **Position:** Client is supine with the involved hip flexed, externally rotated, and abducted to the resistance barrier. If this position is painful, place your flexed knee on the table, and have the client rest his or her leg on your thigh, or place a pillow under the abducted thigh.

▨ **Action:** Place one hand on the distal thigh and the other hand on the opposite ASIS, and have the client resist as you press outward at the knee, attempting to move the hip into further abduction for approximately 5 seconds. Have client relax, and then slowly move the hip into further abduction to lengthen the adductors and pectineus. Repeat several times (Fig. 8-19).

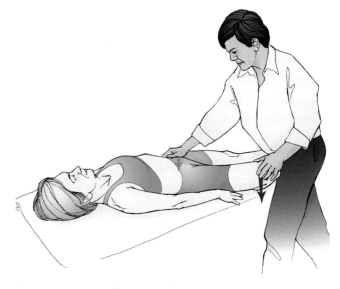

Figure 8-19. CR and PIR MET for the pectineus and adductors.

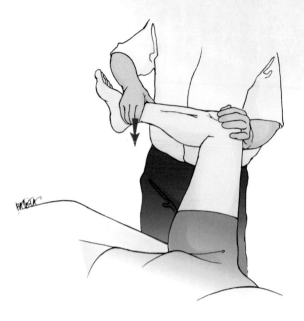

Figure 8-20. CR MET for the rectus femoris.

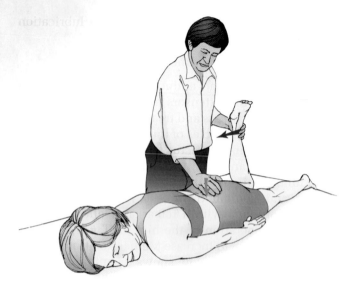

Figure 8-21. PIR MET for the medial and lateral rotators.

3. *Contract-Relax Muscle Energy Technique for the Rectus Femoris*

- **Intention:** The intention is to release the rectus femoris, which is typically short and tight. Because it interweaves with the joint capsule, tightness can cause limited motion in the joint.

- **Position:** Client is supine with the hip and knee flexed to 90°.

- **Action:** Place one hand on the client's distal leg and the other hand on the client's knee. Have the client resist as you attempt to flex the knee by pressing the leg back to the table. Relax for a few seconds. Perform RI MET by having the client resist as you attempt to pull the foot away from the table. This contracts the hamstrings, reciprocally inhibiting the quadriceps. Repeat several times (Fig. 8-20).

4. *Postisometric Relaxation Muscle Energy Technique for Medial and Lateral Rotators*

- **Intention:** If the assessment determined a decrease in medial or lateral rotation of the hip, the intention is to release the medial and lateral rotators. One contributing factor to decreased hip rotation can be hypertonicity of the muscles.

- **Position:** Client is prone, with one knee flexed. Hold the distal leg with one hand, and place your other hand over the sacrum to stabilize the pelvis to prevent it from rotating.

- **Action:** *To release the lateral rotators,* move the client's leg laterally, medially rotating the hip, to the resistance barrier. Have the client resist as you pull out at the ankle for approximately 5 seconds. Have the client relax; then move the leg laterally to a new resistance barrier. Relax and repeat. *To release the medial rotators,* move the client's leg medially, laterally rotating the hip. Ask the client to resist as you push the leg toward the opposite leg (i.e., into further lateral rotation). Have the client relax; then move the leg medially to a new resistance barrier. Relax and repeat (Fig. 8-21).

5. *Contract-Relax Muscle Energy Technique for the Hamstrings*

- **Intention:** The hamstrings are typically hypertonic, and the intention is to reduce their hypertonicity. CR MET in conjunction with the massage strokes is a simple way to accomplish this.

- **Position:** Client is prone, with the feet resting on a pillow. Lift one leg slightly off the pillow. Place one hand on the hamstrings for a sensory cue and your other hand on the back of the heel.

- **Action:** Have the client resist as you attempt to extend the knee by pressing the foot toward the pillow for approximately 5 seconds. Have the client relax; then rest the foot on the pillow. To reciprocally inhibit the hamstrings, have the client resist as you attempt to pull the foot off the pillow for approximately 5 seconds. Relax and repeat (Fig. 8-22).

6. *Assessment of Muscle Firing Pattern for Hip Extension*

- **Intention:** The intention of this test is to assess whether the gluteus maximus contracts in the

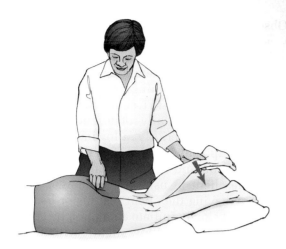

Figure 8-22. CR MET for the hamstrings.

proper sequence and with adequate strength in hip extension. The firing sequence should be hamstrings and gluteus maximus, contralateral lumbar paraspinals, and ipsilateral paraspinals.[5] If the gluteus maximus does not have adequate strength, the trunk will rotate while the hip is being extended. Because the gluteus maximus is typically weak, the hamstrings become dominant, forcing the head of the femur anteriorly during hip extension, stressing the anterior joint capsule.[12] The therapist monitors whether the gluteus maximus fires with the hamstrings and before the paraspinals. If contraction does not occur in the proper sequence, the therapist instructs the client in in the proper sequence and encourages hip extension as a home exercise.

▦ **Position:** Client is prone. Therapist places one hand on the hamstrings and the other on the gluteus maximus (Fig. 8-23).

▦ **Action:** Have the client extend the hip by slowly lifting one leg off the table (only about 10°). Feel the

hamstrings and gluteus maximus to determine whether the gluteus maximus is contracting with the hamstrings. Observe the lumbar paraspinals to determine whether they contract before the gluteus maximus. If the parapsinals contract before the gluteus maximus, instruct the client to contract the gluteus maximus first with the hamstrings, before the paraspinals. If the gluteus maximus is weak, refer to isotonic exercise for the gluteus maximus on p. 132 in Chapter 3).

7. Contract-Relax Muscle Energy Technique for the Adductors in the Side-Lying Position

▦ **Intention:** The adductors are typically hypertonic, and the intention is to reduce this hypertonicity. This position is an easy way to release the adductors in conjunction with performing the massage strokes.

▦ **Position:** Client is side-lying near the edge of the table, with the top hip and knee flexed resting on a pillow and the bottom leg straight on the table.

▦ **Action:** Have the client raise the straight leg off the table for approximately 5 seconds. Make sure the foot is parallel to the table and that the client keeps the trunk from rotating. Have the client resist as you gently attempt to press the leg back to the table. Have the client relax the leg back on the table for a few seconds. To perform RI, have the client resist as you attempt to lift the leg off the table. Relax and repeat several times, and perform on the other side (Fig. 8-24).

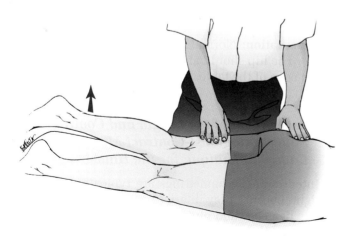

Figure 8-23. Assessment of muscle firing pattern for hip extension.

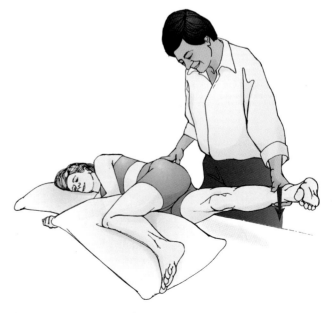

Figure 8-24. CR MET (side-lying position) for the adductors.

FUNCTIONAL TESTING AND MUSCLE ENERGY TECHNIQUE

8. Assessment of the Muscle-Firing Pattern and Contract-Relax Muscle Energy Technique for the Gluteus Medius and Minimus

▨ **Intention:** The gluteus medius is often weak, and to compensate for its weakness, the TFL will contract first to abduct the hip, causing the hip to flex and internally rotate or the trunk to rotate backward to allow the TFL to work more efficiently. The intention is to assess the firing pattern of the gluteus medius and to increase gluteus medius strength.

▨ **Position:** Client is lying on his or her side, without any forward or backward rotation of the trunk. The leg next to the table is flexed to approximately 90°. Stand behind the client.

▨ **Action:** To assess hip abduction, ask the client to slowly abduct the hip. To perform CR MET on the gluteus medius, the hip is abducted approximately 35° in slight extension and external rotation. Rest the client's leg on your flexed elbow, with your hand under the client's knee. Ask the client to slowly lift the leg off your arm. An alternative position is to place one hand near the ankle and your other hand on the gluteus medius and TFL. Have the client resist as you press toward the table (toward adduction). To perform CR MET on the gluteus minimus, the hip is in neutral (i.e., the foot is parallel to the table) and not externally rotated. To perform RI MET, have the client straighten the leg, and place it on the table and resist as you attempt to lift it off the table (Fig. 8-25).

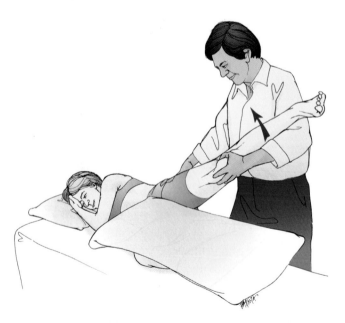

Figure 8-25. CR MET and assessment of the muscle-firing pattern of the gluteus medius.

▨ **Observation:** The gluteus medius is typically weak. To compensate for this weakness, the client will substitute the stronger flexors but rotating the trunk as he or she is attempting to resist. It is important to observe two things: (1) an abnormal firing pattern in which the TFL contracts first, causing the hip to flex and internally rotate, and (2) whether the trunk rotates posteriorly, allowing for the TFL to flex the hip, substituting for the weak gluteus medius. If you find either one of these patterns, educate the client in using the gluteus medius correctly by having the client rest his or her leg on a pillow and slowly initiate abduction by attempting to lift the leg off the pillow slightly without rotating the trunk.

9. Assessment of the Length and Postisometric Relaxation Muscle Energy Technique for the Medial Hamstrings and Adductors

▨ **Intention:** The medial hamstrings and adductors are typically short and tight, and the intention of this technique is to assess their length and to increase their length if they test short.

▨ **Position:** Client is supine with the heel of the supporting leg over the edge of the table to stabilize the body.

▨ **Action:** Abduct the client's leg, and move your body between the table and the tested leg. Keeping the knee extended and the foot in neutral, abduct the client's leg to the tension barrier by moving the leg with your body. Perform PIR MET by having the client resist as you attempt to move the leg into further abduction for approximately 5 seconds. Have the client relax for a few seconds; then slowly abduct the hip to a new tension barrier. Relax, and repeat several times, then perform on the other side (Fig. 8-26).

▨ **Observation:** Normal abduction is approximately 45°. The hip should abduct approximately 25° from the edge of the table.

10. Assessment of the Length and Contract-Relax-Antagonist-Contract Muscle Energy Technique for the Hamstrings

▨ **Intention:** The hamstrings are typically short and tight. Because they interweave with the sacrotuberous ligament and gluteal fascia, tightness prevents full mobility of the lumbopelvic region. The intention of this contract-relax-antagonist-contract (CRAC) MET is to lengthen the hamstrings. This technique is for chronic conditions only.

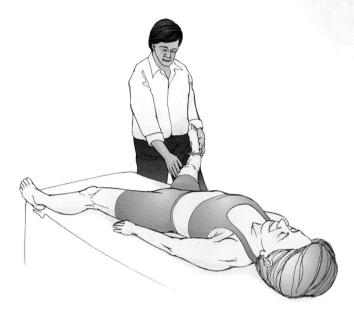

Figure 8-26. PIR MET and assessment of the length of the medial hamstrings and adductors.

■ **Position:** Client is supine. Place the client's ankle over your shoulder, and rest your hands over the client's knee to keep the knee extended.

■ **Action:** To assess the length of the hamstrings, perform a modified SLR test by slowly lifting the leg to the resistance barrier. To perform CRAC MET, have the client resist by pressing his or her leg into your shoulder as you attempt to lift the leg toward the client's head for approximately 5 seconds. Have the client relax, and after a few seconds, have the client actively lift the leg headward while keeping the knee straight. Have the client relax. Repeat the procedure several times, and then perform it on the other leg (Fig. 8-27).

■ **Observation:** The normal length of the hamstrings should allow for approximately 70° of hip flexion

with the opposite leg on the table. With the opposite knee flexed, the range is approximately 90°.

11. Contract-Relax and Eccentric Muscle Energy Technique for Tensor Fascia Lata

■ **Intention:** The TFL is typically tight and short. The intention is to reduce the muscle hypertonicity and to lengthen the fascia. CR and eccentric MET are effective methods to accomplish this goal.

■ **Position:** Client is supine. Hold the client's leg just above the ankle, and assist the client as he or she flexes the hip approximately 45° with slight abduction and medial rotation. Place your other hand on the TFL to give a sensory cue when the muscle is contracting.

■ **Action:** To perform CR for more acute conditions, have the client resist as you press toward extension and adduction, that is, toward the other leg. Relax and repeat. To perform eccentric MET for chronic conditions, have the client continue to offer some resistance, but instruct the client to "let me move your leg very slowly." Then slowly move the leg toward the opposite leg. To perform RI MET, have the client hold one foot against the other on the table and resist as you attempt to pull the leg up into flexion and abduction (i.e., to pull the leg back to the beginning position) (Fig. 8-28). An alternative RI is to have the client's leg remain in the starting flexed and abducted position and have the client resist as you attempt to pull up into greater flexion and abduction.

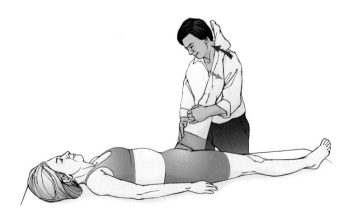

Figure 8-27. CRAC MET and assessment of the length of the hamstrings.

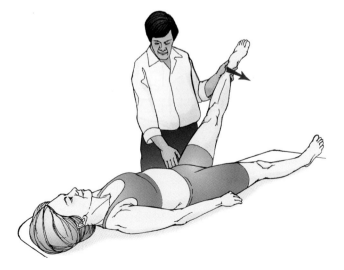

Figure 8-28. CR and eccentric MET for the TFL.

12. *Postisometric Relaxation Muscle Energy Technique for the Tensor Fascia Lata, the Iliotibial Band, and the Quadratus Lumborum for Chronic Conditions*

- **Intention:** The intention is to release the TFL and ITB. The TFL is typically short and tight, and the ITB is typically thick and fibrous, contributing to genu valgus (knock-knees) and patellar tracking dysfunction.
- **Position:** Client is supine with the feet over the edge of the table. To treat the left side, flex the client's right knee and place the right foot on the table on the outside of the left knee. Stretch the left leg toward the right until you feel tissue tension. Place the side of your thigh against the outside of the client's left ankle. Place your right hand on the client's right knee, pressing it to her left, and your left hand on the distal left leg.
- **Action:** Have the client resist as you use your leg to press the client's left leg toward his or her right side for approximately 5 seconds. Have the client relax for a few seconds, and then slowly press the leg further toward the client's right side to a new tension barrier. Relax, and repeat several times. Perform on the other side (Fig. 8-29).

13. *Contract-Relax-Antagonist-Contract Muscle Energy Technique for the Pectineus and Adductors and to Increase Hip Abduction*

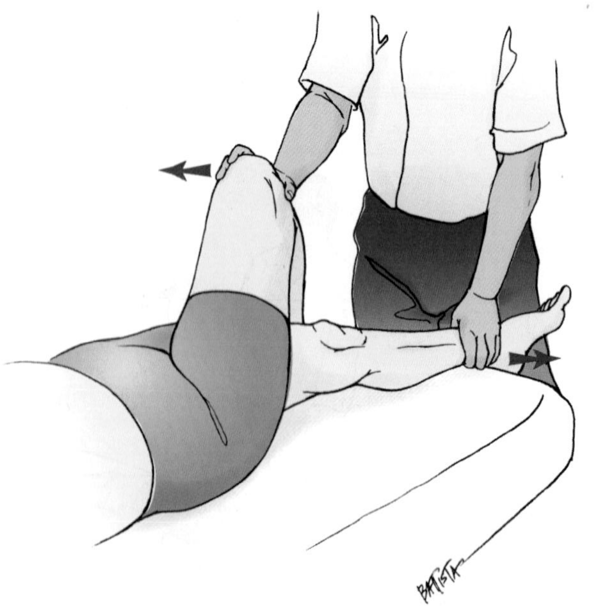

Figure 8-29. PIR MET for the tensor fascia lata, iliotibial band, and quadratus lumborum.

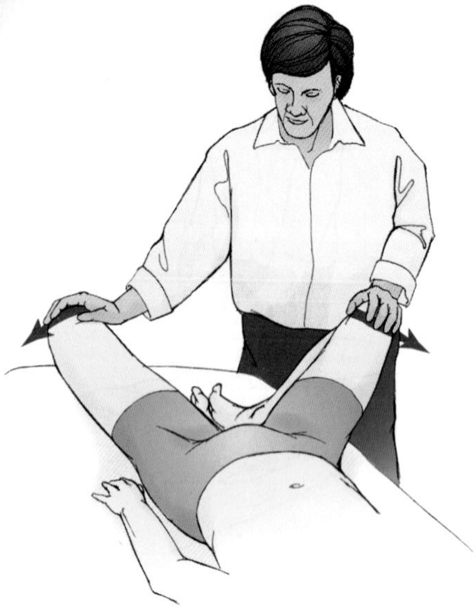

Figure 8-30. CRAC MET for the pectineus and adductors and to increase abduction of the hip.

- **Intention:** The intention is to release the short adductors, which are typically tight in degenerative conditions of the hip, causing limitation of abduction.
- **Position:** Client is supine with both hips flexed, externally rotated, and abducted to their comfortable limit, with the feet on the table in the midline and the soles of the feet touching. Have the client flatten the low back on the table to prevent excessive lordosis. Because the hip is much more limited in its ability to abduct with hip dysfunction or degeneration, begin the MET by placing the "good" hip at the same degree of abduction as the limited hip.
- **Action:** Place both hands on the distal thighs, and ask the client to resist as you attempt to press the knees toward the table for approximately 5 seconds. Relax for a few seconds, and then ask the client to squeeze the buttock muscles (gluteals and external rotators) to pull the knees further toward the table. Typically, only about 1 inch of new movement is achieved. Have the client relax. Repeat the CRAC cycle several times (Fig. 8-30).

MUSCLE ENERGY TECHNIQUE FOR CAPSULITIS AND HIP DEGENERATION

14. *Muscle Energy Technique to Increase Medial and Lateral Rotation*

> ! *CAUTION: This procedure is contraindicated after total hip replacement.*

Intention: The primary intention is to help restore medial rotation, which is the first motion that is lost in capsulitis and joint degeneration (arthritis), by stretching the joint capsule and stimulating the secretion of lubrication (synovial fluid) within the joint. This technique is remarkably effective in restoring function to a hip with mild to moderate degeneration. This MET can also be used to help restore lateral rotation if indicated.

Position: Client is supine. Bring the involved hip into 90° of hip flexion and 90° of knee flexion. Do not allow the hip to adduct or abduct. Place one hand on the lateral aspect of the knee, and hold the leg just proximal to the ankle.

Action: Pull the leg laterally into the comfortable limit of medial rotation of the hip. Have the client resist as you pull laterally at the ankle, attempting to move the hip into further medial rotation, and press at the knee to stabilize it. Have the client relax. After a few seconds, slowly move the leg laterally into a new tension or pain barrier, increasing medial rotation of the hip. Repeat three to five times (Fig. 8-31). After three to five contract-relax-stretch cycles, gently oscillate the hip in small arcs of medial-lateral rotation to sweep the joint with synovial fluid. Bring the hip to the resistance barrier of medial rotation, and repeat the contract-relax-stretch treatment for several minutes. To increase lateral rotation, perform the same technique described above. Move the client's leg toward the resistance barrier of lateral rotation, and have the client resist as you press on the ankle, attempting to move the hip into greater lateral rotation.

15. Muscle Energy Technique to Stretch the Anterior Capsule and to Increase Hip Extension

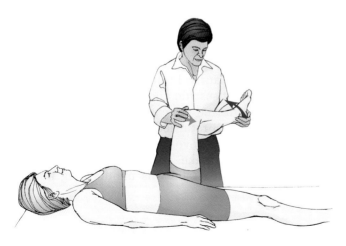

Figure 8-31. MET to increase medial rotation.

Intention: The intention is to lengthen the anterior capsule, which shortens in chronic capsular conditions and hip joint degeneration.

Position: This is the same position as the one that is used in the assessment of passive extension. Client is prone. Assume either of two positions: Tuck one hand under the client's distal thigh, or place your flexed thigh on the table and rest the client's thigh on your thigh.

Action: Pull the thigh into the limit of passive extension (see Fig. 8-14). Have the client resist as you attempt to pull the thigh farther off the table, into further extension. Have the client relax. Then lift the client's thigh into further extension. If your flexed thigh is on the table, move it headward under the client's thigh, bringing the client's hip into further extension. Repeat several times.

SOFT TISSUE MOBILIZATION

BACKGROUND

A thorough discussion of the clinical application of STM can be found on p. 68. In the Hendrickson Method of manual therapy described in this text, the STM movements are called *wave mobilization* and are a combination of joint mobilization and STM performed in rhythmic oscillations with a frequency of 50 to 70 cycles per minute, except when performing brisk transverse friction massage (TFM) strokes, which can be two to four cycles per second. These mobilizations are presented in a specific sequence, which has been found to achieve the most efficient and effective results. This allows the therapist to "scan" the body to determine areas of tenderness, hypertonicity, and decreased mobility. It is important to "follow the recipe" until you have mastered this work. The techniques described below are divided into two sequences: Level I and Level II. Level I strokes are designed for every client, from acute injury to chronic degeneration, to enhance health and bring the body to optimum performance. Level II strokes are typically applied after Level I strokes and are designed for chronic conditions. Guidelines for treating acute and chronic conditions are listed below.

GUIDELINES FOR THE THERAPIST

Acute

The primary intention of treatment is to decrease pain and swelling as quickly as possible, maintain as much pain-free joint motion as possible, and induce relaxation. In this method of treatment, the soft tissue is compressed and decompressed in rhythmic cycles. This provides a pumping action that helps to promote fluid exchange, reducing swelling. The strokes that are applied to the client who is in acute pain need to be performed with a very gentle touch, a very slow rhythm, and small amplitude. There is no uniform "dose" or depth of treatment. The depth of treatment is based on the client's level of pain. If the soft tissue does not begin to relax, use more METs to help reduce discomfort, swelling, and excessive muscle tension. As was mentioned previously, intersperse your STM work with MET. Remember that **stretching is contraindicated** in acute conditions.

Clinical Example: Acute

Subjective: CS is a 51-year-old female office worker who presented to my office complaining of acute hip and groin pain. She reported that the pain had begun about a week previously. She reported that there was no specific injury but that she had started running again about a month earlier. She described the pain as a severe ache and burning, worse at the front of the hip region (she pointed to the ASIS), with the the burning extending into the anterior thigh. She said that the pain was keeping her up at night.

Objective: Examination revealed an unleveled ilium, with the right iliac crest higher than the left. Active lumbar motion was pain free and of normal range. Active hip flexion elicited pain at the anterior hip region. Active hip extension and abduction were weak. Passive motion was full and pain free. Palpation revealed spastic and tender TFL and iliopsoas. Motion palpation revealed a limitation of posterior glide of the head of the femur, indicating an anterior fixation of the femoral head. Palpation of the fascia above the ASIS revealed fibrotic tissue in the area of the exit point of the lateral femoral cutaneous nerve. Digital compression of the area elicited mild pain in the anterior thigh.

Assessment: Spastic and tender TFL and iliopsoas, with anterior fixation of the femoral joint, and entrapment of the lateral femoral cutaneous nerve.

Treatment (Action): Treatment began with the client supine. CR and RI METs for the TFL (MET #11) and iliopsoas (METs #6 and #7 from Chapter 3) were performed to reduce the hypertonic tissue and to reduce the ischemic congestion and swelling in those muscles. The hip was gently mobilized with the soft tissue work to help normalize the articular motion and to induce a relaxation response in the surrounding muscles. The client was placed in the side-lying position, and MET #8 was performed to help recruit (strengthen) the gluteus medius. The client was instructed in how to do this as a home exercise. The other gluteal and lumbar muscles were released with STM (Level I, Lumbosacral Spine). The other side was treated, and then the client was placed supine. Gentle A–P glide mobilization was performed on the right hip. After several oscillations, the hip joint had normal passive glide. I next performed gentle release of the lateral femoral cutaneous nerve (Level II, third series). The treatment was completely comfortable, even though the work created some mild tingling in the anterior thigh. I had the client walk around the treatment room. She said that the pain was completely gone and that active hip motion was also pain free.

Plan: I recommended weekly visits for one month. CS returned to our office in a week and stated that she continued to feel significantly less pain. However, she reported that when she began running again, the pain returned slightly. She described that she had to run with her toes pointing inward to avoid knee pain, a piece of her history that she had failed to mention at the first visit. On palpation and length testing, the ITB was very tight. The TFL and iliopsoas were mildly hypertonic, and the hip was slightly fixed anteriorly. I repeated the treatment described in the first session and added PIR for the ITB (MET #12). I reviewed the exercise to strengthen the gluteus medius. CS returned to my office one week later, symptom free, even with running. I recommended that she make a follow-up visit in one month to ensure that she was maintaining normal function in the hip.

Chronic

The typical exam findings in clients with chronic hip problems are decreased medial rotation; tight flexors, including rectus femoris, iliopsoas, TFL, and ITB; and weakness in the extensors and abductors, including the gluteus maximus and medius, respectively. The hip joint is typically hypomobile, and fixed anteriorly, with thick, fibrous ligaments and capsular tissues limiting flexion, adduction, and medial rotation. Some patients demonstrate the opposite: unstable joints; weak, deconditioned muscles; and atrophied ligaments and capsular tissues. The primary treatment goals depend on the patient. For patients who are hypomobile, the treatment goals are to reduce the hypertonicity of the muscles; promote mobility and extensibility in the connective tissue by dissolving the adhesions in the muscles, tendons, ligaments, and capsular tissues surrounding the joints; rehydrate the cartilage of the joint; reestablish normal joint play and ROM in the joints; and restore normal neurological function by stimulating the proprioceptors and reestablishing the normal firing patterns in the muscles. Patients who are unstable need exercise rehabilitation. Our treatments can support their stability by reducing tension in the tight muscles with STM and MET, strengthening weak muscles, reestablishing normal firing patterns, and rehabilitating the proprioceptors with MET. With chronic hip conditions, it is also important to treat tightness in the lumbosacral spine. With chronic conditions, we use stronger pressure on the soft tissue and more vigorous mobilizations on the joints. In the Level II sequence, we add deeper soft tissue work and work on attachment points, using transverse friction strokes if we find fibrosis (thickening). As was mentioned in the "Acute" section above, intersperse your soft tissue work with METs.

Clinical Example: Chronic

Subjective: KP is a 48-year-old, 5'9", 150-pound, male psychotherapist who presented to my office with pain in the right groin. He described the pain as a diffuse, deep ache that could increase to a moderate sharp pain after a long hike. He stated that the pain had begun a few weeks prior to his visit, without any particular incident. His history included a minor car accident approximately 10 years previously. He stated that he did not have any prior symptoms in his groin and denied any history of back pain or injury to his hip or low back.

Objective: Examination revealed an unleveling of the pelvis, with the ilium high on the right side. Active ROM was full and pain free in all motions, except medial rotation. Passive ROM testing showed an approximately 50% loss of medial rotation, eliciting tenderness in the groin and a capsular end feel, and a loss of A–P glide of the hip joint. Length testing revealed shortness in the iliopsoas, rectus femoris, and TFL, but they were painless with CR MET. The gluteus medius was weak to isometric challenge. Palpation revealed thick, fibrotic tissue below the inguinal ligament in the area of the hip joint at the hip flexor attachments.

Assessment: An assessment was made of capsular fibrosis, hypertonicity of the hip flexors, weakness of the gluteus medius, loss of medial rotation, and anterior fixation of the hip.

Treatment: The goals of treatment were to reduce pain, decrease muscle hypertonicity, and improve joint play and ROM in the joint to restore pain-free function. Treatment began with CR MET for the iliopsoas (METs #6 and #7 from Chapter 3), rectus femoris (MET #3), and TFL (MET #11). MET #8 was performed to help recruit the gluteus medius. STM was then performed on each of these muscles, concentrating on the Level I, fourth and fifth series, and Level II, fifth series, to dissolve the adhesions and restore the extensibility to the tissue. MET #14 was performed to increase medial rotation and to stimulate the secretion of synovial fluid. Grade I and II joint mobilization was performed in oscillating cycles of internal/external rotation to sweep the head of the femur across the acetabulum, spreading the newly secreted synovial fluid. Gentle A–P mobilizations were then performed on the hip. The client was placed in the side-lying position, and the lumbar muscles were released with MET and STM. MET, STM, and joint mobilization were performed on the non-involved side. Tight and tender hip flexors and lumbar erectors were palpated and released.

Plan: I recommended a series of weekly visits for one month. KP returned in a week reporting that the pain was a little less in the groin and more localized in the "crease," that is, the area under the inguinal ligament. He pointed to the AIIS. Examination showed a slight increase in passive medial rotation. CR MET was performed on the RF, TFL, and short adductors (MET #2). The client was then asked to sit on the end of the table, and PIR MET was performed on the iliopsoas and RF (MET #8 from Chapter 3). The client was returned to the supine position, and PIR MET was performed on the long adductors (MET #9). MET #14 to increase medial rotation was repeated for approximately 10 cycles. I repeated the same STM series that was performed at the first visit for the hip and lumbar spine.

KP returned a week later, stating that the pain was slightly better. Examination showed that there was approximately a 50% improvement in passive medial rotation. The same treatment of MET, joint mobilization, and STM was applied as in the previous visit.

On his fourth visit, examination showed that the client had maintained his 50% improvement in me-

dial rotation. The same treatment described above was applied. I recommended two additional treatments at weekly intervals. On his sixth visit, he stated that he had taken a long hike without any discomfort. Examination showed that the ROM was normal in medial rotation. The patient elected to schedule two additional treatments. He had maintained normal ROM and was pain free. The patient was discharged from ongoing treatments and was encouraged to make a follow-up appointment in approximately three months to assess whether he had maintained full ROM.

Table 8-3 lists some essentials of treatment.

LEVEL I: HIP

1. Release of the Gluteus Medius and Minimus

■ **Anatomy:** Gluteus medius and minimus (Fig. 8-32).

■ **Dysfunction:** The gluteus maximus tends to be weak and is usually best treated with MET. The gluteus medius and minimus tend to develop tightness-weakness. If they test significantly weak, perform MET for the adductors first, as they are usually short and tight and might be inhibiting the gluteus medius. Attachment points usually become fibrotic after injury or sustained overuse. The positional dysfunction is for the gluteals to roll into an inferior torsion.

Position
■ **Therapist Position (TP):** standing, facing the direction of the stroke

■ **Client Position (CP):** side-lying, fetal position

MET
As a way to assist palpation, place your fingertips on the superior lateral aspect of the iliac fossa, and

perform CR MET on the gluteus medius (MET #8). This MET will also reduce hypertonicity and discomfort in the soft tissue.

Strokes
We have released this area before: in Chapter 3, "Lumbosacral Spine" (Level I, first series). The series of strokes that is presented here gives the therapist another way to release the gluteal muscles. In this series, we release the muscles from origin to insertion. Because attachment points are usually more tender than mid-belly, they are typically not treated in acute conditions. Release this area with short, scooping strokes, perpendicular to the line of the fiber. The closer you are to the attachment points, the shorter and more brisk your strokes should be. Use double thumb, braced thumb, or the fifth metacarpophalangeal joint (knuckle) of a soft fist.

1. Have the client lie in the fetal position. Perform a series of short, scooping strokes in 1-inch segments, moving transverse to the line of the fiber, medially to laterally on the gluteus medius (Fig. 8-33). Begin your strokes at the most superior portion of the muscle at its attachment under the iliac crest. Continue the strokes to its insertion on the top of the lateral portion of the trochanter. Begin the next line of strokes on the gluteus medius just posterior to the previous line, from the iliac crest to the trochanter. Cover the entire muscle. If the muscle remains hypertonic, perform another series of CR MET on the gluteus medius and the adductors, then come back to the strokes.
2. Palpate the gluteus minimus at its insertion on the anterior aspect of the top of the trochanter as you have your client abduct his or her leg in neutral (i.e., with the foot parallel to the floor).
3. To release the gluteus minimus, perform a series of M–L scooping strokes, beginning at the outer surface

Table 8-3	Essentials of Treatment

■ Rock the client's body while performing the strokes.
■ Shift your weight while performing the strokes.
■ Perform the strokes rhythmically.
■ Perform the strokes about 50 to 70 cycles per minute.
■ Keep your hands and whole body relaxed.

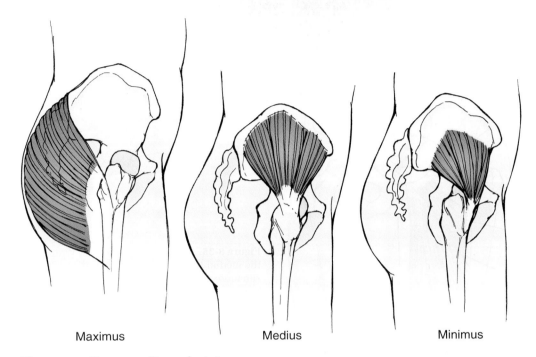

Maximus   Medius   Minimus

Figure 8-32. Gluteus medius and minimus.

of the ilium just posterior to the ASIS, and continue to the anterior-superior surface of the trochanter. Because the minimus is under the medius except at its insertion, you need to penetrate through the medius to address the minimus.

2. *Release of the Adductors*

▨ **Anatomy:** Adductor magnus, brevis, and longus (Fig. 8-34).

▨ **Dysfunction:** The adductors usually become tight and short, typically held in a sustained medial tor-

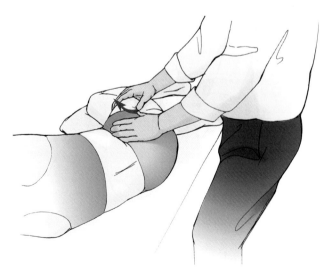

Figure 8-33. Double-thumb release of the gluteus medius and minimus.

sion. This contributes to anteverted hips and genu valgus knees.

Position

▨ **TP:** standing, facing table, or facing headward or standing on opposite side of extended leg to move posterior portion of medial thigh more posteriorly

▨ **CP:** side-lying, with the leg on the table extended and top leg flexed, resting on a pillow; have the client's trunk remain in neutral, not allowing it to rotate forward

MET

You can perform MET on the adductors (MET #7) to reduce hypertonicity and discomfort in the soft tissue. To lengthen the adductors in chronic conditions, perform MET #9.

Strokes

The intention in using these strokes is to "part the midline" of the medial thigh. That is, we move the soft tissue on the posterior half of the medial thigh posteriorly and the tissue on the anterior half of the medial thigh anteriorly. We use fingertips, braced fingertips, and braced thumb.

1. Facing 45° headward, wrap your hands around the thigh several inches below the pubic bone, placing your thumbs on the midline of the medial thigh (Fig. 8-35). Perform a short, scooping A–P stroke on the posterior portion of the medial thigh. Begin another stroke just inferior to your last stroke, and

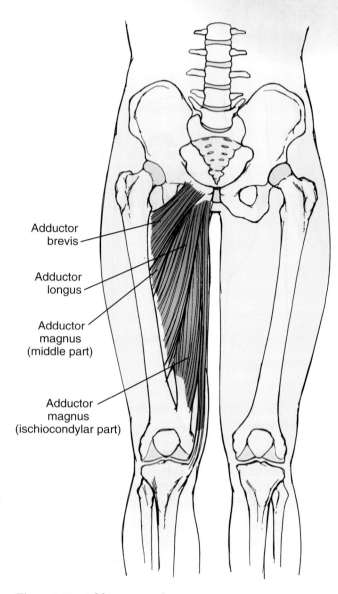

Figure 8-34. Adductor muscles.

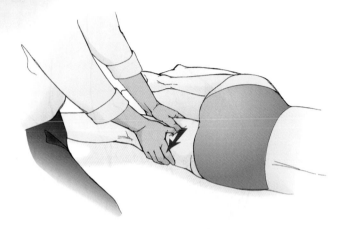

Figure 8-35. Release the adductors. Wrap both hands around the medial thigh, and part the midline. Take the posterior tissue more posteriorly and the anterior tissue more anteriorly.

3. Release of the Hamstrings

▨ **Anatomy:** Semimembranosus, semitendinosus, and long head of the biceps (Fig. 8-37).

▨ **Dysfunction:** Attachment points at the ischial tuberosity and knee tend to thicken and become fibrotic from chronic irritation or injury. The hamstrings are typically tight and short and pull toward the midline in chronic tension. The hamstrings stay in a sustained contraction to counterbalance a forward-tilting pelvis.

Position

▨ **TP:** Standing, facing headward, or facing the table for alternative technique

▨ **CP:** Prone, with a pillow under the ankles

continue to the adductor tubercle, a bony prominence on the superior surface of the medial condyle of the femur.

2. To release the anterior portion of the medial thigh, perform a series of short, scooping strokes from posterior to anterior on the soft tissue of the anterior portion of the medial thigh (Fig. 8-36). Work from the proximal thigh to just above the knee.

3. An alternative method to release the posterior portion of the medial thigh is to move to the opposite side of the table. Bring the client as close to you as is comfortable to minimize your reach. Face the table, and use a braced-thumb technique as described above to stroke anterior to posterior on the soft tissue of the posterior portion of the medial thigh.

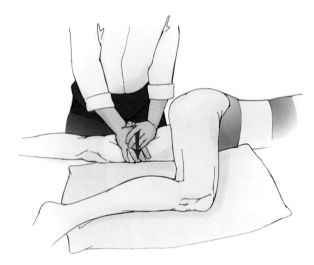

Figure 8-36. To release the anterior half of the medial thigh, the therapist faces the table and uses a braced-thumb technique to move the soft tissue anteriorly.

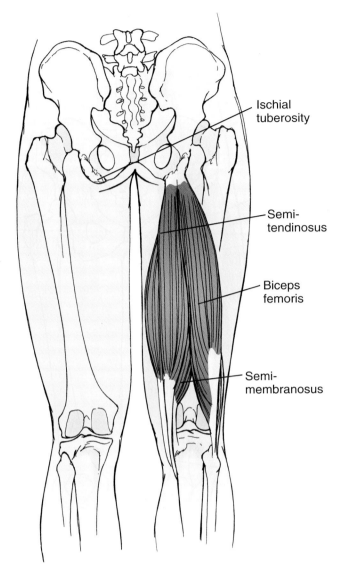

Figure 8-37. Hamstrings, which include the semimembranosus, semitendinosus, and biceps femoris.

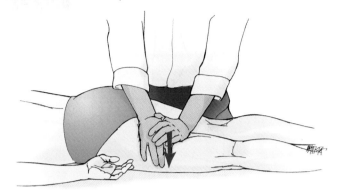

Figure 8-38. Alternative method to release the lateral side of the posterior thigh is to use a braced-thumb technique to move the soft tissue more laterally.

MET

You can perform MET on the hamstrings (MET #5) to reduce hypertonicity and discomfort in the soft tissue. To lengthen the hamstrings in chronic conditions, perform MET #10.

Strokes

Our intention is to "part the midline" to release the torsion developed through chronic tension. Use double-thumb or braced-thumb technique.

1. Facing 45° headward, place your thumbs on the midline of the thigh several inches distal to the ischial tuberosity, using the same hand position as is shown in Fig. 8-35. Perform broad, scooping strokes, unwinding the soft tissue in an M–L direction. Pro-ceed down the entire posterior thigh, following the biceps femoris to its attachment on the fibula.

2. Perform the same scooping strokes from the midline in a lateral-to-medial direction to release the semimembranosus and semitendinosus. Begin several inches below the ischial tuberosity, and continue to the knee.

3. An alternative position to release the medial hamstrings and medial thigh is for you to face the table as shown in the adductor series (see Fig. 8-36). Place your thumb on the midline of the thigh closest to you just below the ischial tuberosity. Using a braced-thumb technique, perform a series of scooping strokes in a medial direction, beginning just below the ischial tuberosity and continuing to the knee.

4. An alternative position to release the biceps femoris and lateral thigh is to stand on the opposite side, facing the table (Fig. 8-38). Place your thumbs on the midline of the thigh. Using a braced thumb, perform a series of strokes in a lateral direction. Begin just below the ischial tuberosity, and continue to the lateral knee.

5. To release the hamstring attachments on the ischial tuberosity, face 45° headward again and use a braced-thumb technique or braced fingertips to perform back and forth strokes on any thickened tissue you palpate (Fig. 8-39). To "clean the bone," cover the entire area just distal to the bone and on the ischial tuberosity itself.

4. Unwinding the Torsion of the Thigh and Release of the Quadriceps and Adductors

Anatomy: Iliopsoas; adductor magnus, longus, and brevis; quadriceps; pectineus; and sartorius (Fig. 8-40).

Dysfunction: The soft tissue tends to wind into a medial torsion, wrapping toward the midline. This

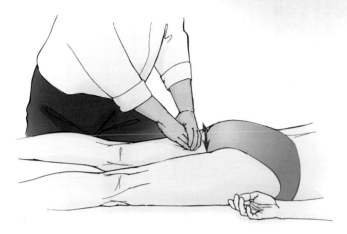

Figure 8-39. Back-and-forth strokes, with braced fingertips on the hamstrings attachment to the ischial tuberosity.

winding is due to the common postural dysfunction ("collapse") of the body in response to gravity. The feet collapse (flatten), the ankles pronate, and the knees migrate toward each other (genu valgus, or knock-knees), winding the soft tissue of the thigh medially. If you are working with a client who has retroverted hips or a client whose hips are held in external rotation, you need to reverse the stroke direction, unwind the leg in the opposite direction as described, and perform PIR on the external rotators.

Position

▨ **TP:** Standing, facing patient, with inferior leg bent at the knee and resting on the table

▨ **CP:** Supine; begin your strokes with the leg extended or a pillow under the knee, and proceed to greater flexion of the hip and knee to allow for deeper work

MET

You can perform MET on the quadriceps (MET #3) and adductors (MET #2) to reduce hypertonicity and discomfort in the soft tissue.

Strokes

This series of strokes helps to accomplish three main intentions: to unwind the torsion of the soft tissue of the thigh, to reset specific muscles in an M–L direction, and to perform back-and-forth strokes to dissolve adhesions as needed.

1. With the client's leg extended or with a pillow under the client's knee, wrap both hands around the proximal thigh, and use broad strokes to unwind the muscles around the femur in a counterclockwise direction on the right leg and clockwise on the left (Fig. 8-41). Begin a few inches below the inguinal ligament. Work down the entire thigh to a

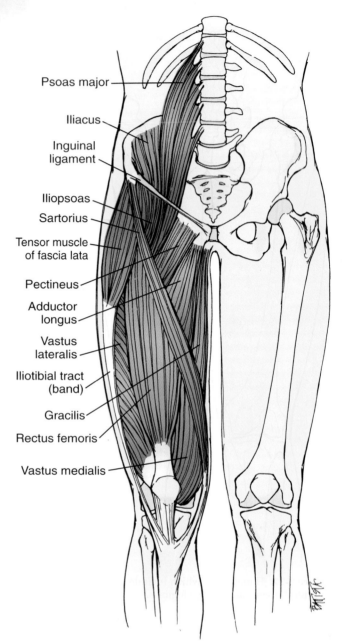

Figure 8-40. Muscles of the anterior and medial thigh.

few inches above the patella. As you work close to the inguinal ligament, use braced-thumb, supported-thumb, or fingertips-next-to-thumb techniques for the medial hand to avoid uncomfortable pressure near the genital and perineal region (see Fig. 8-44 below).

2. Rest the client's hip in a figure-four position by resting the client's thigh and leg on the table in an abducted and externally rotated position. If this is uncomfortable, place a pillow between the table and the client's thigh. Using a braced-thumb technique, begin at the midline of the medial thigh, and perform a series of scooping strokes in an M–L,

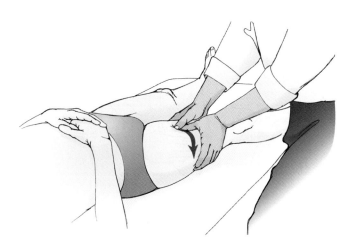

Figure 8-41. Unwinding the muscles of the anterior thigh.

P–A direction on the adductors (Fig. 8-42). Place your thigh against the client's shin just below the knee, and press the leg headward as you stroke. Cover the entire medial thigh.

5. *Release of the Soft Tissue Below the Inguinal Ligament*

▨ **Anatomy:** From medial to lateral, pectineus, iliopsoas, rectus femoris, and sartorius (Fig. 8-43).

▨ **Dysfunction:** Muscle attachments, ligaments, and capsular tissue of the anterior hip tend to become thick and fibrotic because of repetitive stresses such as excessive sitting or prior injury. The flexors become short and tight, pulling the femur forward, irritating the soft tissue in the anterior hip, contributing to fibrotic changes.

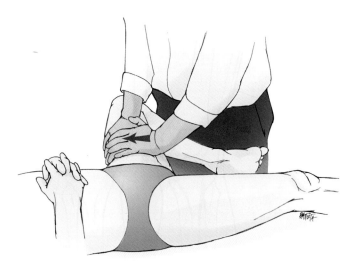

Figure 8-42. Release of the adductors in the figure-four position. The therapist's body rocks the client's hip into flexion (headward) with each stroke.

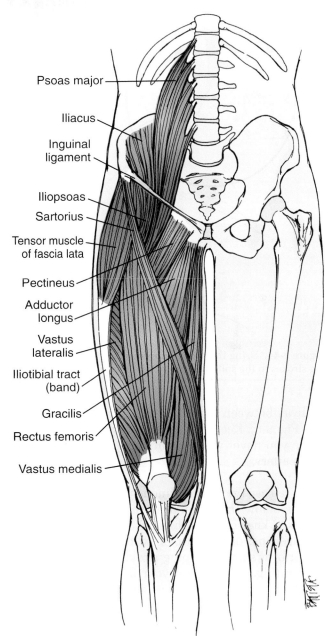

Figure 8-43. Sartorius, rectus femoris, iliopsoas, and pectineus.

Position
▨ **TP:** Standing, facing 45° headward

▨ **CP:** Supine

MET
You can perform MET on the pectineus (MET #2) and rectus femoris (MET #3) and iliopsoas (MET #6 from Chapter 3) to reduce hypertonicity and discomfort in the soft tissue.

Strokes
Find the pulse of the femoral artery by placing your fingertips just below the inguinal ligament approximately

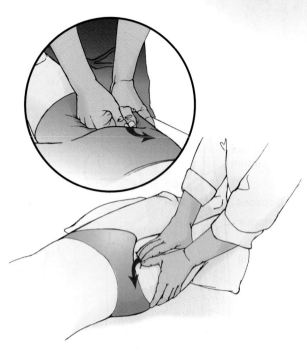

Figure 8-44. Using thumb and fingertips, perform M–L scooping strokes to the soft tissue below the inguinal ligament.

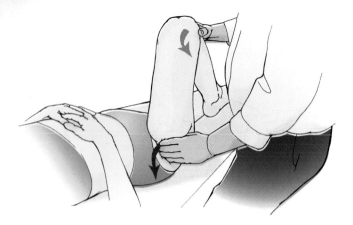

Figure 8-45. Fingertips release of the soft tissue below the inguinal ligament. With each stroke, rock the leg in the direction of the stroke.

midway between the ASIS and the pubic symphysis (see Fig. 8-6). Keep this spot in mind as you work, because you never want to put strong pressure directly on an artery.

1. To release the myotendinous junctions of the muscles below the inguinal ligament, rest the client's flexed knee on your thigh. With fingertips, braced-fingertips, or fingertips-next-to–thumb technique, perform short, scooping strokes in an M–L direction (Fig. 8-44). Begin your first stroke below the ASIS, and begin each new stroke a little more medially, continuing to the adductor longus. If the tissue is fibrotic, perform back-and-forth strokes in the M–L plane.

2. Next, using the fingertips of your superior hand, perform short, scooping strokes in an M–L direction inferior to the inguinal ligament (Fig. 8-45). Your inferior hand holds the knee and rocks the leg in small circles of circumduction with each stroke. Move the hip counterclockwise on the right and clockwise on the left. Cover the entire area under the inguinal ligament.

6. *Release of the Tensor Fascia Lata, Iliotibial Band, and Trochanteric Bursa*

▨ **Anatomy:** TFL, vastus lateralis, ITB (Fig. 8-46), and trochanteric bursa (see Fig. 8-5).

▨ **Dysfunction:** The anterior aspect of the TFL and the anterior band of the fascia lata tend to roll anteriorly and must be reset posteriorly. This is one cause of

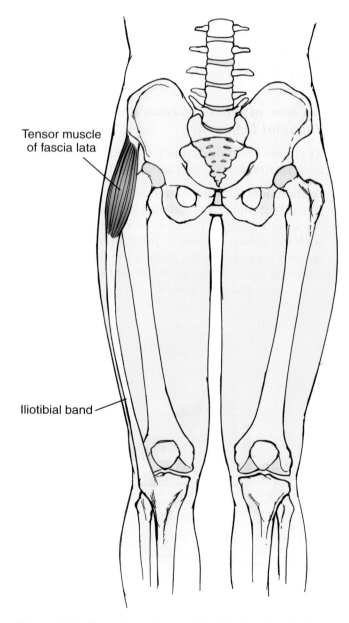

Tensor muscle of fascia lata

Iliotibial band

Figure 8-46. Tensor fascia lata and iliotibial band of the lateral thigh.

"snapping hip syndrome." If the TFL is held in a sustained contraction, the muscle belly shortens and tightens, creating sustained tension on the ITB, causing it to become thick and fibrotic. The trochanteric bursa swells with acute conditions and develops adhesions in chronic conditions.

Position

▨ **TP:** Standing, facing head ward

▨ **CP:** Supine or side-lying

MET

You can perform MET on the TFL (MET #11) and ITB (MET #12) to reduce hypertonicity and discomfort in the soft tissue.

Strokes

1. Use your thumb, fingertips, or fingertips next to thumb to roll the TFL and the fascial bands between the ASIS and the greater trochanter posteriorly in brisk, short, scooping motions (Fig. 8-47). If the area is fibrous, rock the leg into external rotation with each stroke. With less fibrous tissue, hold distal to the knee with your lower hand, and use a shearing stroke by rocking the leg medially as you stroke laterally and posteriorly with your superior hand.

2. An alternative method is to bring the hip into 90° of flexion and hold the leg at the knee with your inferior hand as shown in Figure 8-45. Use the fingertips or thumb of your superior hand to scoop the TFL and ITB in an M–L and A–P direction. Rock the leg laterally with each stroke.

3. If the ITB is fibrous, place the client in a side-lying, fetal position, and stand on the side of the table facing the front of the client's body (Fig. 8-48). Using a double-thumb technique, perform a series of scooping strokes in an A–P direction on the ITB of the top leg to a few inches above the knee.

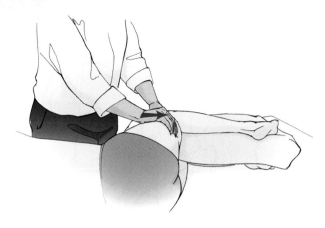

Figure 8-48. Alternative position to release the ITB. Using double-thumb or braced-thumb technique, stroke the ITB from anterior to posterior.

4. To help normalize the trochanteric bursa, face the leg as described in the previous stroke. Apply a little lotion to the lateral thigh. Using the webspace between the thumb and the index finger of one or both hands, begin several inches below the greater trochanter, and stroke up the lateral and posterior shaft of the femur with very gentle pressure in one continuous stroke (Fig. 8-49). Continue to the top of the trochanter. For acute bursitis, these strokes must be extremely gentle. Begin at the most superior aspect of the bursa first, and slowly perform 1-inch strokes, milking the fluid out. Proceed in 1-inch segments more distally.

LEVEL II: HIP

1. *Release of the Sciatic Nerve at the Greater Sciatic Notch*

▨ **Anatomy:** The superior border of the sacrospinous ligament and the medial border of the ischium

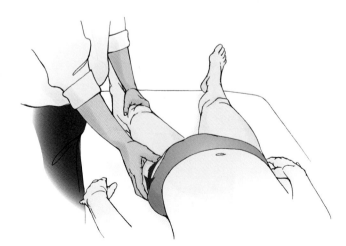

Figure 8-47. Rolling the TFL and the anterior portion of the ITB from anterior to posterior.

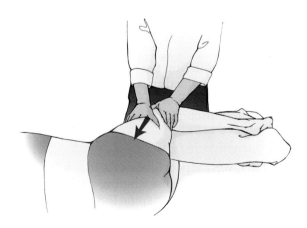

Figure 8-49. To release the trochanteric bursa, use the webspace between the thumb and the index finger and slowly stroke up the shaft of the femur.

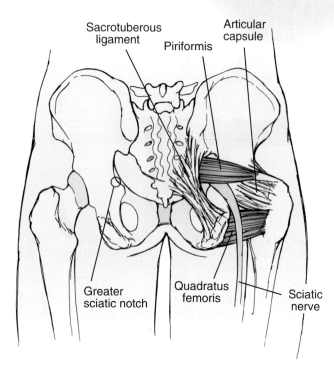

Figure 8-50. Sciatic nerve as it exits from the greater sciatic notch.

> *CAUTION: Do not perform these strokes if your client has a positive SLR test. These strokes are for a client who has chronic, mild, diffuse numbing and tingling in the thigh.*

1. Perform a series of deep, lifting, scooping strokes in a superior-lateral direction (toward the shoulder) to release the sciatic nerve at the greater sciatic notch (Fig. 8-51). The notch might feel fibrous if there has been an injury in the gluteal region or if the nerve has been previously inflamed. If the nerve is entrapped, it is normal for the client to feel a slight tingling down the leg as you are working. Do not proceed if pain refers back up toward the spine, because this can indicate a nerve root problem such as an inflamed disc. Perform this stroke for only about 1 minute, covering the entire area of the greater sciatic notch.

2. Perform a series of deep, lifting strokes from inferior to superior on the superior-lateral aspect of the ischial tuberosity. Feel for thick adhesions on the bone, which might be binding (tethering) the sciatic nerve. You need to penetrate through the deep external rotators to "clean the bone."

form the sciatic notch. The sciatic nerve leaves the pelvis through the greater sciatic notch. The nerve passes over the notch in the form of a thick ribbon but quickly takes its more rounded shape (Fig. 8-50).

▨ **Dysfunction:** A sustained hip flexion posture tightens the sciatic nerve against the notch. Hypertonicity of the hip rotators can also contribute to this entrapment syndrome.

Position

▨ **TP:** Standing

▨ **CP:** Side-lying, fetal position; additional pillows can be placed between the knees to bring the superficial tissue in the gluteal region into more slack

MET

You can perform MET on the piriformis (MET #4 from Chapter 3), gluteus medius and minimus (MET #8), and medial and lateral rotators (MET #4) to reduce hypertonicity and discomfort in the soft tissue.

Strokes

Palpate the lowest aspect of the sciatic notch in the intersection of two lines: one running slightly lateral to the posterior superior iliac spine (PSIS) in the inferior to superior plane and the other running M–L at the level of the most superior aspect of the greater trochanter.

2. *Release of the Muscle Attachments and Posterior Joint Capsule on the Posterior and Medial Femur*

▨ **Anatomy:** Vastus lateralis, adductor longus, gluteus maximus, pectineus, adductor magnus, vastus medialis, posterior joint capsule (Fig. 8-52).

▨ **Dysfunction:** Attachment points usually become fibrotic. This fibrosis inhibits the normal extensibility of the myofascia, preventing normal muscle

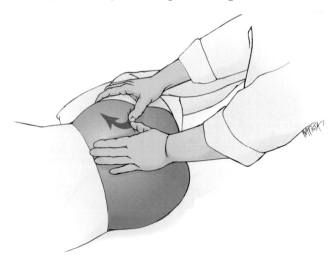

Figure 8-51. Double-thumb release of the sciatic nerve at the greater sciatic notch.

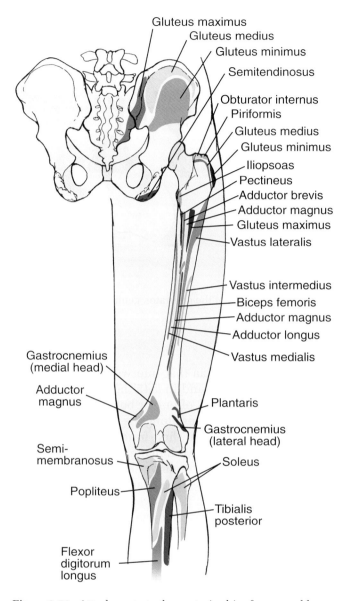

Figure 8-52. Attachments to the posterior hip, femur, and knee.

function. The posterior capsule can shorten, pulling the hip into a sustained external rotation. The muscles of the posterior thigh thicken if they are held in an eccentric contraction trying to counterbalance anterior pelvic tilt (increased lordosis).

Position

■ **TP:** Standing

■ **CP:** Prone; place a pillow under the client's ankle to relax the hamstrings, or place your flexed knee on the table and rest the client's leg on your thigh.

MET

You can perform MET on the hamstrings (MET #5), and adductors (METs #2 and #9) to reduce hypertonicity and discomfort in the soft tissue.

Strokes

Work three lines of strokes down the entire shaft of the femur, using short, scooping strokes; use brisker, transverse strokes with fingertips over thumb or fingertips over fingertips. Keeping your hands relaxed, rock your fingertips back and forth in the M–L plane to allow the muscle fibers to move out of your way so that you can get to the bone.

1. To release the posterior joint capsule, have the client lie prone with a pillow under the ankles. Face 45° headward, and place double thumbs or fingertips next to thumb approximately 2 inches medial to the lateral aspect of the greater trochanter. Perform back-and-forth strokes in a superior-to-inferior plane on the posterior surface of the greater trochanter. Continue 2 to 3 inches more medially.
2. To release the vastus lateralis and intermedius on the lateral aspect of the posterior surface of the femur, place your flexed knee on the table, and rest the client's leg on your thigh (Fig. 8-53). Begin just below the greater trochanter, and using fingertips over thumb or fingertips over fingertips, perform 1-inch, back-and-forth strokes in the M–L plane. Proceed down the entire femur to just above the knee. (Techniques for the knee will be discussed in Chapter 9, "The Knee.")
3. Begin a second line of strokes just below the greater trochanter in the middle of the posterior femur. Perform 1-inch, back-and-forth strokes on the attachments of the biceps femoris, adductor magnus, and gluteus maximus.
4. Beginning just below the gluteal crease, release the third line on the most medial aspect of the posterior femur for the pectineus, vastus medialis, and adductor longus.

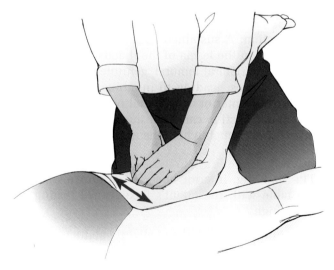

Figure 8-53. Prone release of the attachments to the posterior and medial femur.

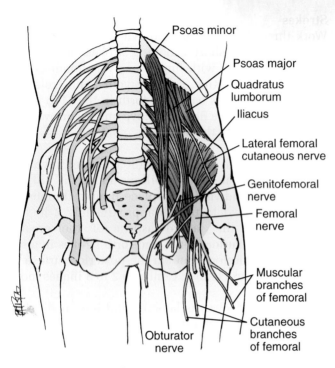

Figure 8-54. Anterior hip region nerves.

5. To release the attachments on the medial femur, put the client in the side-lying position, with the lower leg extended and with the top leg flexed, resting on a pillow (see Fig. 8-36). Either face the table, or stand 45° headward. Using the same hand position as was described above, perform back-and-forth strokes in the M–L plane from the proximal femur to just above the knee.

3. *Release of the Nerves of the Anterior Hip Above the Inguinal Ligament*

■ **Anatomy:** Femoral, genitofemoral, lateral femoral cutaneous, obturator nerves (Fig. 8-54), and iliopectineal bursa (see Fig. 8-5).

■ **Dysfunction:** A sustained contracture in the psoas or fibrosis in the fascia of the iliacus can compress the femoral, lateral femoral, genitofemoral, and obturator nerves, leading to numbing, tingling, and pain in the anterior and medial pelvic region. Sustained contraction can also cause adhesions in the myofascia through which the nerves travel.

Position
■ **TP:** Standing, inferior knee flexed and resting on the table with the client's flexed knee resting on your thigh

■ **CP:** Supine, hip flexed and slightly abducted

MET
You can perform MET on the iliopsoas (MET #6 from Chapter 3) to reduce hypertonicity and discomfort in the soft tissue.

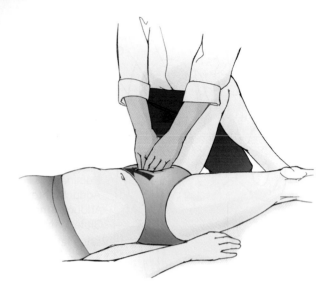

Figure 8-55. Release of the obturator, genitofemoral, and femoral nerves.

Strokes
1. To release the fascia that interweaves with the inguinal ligament, stand in a 45° headward position. Using the fingertips of one or both hands, perform back-and-forth strokes along the superior border of the inguinal ligament, first from anterior to posterior and then in the M–L plane.
2. To release the obturator nerve above the inguinal ligament, stand in the 45° headward position, and place the fingertips of one hand over the fingertips of the other hand just above the inguinal ligament, at the midline of the body (Fig. 8-55). Gently sink your hands into the client's abdomen, and perform a series of short, scooping strokes in the M–L direction. To release the genitofemoral nerve, move your hands 1 inch more laterally, keeping your hands close to the inguinal ligament, and perform another series of M–L scooping strokes, just medial to the psoas.
3. The femoral nerve lies in a trough between the iliacus and the psoas, superior to the inguinal ligament, approximately midway between the ASIS and the pubic symphysis. Place your fingertips just above the inguinal ligament midway between the ASIS and the pubic symphysis, and perform a series of M–L scooping strokes to release the femoral nerve.
4. Release the lateral femoral cutaneous nerve by performing short, scooping strokes in an M–L direction, in the area just superior to the inguinal ligament's attachment to the ASIS (Fig. 8-56). Flex your fingertips, and allow them to follow the contour of the bone.

Note: Strokes 1 to 4 can also be done with the hip flexed to 90° and by scooping medially to laterally with one hand as the hip is being circumducted with the other hand, as shown in Fig. 8-45.

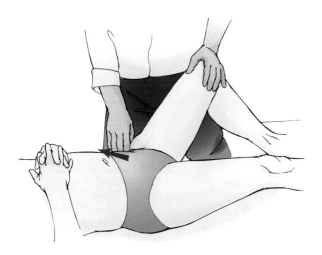

Figure 8-56. Release of the lateral femoral cutaneous nerve. Flex your fingertips over the ASIS, and perform M–L strokes.

5. Iliopectineal bursae: Place a flat thumb parallel to the inguinal ligament and several inches inferior to it. Perform a series of strokes in the superior direction while gently pumping the hip toward the opposite shoulder with each stroke.

6. To help release the inguinal lymphatics, first place some lotion on the proximal thigh. With the leg in extension, gently perform a series of long, continuous strokes from the upper thigh to the inguinal ligament. As your hand is just below the inguinal ligament, add a gentle impulse at the end of your stroke.

4. *Release of the Muscle Attachments to the Pubic and Ischial Ramus*

▓ **Anatomy:** From inferior to superior: adductor magnus, gracilis, adductor brevis, adductor longus, pectineus, obturator nerve (Fig. 8-57).

▓ **Dysfunction:** The myotendinous and tenoperiosteal junctions are commonly injured sites. These sites usually become fibrotic after overuse or injury. The obturator nerve can become entrapped in the fibrous expansions of the adductors, especially the pectineus and adductor longus.

Position

▓ **TP:** Standing, with knee of inferior leg flexed and resting on table

▓ **CP:** Supine, with hip flexed and abducted and knee flexed and resting on your thigh or on a pillow; rock the entire leg with each stroke

MET
You can perform MET on the adductors (METs #2 and #9) to reduce hypertonicity and discomfort in the soft tissue.

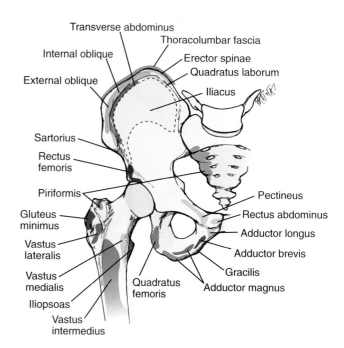

Figure 8-57. Muscle attachments to the ramus of the pubic bone and ischium.

Strokes
To assist palpation, have the client's hip abducted and flexed. The adductor longus typically becomes prominent on the medial thigh. If it does not become prominent, have the client resist as you press at the knee toward further abduction, bringing up the adductor longus. The pectineus lies immediately lateral to the adductor longus, and the adductor brevis attachment lies just inferior to the longus. Flexing the knee emphasizes the gracilis, which lies immediately medial to the adductor brevis. To palpate the gracilis, have the client pull his or her heel into table as you palpate the pubic ramus. The adductor magnus attaches just below the gracilis, on the lowest portion of the bone.

1. Place your flexed knee on the table, and rest the client's leg on your thigh (Fig. 8-58). With your forearm contacting the client's thigh to stabilize it, place your fingertips or braced fingertips on the attachment of the adductor longus at the superior pubic ramus. Perform short, back-and-forth strokes on the adductor longus as you rock your entire body with each stroke.

2. Using the same technique described above, release the gracilis and adductor brevis from the inferior ramus of the pubis, just inferior to adductor longus attachment.

3. Use fingertips or braced fingertips, and perform short, back-and-forth strokes to release the adductor magnus from the lower portion of the inferior pubic ramus and the ischial tuberosity.

4. To release the pectineus attachments from the superior pubic ramus, place your fingertips just lateral

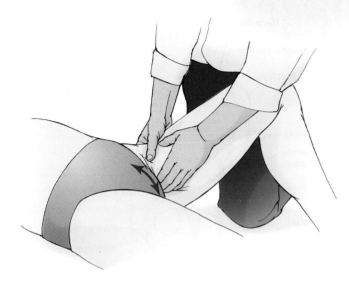

Figure 8-58. Release of the attachment of the adductor longus.

to the proximal part of the adductor longus. Perform short, back-and-forth strokes in the M–L plane, covering the entire area of the medial portion of the superior pubic ramus.

5. The obturator nerve enters the thigh under the pectineus. To release the obturator nerve, perform a series of back-and-forth scooping strokes in the M–L plane, through the pectineus. Then perform back-and-forth strokes on the medial side of the adductor longus and under the longus to release the branches of the nerve. This stroke is performed only if the client has numbing, tingling, or burning on the medial thigh.

5. Release of the Muscle Attachments to the Medial and Anterior Femur and the Anterior Joint Capsule

▨ **Anatomy:** From medial to lateral on the proximal femur: iliopsoas, vastus intermedius, vastus lateralis, and gluteus minimus; from medial to lateral on the anterior ilium: sartorius, and rectus femoris (Fig. 8-59).

▨ **Dysfunction:** Attachment points thicken because of chronic overuse, postural asymmetry, or sustained hip flexion from back pain or after an acute injury. The reflected head of the rectus femoris and the gluteus minimus interweave with the joint capsule. Injury to these muscles and the joint capsule can lead to problems of coordination and balance because of the high population of proprioceptors in the capsule.

Position

▨ **TP:** Standing

▨ **CP:** Supine, with the hip and knee flexed for the work on the lesser trochanter, the joint capsule, and

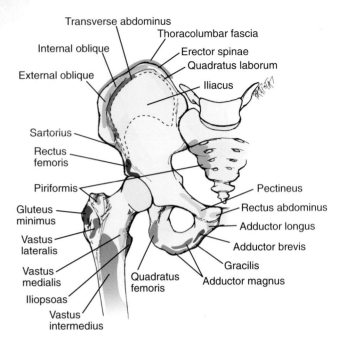

Figure 8-59. Muscle attachments to the pubic ramus and ischium.

the attachment points. Strokes 1 to 5 can also be done with the hip flexed to approximately 90° and by scooping medially to laterally with one hand as the hip is being circumducted or rocked M–L with the other hand, as shown in Fig. 8-45.

MET
You can perform MET on the iliopsoas (MET #6 from Chapter 3), and quadriceps (MET #3) to reduce hypertonicity and discomfort in the soft tissue.

Strokes
1. To release the attachments of the sartorius on the ASIS, use short, back-and-forth strokes with fingertips, braced fingertips, or double thumbs (Fig. 8-60).

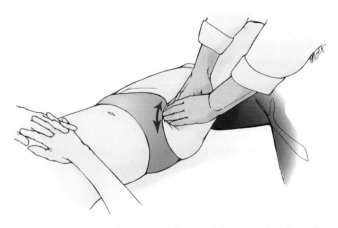

Figure 8-60. Braced-fingertips release of the sartorius from the ASIS and the rectus femoris from the AIIS.

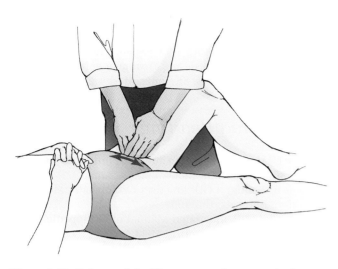

Figure 8-61. Release of the iliopsoas attachment at the lesser trochanter.

Move your hands just lateral and posterior to the sartorius attachment to release the TFL using the same back-and-forth strokes.

2. Using the same hand positions as were described above, release the rectus femoris from the AIIS. The AIIS can be located 1 inch inferior and 1 inch medial to the ASIS.

3. Release the iliopsoas from below the inguinal ligament to its attachment at the lesser trochanter (Fig. 8-61). With the client's thigh flexed and abducted and resting on your thigh, the iliopsoas is located by first grasping the adductor longus in one hand and the sartorius and rectus in the other. The psoas lies between your hands. The lesser trochanter is on the medial-posterior shaft of the femur in a line that is formed from the greater trochanter 45° inferiorly. Using fingertips, perform a series of back-and-forth strokes in the M–L plane, from below the inguinal ligament to the lesser trochanter. Rock your entire body with your strokes. Exercise caution with your strokes so that you do not work on a pulse. The femoral artery typically lies medial to the iliopsoas.

4. To release the anterior joint capsule, flex the hip to approximately 90°. Hold the knee with one hand, and place the fingertips of your superior hand just inferior to the previous stroke. Press deep into the tissue, through the rectus femoris, to the bone. Rock the thigh back and forth in the M–L plane as you perform back-and-forth strokes with your fingertips in the M–L plane. Cover the area between the AIIS and the intertrochanteric line, that is, the area between the medial aspect of the greater trochanter and the lesser trochanter.

5. Straighten the leg. Using the fingertips technique, release the gluteus minimus attachment from the anterior-superior trochanter and the vastus later-

alis immediately distal and medial to it. You can rock the leg with your stroke or in the opposite direction of your stroke.

6. Using fingertips, braced fingertips, or thumbs, perform a series of back-and-forth strokes in the M–L plane to release the vastus intermedius on the anterior shaft of the femur. Continue these strokes to the knee.

Study Guide

Level I

1. Describe the origin, insertion, and action of the following muscles: psoas, gluteus medius, adductor longus, hamstrings, TFL, and rectus femoris.
2. Describe the signs and symptoms of tendinitis of the gluteus medius, adductors, quadriceps, hamstrings, and iliopsoas.
3. Describe the positional dysfunction of the psoas, TFL, and adductors, and describe the stroke direction to correct them.
4. Describe an MET for acute hip pain and the MET to increase medial rotation of the hip.
5. Describe the first motion to be lost in capsulitis and in arthritis of the hip.
6. Describe the MET for the following muscles: gluteus maximus, medius, and minimus; medial and lateral rotators; hamstrings; adductors; and TFL.
7. Describe which muscles of the hip are typically tight and short and which muscles are typically weak, as described in lower (pelvic) crossed syndrome.
8. Describe the symptoms of capsulitis and arthritis of the hip.
9. Describe anteverted and retroverted hips and how the ROM of the hip is affected in each condition.
10. Describe the signs and symptoms of trochanteric bursitis, iliopectineal bursitis, entrapment of the lateral cutaneous nerve of the thigh, entrapment of the obturator nerve, and entrapment of the femoral nerve.

Level II

1. Describe the origin and insertion of the pectineus, sartorius, and gracilis.
2. Describe the stroke direction to release the sciatic nerve in the gluteal region.
3. List three common sites of entrapment of the sciatic nerve in the hip region.
4. Describe the difference in symptoms among an iliopsoas tendinitis, an iliopectineal bursitis, and an entrapment of the femoral nerve.
5. Describe the typical ranges of motion of the hip.
6. Describe the anatomy, function, dysfunction, and injury of the labrum.
7. List the muscle attachments on the pubic ramus and ischial ramus.
8. Describe the sites of entrapment of the obturator, femoral, and lateral femoral cutaneous nerves and the stroke direction to release them.

9. List three factors that contribute to hip pain.
10. Describe Trendelenburg's test. Describe a positive test.

11. Hammer W. The hip. In Hammer W (ed): Functional Soft Tissue Examination and Treatment by Manual Methods. Gaithersburg, MD: Aspen, 1999.
12. Sahrmann S. Diagnosis and Treatment of Movement Impairment Syndromes. St. Louis: Mosby, 2002.

■ References

1. Beattie P. The hip. In Malone T, McPoil T, Nitz A (eds): Orthopedic and Sports Physical Therapy, 3rd ed. St. Louis: Mosby, 1997, pp 459–508.
2. Hertling D, Kessler R. Hip. In Hertling D, Kessler R (eds): Management of Common Musculoskeletal Disorders, 4th ed. Baltimore: Lippincott Williams & Wilkins, 2006, pp 441–486.
3. Grieve G. The hip. Physiotherapy 1983;69:196–204.
4. Oatis CA. Kinesiology: The Mechanics and Pathomechanics of Human Movement. Philadelphia: Lippincott Williams & Wilkins, 2004.
5. Norris CM. The hip. In Norris CM (ed): Sports Injuries: Diagnosis and Management for Physiotherapists. Oxford: Butterworth-Heinemann, 1993, pp 160–163.
6. Janda V, Frank C, Liebenson C. Evaluation of muscular imbalance. In Liebenson C (ed): Rehabilitation of the Spine, 2nd ed. Baltimore: Lippincott Williams & Wilkins, 2007, pp 203–225.
7. Garaci MC. Rehabilitation of the hip, pelvis, and thigh. In Kibler WB, Herring SA, Press JM (eds): Functional Rehabilitation of Sports and Musculoskeletal Injuries. Gaithersburg, MD: Aspen, 1998, pp 216–243.
8. Kendall F, McCreary E, Provance P, Rodgers, M, Romani, W. Muscles: Testing and Function, 5th ed. Baltimore: Lippincott Williams & Wilkins, 2005.
9. Grofton JP. Studies in osteoarthritis of the hip: Part IV. Biomechanics and clinical considerations. CMAJ 1971;104:1007–1011.
10. Brukner P, Khan K. Clinical Sports Medicine, 3rd ed. Sydney: McGraw-Hill, 2006.

■ Suggested Readings

Chaitow L. Muscle Energy Techniques, 3rd ed. New York: Churchill Livingstone, 2006.

Corrigan B, Maitland GD. Practical Orthopaedic Medicine. London: Butterworths, 1983.

Cyriax J, Cyriax P. Illustrated Manual of Orthopedic Medicine. London: Butterworths, 1983.

Garrick J, Webb D. Sports Injuries, 2nd ed. Philadelphia: WB Saunders, 1999.

Greenman PE. Principles of Manual Medicine, 2nd ed. Baltimore: Williams & Wilkins, 1996.

Hertling D, Kessler R. Management of Common Musculoskeletal Disorders, 4th ed. Baltimore: Lippincott Williams & Wilkins, 2006.

Hoppenfeld S. Physical Examination of the Spine and Extremities. New York: Appleton-Century-Crofts, 1976.

Kendall F, McCreary E, Provance P, Rodgers, M, Romani, W. Muscles: Testing and Function, 5th ed. Baltimore: Lippincott Williams & Wilkins, 2005.

Levangie P, Norkin C. Joint Structure and Function, 3rd ed. Philadelphia: FA Davis, 2001.

Magee D. Orthopedic Physical Assessment, 3rd ed. Philadelphia: WB Saunders, 1 997.

Platzer W. Locomotor System, vol. 1, 5th ed. New York: Thieme Medical, 2004.

Reid DC. Sports Injury and Assessment. New York: Churchill Livingstone, 1992.

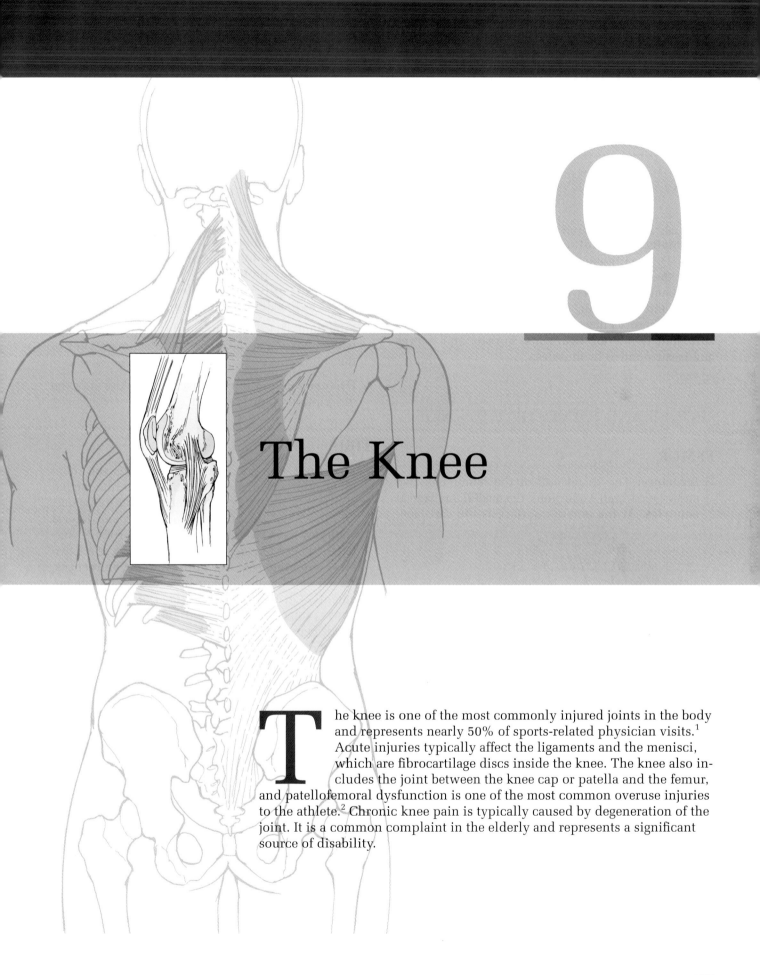

9

The Knee

The knee is one of the most commonly injured joints in the body and represents nearly 50% of sports-related physician visits.[1] Acute injuries typically affect the ligaments and the menisci, which are fibrocartilage discs inside the knee. The knee also includes the joint between the knee cap or patella and the femur, and patellofemoral dysfunction is one of the most common overuse injuries to the athlete.[2] Chronic knee pain is typically caused by degeneration of the joint. It is a common complaint in the elderly and represents a significant source of disability.

Anatomy, Function, and Dysfunction of the Knee

GENERAL OVERVIEW

The knee joint comprises two separate articulations: the **tibiofemoral joint** and the **patellofemoral joint** (Fig. 9-1). The tibiofemoral joint is the articulation between the distal femur and the proximal tibia. The patellofemoral joint is the articulation between the patella and the femur. The knee is a synovial joint with two fibrocartilage **menisci**, a **patella**, a **joint capsule**, and numerous **ligaments, bursae,** and **nerves** and is surrounded by **muscles.**

BONES AND JOINTS OF THE KNEE

FEMUR

■ **Structure:** The distal end of the femur has two cartilage-covered expansions: the **medial** and **lateral condyles.** At the anterior surface is the cartilage-

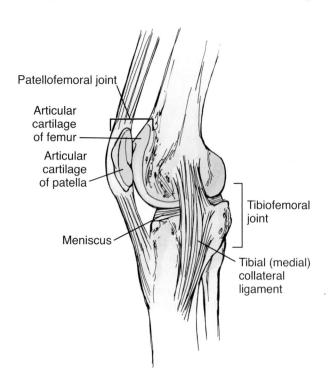

Patellofemoral joint

Articular cartilage of femur

Articular cartilage of patella

Meniscus

Tibiofemoral joint

Tibial (medial) collateral ligament

Figure 9-1. Knee consists of two joints. The tibiofemoral joint is the articulation of the distal end of the femur and the proximal tibia. The patellofemoral joint is the articulation of the femur and patella.

covered patellar surface (trochlear groove) upon which the patella glides. The anterior surface of the lateral condyle extends further anteriorly than the medial condyle and helps to prevent lateral dislocation of the patella.[3] Both condyles have expansions extending from the sides called **epicondyles.** A small bony protuberance above the medial epicondyle is called the *adductor tubercle,* which serves as the attachment for the adductor magnus.

■ **Function:** The distal end of the femur serves as a weight-bearing surface and for attachment sites of the soft tissue.

■ **Dysfunction and injury:** Discussed below after the description of the knee joint.

TIBIA

■ **Structure:** The proximal tibia contains the tibial plateau for articulation with the femur, the medial and lateral condyles, the intercondylar eminence, and the tibial tuberosity. The **medial** and **lateral condyles** have two cartilage-covered articular surfaces. In between these articulating surfaces are two bony prominences, the **intercondylar eminences,** which serve as attachment sites for the cruciate ligaments. On the anterior surface of the tibia is a bony projection, the **tibial tubercle,** where the quadriceps attach.

■ **Function:** The proximal tibia serves as a weight-bearing surface and for attachment sites of the soft tissue.

KNEE JOINT (TIBIOFEMORAL JOINT)

■ **Structure:** The distal end of the femur and the proximal end of the tibia form the tibiofemoral joint (see Fig. 9-1). The fibula does not form part of the knee and will be considered in Chapter 10, "The Leg, Ankle, and Foot." The knee joint is the largest joint in the body, formed by the two largest bones in the body. The knee is a synovial joint with two fibrocartilage menisci. The knee also contains an **infrapatellar fat pad,** which causes the skin to bulge on both sides of the infrapatellar ligament.

■ **Function:** The knee is considered a modified hinge joint, because in addition to the primary motions of flexion and extension, the joint has the ability to rotate. Also, some degree of adduction and abduction is present. The key motion of the tibiofemoral joint is a spiral (i.e., a winding and an unwinding of the tibia relative to the femur). The open (most relaxed) position of the knee is slight flexion, a position in which the joint capsule, quadriceps, and hamstrings are most relaxed. The closed-packed position is extension.

■ **Dysfunction and injury:** Acute injuries to the knee typically involve soft tissue. Dysfunctions and injuries of the specific soft tissue structures are discussed separately below. Chronic conditions of the knee joint typically involve misalignment (see below) and loss of full flexion and extension as well as restricted external rotation of the tibia. The articular cartilage of the femur and tibia are common sites for degeneration, leading to osteoarthritis. This degeneration could result from a specific traumatic episode or from cumulative stress. Severe knee injuries are associated with edema in the subchondral bone, the bone under the cartilage. This injury is known as a *bone bruise* and is visible on an MRI.[4] It indicates significant damage to the articular cartilage and will present as pain, swelling, and delayed recovery.

■ **Treatment implications:** Osteoarthritis of the knee initially manifests as decreased flexion. In the early stages, passive flexion has a reduced range of motion (ROM) and a capsular end feel, representing fibrosis or thickening of the joint capsule. Advanced osteoarthritis has painful restriction of passive flexion with a bony end feel, as well as a loss of full extension. Muscle energy technique (MET) is used to increase flexion, rehydrate the joint, increase joint capsule length, and balance the muscular forces that act on the knee. Because flexion of the tibiofemoral joint includes medial rotation of the tibia and extension requires external rotation of the tibia, MET is performed to normalize these motions. Soft tissue mobilization (STM) is performed to dissolve fibrosis in the capsule and surrounding soft tissue.

PATELLA AND THE PATELLOFEMORAL JOINT

■ **Structure:** The patella, or knee cap, is the largest sesamoid bone in the body. A **sesamoid bone** is a cartilage-covered bone that grows in tendons that cross the ends of bones. The posterior surface of the patella has a central, vertical ridge that divides it into medial and lateral facets. A third "odd" facet is located at the most medial aspect of the patella. This surface is covered with hyaline cartilage, which articulates with the patellar surface (trochlear groove)

on the distal femur, forming the **patellofemoral joint.** This cartilage is the thickest in the human body.[5]

■ **Function:** The functions of the patella are to protect the knee, to help distribute the compressive forces of the quadriceps tendon to prevent the tendon fibers from digging into the articular cartilage of the femur, and to lengthen the quadriceps, increasing its leverage and therefore allowing the quadriceps to develop greater force. During flexion and extension, the patella slides on the femur. To function normally, the patella must have adequate mobility to accept the contractile forces in different positions of the knee, and it must have adequate stability to ensure that the cartilage surfaces are not overly stressed. During extension of the knee, the patella is designed to move upward in line with the central groove of the femur. The line of movement is determined by the combined actions of the vastus medialis obliquus (VMO) and the vastus lateralis. In standing with normal alignment, the patella should face straight forward.[6]

■ **Dysfunction and injury:** There are two common dysfunctions of the patellofemoral joint: becoming too compressed and moving too far laterally in the intercondylar groove. Both conditions cause abrasion of the cartilage, leading to inflammation and degeneration.

☐ The patellofemoral joint becomes too compressed because of increased flexion of the knee, which is caused by sustained tension in the hamstrings, iliotibial band (ITB), and gastrocnemius or by a shortened joint capsule. This compressive force is dramatically increased when a person climbs stairs or gets up from a chair.

☐ If the patella is pulled laterally in the trochlear groove it is called *patellar tracking dysfunction.* Two potential causes are (1) genu valgum ("knock-knees"), which is associated with an anteverted hip, lateral tibial torsion, and pronated ankle, and (2) a weakening of the VMO and an overdevelopment of the vastus lateralis, lateral retinaculum, and tensor fascia lata (TFL). The weakening of the VMO can be caused by two mechanisms. The first is a previous knee injury. When the knee has been injured, it is often difficult to extend it fully because any swelling causes the knee to assume some flexion. Because the VMO functions primarily during the last 15° of extension, the loss of terminal extension causes an atrophy of the VMO. The second cause is the knee's *arthrokinetic reflex.* With this reflex, any irritation of the joint leads to neurological inhibition and weakening of the VMO.

Treatment implications: MET is performed to reduce the hypertonicity of the TFL, ITB, hamstrings, and gastrocnemius and to facilitate or strengthen the VMO and adductors. STM is used to reduce the fibrosis that typically develops around the periphery and undersurface of the patella.

KNEE ALIGNMENT

Structure: The alignment of the femoral shaft to the center of the knee is normally approximately 10° lateral to the mechanical axis and is called the *normal valgus angle* or the **Q-angle** (quadriceps angle). This is because the femoral head and the hip joint are medial to the shaft. The mechanical axis describes the normal line of force that travels from the center of the hip joint through the center of the knee to the center of the ankle.[7] Because of the wider pelvis, women have larger Q-angles than men. An increased Q-angle indicates increased lateral pull on the patella and a greater risk for patellar tracking dysfunction.[3]

Dysfunction: An increase in the normal valgus angle is called **genu valgum** (knock-knees) and causes compressive forces on the lateral side of the joint, including the lateral side of the patella, and tensile forces on the medial side. It can be caused by ITB tightness, femoral anteversion, and pronation of the foot. **Genu varum,** or bow legs, describes a decrease in the normal valgus angle and causes compression on the medial side of the knee and tensile stresses on the lateral side.

Treatment implications: Assessing alignment of the knee is complex and involves assessment and treatment of the feet, hips, and lumbopelvic region as well as structures in the knee itself. For the massage therapist, the goals are to reduce the muscle hypertonicity and to facilitate the weak muscles with MET. All clients who have chronic knee pain or signs of knee misalignment need to be referred to a chiropractor, osteopath, physical therapist, or podiatrist.

SOFT TISSUE STRUCTURES OF THE KNEE

MENISCI

Structure: The knee contains the **medial** and **lateral menisci.** The menisci are C-shaped fibrocartilage discs. They are wedge shaped, and the outer margin is thicker than the inner margin. Both menisci are firmly attached to bony protuberances

called the *intercondylar tubercles* in the middle portion of the tibial plateau. They are also attached along the periphery of the tibia by expansions of the joint capsule called the **coronary ligaments**. The menisci are also attached to the fascial expansion of the quadriceps. As the quadriceps contract, the menisci are drawn forward.[5]

☐ The **medial meniscus** is far less mobile than the lateral meniscus because it is firmly attached to the tibial plateau. It is interwoven with the medial (tibial) collateral ligament, the joint capsule, the coronary ligament, and the anterior cruciate ligament (ACL). It is also attached to the semimembranosus muscle, which pulls the meniscus posteriorly during knee flexion.[5]

☐ The **lateral meniscus** has much more mobility than does the medial meniscus and is therefore much less susceptible to injury. The lateral meniscus has attachments to the posterior cruciate ligament (PCL), the joint capsule, the coronary ligaments, and the popliteus muscle, but it is not attached to the lateral (fibular) collateral ligament. The popliteus assists in drawing the meniscus posteriorly during knee flexion.[6]

Function: The medial and lateral menisci form joint sockets for the femoral condyles. This adds stability to the articulation of the asymmetric, concave tibial plateau and the asymmetric, convex femoral condyles. They increase lubrication and nutrition and reduce friction. The menisci are weight-bearing structures designed to be shock absorbers. They help to carry as much as 50% of the load, which increases with knee flexion. The menisci also play a role in proprioception.[8] The anterior portion of the menisci are somewhat mobile. As the knee extends, the anterior aspects of the menisci glide forward; and as the knee flexes, the menisci are drawn back.

Dysfunction and injury: As with all fibrocartilage, the menisci are susceptible to cumulative stresses and to an acute traumatic episode. Acute injury usually involves a twisting motion to a weight-bearing knee; a blow to the side of the knee, called *traumatic valgus stress*; or full flexion combined with external rotation. The cartilage injury can range from a bruise to a complete tear. An acute tear can cause a fraying of the menisci, and fragments can eventually dislodge. These fragments can cause the knee to "lock," as it interrupts the normal glide of the tibia and femur. Small tears can occur with minimal trauma in the older knee because of weakened, degenerated cartilage. Any injury to the meniscus increases the amount of weight carried by the articular cartilage and increases the risk of degeneration (arthritis). The medial meniscus is much more susceptible to injury than is the lateral meniscus because it is far less mobile.

▨ **Treatment implications:** Injury causes swelling and potential subluxation, that is, misalignment. Assessment reveals a loss of active and passive extension. Lauren Berry, RPT, taught that if the torn tissues in the meniscus could maintain contact with each other and not separate, there would be an increased likelihood of repair. Because the outer one-third of the meniscus has a blood supply, tears in this region can heal.[4] A mobilization in the treatment protocol described in the text was taught by Berry and has proved remarkably effective in normalizing the menisci position to allow proper healing.

JOINT CAPSULE

▨ **Structure:** The joint capsule of the knee encloses the tibiofemoral and the patellofemoral joints (Fig. 9-2). It is attached to the femur approximately two finger widths above the patella and to the proximal tibia. The anterior part of the joint capsule can be divided into superficial and deep portions. The superficial portion is wide and loose, is thin in the front and sides, and is reinforced by the fascial ex-

pansion of the quadriceps muscle, called the **patellar retinaculum**. The retinaculum has several thickenings that are called the **patellofemoral** and **patellotibial ligaments.**[5] The deep portion of the joint capsule has two parts: (1) a deep transverse thickening of the retinaculum from the medial and lateral epicondyles to the patella and (2) the **meniscotibial ligaments,** also called the **coronary ligaments,** which help to stabilize the meniscus to the tibial plateau. The posterior capsule is strengthened by the tendinous expansions of the semimembranosus, popliteus, and gastrocnemius muscles. The oblique popliteal ligament, an expansion of the semimembranosus, interweaves with the arcuate popliteal ligament, a thickening in the posterior wall of the capsule. The synovial lining of the joint capsule has a thickening or fold, referred to as a **plica,** in the medial suprapatellar aspect of the knee in 20% to 60% of the population. If it becomes irritated, thickened, and fibrotic, it impinges on the medial edge of the medial femoral condyle.

▨ **Function:** The joint capsule provides stability to the joint and menisci, serves to lubricate the articulating surfaces, and provides a neurosensory role.[6] Tension is placed on the menisci through the ligaments that form part of the joint capsule when the quadriceps, semimembranosus, and popliteus contract.

▨ **Dysfunction and injury:** Joint capsule dysfunctions and injuries have connective tissue, muscular, and neurological consequences. Injury, repetitive stress, and surgery lead to synovitis, an inflammation of the synovial lining. When the knee is inflamed, it assumes a slightly flexed position as the capsule becomes relaxed and allows more fluid. A common result of prior inflammation is capsular tightness, and adhesions that develop between the joint capsule and bone, causing loss of normal ROM of the knee in a typical pattern. The knee loses about 20° of extension, and flexion is often restricted to only 90° to 100°. Since the normal lubricant (synovial fluid) is secreted only with joint movement, the joint becomes stiff and dehydrated. Restricted flexion leads to articular nerve dysfunction, which decreases sensory input from the mechanoreceptors and leads to arthrokinetic reflexes. Arthrokinetic reflexes typically inhibit (weaken) the quadriceps, especially the VMO, and tighten the hamstrings, especially the biceps femoris, and the ITB. These muscular imbalances lead to joint dysfunction and potential degeneration. The capsule can also develop *plica syndrome,* an irritation to the plica from repetitive stresses, such as running or swimming the breaststroke, or from trauma; this irritation causes pain, snapping, and stiffness at the anteromedial knee.[6]

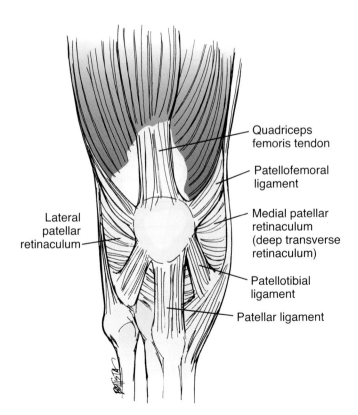

Quadriceps femoris tendon

Patellofemoral ligament

Medial patellar retinaculum (deep transverse retinaculum)

Patellotibial ligament

Patellar ligament

Lateral patellar retinaculum

Figure 9-2. Anterior knee showing the patellar retinaculum. The superficial portion of the joint capsule interweaves with the retinaculum. The retinaculum has distinct thickenings, the patellofemoral and patellotibial ligaments.

The capsule and associated ligaments can also become too slack because of injury, losing their stabilizing function and allowing for excessive joint movement, potential inflammation, and early joint degeneration resulting from the associated muscular inhibition caused by the arthrokinetic reflex.

▨ **Treatment implications:** Because full knee extension is essential to normal gait and because decreased flexion interferes with many daily activities, the therapist's primary intention is to normalize the ROM. This normalization is accomplished through contract-relax (CR) MET. The CR cycle pumps excess fluid out of the joint, reduces muscle hypertonicity, and helps to reestablish normal neurological communication to the surrounding muscles. For chronic thickening in the joint capsule, the therapist's intention is to increase the joint capsule extensibility and rehydrate the joint. Perform MET to increase knee flexion and perform STM to reduce sustained hypermobility in the hamstrings, quadriceps, ITB, gastrocnemius, and popliteus. Plica syndrome is treated with MET and STM. If the joint capsule and ligaments are too slack, the client needs exercise rehabilitation.

INFRAPATELLAR FAT PAD

▨ **Structure:** The infrapatellar fat pad is a small amount of fat located behind and to either side of the patellar tendon. During flexion, the fat pad is drawn deeply into the interior of the joint. The fat pad moves forward and bulges on either side of the infrapatellar tendon on extension of the knee. The back of the pad is lined with synovium.

▨ **Function:** The fat pad brushes against the femoral condyles during flexion and extension, spreading fluid to lubricate the joint.

▨ **Dysfunction and injury:** Impingement of the fat pad between the patella and the femoral condyle can occur because of a direct blow but more commonly occurs from repetitive or uncontrolled hyperextension.[4] Clients experience pain at the inferior pole of the patella, especially with extension.

▨ **Treatment implications:** MET for the hamstrings and joint mobilization will help to reduce the pressure on the fat pad.

LIGAMENTS

▨ **Structure:** The supporting structures, classified by function, are divided into the **static** and **dynamic stabilizers.** The static stabilizers are the superficial fascia, called the *crural fascia*; the joint capsule;

and the ligaments. The dynamic stabilizers are the muscles and their fascial expansions.

As was mentioned, many thickenings of the joint capsule can also be classified as ligaments. Classification of the ligaments by location divides the structures into anterior, posterior, medial, lateral, or internal. The **anterior ligaments** include the patellar ligament (infrapatellar tendon), which is the portion of the quadriceps that attaches to the tibial tuberosity; the medial and lateral patellofemoral and patellotibial ligaments (patellar retinaculum), which are broad tendinous thickenings of the fascial expansion of the quadriceps that connect the VMO and the vastus lateralis to the patella and tibia; the medial and lateral meniscopatellar ligaments, which are thickenings of the quadriceps fascia that place tension on the menisci when the quadriceps contract, drawing them forward; and the medial and lateral coronary ligaments (meniscotibial ligaments). The **posterior ligaments** include the posterior oblique popliteal ligament and the arcuate popliteal ligament. The **medial ligament** is the medial collateral ligament (MCL). **The lateral ligament** is the lateral collateral ligament (LCL). The **internal ligaments** include the ACL and the PCL.

▨ Medial patellofemoral and patellotibial ligaments (medial patellar retinaculum) (Fig. 9-3).

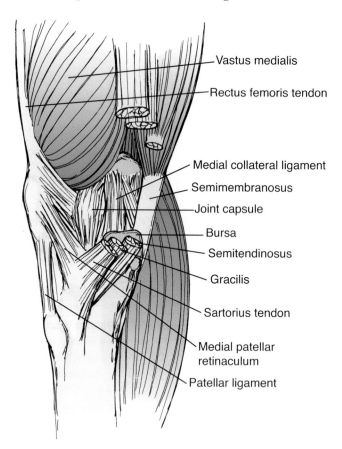

— Vastus medialis

— Rectus femoris tendon

— Medial collateral ligament

— Semimembranosus

— Joint capsule

— Bursa

— Semitendinosus

— Gracilis

— Sartorius tendon

— Medial patellar retinaculum

— Patellar ligament

Figure 9-3. Medial knee showing the ligaments, joint capsule, retinaculum, interweaving tendons, and pes anserinus bursa.

□ **Origin:** These ligaments are thickenings of the patellar retinaculum. Superficial fibers are from the VMO; deep (transverse) fibers are from the adductor tubercle of the medial epicondyle.

□ **Insertion:** The medial patellofemoral and patellotibial ligaments insert on the superior portion of the medial patella and continue to insert on the tibial tuberosity.

■ Lateral patellofemoral and patellotibial ligaments (lateral patellar retinaculum) (Fig. 9-4)
□ **Origin:** Superficial fibers of the vastus lateralis, some fibers from the rectus femoris (RF), and deep fibers from the lateral epicondyle of the femur form these ligaments. Fibers from the ITB insert into and strengthen it.

□ **Insertion:** The lateral patellofemoral and patellotibial ligaments insert on the superior portion of the lateral patella and continue to insert on the tibial tuberosity.

■ Medial and lateral meniscopatellar ligaments
□ **Origin:** Thickening in the quadriceps expansion (retinaculum) from the medial and lateral borders of the patella.

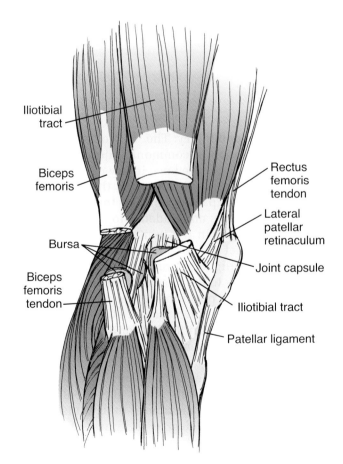

Iliotibial tract

Biceps femoris

Bursa

Biceps femoris tendon

Rectus femoris tendon

Lateral patellar retinaculum

Joint capsule

Iliotibial tract

Patellar ligament

Figure 9-4. Lateral knee showing the ligaments, joint capsule, retinaculum, interweaving tendons, bursae under the iliotibial tract, and biceps femoris.

□ **Insertion:** Into the anterior one-third of the menisci.

■ Posterior oblique popliteal ligament (Fig. 9-5)
□ **Origin:** A tendinous expansion of the semimembranosus muscle and thickening of the posterior joint capsule.

□ **Insertion:** The posterior oblique popliteal ligament attaches to the posterior aspect of the medial tibial condyle and the medial meniscus and to the posterior joint capsule. Contraction of the semimembranosus pulls the medial meniscus posteriorly during knee flexion.

■ Arcuate popliteal ligament (see Fig. 9-5)
□ **Origin:** Considered a thickening of the posterolateral joint capsule, the arcuate popliteal ligament arises from the posterior aspect of the head of the fibula.

□ **Insertion:** The arcuate popliteal ligament attaches to the fascia of the popliteus, the lateral epicondyle of the femur, the posteriolateral capsule, and the lateral meniscus.

■ Medial collateral ligament (MCL) (see Fig. 9-3)
□ **Origin:** A flat and triangular ligament, the MCL blends into the fibrous membrane of the capsule and fuses with the medial meniscus. It originates at the superior aspect of the medial femoral condyle at the adductor tubercle and has superficial and deep fibers.

□ **Insertion:** The MCL inserts into the medial tibia approximately 4 inches below the joint line.

■ Lateral collateral ligament (LCL) (see Fig. 9-4)
□ **Origin:** From the lateral epicondyle of the femur, the LCL, a round, cordlike structure, is neither fused with the capsule nor attached to the lateral meniscus.

□ **Insertion:** The LCL inserts into the fibular head, traveling underneath the biceps femoris tendon.

■ Coronary (meniscotibial) ligaments (Fig. 9-6)
□ Coronary ligaments are the deep, inferior portions of the joint capsule that attach the menisci to the tibia. This deep part of the joint capsule helps to bind the periphery of the medial and lateral menisci to the tibia.

■ Anterior cruciate ligament (ACL) (see Fig. 9-6)
□ **Origin:** The ACL originates from the anterior tibial plateau.

□ **Insertion:** The ACL inserts on the inner portion of the lateral condyle of the femur. It primarily restricts forward movement of the tibia relative to the femur and internal rotation of the tibia.

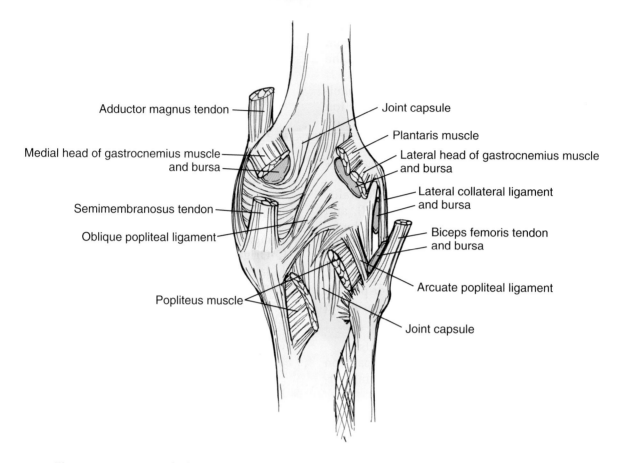

Figure 9-5. Joint capsule, ligaments, bursae, and muscles of the posterior knee.

- Posterior cruciate ligament (PCL) (see Fig. 9-6)
  - □ **Origin:** The PCL originates on the lateral surface of the medial condyle of the femur.
  - □ **Insertion:** The PCL inserts into the posterior tibial plateau and primarily restricts posterior movement of the tibia relative to the femur and internal rotation of the tibia on the femur.

- **Function:** The ligaments of the knee control joint movement more than any other joint in the body.[5] The ligaments are extremely dense, and dislocations are rare. As with all other synovial joints, the ligaments play an important neurosensory role. Ligaments provide vital information about joint position, movement, pressure, and pain and have reflex connections to the surrounding muscles. The ACL prevents forward movement of the tibia relative to the femur. The PCL prevents the femur from sliding forward off the tibial plateau. The MCL prevents excessive medial opening, and the LCL prevents lateral opening of the knee. The cruciate and collateral ligaments provide essential stability to the joint.

- **Dysfunction and injury:** The ligaments of the knee are some of the most commonly injured structures in the body. The acute knee injury of greatest concern, especially to the athlete, is the ACL, which typically accompanies damage to the menisci.[4] Ligament injuries are graded 1 to 3, based on the amount of laxity in the joint. Lauren Berry, RPT, discovered that the collateral ligaments develop a posterior misalignment or positional dysfunction after any injury to the knee that involves swelling. The knee takes a position of sustained flexion after injury, as flexion allows for more fluid in the knee. If the knee is held in flexion for a period of time, the collateral ligaments develop adhesions holding them in a posterior misalignment. As was mentioned, the knee also maintains a sustained flexion after a meniscus injury. If a client hears a "pop" in the knee at the time of injury, it is usually an ACL injury. The degree and onset of swelling are clues to the structures that have been injured. If a bruise develops with swelling within 1 to 2 hours, it is usually an ACL or PCL injury. If swelling develops a few hours later or the next

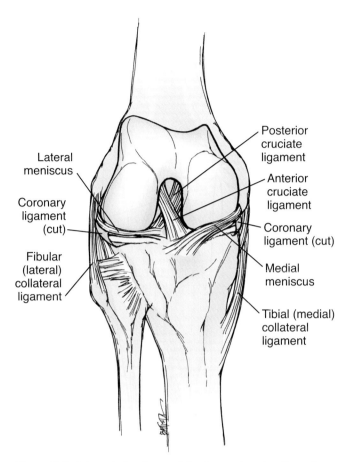

Figure 9-6. Internal structures of the knee, showing the anterior cruciate ligament; the posterior cruciate ligament; the medial and lateral menisci; and the coronary ligament, a part of the deep joint capsule.

Labels in figure:
Lateral meniscus
Coronary ligament (cut)
Fibular (lateral) collateral ligament
Posterior cruciate ligament
Anterior cruciate ligament
Coronary ligament (cut)
Medial meniscus
Tibial (medial) collateral ligament

day, this suggests a mild to moderate ligament injury, capsular irritation, or an injured meniscus. Damage to the ligaments, especially the ACL, leads to excessive and abnormal motion on the articular surfaces and predisposes the joint to early degeneration.[3]

- **Treatment implications:** The collateral ligaments need to be lifted in a posterior-to-anterior direction. The other ligaments do not have a positional dysfunction and need to be released transverse to the line of the fiber. As with the joint capsule, injury and dysfunction to the ligaments have two possible outcomes. In one, the ligaments become too slack, leading to instability, irritation, and degeneration. These ligaments are treated with exercise rehabilitation. In the other, the ligaments can become too tight and fibrotic, decreasing joint movement and leading to degeneration. If the ligaments are external, they are treated with STM to dissolve the fibrosis and rehydrate the tissue and

with MET to help normalize the neurological function.

BURSAE

- **Structure:** A bursa is a synovial-lined sac filled with synovial fluid (see Figs. 9-2 to 9-5). More than 24 bursae are located in the knee area. Three are recesses in the joint capsule that form the suprapatellar pouch, the semimembranosus, and the gastrocnemius bursae. Bursae are also under the muscles of the knee, including the biceps femoris, the semimembranosus, the ITB, and the pes anserinus tendons (see below).

- **Function:** Bursae function to decrease friction.

- **Dysfunction and injury:** Three areas are commonly involved clinically: the bursae of the anterior knee, including the prepatellar, infrapatellar, and suprapatellar bursae; the pes anserine bursa of the medial knee; and the semimembranosus and medial gastrocnemius bursae in the posterior knee. Joint swelling of the posterior knee is also called a **Baker's cyst,** which is chronic swelling that migrates between the two heads of the gastrocnemius. It is commonly associated with injury to the meniscus or degeneration. The bursae of the anterior knee are susceptible to direct impact and to prolonged kneeling, called "housemaid's knee." The bursae under the ITB and the pes anserinus tendons are commonly irritated because of excessive friction, such as running.

- **Treatment implications:** Bursae can be manually drained. The treatment involves gentle, slow, broad strokes toward the heart. Active or passive knee flexion and extension also assist in reducing the swelling by pumping the fluid out of the joint.

NERVES

- **Structure:** Innervation of the knee is from the **tibial, common peroneal,** and **saphenous nerves** (Figs. 9-7 and 9-8). The sciatic nerve divides into the tibial and common peroneal nerves in the distal third of the posterior thigh. The tibial nerve travels through the center of the popliteal fossa of the posterior knee, and the common peroneal nerve travels posterior to the fibular head between the biceps femoris and the lateral head of the gastrocnemius (see Fig. 10-3). The saphenous nerve is the terminal branch of the femoral nerve and gives off the infrapatellar branch, which travels superficially in the medial knee between the tendons of the sartorius and the gracilis.

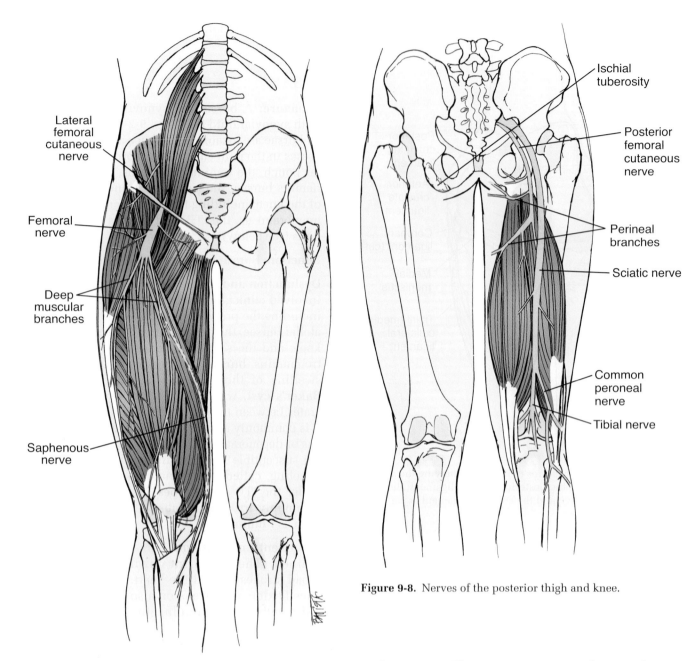

Lateral
femoral
cutaneous
nerve

Femoral
nerve

Deep
muscular
branches

Saphenous
nerve

Ischial
tuberosity

Posterior
femoral
cutaneous
nerve

Perineal
branches

Sciatic nerve

Common
peroneal
nerve

Tibial nerve

Figure 9-8. Nerves of the posterior thigh and knee.

Figure 9-7. Nerves of the anterior and medial thigh and knee.

▨ **Function:** The tibial and common peroneal nerves have articular, muscular, and cutaneous branches (the sural nerve). The saphenous nerve is a cutaneous nerve that innervates the skin in front of the patella and the skin of the leg and foot.

▨ **Dysfunction and injury:** The common peroneal and saphenous nerves are susceptible to irritation because of the friction of the contracting muscles through which they travel. Excessive running or jumping creates vigorous flexion, compressing the nerves. The common peroneal nerve is susceptible to trauma because it is exposed at the neck of the fibula. Impact injuries from falls or kicks, as in soccer, can injure the nerve. Irritation of this nerve can cause a sharp, local pain, numbing, or tingling that starts at the fibular head and travels down the lateral leg to the dorsum of the foot. Irritation of the saphenous nerve can create anterior and medial knee pain, numbing, or tingling.

▨ **Treatment:** Treatment for peripheral nerves involves stroking transverse to the nerve. These are gentle scooping strokes, not brisk friction strokes.

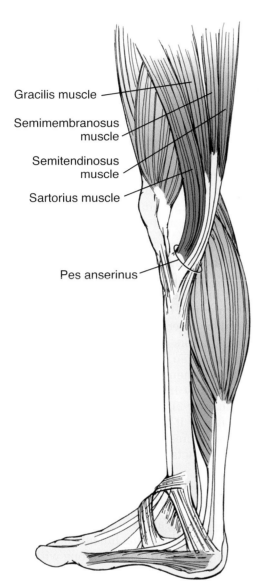

Gracilis muscle

Semimembranosus muscle

Semitendinosus muscle

Sartorius muscle

Pes anserinus

Figure 9-9. Muscles and fascia of the medial knee. The tendons of the sartorius, gracilis, and semitendinosus interweave at their insertion to form the pes anserinus ("goose's foot").

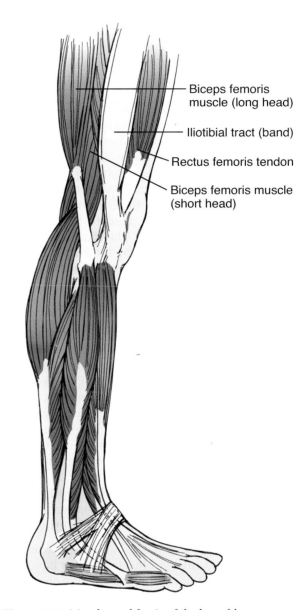

Biceps femoris muscle (long head)

Iliotibial tract (band)

Rectus femoris tendon

Biceps femoris muscle (short head)

Figure 9-10. Muscles and fascia of the lateral knee.

MUSCLES

▦ **Structure:** The muscles that move the knee are located in the thigh and in the leg. The thigh muscles that move the knee can be divided into the anterior and posterior groups. The **anterior muscle group** extends the knee and includes the sartorius and the four muscles of the quadriceps, which are the RF, vastus lateralis, intermedius, and medialis (Fig. 9-9). The **posterior group** consists of knee flexors and medial and lateral rotators of the tibia. It includes the three hamstrings (biceps femoris, semimembranosus, and semitendinosus), popliteus, and gastrocnemius (see Fig. 9-9). The muscles can also be classified by location into the medial and lateral compartments. The **medial compartment** includes the medial head of the gastrocnemius; the sartorius, gracilis, and semitendinosus tendons, collectively called the **pes anserinus;** the semimembranosus; and the quadriceps retinaculum from the vastus medialis (see Fig. 9-9). The pes anserinus muscles are the longest muscles in the anterior, medial, and posterior regions and act like a tripod to stabilize the knee. The **lateral compartment** includes the ITB, biceps femoris, popliteus, and quadriceps expansion from the vastus lateralis (Fig. 9-10).

▦ **Function:** Muscles and their fascial expansions are the **dynamic stabilizers** of the knee. It is important to remember that the body is a tensegrity structure, that is, the muscles (tension members), not the bones (compression members), keep the body upright. This is critical information when applied to the knee. It is muscles that "decompress" the knee by lifting the body weight off the bones. Weak muscles allow the body weight to collapse onto the bones, leading to pain and accelerated degeneration. It is essential to maintain strength in the muscles that cross the knee, including the quadriceps and hamstrings, especially with degeneration or after an injury because there are reflex inhibitions to the muscles that need to be overcome through consistent exercise. The muscles also dynamically stabilize the knee by interweaving with the joint capsule. Muscle contraction tenses the capsule, increasing joint stability. Anteriorly, the quadriceps reinforce the capsule through the medial and lateral retinacula, which are fascial expansions of the quadriceps. Laterally, the capsule in reinforced by the ITB. Medially, the capsule in supported by the pes anserinus tendons (semitendinosus, gracilis, and sartorius). Posterolateral support is provided by the biceps femoris. Posterior dynamic stabilization is provided by gastrocnemius and popliteus muscles. The hamstrings cross two joints and not only flex the knee but also rotate the tibia and pelvis. The semimembranosus muscle attaches to the medial meniscus and retracts it during knee flexion. The popliteus attaches to the lateral meniscus and contributes to posterior movement of the meniscus during knee flexion.

■ **Dysfunction and injury:** Muscle injuries have two categories: acute trauma and cumulative stress. As with the hip, the most commonly injured knee muscles are the two-joint muscles, especially the RF and the biceps femoris, the lateral hamstring. One of the main functions of these muscles is eccentric contraction (i.e., to contract while the muscle is lengthening), during which muscles are much more prone to injury. The RF must eccentrically contract to decelerate the hip and knee, and the hamstrings eccentrically contract as the knee comes to full extension at heel strike.[9] The ITB is often irritated because of repetitive friction against the lateral femoral condyle. This condition is called *iliotibial band friction syndrome.* Another common condition is tendinitis of the pes anserinus insertions at the medial knee. Muscle dysfunction has two categories: muscle imbalance and positional dysfunction. Muscle imbalance describes a condition in which certain muscles are weak and others are short and tight. Muscle imbalance alters move-

ment patterns and therefore adds a continuing stress to the joint system. Positional dysfunction describes a condition in which muscles misalign and develop an abnormal torsion.

Muscle Imbalances of the Knee

■ **Muscles that tend to be tight and short:** Iliopsoas, TFL and ITB, RF, quadratus lumborum, pectineus, gracilis, adductors, hamstrings (biceps femoris more than semitendinosus or semimembranosus), soleus and gastrocnemius (plantar flexors of the ankle), piriformis, and other external rotators of the hip.

■ **Muscles that tend to be weak (inhibited):** Gluteus maximus; hip abductors (gluteus minimus and medius); hip internal rotators vastus lateralis, vastus intermedius, and especially VMO; dorsiflexors of the ankle, especially the tibialis anterior.

☐ The adductors are typically short and tight, but they are often weak because of the tightness-weakness phenomenon, in which a muscle that is habitually in its shortened position is weak (see Chapter 2). The VMO attaches to the adductor magnus; it is important to facilitate the adductors to create a stable base from which the VMO contracts.[10]

Positional Dysfunction of Knee Muscles

■ Gracilis, sartorius, and semitendinosus (pes anserinus tendons) at their attachments on the tibia tend to roll into a posterior torsion along with the MCL.

■ ITB at the knee tends to roll into a posterior torsion along with the LCL.

■ Hamstrings, gastrocnemius, and soleus tend to shorten and roll toward the midline.

The classic postural dysfunction of the lower extremity is a genu valgus deformity, with an internally rotated femur, externally rotated tibia, pronated ankles, and laterally positioned patella on the femur. This is a collapsed position that expresses gravity's toll on the body.

ANATOMY OF THE KNEE MUSCLES

See Table 9-1.

MUSCULAR ACTIONS OF THE KNEE

See Table 9-2.

Table 9-1 Anatomy of the Knee Muscles

Muscle	Origin	Insertion	Action	Dysfunction
Quadriceps				
Rectus femoris (the only quadriceps that crosses two joints)	Arises by two tendinous heads: a straight head from the anterior inferior iliac spine and a reflected head that arises from a groove above the acetabulum and from the fibrous capsule of the hip	Ends in a broad, thick aponeurosis and flattened tendon attached to the upper surface of the patella; central, superficial part of the quadriceps tendon	Extends the knee and assists in flexion and abduction of the hip	The rectus femoris (RF) is typically tight and short, contributing to an anterior pelvic tilt. Tightness of the RF and the other hip flexors inhibits the gluteus maximus.
Vastus lateralis	From the lateral surface of the greater trochanter and the lateral lip of the linea aspera	Quadriceps tendon, which forms the lateral patellar retinaculum attaching to the lateral pole of the patella and the tibial tuberosity	Knee extension. Both the rectus femoris and vastus lateralis exert a lateral pull on the patella	Vasti are typically weak, inhibited by hamstring tightness. Quadriceps weakness is a strong predictor of anterior knee pain. The weakness causes difficulty in climbing stairs and in getting up from and down into a seated position.[11] Tightness of the vastus lateralis adds a compressive load to the lateral patella against the femur.
Vastus intermedius	Anterior and lateral surfaces of the femur	Quadriceps tendon; it covers the articular muscle of the knee (genu articularis), which inserts into the capsule of the knee	Extends the knee	
Vastus medialis	Medial aspect of the linea aspera and intertrochanteric line. The vastus medialis obliquus (VMO) arises from the tendon of the adductor magnus	Quadriceps tendon, forming the medial patellar retinaculum; consists of two parts: the vastus medialis longus and the VMO; whereas the fibers of the longus portion are directed vertically, the fibers of the oblique portion are directed almost horizontally; both attach to the medial border of the patella	Extends the knee and stabilizes the patella during extension	The VMO is the only primary dynamic stabilizer of the medial patella and is typically weak, allowing lateral displacement of the patella during the last phase of knee extension, called *patellar tracking dysfunction.*
Popliteus	On the posterior aspect of the lateral femoral condyle and the lateral meniscus, travelling under the lateral head of the gastrocnemius	Attaches to the posteromedial border of the proximal tibia	Medially rotates the tibia on the femur and flexes the knee when the foot is not fixed (open kinetic chain) and laterally rotates the femur on the tibia in a closed kinetic chain; assists the posterior movement of the lateral meniscus in knee flexion.	Popliteus weakness will inhibit normal posterior glide of the meniscus during knee flexion and lateral rotation of the tibia at the last part of knee extension (terminal extension)

See also the hamstrings, sartorius, and gracilis in Chapter 8 and the gastrocnemius and plantaris in Chapter 10.

Table 9-2	Muscular Actions of the Knee

Twelve muscles contribute to knee flexion and extension and to leg rotation.

Flexion

- Semimembranosus
- Semitendinosus
- Biceps femoris
- Gracilis
- Sartorius
- Popliteus—also medially rotates the lower leg
- Gastrocnemius—also plantar flexes the ankle
- Plantaris—also plantar flexes the ankle

Extension

- Rectus femoris
- Vastus medialis
- Vastus intermedius
- Vastus lateralis

Lower Leg Rotation

Medial Rotation	Lateral Rotation
Semimembranosus	Biceps femoris
Gracilis	
Popliteus	
Semitendinosus	
Sartorius	

Knee Dysfunction and Injury

FACTORS THAT PREDISPOSE TO KNEE PAIN

- Leg-length inequality

- Abnormal position of the patella

- Instability caused by weakness in the static or dynamic stabilizers

- Muscle imbalances (tight flexors, including the hamstrings, ITB, and gastrocnemius, and weak extensors, especially the VMO)

- Altered gait, such as toe-out gait

- Soft tissue fibrosis (adhesions), especially in the joint capsule or lateral retinaculum

- Abnormal alignment, including knock-knees (genu valgum), bow legs (genu varum), or hyperextended knees (genu recurvatum)

- Femoral anteversion

- Internal tibial torsion

- Pronation or an unstable ankle

- Rigid foot, or flat foot, which decreases shock-absorbing capacity[10]

- Immobilization, previous surgery

- Recent change in exercise. A change of more than 10% in an exercise routine is associated with greater injuries.[12]

- Fatigue. Most knee injuries happen at the end of the day, at the end of a performance, at the end of a ski run, and so on.

- Previous injury

DIFFERENTIATION OF KNEE PAIN

- It is important to realize that knee pain can come from structures other than the neuromusculoskeletal system. See the section "Contraindications to Massage Therapy: Red Flags" in Chapter 2, "Assessments and Technique," for guidelines on when massage is contraindicated and when referral is necessary. Assuming that knee pain is not pathological, differentiation can be categorized according to structures involved.

- The knee joint is innervated from L3–S2 nerves, and pain in the knee area can be referred from irritation of the nerve roots from the lumbosacral spine. Typically, the pain is described as a deep ache, numbing, or tingling in the anterior or medial knee. The straight-leg-raising test or passive hip extension increases the pain with nerve root involvement. (See Chapters 3, "Lumbosacral Spine," and 8, "The Hip," for those tests.)

- The hip and the knee joints have common innervation, and knee pain can be referred from the hip. Painful, decreased passive flexion and medial rotation of the hip suggests hip osteoarthritis, also called *degenerative joint disease*.

- Myofascial pain of acute onset is described as a sharp, localized pain that is often associated with swelling, heat, and redness. It is increased with isometric contraction, performed during CR MET, and is better with rest.

- Acute knee pain is typically the result of trauma. The most commonly injured structures are the ACL, MCL, or medial meniscus. With a severe injury, the knee swells immediately. With a less severe injury, the swelling takes 6 to12 hours to develop.[6] The pain is typically localized at the medial joint line, and usually, the client is unable to straighten the knee fully.

- Chronic pain is typically osteoarthritis, caused by degeneration of the cartilage. In the elderly, complaints of stiffness and diffuse pain implicate this condition. Besides injury, the most common area of pain is the anterior knee, usually as a result of tracking disorders of the patellofemoral joint. The pain arises or is worsened with prolonged sitting or going down stairs. In chronic knee dysfunction, the knee can buckle or give way, indicating joint instability. This instability is caused by loose ligaments, muscle inhibition, or a torn meniscus.

- Many older patients report that they have been told that their knee pain is just caused by getting older, when in fact in most of those patients, the pain is in one knee only—and obviously, their other knee is just as old. The pain is often caused by functional problems that have resulted from a previous injury or cumulative stress. Problems of function are typically caused by muscular imbalances, which lead to imbalances in knee alignment and function; capsular fibrosis and thickening, which lead to loss of normal lubrication and nutrition; and loss of normal movement or joint play of the articular surfaces. Proper alignment of the pelvis, feet, and ankles is essential for healthy knees.

COMMON TYPES OF KNEE DYSFUNCTION AND INJURY

ANTERIOR CRUCIATE LIGAMENT SPRAIN

- **Cause:** An ACL injury usually results from a twisting motion combined with hyperextension and a varus or a valgus stress, a direct blow to the knee with the foot planted, or if the foot is planted and the body is propelled forward, as in basketball, or catching the tip of a ski.[9]

- **Symptoms:** Pain and swelling in the anterior knee are symptoms of ACL lesion. With chronic ACL lesions, clients experience a feeling of the knee giving way.

- **Sign:** A positive anterior drawer test is a sign of an ACL lesion.

- **Sites:** ACL injuries occur at the tibial or femoral attachments internal to the knee.

- **Treatment:** For **acute** injuries, gently perform MET #1 with pain-free resistance to contract the flexors and extensors of the knee to reduce pain and swelling, and help prevent muscular inhibition. It is important to maintain good functional balance between the flexors and extensors of the knee, as the hamstrings and ITB tend to shorten and the quadriceps, except the RF, tend to weaken. Treatment usually concentrates on the release of the ITB and facilitation (strengthening) of the VMO. Gently perform Level I STM strokes to maintain adequate circulation of nutrients and oxygen and to stimulate cellular synthesis. For **chronic** ACL injuries, the knee tends to be unstable. The client needs exercise rehabilitation as the primary treatment. Manual therapy concentrates on the release of tight muscles, which can inhibit the strengthening of the weak muscles, and on the manual release of thick, fibrous tissue, which prevent the knee from tracking properly. Perform METs for the hip and knee as both assessment and treatment to identify weak muscles and shortened myofascia. Perform CR MET to recruit inhibited muscles and postisometric relaxation (PIR) MET to lengthen shortened tissue. Perform Level I and II STM to identify areas of soft tissue restrictions and to mobilize the soft tissue.

MEDIAL COLLATERAL LIGAMENT SPRAIN

- **Cause:** The most common mechanism of injury is a blow to the lateral knee when the foot is planted. The MCL is the primary stabilizer to valgus stress.

■ **Symptoms:** MCL sprain is the most common ligament disorder in the body. It usually accompanies a history of trauma, leading to well-localized pain at the medial or posteromedial knee. With chronic MCL injuries, clients might experience an ache or a feeling of the ligament giving way during exertion.

■ **Sign:** Pain at the medial knee on valgus stress test at 30° of knee flexion is a sign of MCL sprain.

■ **Site:** MCL sprains occur at three sites. The ligament can tear at the femoral or the tibial insertions or at the joint line in the midbody of the ligament. These tears result in interbody adhesions or adhesions to the femur or tibia.

■ **Treatment:** The treatment of both acute and chronic MCL injuries is similar to what is described above under ACL injuries. The main difference is that treatment for the MCL allows for manual pressure to the ligament, unlike the ACL, which is located deep within the joint. For **acute** injuries, perform gentle transverse release of the ligament, Level I, second series, and Level II, first series. This prevents the formation of adhesions to the bone and adjacent soft tissue, and helps align the newly formed collagen fibers.[6] As the ligament heals, deeper pressures may be applied. Gentle, pain-free, transverse strokes to an acute injury help to realign the healing fibers. For **chronic** conditions, the area of the MCL is either thick and fibrous or atrophied. For thick tissue, use Level II, first series, transverse friction strokes on a chronic MCL injury help dissolve adhesions. It is important to scan the area in chronic conditions by performing the Level I and Level II series to identify areas of hypertonicity and adhesions and to treat what you find. Atrophied ligaments require exercise rehabilitation.

MEDIAL MENISCUS

■ **Cause:** Twisting on a weight-bearing leg is a frequent cause of injury to the medial meniscus.

■ **Symptoms:** Acute injuries involves a sudden onset of severe pain "somewhere inside the knee" and a feeling that the joint is giving way, accompanied with some swelling. If the condition is chronic, clients usually have complaints of knee locking and of a painful snapping or catching sensation inside the knee or a history of the knee suddenly giving way.

■ **Signs:** Joint line tenderness; loss of normal knee movement, usually lost at the end range of either full flexion or full extension; positive McMurray's test; springy-block end feel with passive extension; and inability to actively extend the knee fully. Atrophy of the VMO and mild chronic swelling are typical.

■ **Treatment:** For **acute** injuries gently perform MET #1 with pain-free resistance to contract the flexors and extensors of the knee to reduce pain and swelling, and help prevent muscular inhibition. The degree of reduced flexion and extension measures the extent of the injury. With severe injuries, there is a painful loss of full flexion with an empty end feel and limited and painful passive extension with a springy-block end feel. **Chronic** conditions have a presentation similar to that of chronic ACL injuries in terms of muscle imbalances. Perform MET to release the short and tight muscles and to recruit the weak muscles. Typically, the knee has lost normal glide, and the meniscus is fixated anteriorly. Perform Level I and II STM strokes, concentrating on the medial and anterior joint line. Perform pain-free, figure-eight mobilization of the knee, Level II, fifth series.

LATERAL COLLATERAL LIGAMENT SPRAIN

■ **Cause:** Typically, a blow to the medial knee causes LCL sprain, which is much less common than MCL injuries.

■ **Symptoms:** LCL sprains usually involve a history of trauma, leading to well-localized pain at the lateral knee. With chronic LCL sprains, clients might experience an ache or a feeling of the ligament giving way during exertion.

■ **Sign:** Pain at the ligament on varus stress test at 30° of knee flexion is a sign of LCL sprain. An LCL sprain needs to be differentiated from a biceps femoris injury, which would be painful with resisted knee flexion.

■ **Sites:** LCL sprains occur at the femoral or fibular attachments or at the joint line.

■ **Treatment:** The treatment of both acute and chronic LCL injuries is described above under ACL injuries; the exam findings are nearly the same. For **acute** injuries, perform gentle transverse release of the ligament, Level I, second series, and Level II, first series. As the ligament heals, deeper pressures may be applied. Gentle, pain-free, transverse strokes to an acute injury help realign the healing fibers. For chronic conditions, the area of the LCL is either thick and fibrous or atrophied. For thick tissue, use Level II, first series, transverse friction strokes to help dissolve adhesions. It is important to scan the area in chronic conditions by performing the Level I and Level II series to identify areas of hypertonicity and adhesions and to treat what you find.

POSTERIOR CRUCIATE LIGAMENT SPRAIN

■ **Cause:** PCL sprain can be caused by a vigorous whip kick in the breaststroke ("breaststroker's knee"), by a direct blow to a flexed knee, or by hyperflexion or hyperextension injuries.

▨ **Symptoms:** Clients experience pain and swelling around the knee. With chronic PCL sprain, clients experience a feeling of the knee giving way.

▨ **Sign:** A positive posterior sag test is a sign of PCL sprain.

▨ **Sites:** PCL sprain occurs at the tibial or femoral attachments internal to the knee.

▨ **Treatment:** See the treatment described above under "Anterior Cruciate Ligament Sprain."

CORONARY (MENISCOTIBIAL) LIGAMENT SPRAIN

▨ **Cause:** Repetitive twisting, such as when playing tennis, dancing, or prolonged walking downhill, can cause coronary ligament sprain. The ligament often adheres to the anteromedial tibial plateau, restricting the mobility of the meniscus, which should move posteriorly on knee flexion.

▨ **Symptoms:** Clients experience well-localized pain, usually at the medial tibial plateau. Lateral coronary ligament problems are rare.

▨ **Sign:** Pain at the medial tibial plateau to palpation or pain with full passive flexion of the knee during the anterior drawer test or passive lateral rotation is a sign of coronary ligament sprain.

▨ **Treatment:** See the treatment described above under "Anterior Cruciate Ligament Sprain." Perform Level II, first series, which describes transverse massage to the ligament with the strokes directed downward onto the tibial plateau.

JOINT CAPSULE FIBROSIS

▨ **Cause:** Any inflammatory condition, including trauma or surgery, or immobilization can result in capsular fibrosis. Inflammation can also result from chronic irritation that causes a chronic microinflammatory environment that is subclinical, that is, it does not visibly swell, nor is it hot. Inflammation that results from a specific trauma or surgery leads to the usual signs of redness, heat, and swelling.

▨ **Symptoms:** Clients experience pain on either side of the superior portion of the patella after exertion. The knee feels stiff, especially after the client sits for long periods.

▨ **Sign:** Palpation reveals thickened, tender tissue at the sites described above. The ROM is reduced in a typical pattern of about 20° loss of extension and flexion is limited to about 100° with a capsular end feel.

▨ **Treatment:** The treatment goals for this chronic condition are to reduce the hypertonicity of the muscles surrounding the knee, lengthen the joint capsule, and normalize the ROM of the tibiofemoral and patellofemoral joints. Perform MET to lengthen the joint capsule and increase knee flexion (MET #8). Perform Level I and II STM strokes to the retinaculum and joint capsule, which broadens the fibers and helps to dissolve the adhesions within the substance of the capsule and between the bone.

QUADRICEPS TENDINITIS, PATELLAR TENDINITIS/TENDINOPATHY

▨ **Causes:** Irritation of the quadriceps tendon above the patella is referred to as a *quadriceps tendinitis*, and irritation of the tendon below the patella is referred to as a *patellar tendinitis*. As has been mentioned, recent research has found that chronic pain in tendons represents a degeneration of the collagen rather than a chronic inflammation.[4] Current literature prefers the term *tendinopathy* or *tendinosis* rather than *chronic tendinitis*. Repetitive or excessive jumping, running, dancing, or hiking can cause quadriceps tendinitis and patellar tendinitis/tendinopathy.

▨ **Symptoms:** Clients experience pain on the front of the knee after exertion. This pain is well localized to one of three common sites: infrapatellar tendon (jumper's knee), tenoperiosteal insertion at the superior portion of patella, or lateral patellar retinaculum.

▨ **Signs:** Pain on resisted knee extension at site of injury and possible pain on full passive knee flexion are signs of patellar tendinitis/tendinopathy at the knee.

▨ **Treatment:** The primary intention in treating **acute** injuries is to reduce pain, swelling, and muscle spasms. Perform CR and reciprocal inhibition (RI) MET for the quadriceps with light pressure (MET #1 or MET #3, hip). Perform Level I STM first series and the fourth stroke in the fourth series, with gentle pressure and a slow rhythm. As you perform the strokes and the patellar tendon remains tender, perform more MET to reduce the tenderness and excessive tension on the tendon. For **chronic** conditions, assess the length of the RF (Ely's test). Because the RF is typically short and tight, perform PIR MET #6 to lengthen the rectus. Next, perform STM, Level I, fourth series, to dissolve adhesions in the tendon and at the attachment points of the RF at the patella and tibial tuberosity. Transverse friction massage might need to be performed for 3 to 4 minutes, one time a week, for four to six weeks to dissolve the adhesions. Perform joint mobilization for the patellofemoral and tibiofemoral joints, Level II, fifth series, to help normalize joint function.

HAMSTRINGS TENDINITIS/ TENDINOPATHY AT THE KNEE

■ **Causes:** Hamstrings tendinitis/tendinopathy at the knee is common in runners and is associated with pronated ankles and anteverted hips. The hamstrings eccentrically contract as the knee comes to full extension at heel strike, making it vulnerable to injury.

■ **Symptoms:** With biceps femoris injury, clients experience pain at the posterolateral aspect of the knee at the tenoperiosteal insertion at the fibular head. With semimembranosus involvement, clients experience pain at the posteromedial surface of the knee.

■ **Signs:** With hamstrings tendinitis at the knee, clients exhibit the following signs: for biceps femoris injury, pain elicited on resisted knee flexion when performed with lateral rotation of the thigh and leg, and for semimembranosus involvement, pain elicited on resisted knee flexion with medial rotation of thigh and leg.

■ **Treatment:** For **acute** injuries, perform CR and RI MET for the hamstrings to reduce pain, swelling, and muscle spasms (MET #5, hip). Perform Level I, fifth series, STM strokes with gentle pressure and a slow rhythm. As you perform the strokes, if the hamstrings remain tender and hypertonic, intersperse MET with your strokes to reduce the tenderness and hypertonicity in the muscle. For **chronic** conditions, assess the length of the hamstrings (MET #10, hip). Because the hamstrings are typically short and tight, perform contract-relax-antagonist-contract (CRAC) MET #10, hip, and PIR MET #5 to lengthen the hamstrings, and increase the extensibility of the lower tendinous attachments at the knee. Next, perform STM, Level I, third series (hip), and Level I, fifth series (knee), to dissolve adhesions in the hamstrings belly and at the tendon attachments at the posterior knee. Perform joint mobilization for the patellofemoral and tibiofemoral joints, Level II, fifth series, to help normalize joint function.

OSTEOARTHRITIS OF THE KNEE (DEGENERATIVE JOINT DISEASE)

■ **Causes:** A degenerated or osteoarthritic knee means that the cartilage has worn down. Fibrosis, dehydration, and shortening of the joint capsule typically precede the degeneration. Osteoarthritis of the knee results from cumulative stress due to abnormal mechanics, such as genu valgum or genu varum, leg-length inequality, or obesity. It can also result from a specific traumatic event, such as a fall on the knee or an injury to the ACL, MCL, or meniscus.

■ **Symptoms:** Symptoms begin as a dull ache that increases with activity and stiffness in the morning and after long periods of sitting. With advanced degeneration, clients report more severe pain, especially medially, present even at rest, especially with sitting. If the knee also has an inflammatory component, pain can disturb sleep.

■ **Sign:** A decrease in passive flexion with capsular or hard end feel is a sign of arthritis of the knee.

■ **Treatment:** It is critical to restore normal length to the joint capsule, as the inner lining of the capsule is the source of nutrition and lubrication to the joint and a shortened capsule predisposes the joint to degeneration. Perform MET #6 to lengthen the RF, and MET #8 to lengthen the capsule. If the client has an **acute** inflammation with a knee that is also degenerated, the initial treatment goals are to reduce the swelling and pain by performing CR and RI MET #1 for flexion and extension. Also perform MET on the short and tight muscles, which would include the protocol described above for capsulitis/synovitis. For **chronic** conditions, the intention is to identify short and tight muscles, fibrous tissue, and weak muscles and to restore the ROM of the knee, as well as joint play. In addition to a short and tight capsule, the hamstrings, RF, ITB, adductors, and gastrocnemius are short and tight and need to be treated first. The VMO, gluteus medius, and gluteus maximus are typically weak and need to be recruited (strengthened). The knee is typically hypomobile and needs to be mobilized to restore normal joint play (Level II, fifth series).

PLICA SYNDROME

■ **Causes:** The plica is a vestigial remnant of the synovial lining and is normally found in approximately 20% to 60% of the population.[6] Repetitive stress to the anteromedial knee, such as prolonged running or biking, can cause a friction irritation, and the plica can become thickened and fibrotic.

■ **Symptoms:** Clients experience pain at the anteromedial knee with an occasional snapping sensation medial to the patella.

■ **Signs:** The presence of a cordlike structure medial to the patella revealed with palpation and a jump or jog in the patella with active knee extension are signs of plica syndrome.

■ **Treatment:** For **acute** inflammation of the plica, the initial treatment goals are to reduce the swelling and pain and to decrease the muscular tension on the anterior knee. Perform CR and RI MET #1 to gently contact and relax the flexors and extensors of the knee to pump the swelling out of the area. Next, perform gentle Level I STM strokes, first to fourth series, to reduce the swelling in the area through compression and decompression cycles. For **chronic** conditions, perform the protocol described above to help reduce excess muscle tension, and release the patellar retinaculum, which lies superficial to the plica. Next, perform PIR MET for the hamstrings (MET #5) and quadriceps (MET #6) to lengthen the myofascia, reducing the compressive load to the anterior knee. Finally, perform Level II, third series, STM strokes to dissolve fibrous deposits on the plica and adhesions between the plica and the bone.

POPLITEUS TENDINITIS/TENDINOPATHY

▨ **Causes:** Popliteus tendinitis/tendinopathy is often associated with pronated ankles and excessive running or hiking.

▨ **Symptoms:** Clients typically experience pain at the posterolateral corner of the knee at the femoral attachment, especially after walking or running downhill or sitting cross-legged. However, pain may be more diffuse to the posterior knee in the muscle belly or at the lower insertion at the medial tibia. Pain can also arise from the popliteus–arcuate ligament complex at the posterior knee.[4]

▨ **Signs:** Pain with resisted medial rotation of the tibia and pain at the posterior aspect of the knee with passive knee flexion are signs of popliteus tendinitis/tendinopathy. Chronic tendinopathy will manifest either as reduced external tibial rotation if the tissue is short and thick with adhesions or as excessive tibial rotation if the popliteus has atrophied because of a poor repair.

▨ **Treatment:** For **acute** injuries, perform CR and RI MET for the popliteus to reduce pain, swelling, and muscle spasms (MET #7). Perform Level I, fifth series, and Level II, fourth series, STM strokes, with gentle pressure and a slow rhythm. As you perform the strokes, if the popliteus remains tender and hypertonic, intersperse MET with your strokes. For **chronic** conditions, assess the length of the popliteus (MET #4). Because the popliteus can be either short and tight or long and atrophied, your assessment will determine your treatment. For excessive tibial rotation, the client needs resistance exercise for the popliteus (to strengthen internal rotation of the tibia and knee flexion and to increase the density of the posterior ligaments and capsule). If assessment reveals loss of external tibial rotation, perform PIR MET #7 to lengthen the popliteus, and increase the extensibility of the popliteus–actuate ligament complex at the posterior knee. Next, perform Level I, fifth series, and Level II, fourth series, STM strokes to dissolve adhesions. Perform joint mobilization for the patellofemoral and tibiofemoral joints (Level II, fifth series) to help normalize joint function.

ILIOTIBIAL BAND FRICTION SYNDROME

▨ **Cause:** The ITB arises from the gluteus maximus and TFL. It is pulled anteriorly by the TFL in flexion and posteriorly by the gluteus maximus in extension. Repetitive flexion and extension of the knee cause friction of the ITB against the lateral femoral epicondyle, which is common in cyclists and runners. This syndrome is associated with weakness in the hip abductors and flexors and pronated feet.[4]

▨ **Symptoms:** Clients experience pain at the lateral aspect of the knee at the lateral femoral epicondyle.

▨ **Sign:** Pain at lateral femoral epicondyle reproduced while the client extends the knee from 90° flexion to approximately 30° flexion.

▨ **Treatment:** For **acute** conditions perform CR and RI MET for the TFL (MET #11, hip) to reduce pain and swelling and to reduce the tension in the ITB by reducing the muscle tension in the TFL. Perform Level I, hip, sixth series, STM strokes to reduce the tension in the proximal portion of the ITB, and perform Level I, third series, to help reduce swelling and realign the fibers at the knee. As you perform the strokes, if the ITB remains tender, intersperse MET with your strokes. For **chronic** conditions, because the ITB is typically short and tight, perform PIR MET for the ITB (MET #12, hip) to lengthen the ITB and to increase the extensibility of it attachment at the lateral knee. Next, perform Level II, second series, STM strokes to dissolve adhesions between the ITB and the lateral patella, distal femur, and tibia.

BURSITIS

▨ **Cause:** Repetitive contraction of a muscle can irritate the bursa that lies under it and cause swelling and pain. The prepatellar bursa is irritated with prolonged kneeling or from a direct blow to the anterior knee. Swelling in the joint can cause a swelling of the semimembranosus and gastrocnemius bursae. If the swelling is chronic, a bursa can dry out and develop adhesions because of lack of movement due to pain.

▨ **Symptoms:** Clients experience local swelling and achy, throbbing, burning pain. There are three common areas of knee involvement (see "Signs").

▨ **Signs:** With bursitis, signs are particular to the area involved.
  ☐ **Prepatellar ("housemaid's knee"):** Swelling superficial to the patella.

☐ **Pes anserinus:** Lies between the tibial collateral ligament and the tendinous insertions of gracilis, sartorius, and semitendinosus; well-localized swelling approximately 2 inches below the medial joint line.

☐ **Gastrocnemius (Baker's cyst):** Swelling in the posterior knee; lies between medial head of gastrocnemius and semimembranosus tendon; best seen with the knee in extension.

▨ **Treatment:** Bursae respond well to lymphatic massage. In both acute and chronic conditions, perform MET to reduce swelling and tension in the muscle of the involved bursa. In **acute** conditions, perform very slow, gentle, broad continuous strokes toward the heart. Begin at the proximal part of the bursa, and milk the fluid headward. For the prepatellar bursa and suprapatellar pouch, perform Level I, first series; for the pes anserinus bursa, perform Level I, fifth series, and for the gastrocnemius bursa, perform Level II, first series. For **chronic** conditions, perform PIR MET for the involved muscles to incease the extensibility of the tissue over the bursa. Next, perform the same series of strokes described above. If the bursa feels swollen, use light pressure. If the area of the bursa is thick and fibrous, deeper pressures may be applied to help stimulate the bursa to restore its fluid.

PATELLAR TRACKING DYSFUNCTION (PATELLOFEMORAL JOINT DYSFUNCTION)

▨ **Cause:** Medial rotation (anteversion) of the femur; lateral tibial rotation; pronation; excessive genu valgum; weakness of the VMO (which reduces medial stabilization) and tightness of the ITB creating a bowstring effect, pulling the patella laterally. As the patella is pulled laterally, it creates a thickening of the lateral patellar retinaculum and excessive tensile (pulling) forces on the medial retinaculum, creating pain on the medial side and thickened restrictions on the lateral side of the patella.

▨ **Symptoms:** Clients experience a gradual onset of a diffuse ache in the anterior and medial knee and pain behind the patella, especially after prolonged sitting or going down stairs, and might have cracking and popping noises (crepitation).

▨ **Signs:** Pain behind the patella on resisted knee extension and while performing the squat test, pain on patellar compression, weak VMO and adductors, tight ITB and biceps femoris, and fibrosis of the lateral patellar retinaculum to palpation are signs of patellar tracking dysfunction.

▨ **Treatment:** For **acute** conditions, perform CR and RI MET #1 to contract the flexors and extensors of the knee to reduce pain and swelling in the anterior knee. Next, perform gentle CR and RI MET for the TFL (MET #11, hip) and for the hamstrings to reduce tension in the ITB by reducing the muscle tension in the TFL and biceps femoris. Perform Level I, first to fourth series, STM strokes to reduce the tension and swelling, and help to realign the fibers in the distal thigh and anterior, medial, and lateral knee. As you perform the strokes, if the area remains tender, intersperse MET with your strokes. For **chronic** conditions, it is important to help strengthen the VMO and adductors, because the weakness of the medial musculature allows a tight ITB and biceps femoris to pull the patella laterally. However, the tight and short muscles must be released first, because they have an inhibiting effect on their antagonists. Because the ITB is typically short and tight, perform PIR MET for the ITB (MET #12, hip) to lengthen the ITB and increase the extensibility of it attachment at the lateral knee. Next perform, CRAC MET for the hamstrings (MET #10, hip). Because the VMO attaches to the adductor magnus, perform MET #7 (hip) to recruit the adductors. Finally, perform Level II, second series, STM strokes to dissolve adhesions between the ITB and the lateral patella, distal femur, and tibia. To strengthen the VMO, instruct the client in supine straight-leg raises with external rotation of the leg as home exercises.

CHONDROMALACIA PATELLA (PATELLOFEMORAL ARTHRITIS)

▨ **Cause:** Chondromalacia patella is usually the result of a fall onto the flexed knee, creating inflammation that releases enzymes causing a softening of the hyaline cartilage of the patella, with loosening of the fiber matrix (fibrillation) and consequent calcium deposits. The inflammation leads to fibrosis in the patellar retinaculum (quadriceps expansion), which adds a compressive load to the patellofemoral joint. This condition often leads to patellofemoral arthritis. A contributing factor is sustained tightness in the hamstrings and gastrocnemius, which pulls the knee toward flexion, adding a compressive load to the joint.

▨ **Symptoms:** Clients experience a deep-seated ache under the patella, especially going up and down stairs or after sitting for long periods.

▨ **Sign:** Pain reproduced by compressing the patella against the femur, called the *patellar grinding test*.

▨ **Treatment:** To release the sustained tension on the patella, the hamstrings and gastrocnemius need to be released first. Perform MET #5 (hip) to reduce the hypertonicity, and CRAC MET #10 (hip) for hamstrings and CRAC MET #3 for the gastrocnemius. Perform PIR MET #5 to release the attachment points of the hamstrings at the posterior knee. Next, perform Level I, first to fifth series, and Level II, first to fourth series, STM strokes to release the soft tissue adhesions to the patella and posterior knee. Finally, perform conservative mobilization of the patella (Level II, fifth series, first stroke).

SAPHENOUS NERVE ENTRAPMENT

▧ **Causes:** Excessive knee extensions and contracted adductors.

▧ **Symptoms:** Clients experience medial and anterior knee pain.

▧ **Sign:** Medial knee pain with digital compression in adductor canal area; pressure over the adductor canal can radiate pain to the medial knee and down to the ankle.

▧ **Treatment:** Perform Level I, first series, STM strokes transverse to the nerve at the medial thigh and knee.

Knee Assessment

HISTORY QUESTIONS FOR THE CLIENT WHO HAS KNEE PAIN

▧ Have you had an injury recently?
  ☐ If there has been an injury, have the client describe the injury. Did the client feel a "pop" or feel a tear? Did swelling occur? If so, how long did the swelling take to develop?

▧ Is it painful to walk?
  ☐ The degree of disability is simply determined by the ability to walk. How far can the client walk? Can the client walk up and down hills or climb up and down stairs?

▧ Describe the pain or disability, and point to the pain or area of stiffness.
  ☐ The first task for the therapist is to differentiate acute from chronic problems. In acute problems, your intention is to reduce muscle spasms, increase joint ROM, and stimulate normal muscle firing in cases in which the muscle might be inhibited. For the client who has chronic knee pain or stiffness, your goal is to restore proper alignment and muscle function to reduce cumulative stresses to the knees. Carefully observe the alignment of the pelvis, hip, knees, ankles, and feet; and assess the length of the ITB, hamstrings, adductors, and gastrocnemius and the strength of the VMO, TFL, and abductors.

OBSERVATION AND INSPECTION

GAIT

▧ Observe as the client walks around the treatment room. Indications that there might be a knee problem are a limp and an inability to straighten the knee at toe-off phase. Are the knees in a genu valgus or varus alignment in walking? Note if the ankles are pronated or supinated and whether the feet are inverted or everted.

ALIGNMENT (FOR CHRONIC CONDITIONS ONLY)

▧ **Position:** Client is standing, facing the therapist, with the knees and ankles as close together as possible.

▧ **Action:** First observe the alignment of the knees, including the distance between the knees, and the facing of the patellae (Fig. 9-11). Place your thumb and index finger on either side of the patella to help determine the direction in which it faces. Next, ask the client to tighten the quadriceps to lift the knee cap, and observe the medial part of the distal thigh to see whether the VMO contracts and creates a bulge just above and medial to the superior pole of the patella when it contracts.

▧ **Observation:** If the knees touch and the ankles do not, the client has genu valgum (knock-knees). If the ankles touch and there is more than two finger widths between the knees at the joint line, the client has genu varum (bow legs). The facing of the patella is primarily dictated by the rotation in the femur. With the ankles and knees as close together as possible, the patella should face forward. With femoral anteversion, the femur is rotated internally, and the patella faces inward ("squinting patella"). The VMO is often atrophied after a knee injury or chronic knee dysfunction, caused by an arthrokinetic reflex from irritation in the joint. Atrophy also occurs because of the loss of full extension for a time after an injury. Because the VMO is a key muscle for terminal extension of the knee, it often atrophies after a knee injury.

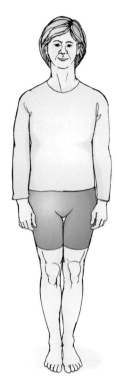

Figure 9-11. Observe the alignment of the knees by having the client bring the feet together. The patellae should point straightforward.

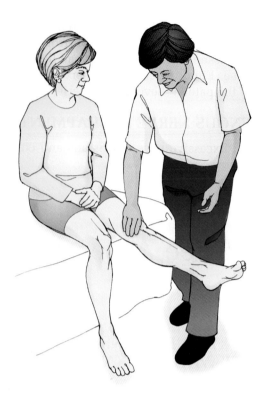

Figure 9-12. Active extension. First, observe the movement of the patella. Next, place one hand on the patella, and have the client repeat knee extension. Feel for noise (crepitus) and whether the movement of the patella is smooth.

OBSERVATION FOR SWELLING

▨ **Position:** Client is sitting, with the knees over the edge of the table.

▨ **Action:** Observe for swelling.

▨ **Observation:** Check for the normal concavity at the anteromedial joint line that is obliterated with swelling.

ACTIVE MOVEMENTS

EXTENSION

▨ **Position:** Client is sitting, with the knees over the edge of the table.

▨ **Action:** Have the client extend the knee from the 90° flexed position (Fig. 9-12). Repeat extension as you place your hand on the patella.

▨ **Observation:** Observe and feel how the patella moves. Normally, the patella moves straight upward until the end of extension, when it is pulled slightly laterally. Lateral deviation early in knee extension indicates a patellar tracking dysfunction. Crepitus or pain in the anterior knee indicates patellofemoral joint degeneration. If there is a jump or jog in the patella as the client moves from flexion to extension,

it indicates a potential mediopatellar plica. Loss of full extension often indicates a meniscal injury.

SQUAT TEST (FOR CHRONIC CONDITIONS ONLY)

▨ **Position:** Client is standing, with one hand on the table for support.

▨ **Action:** Have the client perform a squat to the comfortable limit and then come to standing again. Ask the client to keep his or her feet parallel and shoulder width apart (Fig. 9-13).

▨ **Observation:** Observe the ROM, and ask whether there is any pain. This procedure is a quick screening test for chronic knee pain and stiffness. There is often pain behind the patella and crepitus with patellofemoral joint dysfunction and a loss of motion and pain with tibiofemoral joint problems.

FLEXION

▨ **Position:** Client is supine, with a pillow under the knee if the condition is acute.

▨ **Action:** Have the client lift his or her thigh toward the chest, pulling the heel toward the buttock as far as possible (Fig. 9-14).

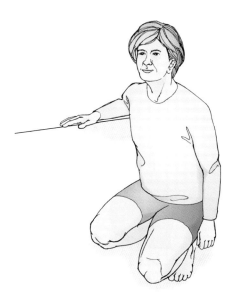

Figure 9-13. Squat test. This is for chronic conditions only.

▨ **Observation:** The normal ROM is approximately 140°. There is a loss of flexion in acute and chronic knee problems. In the acute knee, the loss of motion is caused by swelling; in the chronic knee, it is caused by fibrosis of the joint capsule or loss of joint space resulting from cartilage degeneration.

PASSIVE MOVEMENTS

FLEXION

▨ **Position:** Client is supine, with a pillow under the knee if the injury is acute.

▨ **Action:** First, bring the knee into flexion, and place the foot on the table. Next, place one hand on the knee, and hold the distal leg with the other hand. Slowly bring the hip to 90° of flexion, with the hip in neutral and not internally or externally rotated. Slowly press the knee into the comfortable limit of flexion. If there is no pain, you may press further to assess the end feel (Fig. 9-15).

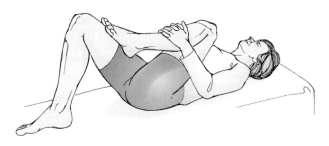

Figure 9-14. Active flexion. This test is for acute conditions to determine the knee ROM.

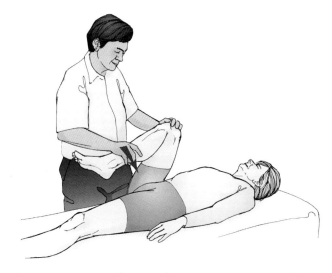

Figure 9-15. Passive flexion. The intention is to assess the ROM and the end feel, the quality of resistance at the end of the passive ROM.

▨ **Observation:** The heel should touch the buttock with overpressure. Flexion is the first motion that is lost in capsular fibrosis (leathery end feel) and in degenerative joint problems (hard end feel). Passive flexion is painful and limited with acute injuries to the knee. Swelling will be extensive with injuries to the menisci or cruciates and passive flexion will have an empty end feel, that is, the patient will feel pain before the therapist feels tissue tension. Tight quadriceps have a tissue stretch end feel.

EXTENSION

▨ **Position:** Client is supine.

▨ **Action:** Perform passive flexion (see Fig. 9-15), and then move your superior hand and place it behind the knee. Slowly lower the knee into extension. If you can achieve full painless extension, flex the knee approximately 10°, and let the knee fall into the last 10° of extension (Fig. 9-16).

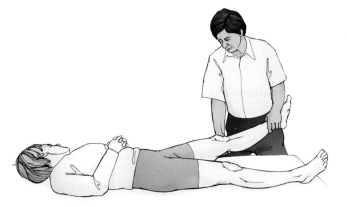

Figure 9-16. Passive extension. Loss of extension with pain and a springy-block end feel often indicate a meniscus injury.

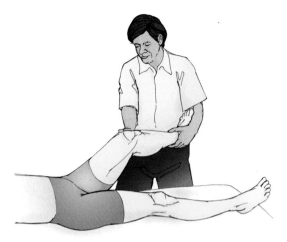

Figure 9-17. McMurray's test to assess the medial meniscus.

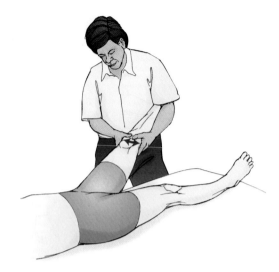

Figure 9-18. Valgus and varus stress tests to assess the MCL and LCL.

■ **Observation:** Normally, the knee has a solid, bony end feel if it drops into full passive extension. Loss of motion in passive extension is a key finding in meniscus injuries, although any acute injury to the knee causes a loss of full extension. With an injury to the meniscus, the end feel is described as a "springy block" during the end stage of passive extension. That means that the knee will reflexively "bounce" into slight flexion and not allow full extension. Hyperextension could indicate an ACL or PCL tear if extension is greater than that of the other knee. The position shown in Fig. 9-16 can also be used as an MET to increase the terminal extension. The therapist asks the client to resist as the therapist attempts to lift up at the heel to pull the knee into greater extension. Relax and repeat.

McMURRAY TEST

■ **Intention:** To assess the medial meniscus (Fig. 9-17).

■ **Position:** Client is supine.

■ **Action:** Place one hand over the knee, and hold the distal leg with the other hand. Slowly flex the knee as far as possible; then exert a lateral to medial pressure on the knee (valgus stress) as you externally rotate the foot and tibia and extend the knee.

■ **Observation:** This is a screening test for injuries to the medial meniscus. With a meniscus injury, the client might be unable to allow full knee extension because of pain, or experience a painful pop or click along the joint line.

VALGUS AND VARUS STRESS TEST

■ **Intention:** To assess the MCL and LCL ligaments (Fig. 9-18).

■ **Position:** Client is supine. Two positions are used to assess the MCL and LCL, one in flexion and the other in extension. First, bring the knee into approximately 20° to 30° of flexion, and place the client's leg in your axilla with both of your hands around the knee. The second position is to bring the client's leg to full extension. Do not allow internal or external rotation of the femur.

■ **Action:** To assess the MCL, attempt to pull the lower leg laterally by rotating your body and pressing the outside of the knee with the superior hand. The same action is performed with the knee in full extension, with the client's leg in your axilla or resting on the table. To assess the LCL, rotate your body the opposite direction, pressing on the inside of the knee. Compare both sides.

■ **Observation:** Pain at the medial knee typically indicates an MCL injury. Pain at the lateral knee indicates an LCL injury. An increased gapping compared with that of the uninjured knee indicates a tear of the ligament. There should be no gapping at all with the knee in full extension. Any lateral movement in knee extension in the valgus stress test indicates a much worse injury and involves the MCL and joint capsule.

POSTERIOR SAG SIGN

■ **Intention:** To assess the integrity of the PCL.

■ **Position:** Client is supine, with the hip and knee flexed and feet on the table.

■ **Action:** Observe from the side to see whether the tibia drops posteriorly relative to the femur. Compare both sides.

■ **Observation:** Normally, the tibia extends slightly anterior to the femoral condyles. If the tibia drops

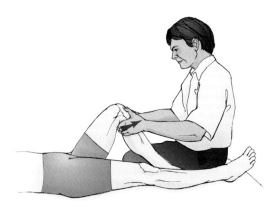

Figure 9-19. Anterior drawer test to assess the integrity of the ACL.

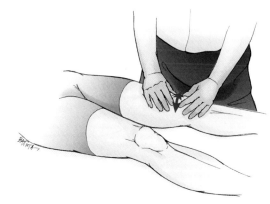

Figure 9-20. Patellar mobility test. Loss of patellar glide is a common clinical finding and is a sign of adhesions in the retinaculum.

posteriorly relative to the femur, it indicates an injury to the PCL. It is important to perform this test prior to the anterior drawer test described below, because if the tibia is sagging posteriorly, you might get a false-positive anterior drawer test.

ANTERIOR DRAWER TEST

▨ **Intention:** To assess the ACL (Fig. 9-19).

▨ **Position:** Client is supine, feet on the table, with the hip flexed 45°, the knee flexed 90°, and the tibia in neutral (i.e., with the feet pointed straight ahead). Therapist sits on the table, facing headward.

▨ **Action:** Stabilize the foot by sitting gently on the toes. Wrap both hands around the proximal tibia with your thumbs on either side of the infrapatellar tendon. Your fingers can sense whether the hamstrings are relaxed, which is necessary for this test to be accurate. Pull the tibia anteriorly. Repeat several times.

▨ **Observation:** Compare both sides. A normal ACL gives a firm, tight end feel rather than a soft, gradual end feel. An increased movement of the tibia relative to the femur compared with that of the uninjured knee is one indication that there might be a tear in the ACL.

PATELLA LATERAL PULL TEST

▨ **Intention:** To assess patellar tracking dysfunction.

▨ **Position:** Client is supine, with the knee extended.

▨ **Action:** Have the client contract the quadriceps.

▨ **Observation:** Normally, the patella moves straight headward (superiorly) in the initial phase of quadriceps contraction, or it moves superiorly and laterally in equal proportions. Patellar movement in a primarily lateral direction indicates patellofemoral dysfunction and typically a weak-

ness of the VMO. A simple yet effective exercise to retrain the VMO is to have the client perform straight-leg raises with the femur externally rotated. Have the client "set" the quads by tightening them first before lifting. Repeat until fatigue. It is also important to release the TFL and ITB, because they are typically tight and short.

PATELLAR MOBILITY TEST

▨ **Intention:** To assess adhesions in the patellar retinaculum.

▨ **Position:** Client is supine, with the knee extended.

▨ **Action:** Hold the patella with your thumb and index finger, and move the patella medially and laterally and then proximally and distally (Fig. 9-20).

▨ **Observation:** The patella should move one-half the width of the patella medially to laterally; check for a decrease or an increase in movement. Be cautious pushing laterally. With a history of subluxation or dislocation, there could be apprehension, as nearly all dislocations are lateral.

PATELLAR GRINDING TEST

▨ **Intention:** To assess calcium depositions in the patellofemoral joint.

▨ **Position:** Client is supine, with the knee extended.

▨ **Action:** Stabilize the leg in neutral so that the femur is not internally or externally rotated. Stabilize the patella with the thumb and index finger of your superior hand, and place the palm of the inferior hand over the patella. Press the patella into the femur, and move the patella superiorly and inferiorly several times to feel and listen for calcium deposits (Fig. 9-21).

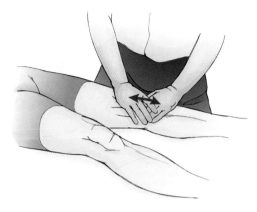

Figure 9-21. Patellar grinding test.

▨ **Observation:** Crepitation (grinding noise) or pain suggests patellofemoral joint degeneration, also called chondromalacia patella.

PALPATION

Most of the soft tissue palpation is done while performing the strokes. As you perform each stroke, feel for temperature, texture, tenderness, and tone. Before you begin the STM, feel for heat in the knee by placing your hands on the same areas on both knees to compare the temperature. Heat is an indication of inflammation and requires much less pressure in your strokes.

Techniques

GUIDELINES TO APPLYING TECHNIQUES

A thorough discussion of treatment guidelines can be found on p. 86 in Chapter 2. In the method of treatment described in this text we make two underlying assumptions. First, we assume that pain or dysfunction in one localized area affects the entire region, so we assess and treat an entire region rather than localized pain. An osteoarthritic knee, for example, is not an isolated condition but typically affects the hip joint and low back as well as the muscles of the thigh and lumbosacral region. The second assumption is that pain and dysfunction that localize in one tissue affect many other tissues in the area. ITB friction syndrome, for example, typically involves not only the lower fascial expansion of the ITB, but also the LCL, lateral patellar retinaculum, and lateral joint capsule. It also has an inhibiting effect on the muscles of the medial knee and the alignment and motion of the patellofemoral joint. The treatments that are described in this text address all the structures of the region through three techniques: muscle energy technique (MET), soft tissue mobilization (STM), and joint mobilization. These techniques can be applied to every type of knee pain, but the "dose" of the technique varies greatly, from slow movements and light pressures for acute conditions to stronger pressures and deeper amplitude mobilizations for chronic problems. Each aspect of the treatment is also an assessment to determine pain, tenderness, hypertonicity, weakness, and hypomobility or hypermobility. We use the philosophy of treating what we find when we find it. Remember that the goal of treatment is to heal the body, mind, and emotions. Keep your hands soft, keep your touch nurturing, and work only within the comfortable limits of your client so that he or she can completely relax into the treatment.

THE INTENTIONS OF TREATMENT FOR ACUTE CONDITIONS ARE AS FOLLOWS

▨ To stimulate the movement of fluids to reduce edema, increase oxygenation and nutrition, and eliminate waste products.

▨ To maintain as much pain-free joint motion as possible to prevent adhesions and maintain the health of the cartilage, which is dependent on movement for its nutrition.

▨ To provide mechanical stimulation to help align healing fibers and stimulate cellular synthesis.

▨ To provide neurological input to minimize muscular inhibition and help to maintain proprioceptive function.

 *CAUTION: Stretching is **contraindicated** in acute conditions*

THE INTENTIONS OF TREATMENT FOR CHRONIC CONDITIONS ARE AS FOLLOWS

▨ To dissolve adhesions, and restore flexibility, length, and alignment to the myofascia.

▨ To dissolve fibrosis in the ligaments and capsular tissues surrounding the joints.

▨ To rehydrate the cartilage and restore mobility and ROM to the joints.

▨ To eliminate hypertonicity in short and tight muscles, strengthen weakened muscles, and reestablish the normal firing pattern in dysfunctioning muscles.

▨ To restore neurological function by increasing sensory awareness and proprioception.

Clinical examples are described below under "Soft Tissue Mobilization."

MUSCLE ENERGY TECHNIQUE

THERAPEUTIC GOALS OF MUSCLE ENERGY TECHNIQUE (MET)

A thorough discussion of the clinical application of MET can be found on p. 76 in Chapter 2. The MET techniques that are described below are organized into one section for teaching purposes. In the clinical setting, the METs and STM techniques are interspersed throughout the session. METs are used for assessment and treatment. A healthy muscle or group of muscles is strong and pain free when isometrically challenged. MET will be painful if there is ischemia or inflammation in the muscles or their associated joints. The muscle will be weak and painless if the muscle is inhibited or the nerve is compromised. During treatment, MET is used as needed. For example, when you find a tight and tender biceps femoris, use CR MET to reduce the hypertonicity and tenderness. If the biceps femoris is painful while contracting, perform an RI MET, contracting the RF, inducing a neurological relaxation in the biceps. If the knee extensors are weak and inhibited, first release the tight knee flexors, then use CR MET to recruit and strengthen the knee extensors.

MET is very effective for an acute, painful knee, but the pressure that is applied must be very light so as not to induce pain. Gentle, pain-free contraction and relaxation of the knee flexors and extensors provide a pumping action to reduce swelling, promote the flow of oxygen and nutrition, eliminate waste products, and improve pain-free ROM.

THE BASIC THERAPEUTIC INTENTIONS OF MET FOR ACUTE CONDITIONS ARE AS FOLLOWS

▨ Provide a gentle pumping action to reduce pain and swelling, promote oxygenation of the tissue, and remove waste products.

▨ Reduce muscle spasms.

▨ Provide neurological input to mimimize muscular inhibition.

▨ Help to maintain as much pain-free joint motion as possible.

THE BASIC THERAPEUTIC INTENTIONS OF MET FOR CHRONIC CONDITONS ARE AS FOLLOWS

▨ Decrease excessive muscle tension.

▨ Strengthen muscles.

▨ Lengthen connective tissue.

▨ Increase joint movement and increase lubrication to the joints.

▨ Restore neurological function.

The hamstrings, RF, ITB, gastrocnemius, and adductors are typically short and tight, and the quadriceps (except RF) and abductors are typically weak. Refer to Chapter 8 for METs for the adductors, TFL, ITB, an alternative MET for RF, and a CRAC MET to lengthen the hamstrings in chronic conditions.

The MET section below shows techniques that are used for most clients. In acute conditions, use MET #1 to reduce swelling and pain in the joint. METs #6 and #7 are for chronic conditions only, because they involve increasing the length of the myofascia. Remember that stretching is **contraindicated** in acute conditions.

MET should not be painful. Mild discomfort as the client resists the pressure is normal if the area is irritated or inflamed. Refer to Chapter 8 for METs for the hip, which directly influences the knee.

MUSCLE ENERGY TECHNIQUES FOR ACUTE PAIN

1. *Contract-Relax Muscle Energy Technique for Acute Knee Injury*

▨ **Intention:** The primary intentions are to reduce swelling, decrease pain, and increase the ROM.

▨ **Position:** Client is supine. Place one hand under the knee and the other hand at the ankle.

▨ **Action:** Gently flex the knee to its comfortable limit. If it is too painful to lift the foot off the table, place a pillow under the knee. Have the client resist as you use light pressure to attempt to flex the knee. Have the client relax, then have the client resist as you gently attempt to extend the knee. Alternate performing resisted flexion and extension for several cycles. After several cycles, slowly pump the

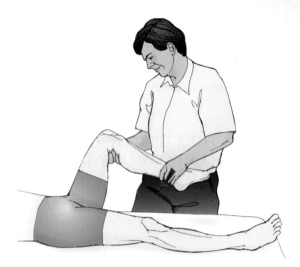

Figure 9-22. CR MET for acute knee injury.

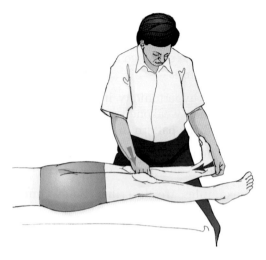

Figure 9-23. Length assessment of the gastrocnemius.

knee in small arcs of flexion and extension to pump the excess fluid out of the knee. Slowly move the client's knee into greater flexion until you encounter the next resistance barrier. Remember that it should not be painful. Repeat this series several more times. (Fig. 9-22).

LENGTH ASSESSMENT AND MUSCLE ENERGY TECHNIQUES FOR HYPERTONICITY

2. *Length Assessment of the Gastrocnemius*

▦ **Intention:** The gastrocnemius is typically short and tight. A tight gastrocnemius prevents normal dorsiflexion of the ankle and compromises the Achilles tendon and plantar fascia.

▦ **Position:** Client is supine, with the knee extended. Place one hand on the client's knee to keep it extended and the other hand on the ball of the foot.

▦ **Action:** Pull the ball of the foot toward client's head (Fig. 9-23).

▦ **Observation:** The normal length of these muscles should allow the foot to reach 90° (i.e., perpendicular to the leg).

3. *Contract-Relax-Antagonist-Contract Muscle Energy Technique for the Gastrocnemius*

▦ **Intention:** Because this muscle is usually short and tight, we typically want to lengthen it. This MET is also important in chronic ankle conditions to increase dorsiflexion of the ankle.

▦ **Position:** Client is supine, with the knee extended. Place one hand on the client's knee with the other hand holding the heel and the forearm resting on the ball of the foot.

▦ **Action:** Have the client pull the foot into dorsiflexion, relax in this position, and then resist as you attempt to pull the foot further into dorsiflexion. Hold for 5 seconds. Have the client relax and then move the foot headward. Repeat the CRAC cycle several times. Repeat on the other side (see Fig. 9-23).

4. *Assessment of Tibial Rotation and MET to Increase Tibial Rotation*

▦ **Intention:** The tibia normally externally rotates in the final stage of knee extension and internally rotates with knee flexion. This assessment and MET ensure normal tibial rotation.

▦ **Position:** Client is supine, with the hip and knee in 90° of flexion. Place one hand on the client's knee to stabilize the femur, the other hand holding the client's foot. Dorsiflex the ankle to lock the foot to the ankle.

▦ **Action:** Slowly move the foot into the limits of internal and external rotation (Fig. 9-24). In 90° of knee flexion permits about 15° of internal rotation and 30° of external rotation. Compare both sides.

▦ **Observation:** If there is limited external rotation, have the client resist as you attempt to turn the foot (and tibia) into greater external rotation for about 5 seconds. Relax, and turn the tibia to a new degree of external rotation. Repeat three to five times.
  □ **Variations:** To help isolate the popliteus, perform MET #7. The popliteus is an important internal rotator of the knee, and a short and tight popliteus will prevent full external rotation of the tibia.

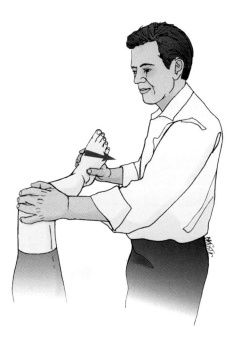

Figure 9-24. Assessment and MET for tibial rotation.

5. Postisometric Relaxation Muscle Energy Technique for the Hamstrings Lower Attachments

Intention: This position is different from the MET shown in Chapter 8, "The Hip," in that it emphasizes contraction of the hamstrings at their attachments to the posterior knee.

Position: Client is supine

Action: Bring the hip to 90° of flexion, and slowly extend the knee to the tension barrier. Have the client resist as you attempt to push the knee into greater extension (i.e., by pushing at the foot for approximately 5 seconds). Relax, wait a few seconds, and while the client is relaxed, extend the knee to a new resistance barrier. Repeat the CR–lengthen cycle several times (Fig. 9-25).

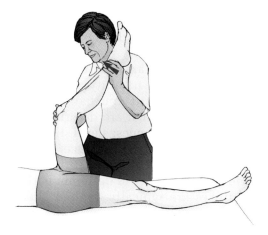

Figure 9-25. PIR MET for the hamstrings lower attachments.

Observation: Normally, the range of knee extension is approximately 70° with the hip flexed to 90°.

6. Length Assessment (Ely's Test) and Postisometric Relaxation Muscle Energy Technique for the Rectus Femoris

Intention: The intention is to assess the length of the RF and to increase its length if the therapist cannot press the client's heel against the buttock with overpressure.

Position: Client is prone. Place one hand on the sacrum to stabilize it and the other hand on the ankle.

Action: Do not allow medial or lateral rotation or abduction or adduction of the hip. If the client is hyperlordotic or has low-back discomfort, place a pillow under the abdomen to flex the lumbar spine. Flex the client's knee by pressing the foot toward the buttock until the resistance barrier is felt. If heel does not touch the buttock, have the client resist as you attempt to press the heel further toward the buttock. Have the client relax, and as client relaxes, flex the knee until a new resistance barrier is encountered. Have the client relax. Repeat this cycle several times (Fig. 9-26).

7. Contract-Relax and Postisometric Relaxation for the Popliteus

Intention: The intention is to recruit an inhibited or atrophied popliteus or lengthen a tight, short muscle and help to restore normal external rotation of the tibia. Normal knee extension requires external rotation of the tibia during the last 10° to 15°. The popliteus is the primary internal rotator of the tibia. A short or tight popliteus or a short posteromedial capsule can cause decreased external rotation. Resisted medial rotation helps to release popliteus hypertonicity and increase tibial external rotation. CR

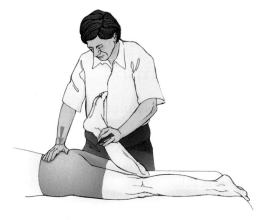

Figure 9-26. Length assessment (Ely's test) and PIR MET for the rectus femoris.

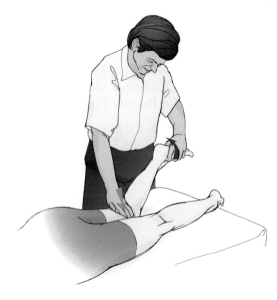

Figure 9-27. PIR MET for the popliteus and to increase external rotation of the tibia.

MET will help to strengthen a weak or atrophied muscle.

▓ **Position:** Client is prone, with the knee flexed approximately 20°. Place one hand on the back of the knee to stabilize it and the other hand on the medial arch of the foot.

▓ **Action:** To release the popliteus, medially rotate the tibia by first dorsiflexing the ankle to lock the foot to the ankle and then by cocking the foot medially (toward the other leg). Have the client resist as you attempt to laterally rotate the tibia by pulling the foot laterally. Instruct the client to relax, and then move the client's tibia more laterally. Have the client relax. Repeat the cycle several times (Fig. 9-27). Another effective method to release the popliteus is with the client prone. With the knee at 90° of flexion, externally rotate the tibia, and have the client resist as you pull on the ankle, attempting to extend the knee. Pain in the posterior knee is a sign of popliteus involvement.[4]

MUSCLE ENERGY TECHNIQUE FOR CHRONIC CAPSULAR FIBROSIS AND LOSS OF KNEE MOTION

8. *Muscle Energy Technique to Increase Knee Flexion*

▓ **Intention:** Chronic loss of flexion is a sign of capsular fibrosis or cartilage degeneration. The end feel of fibrosis is thick and leathery. Degeneration has a hard end feel.

▓ **Position:** Client is supine. Place one hand on the knee and the other hand on the distal leg.

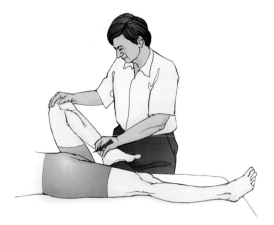

Figure 9-28. MET to increase knee flexion.

▓ **Action:** Lift the client's leg to the comfortable limit of knee flexion. Have the client resist as you attempt to flex it further. Instruct the client to relax, and as the client relaxes, move the knee into greater flexion. Repeat several times (Fig. 9-28).

▓ **Observation:** When performing this MET, ensure that the client's hip is in neutral (i.e., no internal or external rotation, abduction, or adduction).

SOFT TISSUE MOBILIZATION

BACKGROUND

A thorough discussion of the clinical application of STM can be found on p. 68. In the Hendrickson Method of manual therapy described in this text, the STM movements are called *wave mobilization* and are a combination of joint mobilization and STM performed in rhythmic oscillations with a frequency of 50 to 70 cycles per minute, except when performing brisk transverse friction massage strokes, which can be two to four cycles per second. These mobilizations are presented in a specific sequence, which has been found to achieve the most efficient and effective results. This allows the therapist to "scan" the body to determine areas of tenderness, hypertonicity, and decreased mobility. It is important to "follow the recipe" until you have mastered this work. The techniques that are described below are divided into two sequences: Level 1 and Level II. Level I strokes are designed for every client, from acute injury to chronic degeneration, to enhance health and bring the body to optimum performance. Level II strokes are typically applied after Level I strokes and are designed for chronic conditions. Guidelines for treating acute and chronic conditions are listed below.

GUIDELINES FOR THE THERAPIST

Acute

The primary intention of treatment is to decrease pain and swelling as quickly as possible, maintain as much pain-free joint motion as possible, and induce relaxation. In this method of treatment, the soft tissue is compressed and decompressed in rhythmic cycles. This provides a pumping action that helps to promote fluid exchange, reducing swelling. The strokes that are applied to the client who is in acute pain need to be performed with a very gentle touch, a very slow rhythm, and small amplitude. There is no uniform "dose" or depth of treatment. The depth of treatment is based on the client's level of pain. If the soft tissue does not begin to relax, use more METs to help reduce discomfort, swelling, and excessive muscle tension. As was mentioned previously, intersperse your STM work with MET. Remember that **stretching is contraindicated** in acute conditions.

Clinical Example: Acute

Subjective: SM is a 58-year-old lawyer who presented to my office complaining of acute right knee pain. He reported that the pain had begun about a week earlier after he went on a long hike on a very slippery trail. The knee was swollen after the hike and hurt to bear weight. He described the pain as an ache, worse at night and when getting up from a chair.

Objective: Examination revealed a slight limp. The knee was swollen and held in slight flexion. Active knee flexion and extension were limited and elicited pain at the anterior joint line. Passive motion was limited and painful in flexion and extension with an empty end feel in flexion and springy-block end feel in extension. Palpation revealed boggy and warm, soft tissue about the knee and spastic and tender hamstrings, ITB, and gastrocnemius muscles. McMurray's test was positive, indicating involvement of the medial meniscus. The anterior drawer test allowed slightly greater motion in the right knee than in the left, indicating involvement with the ACL.

Assessment: Painful and swollen knee, with loss of ROM in both flexion and extension and spastic and tender muscles.

Treatment (Action): Treatment began with the client supine. CR MET and RI MET #1 were performed to contract the flexors and extensors of the knee to reduce the swelling and pain and prevent muscular inhibition. MET for the hamstrings (MET #5, hip), TFL (MET #11, hip) and gastrocnemius (MET #3) were performed to reduce the hypertonicity and allow for greater extension of the knee. After the METs, the knee was gently mobilized in a comfortable range of flexion and extension. I performed the Level I STM series, with gentle pressure and a slow rhythm. I finally performed a modified version of the figure-eight mobilization for the knee (Level II, fifth series, second stroke). I gently pumped the knee in the limits of pain-free flexion with my forearm behind the knee. The patient felt much better in walking around the exam room and was able to staighten his knee a little bit more.

Plan: I recommended weekly visits for one month. SM returned to my office in a week and stated that he was feeling less pain. Exam findings on the second visit were similar to those of the first visit. Passive flexion and extension were slightly increased, and the tissue was slightly less swollen. On palpation, the medial joint line was very tender. I repeated the treatment described above. The gastrocnemius and medial hamstrings were very tight and tender, so I performed CR MET for those muscles. The third and fourth visits showed better improvement. The patient was continuing to feel better and was not awakened at night with pain. I was able to perform pain-free PIR METs for the hamstrings, popliteus, and gastrocnemius, which allowed the knee to achieve greater extension. The figure-eight mobilization was performed with greater ROM. On the fourth visit, I was finally able to achieve terminal extension. The patient was able to walk without a limp and achieved full ROM. I recommended that he make a follow-up visit in two weeks to ensure that full, pain-free ROM of the knee had been maintained.

Chronic

The typical exam findings in clients with chronic knee problems are decreased flexion; tight RF, hamstrings, adductors, TFL, and ITB; and weakness in the other quadriceps, especially the VMO and abductors, including the gluteus medius. The knee joint is typically hypomobile, with thick, fibrous ligaments and capsular tissues limiting flexion. The patella is typically fixed laterally, with thick, fibrous tissue binding it to the lateral patellar groove of the femur. Some patients demonstrate the opposite: instability in the joints; weak, deconditioned muscles; and atrophy in the ligaments and capsular tissues. The primary goals of treatment depend on the patient. For patients who are hypomobile, the treatment goals are to reduce the hypertonicity of the muscles; promote mobility and extensibility in the connective tissue by dissolving the adhesions in the muscles, tendons, ligaments, and capsular tissues surrounding the joints; rehydrate the cartilage of the joint; reestablish normal joint play and ROM; and restore normal neurological function by stimulating the proprioceptors and reestablishing the normal firing patterns in the muscles. Patients who are unstable need exercise rehabilitation. Our treatments can support their stability by reducing tension in the tight muscles with STM and MET and strengthening weak muscles, reestablishing normal firing patterns, and rehabilitating the proprioceptors with MET. With chronic conditions, we use stronger pressure on the soft tissue and more vigorous mobilizations on the joints. In the Level II sequence, we add deeper soft tissue work and work on attachment points, using transverse friction strokes if we find fibrosis (thickening). As was mentioned in the "Acute" section above, intersperse your soft tissue work with METs.

Clinical Example: Chronic

Subjective: HG is a 22-year-old, 5'8", 150-pound female college student who presented to my office with a chronic painful and slightly swollen left knee. She described the pain as an ache that worsened when she climbed stairs and improved with rest. Her history includes several patellar dislocations since she was 13 years old. She became a competitive diver at an early age, but the dislocations became so frequent that she had to stop. Eight months previously, she had had surgery that involved a tibial tubercle transfer and a lateral release. She had received physical therapy and massage and was working with an athletic trainer.

Objective: Examination revealed an inward facing patella, the left greater than the right, and a pronated ankle on the left. Active ROM and passive flexion were painful and limited to 75% of normal. She showed inadequate recruitment of the VMO on the lateral pull test of the patella, indicating a weakness of the VMO. Decreased passive glide of the patella was also found in the lateral-to-medial direction. Palpation revealed tight hamstrings, especially the biceps femoris, and ITB at the distal attachment site. Palpation also revealed thick, fibrotic tissue at the lateral patellar retinaculum, medial coronary ligament, medial joint capsule, and the undersurface of the patella.

Assessment: An assessment was made of muscular imbalances, fibrosis of the lateral patellar retinaculum, joint capsule and ligaments, and fixation of the patellofemoral joint.

Treatment: Recommendations were made for four treatments on a weekly basis. The goals of treatment were to reduce the pain, decrease the muscle hypertonicity, and improve the joint play and ROM in the joint to restore pain-free function. Treatment began with the client supine. CR MET and RI MET (MET #1) were performed to reduce the swelling and improve flexion. MET for the hamstrings (MET #5), TFL, and ITB (METs #11 and #12, hip) were performed to reduce the lateral pull on the knee and patella and increase the extensibility of the lateral and posterior soft tissue. CR MET for the quadriceps (MET #3, hip) was performed to release the hypertonicity and to increase the extensibility of the quadriceps attachments to the patella. Next, a PIR MET for the RF was performed (MET #6) to lengthen the rectus. Level I STM strokes were performed, especially the Level I, fourth series, to reduce the hypertonicity and dissolve adhesions in the soft tissue of the distal thigh and knee. I then performed Level II series of STM strokes and joint mobilization, concentrating on the lateral retinaculum, the medial coronary ligament, the medial joint capsule, the undersurface of the patella, and mobilization of the patella. I reviewed an isotonic exercise for the VMO with the client.

Plan: I recommended a series of weekly visits for one month. HG returned to the office one week after our initial visit reporting that the knee had been sore to the touch after the treatment but otherwise felt slightly better. Examination findings indicated a slight increase in knee flexion and slightly better glide to the patella. The soft tissue felt less thick at the lateral poles of the patella. I applied the same treatment described above at the beginning of the session. In the second session, I concentrated on lengthening the ITB with PIR MET (MET #12, hip) and the hamstrings with

CRAC MET (MET #10, hip). I concentrated STM on the lateral patella retinaculum and coronary ligament.

HG received weekly treatments for two additional weeks. On her fourth visit, she reported that she continued to improve. Examination revealed less fibrosis and better tracking of the patella on the lateral pull test. Recommendations were made for two additional treatments. The same MET and STM were applied.

After the fifth treatment, she stated that she was feeling much better. Palpation revealed that the fibro-sis was substantially reduced and that the patella was tracking normally. HG returned for follow-up visits on two occasions, the latter approximately one year after her first visit, as she had moved out of the area and made an appointment during her visit. She stated that she had returned to diving with only slight, occasional pain. Examination revealed that the knee had normal ROM, the patella had normal glide, and the soft tissue had only the normal fibrosis associated with a prior surgery.

Table 9-3 lists some essentials of treatment.

LEVEL 1: KNEE

1. *Transverse Release of the Distal Thigh*

▨ **Anatomy:** Gracilis, sartorius, adductor magnus; saphenous nerve, quadriceps expansion of vastus medialis, intermedius, and lateralis; and suprapatellar tendon of the RF, prepatellar bursa, and suprapatellar pouch (Fig. 9-29).

▨ **Dysfunction:** The fascial expansions of the quadriceps can become fibrous because of previous inflammation as a result of a knee injury or because of chronic irritation caused by the cumulative stresses of weight-bearing dysfunctions, such as pronated ankles or genu valgum (knock-knees). The saphenous nerve can become entrapped in the area of the adductor canal in the distal third of the medial thigh. As was mentioned in Chapter 8, "The Hip," if you are working with a client who has retroverted hips, you need to reverse the direction of your strokes and roll the thigh inward from the externally rotated position.

Position

▨ **Therapist Position (TP):** standing, either 45° headward or facing the table

▨ **Client Position (CP):** supine; if the client has an acute knee injury, place a pillow under the knee

Table 9-3	Essentials of Treatment

- Rock the client's body while performing the strokes.
- Shift your weight while performing the strokes.
- Perform the strokes rhythmically.
- Perform the strokes about 50 to 70 cycles per minute.
- Keep your hands and whole body relaxed.

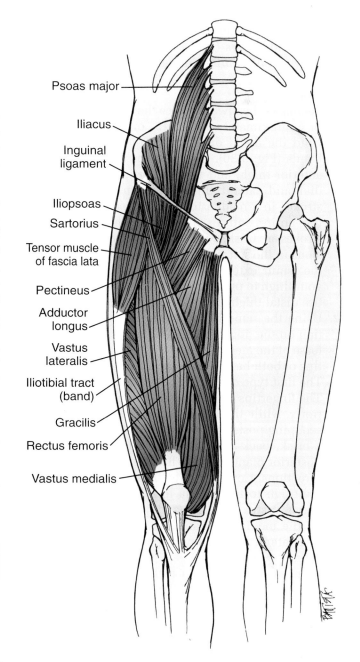

Psoas major
Iliacus
Inguinal ligament
Iliopsoas
Sartorius
Tensor muscle of fascia lata
Pectineus
Adductor longus
Vastus lateralis
Iliotibial tract (band)
Gracilis
Rectus femoris
Vastus medialis

Figure 9-29. Muscles and fascia of the anterior thigh and knee.

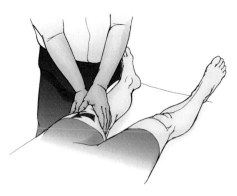

Figure 9-30. Transverse release of the distal thigh by unwinding the soft tissue around the bone in a medial to lateral direction.

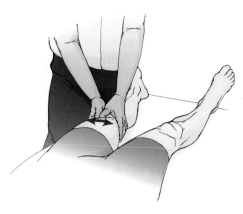

Figure 9-31. Double-thumb technique to release the suprapatellar tendon.

MET

Use METs for the quadriceps (MET #3, hip), RF (MET #6), and adductors (METs #9, hip) to reduce hypertonicity and discomfort in the soft tissue.

Strokes

1. Facing 45° headward, place the femur in neutral or in approximately 10° to 15° of external rotation. Hold the distal one-third of the thigh with both hands (Fig. 9-30). Your thumbs should be on the anterior thigh, and your fingertips are on the medial and lateral thigh. Perform short scooping strokes in a medial to lateral direction to unwind the entire soft tissue around the bone. These strokes are brisk, 1-inch strokes to release the adhesions in the soft tissue of the thigh. Do not to rotate the femur externally. You can brace the leg with your thigh to prevent it from rotating. Cover the entire distal thigh, and continue to the patella.
2. Using the same hand positions, now focus attention on the fingertips of both hands for specific release of the medial and lateral thigh. Use the fingertips of both hands to perform two types of strokes. The first type of stroke is a 1-inch scooping stroke. The fingertips on the medial thigh are lifting anteriorly, while the fingertips on the lateral thigh are scooping posteriorly. The second type of stroke is a brisk, back-and-forth stroke in the anterior-to-posterior plane with the hands moving in opposite directions. Cover the area from the distal third of the thigh to the patella to release the saphenous nerve, vastus medialis, and quadriceps expansion on the medial side and the ITB, vastus lateralis, and lateral quadriceps expansion on the lateral side.
3. Using a double-thumb technique, perform brisk back-and-forth strokes in the media-to-lateral plane, on the suprapatellar tendon of the RF and the vastus intermedius underneath (Fig. 9-31). Begin approximately 6 inches above the patella, and continue to the superior pole of the patella.

4. If the knee is swollen, wrap your hands around the distal thigh as illustrated in Fig. 9-30. Squeeze the thigh, and gently and slowly move your hands several inches headward to milk the suprapatellar pouch, an expansion of the anterior joint capsule. Repeat several times. Move your hands over the patella, and perform the same strokes to disperse fluids in the prepatellar bursa.

2. *Lifting Medial Soft Tissue Anteriorly*

▨ **Anatomy:** Vastus medialis and pes anserinus tendons, which are, from anterior to posterior, the sartorius, gracilis, and semitendinosus (Fig. 9-32).

▨ **Dysfunction:** This soft tissue tends to misalign posteriorly and needs to be lifted anteriorly. In most injuries and dysfunctions of the knee, there is an inability to extend the knee fully, thus keeping the soft tissue in a sustained posterior position relative to the joint. Adhesions can develop within the body of the muscles or between the soft tissue and the bone.

Position

▨ **TP:** Standing, facing perpendicular to the table

▨ **CP:** Supine, usually with the knee extended; if the injury is acute, place a pillow under the knee

MET

Use METs for the quadriceps (MET #3, hip) and adductors (METs #9, hip) to reduce hypertonicity and discomfort in the soft tissue.

Strokes

The first intention is to reset the soft tissue from posterior to anterior; the second is to dissolve any fibrosis that might have developed in response to injury or overuse. The area of the medial knee is divided into three lines from anterior to posterior. Begin your

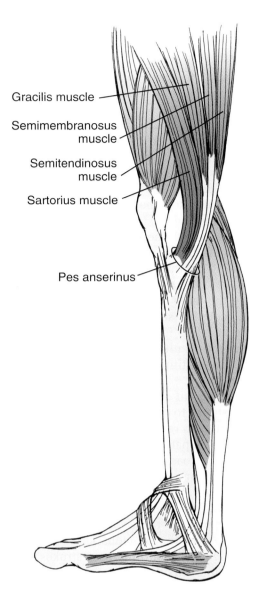

Gracilis muscle

Semimembranosus muscle

Semitendinosus muscle

Sartorius muscle

Pes anserinus

Figure 9-32. Muscles and fascia of the medial knee. The tendons of the sartorius, gracilis, and semitendinosus interweave at their insertion to form the pes anserinus ("goose's foot").

strokes on the first line at the distal thigh a few inches proximal to the patella, and proceed to the proximal tibia. The second line is approximately 1 inch posterior to the first line, and the third line is approximately 1 inch posterior to the second. Cover the entire medial knee.

1. Use the fingertips of both hands to perform broad, 1-inch, scooping strokes in a posterior to anterior direction on the first line for the vastus medialis and medial retinaculum (Fig. 9-33). Begin at the distal thigh, and continue to the proximal tibia. Stabilize the leg with your thumbs and the base of your hands to limit the amount of external rotation of the femur.

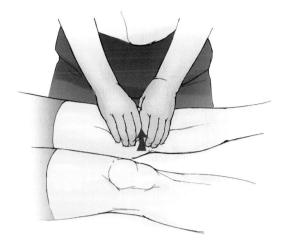

Figure 9-33. Lifting the soft tissue of the medial knee anteriorly.

2. Perform the same series of strokes (as described for stroke 1) on the second line of the thigh, 1 inch posterior to the first line, for the sartorius. Begin your strokes at the distal thigh, and continue to the proximal knee.
3. Perform the same strokes (as described for stroke 1) on the third line for the gracilis, semimembranosus, and semitendinosus.
4. An additional way to release this area is to place the flexed knee of your superior leg on the table and rest the client's leg on your thigh (Fig. 9-34). With your inferior hand holding the client's ankle, keep the leg in neutral, and lift the foot to extend the knee as you use the fingertips of your superior hand to lift the soft tissue anteriorly.

3. *Lifting Lateral Soft Tissue Anteriorly*

Anatomy: ITB, vastus lateralis and lateral patellar retinaculum, biceps femoris, (Fig. 9-35).

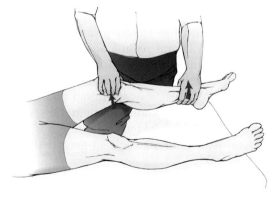

Figure 9-34. Using the fingertips of one hand to lift the soft tissue anteriorly; the other hand lifts the knee into extension with each stroke.

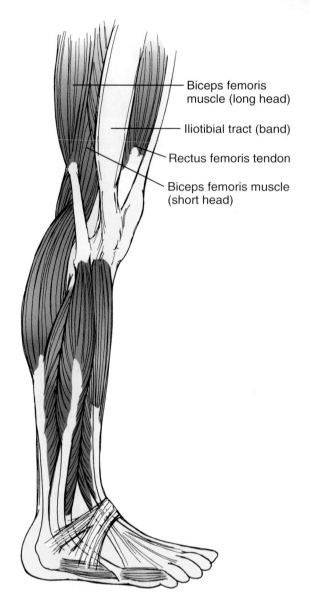

Figure 9-35. Muscles and fascia of the lateral knee.

▨ **Dysfunction:** As was mentioned in the discussion of the previous stroke, the soft tissue of the knee tends to misalign posteriorly. The ITB usually becomes taut, and the lateral retinaculum thickens, anchoring the lateral patella against the lateral femur, creating patellar tracking dysfunction. This condition can be as a response to a knee injury, because the VMO becomes inhibited and the vastus lateralis and ITB get short and tight. Or it can be in response to cumulative tension through weight distribution dysfunction, such as genu valgum and pronated ankles.

Position
▨ **TP:** Standing, facing the table

▨ **CP:** Supine; place a pillow under an acute knee

MET
Use METs for the quadriceps (MET #3, hip), TFL and ITB (METs #11 and #12, hip), and hamstrings (METs #10, hip, and #5, knee) to reduce hypertonicity and discomfort in the soft tissue.

Strokes
Divide the lateral knee into three lines from anterior to posterior. The first line is just lateral to the patella. Begin strokes on the first line at the distal thigh a few inches proximal to the patella, and proceed to the proximal fibula. Roll the thigh into neutral if it is in external rotation, and stabilize it in neutral with the base of your hands. These strokes move the soft tissue relative to the bone rather than externally or internally rotating the thigh or leg.

1. Facing the table and using both thumbs, perform short, scooping strokes from posterior to anterior on the first line for the vastus lateralis and lateral patellar retinaculum (Fig. 9-36). Begin at the distal thigh, and continue this line of strokes to the proximal leg.

2. Begin a second line of strokes approximately 1 inch posterior to the first line at the lateral condyle of the femur to release the ITB and the fascia from the ITB to the patella. Continue to the proximal leg. Begin with broad, scooping strokes approximately 1 inch long, and proceed to more brisk, transverse strokes as you work closer to the bone.

3. Perform a third line of strokes approximately 1 inch posterior to the second line for the biceps femoris. As in the previous strokes, begin at the distal thigh, and continue your strokes to the fibular head and proximal leg.

4. An additional way to release this area is for the therapist to place the flexed knee of your superior leg on the table and rest the client's leg on your thigh (Fig. 9-37). With your inferior hand holding the client's

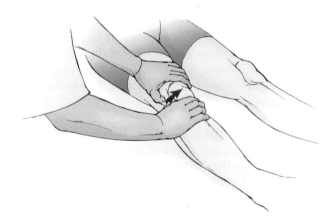

Figure 9-36. Double-thumb technique to lift the lateral soft tissue anteriorly.

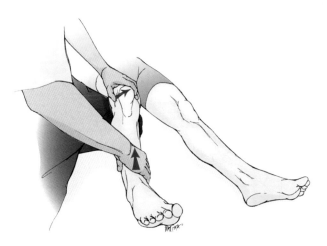

Figure 9-37. To mechanically assist the realigning of the soft tissue, lift the tissue with the thumb of one hand while the other hand lifts the knee into extension with each stroke.

ankle, lift the foot to extend the knee (be sure to keep the leg in neutral), as you use the thumb of your superior hand to lift the soft tissue anteriorly.

4. *Release of the Patellar Retinaculum*

▨ **Anatomy:** The patellar retinacula, which is an expansion of the quadriceps fascia and the thickenings of the superficial joint capsule, attaches at four major points to the superior and inferior margins of the patella. If 12 o'clock is headward, the approximate points of attachment are at 2, 4, 8, and 10 o'clock. The retinacula also attaches to the undersurface of the patella. The ITB interweaves with the lateral patellar retinaculum (Fig. 9-38).

▨ **Dysfunction:** The quadriceps expansion often develops fibrosis at its attachment to the patella, constricting the normal glide of the patella and increasing the pressure of the patellofemoral joint. Typically, the lateral retinaculum is thickest.

Position
▨ **TP:** Standing

▨ **CP:** Supine; place a pillow under the knee if it has been injured

MET
Use METs for the quadriceps (MET #3, hip), RF (MET #6) adductors (MET #9, hip), and TFL and ITB (METs #11 and #12, hip) to reduce hypertonicity and discomfort in the soft tissue.

Strokes
1. Release the superior portion of the medial patella by facing the table and stabilizing the patella with your inferior hand. Perform back-and-forth strokes

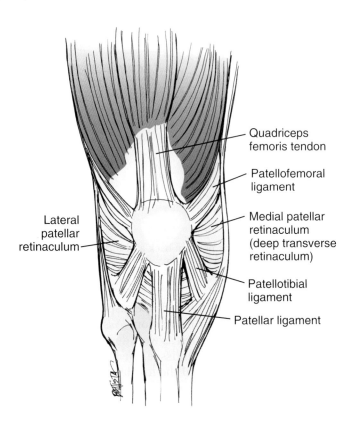

Figure 9-38. Anterior knee showing the patellar retinaculum. The superficial portion of the joint capsule interweaves with the retinaculum and has distinct thickenings, the patellofemoral and patellotibial ligaments.

- Quadriceps femoris tendon
- Patellofemoral ligament
- Medial patellar retinaculum (deep transverse retinaculum)
- Patellotibial ligament
- Patellar ligament
- Lateral patellar retinaculum

with the fingertips of your superior hand on the superior aspect of the medial side of the patella (Fig. 9-39). To release the inferior aspect of the medial patella, switch hands, stabilize with your superior hand, and use the fingertips of your inferior hand. To release the lateral patella, perform back-and-forth strokes with the thumb while stabilizing the medial patella with your fingertips.

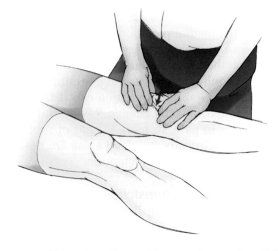

Figure 9-39. Fingertips release of the superior portion of the patellar retinaculum with back-and-forth transverse strokes.

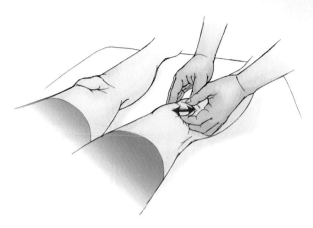

Figure 9-40. Fingertips perform back-and-forth strokes to the undersurface of the lateral patella.

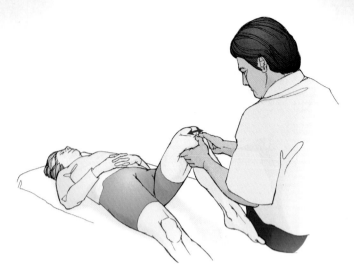

Figure 9-41. Transverse release of the infrapatellar tendon by use of the double-thumb technique.

2. Dissolve adhesions in the deeper aspect of the tissue by applying a shearing motion. Assume the same stance and hand position as were described for stroke 1. To release the medial tissue, push the patella with your thumb as you pull the medial tissue with your fingertips. For the lateral retinacula, reverse your hands, and pull the patella toward you with your fingertips as you scoop into the lateral retinacula with your thumb. Repeat this stroke many times in an oscillating motion. **This is for chronic conditions only.**
3. Release the undersurface of the lateral pole of the patella by facing headward and using the fingertips of one hand to stabilize the medial patella (Fig. 9-40). Move it slightly laterally, and use the fingertips of your other hand to perform brisk strokes in the inferior-to superior-plane, on the edge, and undersurface of the patella.
4. Release the undersurface of the medial superior pole by turning your body to face the table and by pushing the patella medially with your superior hand. Use the fingertips of your inferior hand to perform brisk, back-and-forth strokes in the inferior-to-superior plane, on the edge, and undersurface of the medial patella.
5. Perform transverse strokes in the medial-to-lateral plane on the infrapatellar tendon with fingertips or with a double-thumb or single-thumb technique (Fig. 9-41). Stabilize the knee cap if the leg is in extension, or put the knee in flexion if it has been injured, is in pain, or has a history of subluxation. The most clinically involved areas are the medial and lateral borders of the tendon.

5. *Release of the Hamstrings, Gastrocmenius, Popliteus, and Bursae at the Popliteal Fossa*

■ **Anatomy:** Biceps femoris, semimembranosus, semitendinosus, popliteus (Fig. 9-42), and semi-

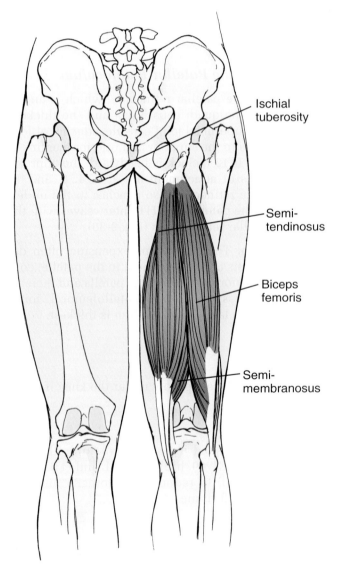

Figure 9-42. Posterior thigh and knee showing the hamstrings.

membranosus and medial gastrocnemius bursae (see Fig. 9-5).

■ **Dysfunction:** The flexors of the knee are typically short and tight, inhibiting the quadriceps. Attachment points usually thicken and become fibrotic with overuse or injury. Sustained flexion due to injury or degeneration shortens and thickens the hamstrings and gastrocnemius attachments. The semimembranosus and medial gastrocnemius bursae communicate with the articular cavity and are often swollen after a knee injury.

Position

■ **TP:** Standing, facing headward

■ **CP:** Prone, with a pillow under the ankle to keep the knee in slight flexion or with your flexed thigh under the client's flexed leg

MET

Use METs for the hamstrings (METs #10, hip, and #5, knee), popliteus (MET #7), and gastrocnemius (MET #3) to reduce hypertonicity and discomfort in the soft tissue.

Strokes

1. Face headward, and place your flexed knee on the table (Fig. 9-43). Flex the client's knee, and rest his or her shin on your thigh. Using a double-thumb technique, roll the biceps femoris laterally and the semimembranosus and semitendinosus medially. As you approach the attachment points, the tissue changes from muscle to tendon and naturally becomes more cordlike. The popliteus is often tender medial to the biceps at the posterolateral corner of the knee. The intention is to release any fibrosis on the body of the tendons. Keep your hands soft, and make your strokes more brisk and of shorter amplitude.

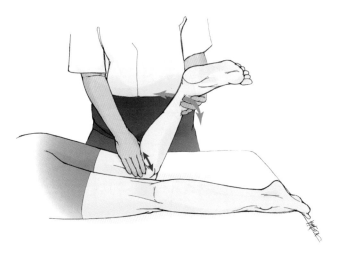

Figure 9-44. Technique to assist the release of distal hamstrings mechanically. Move the client's leg medially and laterally with one hand while the fingertips or thumb of the other hand strokes the tendons.

2. An alternative method is to stand facing the table. Flex the client's knee to 90° (Fig. 9-44). Place your fingertips on the medial tendons with one hand, and hold the client's distal leg or foot with the other hand. Next, move the leg toward and away from you, massaging the tendons under your working hand. You may use a shearing motion and move your fingertips in the opposite or in the same direction as the leg. Next, place your thumb on the lateral tendons, and perform the same strokes as were described for stroke 1.

 CAUTION: *Do not work the center of the popliteal fossa in this manner, because the neurovascular bundle runs through this region and could be bruised with deep work on it.*

3. Release the bursae and lymphatics of the popliteal fossa by placing a pillow under the client's ankle. Apply some lotion or oil on the back of the knee. Face 45° headward. Wrap your hands around the proximal leg just below the knee, using a parallel-thumb technique in the midline of the fossa. Perform a series of long, slow, continuous strokes in a headward direction (Fig. 9-45).

LEVEL II: KNEE

1. Release of the Coronary and Medial Collateral Ligaments and of the Pes Anserinus Bursa

■ **Anatomy:** Coronary ligaments, which are the deep, inferior portions of the joint capsule that attach to

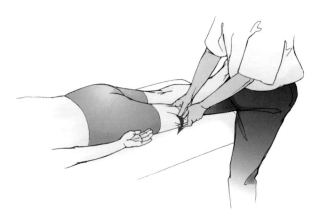

Figure 9-43. Double-thumb technique performing medial to lateral strokes on the biceps femoris.

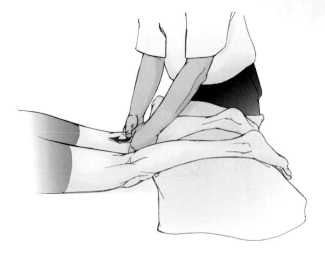

Figure 9-45. Massage of the bursae of the posterior knee with flat thumbs.

the menisci and tibia (Fig. 9-46), MCL (see Fig. 9-1), and pes anserinus bursa (see Fig. 9-3).

▪ **Dysfunction:** The coronary and MCL ligaments are often involved in knee injuries. Fibrosis of the coronary ligament gives local pain, typically at the medial joint line, and prevents the normal movement

of the menisci during knee flexion. The MCL is either thick and fibrotic or slack and weak in the chronic phase after an injury. Deep transverse massage is applied only to thickened ligaments. Rehabilitation for ligaments that are too loose is through exercise. The pes anserinus bursa swells after acute or overuse injuries, with sustained genu valgus posture, or with a pronated foot.

Position
▪ **TP:** Standing, facing work

▪ **CP:** Supine

MET
Use METs for the quadriceps (MET #3, hip), RF (MET #6), and adductors (METs #9, hip) to reduce hypertonicity and discomfort in the soft tissue.

Strokes
1. Release the medial aspects of the coronary ligament by bringing the client's knee into flexion and placing the foot on the table (Fig. 9-47). Turn the foot laterally, which places the tibia into slight external rotation and exposes the medial plateau of the tibia. Using a single-thumb technique, first press down on the tibial plateau and then perform brisk, back-and-forth strokes in the medial to lateral plane for the attachment points of the ligament. Cover the entire area from the patellar tendon to the MCL. To release the lateral portion of the coronary ligament, internally rotate the tibia by turning the foot inward, and repeat the same strokes as were described for stroke 1 on the lateral plateau of the tibia.
2. Place your flexed knee on the table, and rest the client's leg on your thigh. The MCL is attached to the medial condyle of the femur just inferior to the adductor tubercle and on the tibia 2 to 4 inches

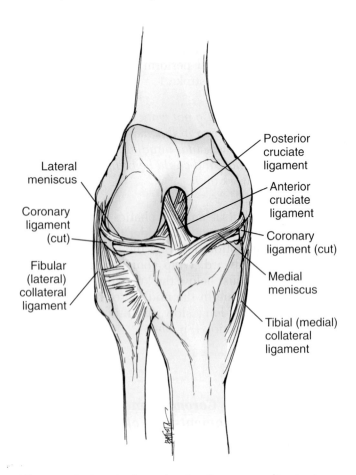

Lateral meniscus

Coronary ligament (cut)

Fibular (lateral) collateral ligament

Posterior cruciate ligament

Anterior cruciate ligament

Coronary ligament (cut)

Medial meniscus

Tibial (medial) collateral ligament

Figure 9-46. Anterior knee showing the coronary ligaments.

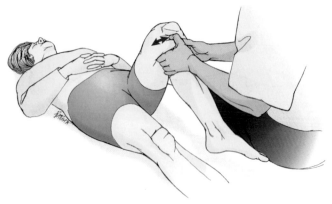

Figure 9-47. Single-thumb technique to release the medial coronary ligament.

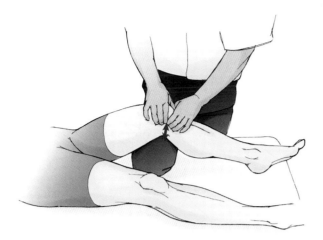

Figure 9-48. Fingertips performing transverse strokes on the MCL.

below the joint line. Using a fingertips technique, perform short back-and-forth strokes in the posterior-to-anterior plane from the proximal to the distal attachment sites (Fig. 9-48).

3. Bring the client's leg to rest on the table again. Place a little lotion on the medial knee, and use a flat index finger to stroke the pes anserinus bursa gently in long, continuous strokes in a superior direction (Fig. 9-49). Begin on the medial leg at the level of the tibial tuberosity, and continue to the distal thigh.

2. *Release of the Soft Tissue Attachments on the Lateral Aspect of the Knee*

▨ **Anatomy:** ITB, lateral joint capsule, and fibular collateral ligament (Fig. 9-50).

▨ **Dysfunction:** Attachment points thicken with overuse or after injury. This series of strokes releases the

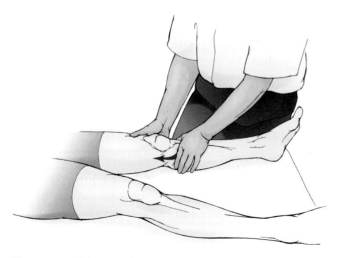

Figure 9-49. Massage of the pes anserinus bursa headward with the flat surface of the fingers.

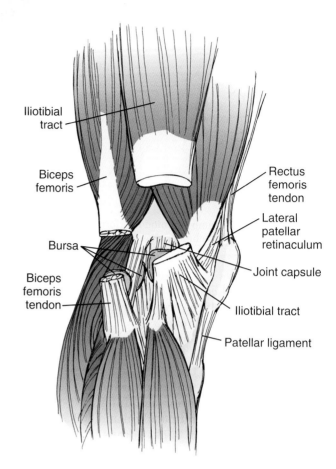

Figure 9-50. Lateral knee showing the ligaments, joint capsule, retinaculum, interweaving tendons, and the bursae under the iliotibial tract, and biceps femoris.

deep portion of the joint capsule and the soft tissue attachments to the periosteum covering the bone.

Position
▨ **TP:** Standing

▨ **CP:** Supine, knee extended

MET
You can perform CR and PIR MET for the TFL and the ITB (MET #11 and #12, hip) to reduce the hypertonicity and tenderness in the tissue.

Strokes
1. Release the attachment sites of the ITB at the femur and the tibia. The ITB inserts on the femoral supracondylar tubercle, the lateral tubercle of the tibia (Gerdy's tubercle), the patella, and the patellar tendon. To assist palpation, place your fingertips at the lateral knee approximately two finger widths lateral to the patella. With the knee extended, have your client lift his or her leg off the table slightly. Feel the ITB come into tension. Using double thumbs or fingertips, perform deep back-and-forth strokes in the posterior-to-anterior plane, starting

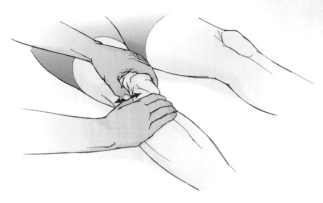

Figure 9-51. Double-thumb technique performing transverse strokes to release the attachment sites of the ITB at the femur and tibia.

from the lateral condyle of the femur to the lateral tibia (Fig. 9-51). If the area feels fibrotic, use brisk, transverse friction strokes.

3. Face 45° headward, and use a double-thumb or a fingertips technique to release the fascial expansion of the ITB and the lateral patellar retinaculum underneath it (Fig. 9-52). Perform these strokes in the anterior-to-posterior and inferior-to-superior planes, because the retinaculum and ITB are at various angles. Feel for thick, fibrous, "thready" tissue. Cover the entire area between the ITB and lateral patella.

4. Palpate the fibular collateral ligament by first placing the knee in a figure-four position (flexed knee, abducted and externally rotated hip). The ligament palpates as a taut cord at the joint line. Bring the leg back onto the table, placing a pillow under the knee. Using a fingertips or a double-thumb technique, perform deep back-and-forth strokes transverse to the line of its fiber, from the lateral epicondyle of the femur to the fibular head (Fig. 9-53). Perform brisk, transverse friction strokes if it feels fibrotic.

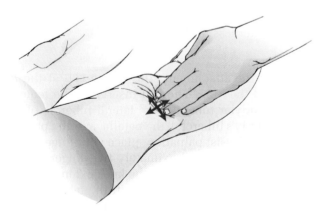

Figure 9-52. Fingertip release of the lateral retinaculum and ITB between the fibula and the lateral pole of the patella.

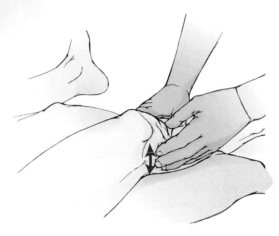

Figure 9-53. Fingertips performing transverse release of the fibular (lateral) collateral ligament.

3. *Release of the Anterior Joint Capsule*

▨ **Anatomy:** The joint capsule of the knee is attached to the femur approximately two finger widths above the patella and to the proximal tibia. It has several deep transverse thickenings from the medial and lateral epicondyles to the patella. The synovial lining of the joint capsule has a thickening or fold, referred to as a **plica,** in the medial suprapatellar aspect of the knee in 20% to 60% of the population (Fig. 9-54).

▨ **Dysfunction:** The joint capsule thickens in response to overuse or injury. The medial side of the capsule is more commonly involved clinically than the lateral side. Chronic irritation of the the plica leads to fibrous thickenings, creating adhesions, leading to impingement on the medial edge of the medial femoral condyle, a condition called *plica syndrome.* Adhesions of the capsule to the periosteum or within the capsule itself decrease its lubrication and normal extensibility. This leads to mechanical and neurosensory dysfunctions. The deep transverse thickenings are often thick and fibrotic after injury or due to degeneration.

Position
▨ **TP:** Standing, facing 45° headward

▨ **CP:** Supine; place a pillow under the knee

MET
Use METs for the quadriceps (MET #3, hip), RF (MET #6), and adductors (MET #9, hip) to reduce hypertonicity and discomfort in the soft tissue.

Strokes
1. Release the medial joint capsule by first stabilizing the lateral knee with one hand. Use fingertips to

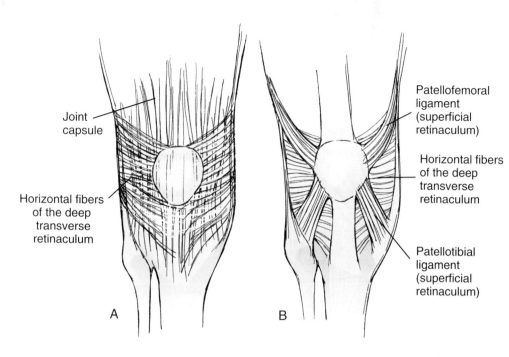

Joint capsule

Horizontal fibers of the deep transverse retinaculum

Patellofemoral ligament (superficial retinaculum)

Horizontal fibers of the deep transverse retinaculum

Patellotibial ligament (superficial retinaculum)

A

B

Figure 9-54. A. The anterior joint capsule and the horizontal fibers of the deep transverse retinaculum. **B.** Patellofemoral and patellotibial ligaments are distinct thickenings in the superficial fibers of the retinaculum (quadriceps extension).

perform deep back-and-forth strokes in the area medial to the patella on the medial femoral condyle (Fig. 9-55). This procedure helps to dissolve fibrosis in the joint capsule. Cover the entire area between the medial edge of the patella and the medial femoral condyle. Use strokes that are transverse to the femoral shaft, strokes that are in the inferior-to-superior plane for the deep transverse retinaculum, and strokes that are random for the joint capsule, because the joint capsule is interwoven in all directions. Feel for any thickening compared with the uninvolved knee, which might indicate capsular fibrosis. You might palpate a cordlike structure in the medial joint capsule. This cordlike structure is a plica. The intention is to cross transverse to the plica and clean any potential fibrotic adhesions to the underlying bone or any other aspects of the capsule.

2. Release the lateral joint capsule of the knee by performing the same strokes as were described for stroke 1 on the lateral femoral condyle. Cover the entire area between the lateral aspect of the patella and the ITB.

3. Release the attachments of the joint capsule on the tibia just below the tibial plateau. Work on either side of the infrapatellar tendon. Use fingertips, and perform deep back-and-forth strokes on the bone. The bone should feel glistening and smooth. **These strokes are for chronic conditions only.**

4. *Release of the Attachments in the Posterior Aspect of the Knee*

▥ **Anatomy:** Medial femur—medial head of the gastrocnemius (Fig. 9-56); lateral femur—plantaris, lateral head of the gastrocnemius, and popliteus; posterior tibia—semimembranosus and popliteus; and posterior fibula—soleus (see Fig. 10-7 in Chapter 10).

▥ **Dysfunction:** The semimembranosus attaches to the medial meniscus. Sustained contraction can create a dysfunction in the position of the medial meniscus. The popliteus attaches to the lateral meniscus, and sustained tension creates a dysfunction in the position of the lateral meniscus. The posterior attachment points are often strained in hyperextension injuries of the knee, or they shorten owing to a sustained contraction after an injury to the knee ligaments or cartilage.

Position

▥ **TP:** Standing, facing 45° headward

▥ **CP:** Prone, placing his or her shin on your thigh

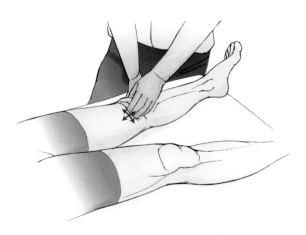

Figure 9-55. Fingertip release of the anterior joint capsule.

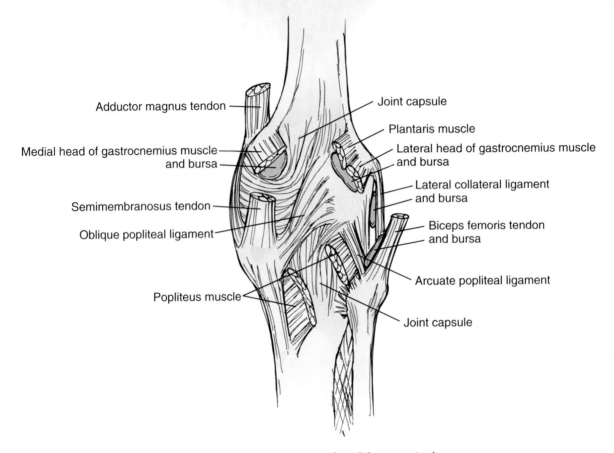

Figure 9-56. Joint capsule, ligaments, bursae, and muscles of the posterior knee.

MET

Use METs for the hamstrings (METs #10, hip, and #5, knee), popliteus (MET #7), and gastrocnemius (MET #3) to reduce hypertonicity and discomfort in the soft tissue.

Strokes

1. Release the plantaris, lateral head of the gastrocnemius, and popliteus from the lateral femur by standing, facing 45° headward. Place the flexed knee of your inferior leg on the table, and rest the client's shin on your thigh. Use a double-thumb technique, wrapping your hands around the distal femur (Fig. 9-57). Medially rotate the femur by moving the lower leg laterally, and place your thumbs on the medial side of the biceps tendons. Press laterally and deeply until your thumbs are in the area of the posterior surface of the lateral femoral condyle. Next, rock the client's entire leg medially and laterally as you perform small back-and-forth strokes in the medial-to-lateral plane. It is difficult to touch these attachments unless these areas have had a great deal of preparation. Next, perform a series of back-and-forth strokes in the inferior to superior plane on the popliteus, from the lateral femur to the medial tibia. Be careful not to work over an area in which you feel the pulse of the artery.

2. Use the same technique as was described for stroke 1 to release the medial aspects of the posterior femur and tibia (Fig. 9-58). First, laterally rotate the femur by moving the lower leg medially, and place your thumbs on the lateral side of the semimembranosus and semitendinosus tendons. Press medially and deeply until your thumbs are on the gastrocnemius, moving toward its attachment on the posterior

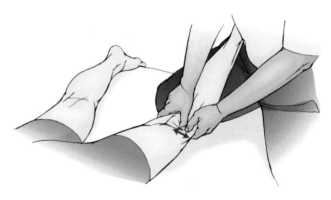

Figure 9-57. Double-thumb release of the attachments to the lateral aspect of the posterior knee.

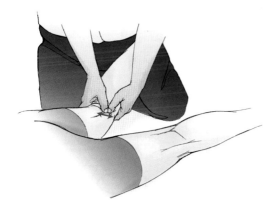

Figure 9-58. Double-thumb release of the attachments to the medial aspect of the posterior knee.

surface of the medial femoral condyle. Next, rock the client's leg into medial and lateral rotation, and perform small back-and-forth strokes in the medial-to-lateral plane. Continue to the medial aspect of the proximal tibia to release the semimembranosus and popliteus attachments.

5. Mobilization of the Knee

Anatomy: Patellofemoral joint and tibiofemoral joint (Fig. 9-59) and the medial and lateral meniscus (see Fig. 9-6).

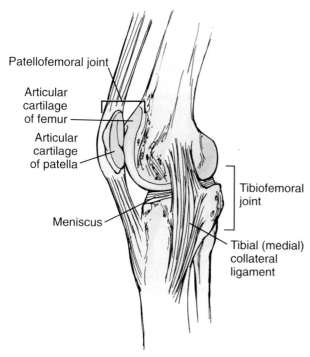

Figure 9-59. Knee consists of two joints. The articulation of the distal end of the femur and the proximal tibia is called the tibiofemoral joint. The articulation of the femur and patella is called the patellofemoral joint.

Dysfunction: Normally, a slight negative pressure exists in the joint cavity, which is lowered even further with joint distraction.[13] The anterior portions of the menisci move anteriorly on extension and posteriorly on flexion. Typically, the menisci get fixated anteriorly, making it difficult to fully extend the knee. Lauren Berry, RPT, taught that a decrease in knee joint pressure would draw the menisci into the joint slightly and help to normalize their position. The figure-eight mobilization would then help to seat the cartilage properly. This is an extremely effective mobilization. The patella can develop a roughened surface from either acute injury or chronic irritation. The inflammation digests the cartilage surface, pitting it, and the cartilage heals with a roughened surface. The menisci are susceptible to adhesions, malposition, abrasion, and tearing, which inhibit their normal gliding characteristics.

Position

TP: Standing

CP: Supine

MET

Use METs for the quadriceps (MET #3, hip), TFL and ITB (METs #11 and #12, hip), adductors (MET #9, hip), and hamstrings (METs #10, hip, and #5, knee) to reduce hypertonicity and allow for greater ROM in the joint.

Strokes

1. Place the patella in the palm of your superior hand. Your inferior hand stabilizes the inferior aspect of the patella (Fig. 9-60). Gently push the patella into the joint, and mobilize in all planes of motion with back-and-forth oscillations. If a high-pitched grinding is heard or felt, perform the grinding for no more than 1 minute per session, because too much

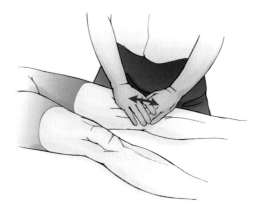

Figure 9-60. Mobilization of the patellofemoral joint.

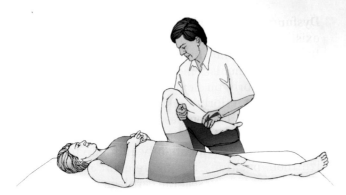

Figure 9-61. Passive flexion of the knee with the forearm in the popliteal fossa decreases the pressure in the joint cavity and draws the menisci toward their resting position.

treatment can irritate the joint. This gentle grinding helps to dissolve calcium spicules, reducing the pain and dysfunction of this joint. A low-toned grinding can indicate a pedunculated calcification (rounded), and the intention is not to dissolve these protuberances but to clean around them with great care. This technique can be safely performed for approximately 1 minute.

2. Help to normalize the function of the menisci by bringing the client's hip into approximately 90° of flexion and placing your forearm in the popliteal space (Fig. 9-61). Hold the client's distal leg with your other hand, and gently press the knee into passive flexion until pain or tissue tension is felt; then exert an overpressure if there is no pain. This gaps the joint. This passive flexion should be painless. If the joint is painful, instead of pressing the knee into flexion, gap the joint by pulling your forearm toward you, distracting the tibia away from the femur. Next, perform a figure-eight motion. Place the lower leg under your axilla, and hold the leg next to your body. Place your thumbs on either side of the patellar tendon at the joint line, with fingertips holding the posterior surface of the knee (Fig. 9-62). Take the knee into a circular motion, first upward and laterally, while you increase the pressure of the thumb on the lateral side. Then bring the knee down and back to the center, placing traction on the knee by leaning back with your body. Repeat the circle and traction to the medial side. Perform this circle, traction, and circle medially and laterally (figure eight) several times, making the circle smaller each time and extending the knee. End with the knee resting on the table in full extension and externally rotated approximately 15°. Place the webspace between your thumb and index finger at the joint space of the client's knee, and press posteriorly as you passively extend the knee slightly.

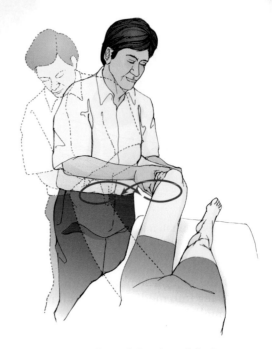

Figure 9-62. Figure-eight mobilization of the knee.

■ *Study Guide*

Level I

1. Describe the MET for an acute knee.
2. Describe genu valgus and three factors that cause it.
3. Describe why the medial meniscus is more commonly injured than is the lateral meniscus.
4. Describe the signs and symptoms of sprains of the MCL and the LCL, the coronary ligament, fibrosis of the joint capsule, and arthritis of the knee.
5. Describe the stroke direction to release the soft tissue of the medial and lateral knee, and explain why that direction is used.
6. List four factors predisposing to knee pain.
7. Describe the structure and function of the coronary ligaments and the stroke direction to release them.
8. List which knee muscles tend to be tight and which tend to be weak.
9. Describe the medial and lateral patellar retinaculum and their attachments.
10. Describe the two possible outcomes of injury to the ligaments and the implications for the massage therapist.

Level II

1. Describe the MET for the popliteus, quadriceps, and lower attachments of the hamstrings.
2. Describe the signs and symptoms of the following conditions: popliteal tendinitis, chondromalacia patella, and injuries of the menisci.
3. List the structures that are released on the medial and lateral aspect of the knee.
4. List the structures that attach onto the posterior aspect of the femur and onto the tibia and fibula at the knee.
5. Describe the knee muscle that is most commonly atrophied after an injury, and explain why.

6. Describe the intention of performing figure-eight mobilization of the knee.
7. Describe patellar tracking dysfunction, and list two causes.
8. Describe the stroke direction to release the joint capsule.
9. Describe the assessment findings of an injury to the meniscus.
10. Describe the test to assess patellar tracking dysfunction.

References

1. Garrick J, Webb D. Sports Injuries, 2nd ed. Philadelphia: WB Saunders, 1999.
2. Shelbourne KD, Rask B, Hunt S. Knee injuries. In Schenck R (ed): Athletic Training and Sports Medicine, 3rd ed. Rosemont, IL: American Academy of Orthopedic Surgeons, 1999, pp 435–488.
3. Oatis CA. Kinesiology: The Mechanics and Pathomechanics of Human Movement. Philadelphia: Lippincott Williams & Wilkins, 2004.
4. Brukner P, Khan K, Kibler WB, Murrel G. Clinical Sports Medicine, 3rd ed. Sydney: McGraw-Hill, 2006.
5. Wallace L, Mangine R, Malone T. The knee. In Malone T, McPoil T, Nitz A (eds): Orthopedic and Sports Physical Therapy. St. Louis: Mosby, 1997, pp 295–325.
6. Hertling D, Kessler R. Knee. In Hertling D, Kessler R (eds): Management of Common Musculoskeletal Disorders, 4th ed. Baltimore: Lippincott Williams & Wilkins, 2006, pp 487–557.
7. Levangie P, Norkin C. The knee complex. In Joint Structure and Function, 3rd ed. Philadelphia: FA Davis, 2001, pp 326–366.
8. Frick H, Leonhardt H, Starck D. Human Anatomy, vol. 1. New York: Thieme Medical, 1991.
9. Press J, Young J. Rehabilitation of the patellofemoral pain syndrome. In Kibler WB, Herring SA, Press JM (eds): Functional Rehabilitation of Sports and Musculoskeletal Injuries. Gaithersburg, MD: Aspen, 1998, pp 254–264.
10. Richards D, Kibler WB. Rehabilitation of knee injuries. In Kibler WB, Herring SA, Press JM (eds): Functional Rehabilitation of Sports and Musculoskeletal Injuries. Gaithersburg, MD: Aspen, 1998, pp 244–253.
11. Kendall F, McCreary E, Provance P, M Rogers, W Romani. Muscles: Testing and Function, 5th ed. Baltimore: Lippincott Williams & Wilkins, 2005.
12. Henning C, Lynch M, Glick K. Physical examination of the knee. In Nicholas J, Hershman E (eds): The Lower Extremity and Spine in Sports Medicine. St. Louis: Mosby, 1986, pp 765–800.
13. Grieve G. Common Vertebral Joint Problems. Edinburgh: Churchill Livingstone, 1981.

Suggested Readings

Corrigan B, Maitland GD. Practical Orthopaedic Medicine. London: Butterworths, 1983.

Cyriax J, Cyriax P. Illustrated Manual of Orthopedic Medicine. London: Butterworths, 1983.

Hammer W. Functional Soft Tissue Examination and Treatment by Manual Methods, 2nd ed. Gaithersburg, MD: Aspen, 1999.

Hertling D, Kessler R. Knee. In Hertling D, Kessler R (eds): Management of Common Musculoskeletal Disorders, 4th ed. Baltimore: Lippincott Williams & Wilkins, 2006, pp 487–557.

Hoppenfeld S. Physical Examination of the Spine and Extremities. New York: Appleton-Century-Crofts, 1976.

Kendall F, McCreary E, Provance P, M Rogers, W Romani. Muscles: Testing and Function, 5th ed. Baltimore: Lippincott Williams & Wilkins, 2005.

Levangie P, Norkin C. The knee complex: In Joint Structure and Function, 3rd ed. Philadelphia: FA Davis, 2001, pp 326–366.

Magee D. Orthopedic Physical Assessment, 3rd ed. Philadelphia: WB Saunders, 1997.

Reid DC. Sports Injury and Assessment. New York: Churchill Livingstone, 1992.

Wallace L, Mangine R, Malone T. The knee. In Malone T, McPoil T, Nitz A (eds): Orthopedic and Sports Physical Therapy. St. Louis: Mosby, 1997, pp 295–325.

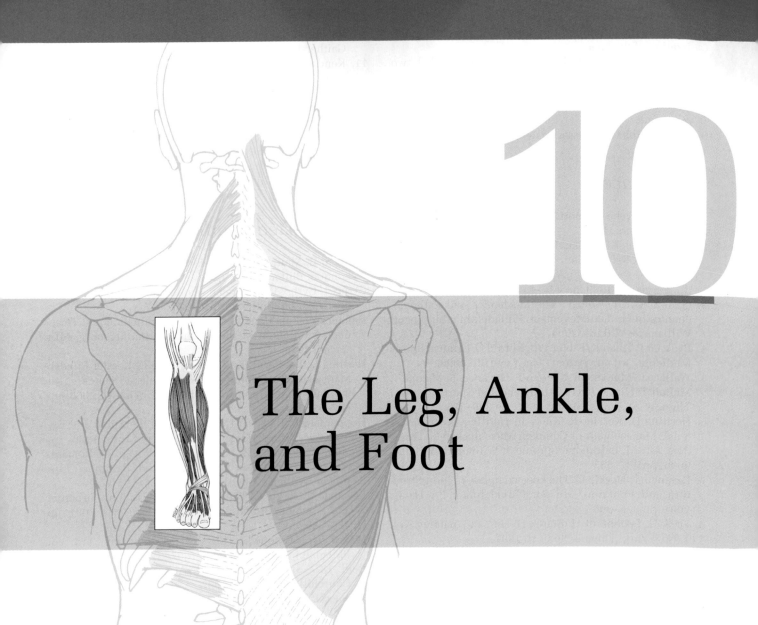

The Leg, Ankle, and Foot

The leg is the fourth most frequently involved region in athletic injuries.[1] Most of these injuries involve a strain of the gastrocnemius and Achilles tendon. The Achilles tendon is the most common site of overuse injury in the lower extremity and the most frequently ruptured tendon in the body.[2] The ankle sprain is probably the most common injury in sports and perhaps the most commonly injured ligament in the body.[3] The foot is more susceptible to degenerative problems than to acute injuries. Most painful conditions in the foot originate in the soft tissue.[4] The function of the ankle and foot has a dramatic influence on the knee, hip, and spine; and misalignment of the foot is involved in many dysfunctions of the lower extremity.

General Overview of the Leg, Ankle, and Foot

The leg consists of the structures between the knee and ankle. The leg bones are the **tibia** and the **fibula.** The distal ends of the tibia and fibula, called the *medial malleolus* and the *lateral malleolus*, respectively, form part of the ankle with the talus bone. The 12 muscles of the leg contribute to foot and ankle movements; 3 of these 12 contribute to knee flexion. The foot contains 26 bones, 30 joints, and 20 intrinsic muscles. The top of the foot is called the **dorsum,** and the bottom of the foot is called the **plantar surface.** To bend the foot toward the ground is called *foot and ankle flexion* or **plantar flexion,** and to bring the top of the foot and ankle toward the anterior leg is called *foot and ankle extension*, also referred to as **dorsiflexion.**

Anatomy, Function, and Dysfunction of the Leg

BONES AND JOINTS OF THE LEG

See Figure 10-1.

TIBIA

▦ **Structure:** The tibia, or shin bone, is a strong, triangular bone that connects the distal femur and the bones of the ankle and foot. The sharp anterior surface has a protrusion on its proximal portion called the **tibial tuberosity** where the quadriceps tendon attaches. The proximal portion of the tibia was discussed in Chapter 9, "The Knee." The distal end of the tibia has an expansion on the medial side called the medial malleolus, and the inferior part of the tibia articulates with the talus, a part of the ankle discussed below. The tibia has a spiral twist from the proximal to the distal end called **tibial torsion,** which is normally approximately 15° of lateral rotation.

▦ **Function:** The tibia bears nearly all the weight from the thigh to the foot. As was mentioned, only the tibia forms the articulation with the femur at the knee, and the tibia is the major weight-bearing surface at the ankle. Along the medial side of the distal tibia is a groove for the tibialis posterior tendon.

▦ **Dysfunction and injury:** Increased lateral tibial torsion is associated with patellar tracking dysfunction and increased Q-angles (see Chapter 9), and increased medial tibial torsion is associated with toe-in posture.[5]

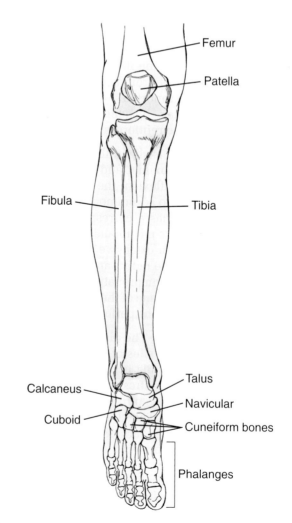

Figure 10-1. Bones of the leg, ankle, and foot.

FIBULA

■ **Structure:** The fibula is a thin bone, composed of a triangular shaft and proximal and distal ends. The distal end has an expansion on its lateral surface called the *lateral malleolus*, which forms part of the ankle and articulates with the talus. The posterior aspect of the lateral malleolus has a groove for the peroneal tendons.

■ **Function:** The fibula is an attachment site for muscles of the foot and ankle and forms part of the ankle joint. The anterior surface serves as an attachment site for the extensor muscles of the foot, the lateral surface for the peroneal muscles, and the posterior surface for the flexors of the foot. It carries approximately one-sixth of the static weight of the body.[6]

TIBIOFIBULAR JOINTS

■ **Structure:** The tibia and fibula form three joints. The first two are the **proximal** and **distal tibiofibular joints;** the third is a **fibrous joint** formed by the **interosseous membrane** connecting the first and second joints. The proximal tibiofibular joint is a synovial joint, with a joint capsule and anterior and posterior ligaments of the fibular head. The distal tibiofibular joint is a fibrous joint, without a synovial membrane, supported by the anterior and posterior tibiofibular ligaments. A strong interosseous membrane reinforces both joints.

■ **Function:** Although it is slight, there is some movement between the proximal and distal tibiofibular joints. With foot dorsiflexion, the distal tibiofibular joint widens slightly to accommodate the talus, and the proximal fibula has a corresponding superior glide. The interosseous membrane connects the two bones and serves as an extensive area for muscular attachments. Unlike the radius and ulna of the forearm, which allow forearm pronation and supination, the interosseous membrane of the leg is so dense that a similar motion cannot be performed.

■ **Dysfunction and injury:** The distal ends of the tibia and fibula are frequent sites of fractures. The *bootstrap fracture* of the fibula is common in the skier, and fatigue fractures or stress fractures in the tibia can occur with excessive or unusual stress, such as long-distance running. The client often walks with a limp and has acute tenderness and redness at the fracture site, usually localized to an area less than 1.5 inches in diameter.[1] The ligaments, retinacula, and fascia thicken after a fracture. The tibiofibular joint consequently has limited dorsiflexion, and the fibula loses its normal gliding characteristics at the proximal joint.

■ **Treatment implications:** Loss of dorsiflexion is a common outcome after ankle sprains or fractures or in the case of weak dorsiflexors from lumbosacral nerve root irritation. Because full dorsiflexion is essential for normal gait, decreased range of motion (ROM) leads to degeneration in the ankle and loss of full extension in the knee and hip, contributing to their degeneration. Perform muscle energy technique (MET) to release the gastrocnemius and soleus, soft tissue mobilization (STM) to the anterior ligaments and capsular tissue, and joint mobilization to restore normal joint play and full dorsiflexion.

SOFT TISSUE STRUCTURES OF THE LEG

FASCIA AND RETINACULUM

See Figure 10-2.

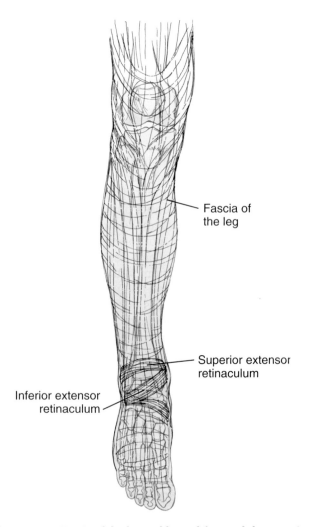

Fascia of the leg

Superior extensor retinaculum

Inferior extensor retinaculum

Figure 10-2. Fascia of the leg, ankle, and foot and the superior and inferior retinacula.

▦ **Structure:** The fascia of the leg is called the **crural fascia** and is a continuation of the fascia lata of the thigh. It is interwoven to the periosteum of the medial surface of the tibia. The anterior and lateral portions are extremely dense and have little ability to expand, whereas the posterior portion is loose and relaxed. The deep crural fascia forms three **intermuscular septa.** With the addition of the interosseous membrane between the tibia and the fibula, there are four compartments of the leg that contain the muscles that are primarily concerned with movement of the foot and ankle. The **anterior compartment** contains the extensor muscles; the **lateral compartment** contains the evertors; and the **superficial** and **deep posterior compartments** contain the flexor muscles. The fascia is reinforced by transverse thickenings called **retinacula.** The retinaculum acts like a strap to prevent the muscles and tendons running under it from lifting off the bone during contraction.

☐ On the distal aspect of the anterior leg are the **superior extensor retinaculum** and the **inferior extensor retinaculum.** The superficial layer of this fascia stabilizes the tendons that extend (dorsiflex) the foot, including the tibialis anterior, extensor hallucis longus, and the extensor digitorum longus.

☐ Between the medial malleolus and the calcaneus is the **flexor retinaculum,** which has a superficial and a deep layer. The deep layer stabilizes the tendons that flex (plantarflex) the foot, including the tibialis posterior, flexor hallucis longus, and flexor digitorum longus. The area between the superficial and deep layers of the flexor retinaculum is called the **tarsal tunnel,** and it contains the **posterior tibial nerve,** which innervates the sole of the foot.

☐ The lateral ankle has fascial expansions called the **superior peroneal retinaculum** and the **inferior peroneal retinaculum,** which stabilize the peroneus longus and peroneus brevis.

▦ **Function:** The fascia of the anterior and lateral compartments is extremely dense to contain the hydrostatic pressure from carrying the body weight. The fascial compartments separate muscle groups, provide lubrication to decrease friction, and guide muscle contraction. The muscles within these fascial compartments normally slide relative to each other and relative to the fascial envelope. The compartments also contain the major arteries and nerves of the leg. During vigorous exercise, there may be a 20-fold increase in blood flow in the leg.[6]

▦ **Dysfunction and injury:** Many factors predispose to fascial stress. Leg-length inequality, muscle imbalances, and pronation are three common factors.[7] With pronation, the muscles of the posterior compartments (gastrocnemius, soleus, tibialis posterior, flexor hallucis longus, and flexor digitorum longus) are placed in a lengthened, weakened position, making them susceptible to injury.[8] Injuries to the fascia of the leg are described with various names by different authors. The basic categories of injury include the acute and chronic compartment syndromes and the shin splint.

☐ An **acute compartment syndrome** is a rare medical emergency that is caused by rapid swelling, venous stasis, ischemia (decreased oxygen) resulting from bone fracture, muscle rupture, or severe overuse of the muscles. Because the dense fascia of the anterior and lateral compartments of the leg expands only slightly, extreme swelling can compress the arteries, veins, and nerves and cut off the blood supply and sensation to the foot.

☐ **Chronic compartment syndrome** describes ischemic muscle pain that can be caused by either static or dynamic stresses. An example of static stress is an occupation that requires standing most of the day. A dynamic stress is typically exercise induced. In the chronic condition, repetitive stress on the fascia causes inflammation, leading to eventual thickening in the superficial and deep layers of the fascia and fibrosis in the muscle's connective tissue layers. Fibrosis prevents the normal expansion of the muscles when they contract, and thickened fascia prevents the normal gliding of the muscles within their compartments, leading to ischemia and pain.

☐ A **shin splint** is a tenoperiosteal tear of the muscle's fascia where it interweaves with the periosteum, called the *tenoperiosteal junction.* This is the acute manifestation of a chronic condition. Excessive stress to the fascia is typically the result of cumulative stresses from vigorous activity, such as running. Shin splints are best described by their anatomical location. An anterolateral shin splint involves the muscles of the anterior compartment. A posteromedial shin splint typically involves the soleus and tibialis posterior.

▦ **Treatment implications:** Perform MET to reduce the hypertonicity of the muscles within the compartments, and perform STM to stretch the superficial and deep layers of the fascia and to dissolve the fibrosis at the tenoperiosteal junction. Postisometric relaxation (PIR) MET is used to lengthen short muscles and their fascia. Identify the weak muscles with the isometric contractions of contract-relax (CR) MET, and strengthen those muscles with MET, or refer the client for exercise rehabilitation. With acute compartment syndrome, the client presents with extreme pain in the leg and a cold foot. Refer the client to an emergency room because the loss of blood supply to the foot can cause permanent damage.

NERVES

See Figures 10-3**A** and 10-3**B** and Figure 10-4.

■ **Structure:** The major nerves of the leg are branches of the sciatic nerve. They are the **superficial** and **deep peroneal, tibial, saphenous,** and **sural nerves.** The superficial and deep peroneal nerves travel through an arcade or opening in the peroneus longus, just distal to the fibular head.[6] The tibial nerve becomes the posterior tibial nerve as it travels through a fibrous arch in the soleus muscle in the proximal calf. It travels behind the medial ankle and becomes the medial and lateral plantar nerves in the foot. The saphenous nerve is a terminal branch of the femoral nerve and becomes superficial at the medial thigh and knee. The sural nerve is a cutaneous nerve from branches of the tibial and peroneal nerves.

■ **Function:** The deep peroneal nerve innervates the muscles in the anterior compartment and gives sensation to the webspace between the first and second toes on the dorsum (top) of the foot. The superficial peroneal nerve innervates the lateral compartment and gives sensation to most of the dorsum of the foot. The posterior tibial nerve innervates the deep posterior compartments and gives sensation to the plantar (bottom) aspect of the foot. The saphenous nerve supplies sensation to the medial leg and foot. The sural nerve supplies sensation to the lateral and posterior distal third of the leg.

■ **Dysfunction and injury:** The nerves can become entrapped in the leg, ankle, or foot. The common peroneal nerve can become entrapped just distal to the head of the fibula and approximately 4 to 5 inches proximal to the lateral ankle. The posterior tibial nerve can become entrapped in the proximal leg as it passes under the soleus or at the tarsal tunnel. The sural nerve can become entrapped proximal to the

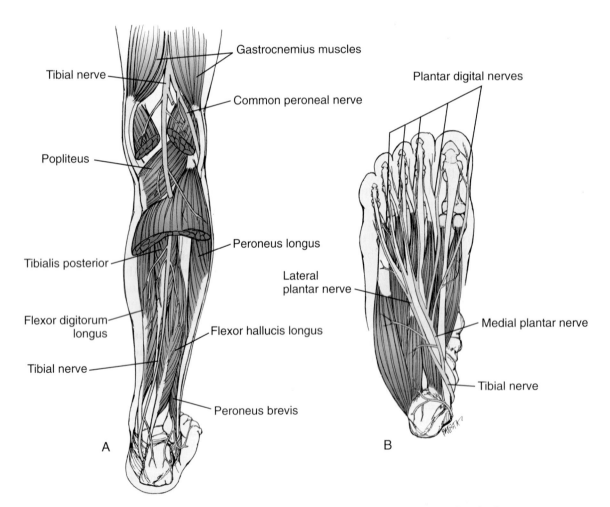

Figure 10-3. **A.** Tibial nerve and the muscles innervated by the tibial nerve. **B.** The tibial nerve continues into the bottom of the foot as the medial and lateral plantar nerves.

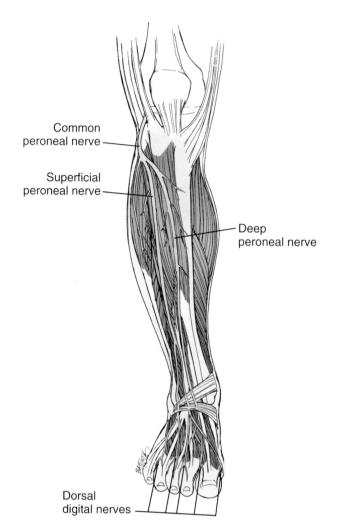

Figure 10-4. Common, superficial, and deep peroneal nerves.

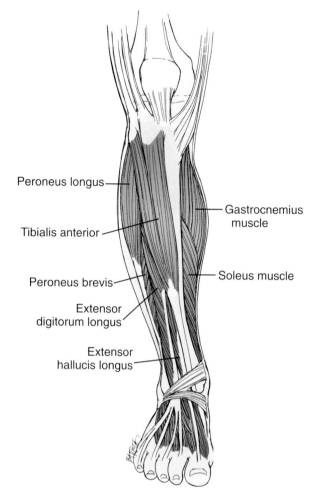

Figure 10-5. Muscles of the anterior compartment of the leg include the tibialis anterior, the extensor digitorum longus, and the extensor hallucis longus.

lateral ankle. The saphenous nerve can become entrapped in the medial thigh.

▍ **Treatment implications:** The nerves of the leg are treated with gentle transverse scooping strokes to reduce the tension in the fascia suspending the nerve and to dissolve the adhesions that restrict the normal gliding characteristics of the nerves.

MUSCLES

▍ **Structure:** Muscles of the leg are broadly categorized by location. The extensor (dorsiflexor) muscles of the ankle and foot lie in the anterior leg. The evertors lie in the lateral leg (Fig. 10-5; see also Fig. 9-10). The flexors (plantarflexors) of the ankle and foot lie in the posterior leg, and the tendons travel around the medial ankle (Figs. 10-6 and 10-7; see also Fig. 9-9). Muscles of the leg are also classified by **fascial compartments**. Four compartments—the anterior, lateral, superficial posterior, and deep

posterior—contain 12 muscles, all of which attach to bones in the foot, except the popliteus.

☐ The **anterior compartment** contains the extensor muscles of the ankle and foot (dorsiflexors) and includes the tibialis anterior, extensor hallucis longus, extensor digitorum longus, and peroneus tertius, a variant of the extensor digitorum longus extending to the fifth toe (see Fig. 10-5). The superficial and deep peroneal nerves serve the anterior compartment.

☐ The **lateral compartment** contains the evertors of the ankle and foot and includes the peroneus longus and brevis. The superficial and deep peroneal nerves serve this compartment as well (see Fig. 9-10).

☐ The **superficial posterior compartment** contains the two heads of the gastrocnemius, the soleus, and the plantaris. The superficial and deep compartments contain the foot and ankle flexors (plantarflexors) and are served by the tibial nerve. The gastrocnemius and soleus form the

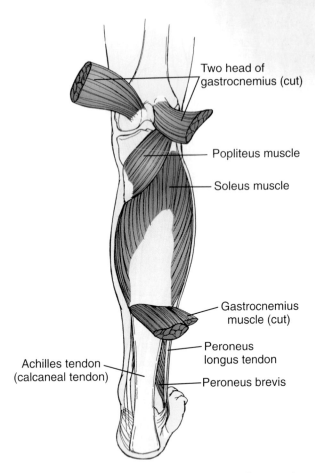

Figure 10-6. Superficial posterior compartment showing the gastrocnemius cut away to reveal the underlying soleus.

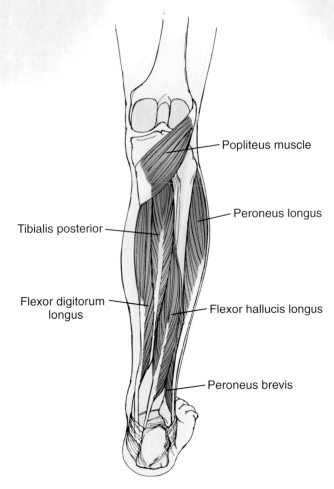

Figure 10-7. Deep posterior compartment showing the tibialis posterior, flexor digitorum longus, and the flexor hallucis longus.

Achilles tendon—the main plantar flexor of the ankle (see Fig. 10-6).

☐ The **deep posterior compartment** contains the popliteus, flexor hallucis longus, flexor digitorum longus, and tibialis posterior (see Fig. 10-7). The tibial nerve also innervates this compartment.

◼ **Function:** The gastrocnemius and soleus must maintain some contraction during relaxed standing posture so that the body does not fall forward, because the center of gravity is in front of the ankle.[4] The Achilles tendon is the strongest tendon in the body and is engaged with every step. The muscles of the leg provide dynamic support to the knee, ankle, and foot and are responsible for balance, coordination, fine postural control, movement of the body, and dynamic stability to the foot and ankle. As with all muscles, they contain muscle spindles and Golgi tendon organs that have reflexive connections to the mechanoreceptors in the soft tissue surrounding the joints, including the ligaments and the joint capsule. The other muscles have functions for the foot and ankle and

are discussed in the section "Muscles of the Ankle and Foot," p. 465.

◼ **Dysfunction and injury:** The most commonly injured muscle of the leg is the gastrocnemius, typically the medial head near the myotendinous junction. This muscle is called a two-joint muscle because it crosses the knee and the ankle. The gastrocnemius is commonly injured because one of the main functions of this muscle is eccentric contraction (i.e., to contract while the muscle is lengthening), which occurs at heel strike during normal walking. Muscles are much more prone to injury during eccentric contraction. *Achilles tendinitis* is the most common tendinitis of the leg. Muscles of the anterior compartment help to lift the foot off the ground during walking. They can become severely weak after a herniated disc in the lumbar spine damages the roots of the nerves innervating these muscles, leading to "*foot drop*"—an inability to dorsiflex the foot. *Muscle cramps* in the gastrocnemius and soleus are also common. The cramps typically occur as a result of salt depletion and after prolonged activity.[6] The exact cause is not clearly understood, and a low calcium level is also implicated.

Muscle Imbalances of the Leg

Two basic categories of muscle dysfunction are muscle imbalance and positional dysfunction. Muscle imbalance describes a condition in which certain muscles tend to be weak and others tend to be short and tight. Muscle imbalances alter movement patterns and therefore add continuing stress to the joint system. Janda and colleagues have described certain predictable patterns of muscle imbalance in the leg.[9] Positional dysfunction describes a condition in which muscles misalign and develop an abnormal torsion.

▌ **Muscles that tend to be tight and short:** The triceps surae (gastrocnemius and soleus) and tibialis posterior tend to be tight, short muscles. Tight plantar flexors restrict ankle dorsiflexion and increase the tendency for excessive pronation.

▌ **Muscles that tend to be inhibited and weak:** The tibialis anterior, extensor hallucis longus, extensor digitorum longus, and peroneals tend to be inhibited, weak muscles.

Positional Dysfunction of the Leg Muscles

The gastrocnemius tends to develop a torsion that pulls the the two heads toward the midline. With a pronated ankle, the triceps surae (gastrocnemius and soleus) is pulled laterally. The other muscles are contained so tightly within their fascial compartments that no other positional dysfunctions occur.

▌ **Treatment implications:** Muscle cramps are treated with passive stretching. Other muscle dysfunctions and injuries are treated with MET, STM, and joint mobilization as described in the "Technique" section below.

MUSCLES OF THE LEG (EXTRINSIC MUSCLES OF THE ANKLE AND FOOT)

See Table 10-1.

Table 10-1 Muscles of the Leg (Extrinsic Muscles of the Ankle and Foot)

Muscle	Origin	Insertion	Action	Dysfunction
Anterior Compartment				
Tibialis anterior	Upper two-thirds of the lateral surface of the tibia.	Medial and plantar surface of the medial cuneiform and the base of the first metatarsal	Prime mover for dorsiflexion and inversion of the foot. Provides dynamic support for medial longitudinal arch	Tibialis anterior resists plantar flexion at heel strike, and susceptible to fatigue and tightness-weakness. Weakness limits ankle dorsiflexion. Tightness produces high medial arch.
Extensor digitorum longus	Lateral condyle of the tibia, the upper three-fourths of the anterior surface of the fibula	Dorsal aspects of the second through fifth toes and their extensor expansions	MTP and toe extension and dorsiflexion and for eversion of the foot	Weakness decreases ability of toes to lift off ground in walking. Tightness leads to claw toe deformity.
Extensor hallucis longus	Anterior surface of the fibula and interosseous membrane, at the middle half of the leg	Dorsal aspect of base of the distal phalanx of the great toe	Prime mover for extension of the great toe; assists with dorsiflexion and inversion of the foot	Weakness causes inability to extend great toe. May reflect disc injury at L5. Tightness pulls MTP into extension, which flexes interphalangeal joint, causing claw toe.
Lateral Compartment				
Peroneus longus	Lateral condyle of the tibia and the upper two-thirds of the lateral aspect of the fibula	Lateral side of the first cuneiform bone and the first metatarsal	Prime mover for eversion; assists with plantar flexion; acts as a bowstring, providing dynamic support of the transverse arch of the foot	Weakness allows the invertors, especially the tibialis posterior, to pull the foot into inversion. Tightness leads to overuse of peroneal tendons, excessive pronation.

(continued)

Table 10-1	Muscles of the Leg (Extrinsic Muscles of the Ankle and Foot) (*Continued*)			
Muscle	***Origin***	***Insertion***	***Action***	***Dysfunction***
Lateral Compartment				
Peroneus brevis	Distal two-thirds of the lateral surface of the fibula	Lateral tubercle at the base of the fifth metatarsal	Prime mover for eversion; assists with plantar flexion	Weakness same as for peroneus longus. Tightness can contribute to eversion of foot.
Superficial Posterior Compartment				
Gastrocne-mius	By two tendons from the posterior aspect of the condyles of the femur; some fibers also arise from the capsule of the knee	Posterior surface of the calcaneus as the Achilles tendon	Prime mover for plantar flexion; assists with knee flexion; stabilizes the femur on the tibia	Tightness limits dorsiflexion. Weakness limits the ability to rise up on the toes, limiting the ability to climb stairs. A strain of the gastrocnemius usually involves the medial head at the musculotendinous junction.
Soleus	Proximal part of the posterior surfaces of the tibia, fibula, and interosseous membrane	By the Achilles tendon into the calcaneus	Prime mover for plantar flexion; stabilizes the lower leg on the tarsus	Poteromedial shin splints often involve the soleus. Same tightness-weakness patterns as gastrocnemius.
Plantaris	Posterior, lateral femoral condyle proximal to gastrocnemius; joint capsule	Blends with the medial edge of the Achilles tendon	Weak assistant for knee and plantar flexion	A small muscle that has not be implicated in clinical problems.
Deep Posterior Compartment				
Popliteus	Lateral condyle of the femur	Posterior medial surface of the tibia	Knee flexion; rotates tibia medially; dynamic stabilizer of the knee; assists in pulling lateral meniscus posteriorly during knee flexion	Tightness limits ability of tibia to externally rotate fully in normal gait. Weakness promotes instability at the knee and lack of normal glide of lateral meniscus.
Flexor hallucis longus	Distal two-thirds of the posterior surface of the fibula and from the interosseous membrane	Plantar surface of the base of the distal phalanx of the great toe	Prime mover for flexion of the great toe; assists with plantar flexion and inversion of the foot	Weakness reduces strength of plantar flexion. Tightness limits extension of great toe and contributes to claw toe deformity.
Flexor digitorum longus	Medial part of the posterior surface of the tibia and from the fascia covering the tibialis posterior	Bases of the distal phalanges of the four small toes; each tendon passes through an opening in the corresponding tendon of the flexor digitorum brevis	Prime mover for flexion of the second through fifth toes; assists with plantar flexion and inversion	Tightness contributes to claw toe deformity. Inflammation leads to pain in plantar aspect of midfoot due to pronation or excessive plantar flexion (e.g., jumping).
Tibialis posterior	Upper half of the posterior surface of the interosseous membrane and the adjacent parts of the tibia and fibula	Tuberosity on the plantar surface of the navicular and the three cuneiform bones	Prime mover for inversion; assists with plantar flexion; dynamic support for the longitudinal arch; important stabilizer of the foot	Weakness lowers medial arch and predisposes to pronation. Tendinitis is most common cause of medial ankle and foot pain.[8]

Anatomy, Function, and Dysfunction of the Ankle

BONES AND JOINTS OF THE ANKLE

TALOCRURAL JOINT (ANKLE MORTISE)

See Figure 10-1.

▨ **Structure:** The ankle is the articulation between the talus and the tibia and fibula and is referred to as the **talocrural joint.** The body weight is transferred from the femur through the tibia and fibula to the talus and then to the calcaneus, the main contact point with the ground. The plantar surface of the calcaneus has a thick *fat pad*, encapsulated in a fibroelastic structure designed to absorb shock. The ankle joint is referred to as a mortise, as the distal ends of the tibia and fibula, called malleoli, form a socket that holds the talus in between them. On the medial side of the talus is a groove for the flexor hallucis longus tendon.

▨ **Function:** The ankle is a synovial joint with two possible motions: flexion and extension. At the ankle, flexion and extension are called *plantar flexion* and *dorsiflexion*, respectively. The foot moves within the ankle because of the contraction of the gastrocnemius–soleus muscles that create plantar flexion and the muscles of the anterior leg that cause dorsiflexion. The ankle joint faces approximately 15° laterally in its neutral position, since the medial malleolus is anterior to the lateral malleolus. It produces a normal toe-out stance, which is referred to as the **Fick angle.** Because of this angle, dorsiflexion elicits an up-and-out movement of the foot, and plantar flexion results in the foot moving down and medially.

▨ **Dysfunction and injury:** If the ankle is in its neutral position, there is a vertical alignment through the tibia, talus, and calcaneus (heel bone). **Pronation** is a common weight-bearing dysfunction in which the talus is positioned anteriorly and medially and the bottom of the heel angles laterally (everts). This changes the contact area on the weight-bearing surfaces of the joints, leading to degeneration of the cartilage. Pronation causes excessive stress on the medial side of the foot, leading to the development of sesamoiditis, bunions, and interdigital neuroma (Morton's neuroma). **Hallux valgus,** or lateral deviation of the great toe, and pain in the great toe can also develop as a result of pronation. Leg pain can also develop from pronation caused by excessive tension of the anterior and posterior tibialis. Knee pain is common because of lateral tracking of the patella from the genu valgus position of the knee associated with pronation.[10] Traumatic injuries to the ankle often leave the pariarticular (i.e., surrounding the joint) soft tissue fibrotic, decreasing the normal ROM in the joint, typically causing a loss of dorsiflexion, leading to degeneration and arthritis, and pain in weight bearing.

▨ **Treatment implications:** Acute ankle sprains are treated initially with CR MET and reciprocal inhibition (RI) MET to reduce swelling and pain, promote nutritional exchange, and minimize muscular inhibition. Gentle passive motion in dorsiflexion and plantarflexion is performed to prevent adhesions on the joint surfaces. Degeneration and loss of joint motion in the ankle are treated initially with MET. MET helps to increase the extensibility of the ligaments and tendinous-fascial insertions and increases the ROM of the joint. PIR MET is performed on the short and tight muscles, especially the gastrocnemius and soleus, which could be inhibiting dorsiflexion. STM is performed on the periarticular soft tissue to dissolve adhesions and to allow for greater extensibility. Mobilization is then performed to stimulate nutritional exchange in the cartilage and help dissolve calcium deposits on the articular surfaces. Perform CR MET to help strengthen the intrinsic muscles of the feet and the anterior and posterior tibialis muscles.

SOFT TISSUE STRUCTURES OF THE ANKLE

JOINT CAPSULE AND LIGAMENTS

▨ **Structure:** The joint capsule of the ankle is thin and provides little support. The ligaments and muscles provide passive and dynamic stability, respectively. The ligaments on the medial and lateral sides can be grouped together as the medial and lateral collateral ligaments.

☐ The **medial collateral ligament** is also called the **deltoid ligament** and consists of fibers that run

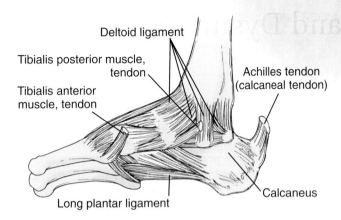

Figure 10-8. Ligaments and tendons of the medial ankle.

from the medial malleolus to the navicular, talus, and calcaneus. These ligament fibers blend into one another, unlike the lateral collateral ligament, which is formed from separate bands (Fig. 10-8).

☐ The **lateral collateral ligament** consists of the anterior and posterior talofibular ligaments and the calcaneofibular ligaments (Fig. 10-9).

▨ **Function:** The joint capsule and ligaments of the ankle provide passive stability to the ankle and foot. In plantar flexion, the anterior talofibular ligament restricts inversion of the talus. The ligaments also have a dense population of mechanoreceptors that function in the control of posture and movement. Arthrokinetic and arthrostatic reflexes exist between these mechanoreceptors and the muscles of the leg that function to provide instantaneous and precise contractions for control of the foot and ankle in movement and fine postural control.[11]

▨ **Dysfunction and injury:** *Ankle sprains* are injuries to the ligaments. The **anterior talofibular** is the

weakest ligament of the ankle, the first ligament to be affected in an inversion stress, and the most commonly injured ligament of the ankle.[11] At least 95% of ankle sprains are to the lateral ligaments.[12] Injury occurs as a result of either acute or cumulative inversion stress for two anatomic reasons: The distal end of the fibula extends further than the tibia and helps to provide lateral stability; and the deltoid ligament is much stronger than the lateral collateral ligaments. After an ankle sprain, two outcomes are possible. In the first, the ankle becomes fibrous and stiff with decreased ROM, especially decreased dorsiflexion at the talocrural joint, and restricted inversion and eversion at the subtalar joint. The ankle can also develop painful impingement at the anterior or anterolateral joint due to thickened synovium. In the second outcome, the ankle becomes unstable due to ligamentous laxity, muscle weakness, and poor proprioceptive control. Studies show that approximately 40% of injuries to the lateral ligament of the ankle lead to the feeling that the foot tends to "give way."[11] Freeman and colleagues[13] suggest that the ankle becomes unstable because of a partial loss of the normal reflex activity between the mechanoreceptors of the capsule, ligaments, and calf muscles.

▨ **Treatment implications:** If the ankle ligaments have become fibrous and thickened because of deposits of excessive collagen after an injury, perform MET to the muscles that cross the ankle, as this increases the extensibility to the ligaments. MET is also used to strengthen the peroneals and to lengthen the gastrocnemius and soleus. Next, perform STM, including transverse friction massage, to the body and attachment points of the ligaments. This combined treatment helps to dissolve adhesions and restore normal extensibility

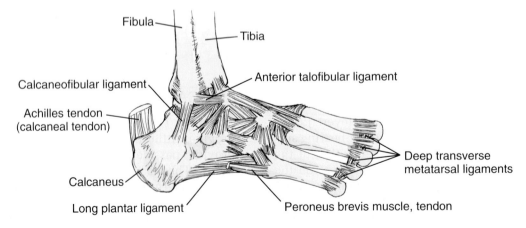

Figure 10-9. Ligaments and tendons of the lateral ankle.

Table 10-2	Ligaments of the Ankle	

The talocrural joint, or ankle joint, is stabilized medially by the medial collateral ligament complex and laterally by the lateral collateral ligament complex. The following ligaments are listed in the order of frequency of injury.

Ligament	Origin	Insertion
Anterior talofibular ligament (part of lateral collateral ligament)	Lateral malleolus (fibula)	Neck of the talus
Calcaneofibular (part of lateral collateral ligament)	Distal fibula	Calcaneus
Calcaneocuboid	Distal aspect of the lateral calcaneus	Lateral surface of the cuboid
Anterior tibiofibular	Distal aspect of the lateral tibia	Distal aspect of the medial fibula
Deltoid ligament (medial collateral ligament)	Comprises the tibionavicular, tibiocalcaneal, and the anterior and posterior tibiotalar ligaments; originates at the distal tibia	Inserts on the navicular, talus, and calcaneus

to the ligaments. Decreased passive glide and impingement of the ankle are treated with mobilization. If the ligaments have become too slack and the ankle is unstable, exercise rehabilitation, including balance and proprioception exercises to restore normal neurological function, is recommended.

LIGAMENTS OF THE ANKLE

See Table 10-2.

NERVES OF THE ANKLE

See Figures 10-3**A** and 10-3**B** and Figure 10-4.

- **Structure:** The deep peroneal nerve passes under the extensor retinaculum of the ankle to the dorsum of the foot. The superficial peroneal nerve travels under the skin on the anterolateral ankle and foot. The posterior tibial nerve travels behind the medial malleolus between the superficial and deep layers of the flexor retinaculum, in what is called the **tarsal tunnel.**

- **Function:** The deep peroneal nerve supplies the anterior compartment and provides sensation to the webspace between the first and second toes. The superficial peroneal nerve supplies the skin to the dorsum of the foot. The posterior tibial nerve supplies the intrinsic muscles of the foot and provides sensation to the bottom of the foot through its branches, the medial and lateral plantar nerves (see "Nerves of the Foot").

- **Dysfunction and injury:** Entrapment of the nerves that cross the ankle is common. The posterior tibial nerve can become compressed in the tarsal tunnel owing to injury to the ankle or to pronation. The deep peroneal nerve can become compressed under the extensor retinaculum because of ankle injury, tight-laced boots, or high heels.

- **Treatment implications:** As in the other areas of the body, the nerves are released by gentle scooping strokes, transverse to the line of the nerve. This treatment releases the adhesions and takes the nerves out of tension.

MUSCLES OF THE ANKLE AND FOOT

- **Structure:** Thirty-one muscles contribute to foot and ankle movements. Of these 31 muscles, 11 originate in the leg and are called *extrinsic muscles* of the foot, and 20 originate in the foot and are called *intrinsic muscles*. All the muscles of the calf cross the ankle as tendons and insert on the foot. They are held in place by the retinaculum, described above. These tendons have tendon sheaths as they cross the ankle and are therefore susceptible to tenosynovitis and stenosing tenosynovitis in this region. The muscles and tendons can be divided into four categories, based on their function and location.
  - ☐ The **flexors** pass behind the medial malleolus and under the flexor retinaculum, and each is contained within its own synovial sheath. The flexors from anterior to posterior (A–P) are the tibialis posterior, flexor digitorum longus, and flexor hallucis longus (see Fig. 9-9). The tendons of these muscles travel with the tibial nerve under the flexor retinaculum through the tarsal tunnel.
  - ☐ The **extensors** cross on the dorsum of the foot under the superior and inferior extensor retinaculum, each within its own synovial sheath. The extensors include the tibialis anterior, extensor hallucis longus, and extensor digitorum longus (see Fig. 10-5).
  - ☐ The **evertors** are the peroneus longus and brevis, and they pass behind the lateral malleolus under the superior and inferior peroneal retinaculum, through a common peroneal sheath. The peroneals

exit the common sheath distal to the inferior retinaculum (see Fig. 9-10).

☐ The **invertors** are the anterior and posterior tibialis.

■ **Function:** Ankle muscles provide dynamic stability to the ankle and foot. The muscles are responsible for postural control, balance, coordination, and movement.

■ **Dysfunction and injury:** With excessive or repetitive ankle stress, such as running, dancing, and hiking, or with chronic postural stress, such as pronation, the synovial lining in the tendon sheaths can become irritated and inflamed where they cross the ankle. In the acute stage, it manifests as local pain and swelling at the involved tendon. In the chronic phase, thickening can develop on the sheath because of fibrous deposition from the inflammation, which leads to a narrowing of the sheath, called **stenosing tenosynovitis.**

■ **Treatment implications:** The tendons of the ankle are treated with STM, stroking transverse to the line of the tendon, joint mobilization, and MET. To reduce the hypertonicity in the muscle–tendon unit, perform CR MET. To lengthen a shortened muscle–tendon unit, perform PIR MET. Adhesions around or in the tendon sheath are treated with transverse friction massage.

MUSCULAR ACTIONS OF THE ANKLE

See Table 10-3.

Table 10-3	Muscular Actions of the Ankle

The ankle is the articulation of the talus bone with the tibia and fibula. It is a hinge-type joint capable of two movements: flexion (plantarflexion) and extension (dorsiflexion).

Plantarflexion

Eight muscles contribute to plantar flexion; seven of these muscles span two joints.
- Gastrocnemius
- Soleus
- Peroneus longus—also causes eversion of the foot and helps maintain the arch of the foot.
- Peroneus brevis—also causes eversion of the foot.
- Flexor digitorum longus—also inverts the foot and flexes the toes.
- Tibialis posterior—also assists in inversion.
- Flexor hallucis longus—flexes the big toe, inverts the foot, plantar flexes the ankle.
- Plantaris

Dorsiflexion

Four muscles contribute to dorsiflexion.
- Tibialis anterior—also inverts the foot.
- Extensor digitorum longus—also extends the toes, and everts the foot.
- Extensor hallucis longus—also extends the great toe.
- Peroneus tertius—also everts the foot.

Anatomy, Function, and Dysfunction of the Foot

BONES AND JOINTS OF THE FOOT

See Figure 10-1.

■ **Structure:** The foot contains 26 bones and 30 joints, and it can be divided into the hindfoot, midfoot, and forefoot. The **hindfoot** consists of the talus and calcaneus. The **midfoot** consists of the navicular, the cuboid, and the three cuneiforms. The **forefoot** consists of the five metatarsals and the fourteen phalanges that make up the five toes.

■ **Function:** The motions of the foot are dorsiflexion, plantar flexion, inversion, and eversion. Inversion is the combination of adduction, supination (elevation of the medial margin), and plantar flexion. Eversion is abduction, pronation (lowering of the medial margin of the foot), and dorsiflexion. The toes may flex, extend, abduct, and adduct. Normal function of the foot is essential for fine postural control. It must have adequate mobility for proper gait and to accommodate uneven surfaces. It must also have stability for sustained weight bearing and strength for dynamic movement of the body. In the following section, the joints are described individually for clarification.

SUBTALAR (TALOCALCANEAL) JOINT

■ **Structure:** The **subtalar** or **talocalcaneal** joint is the articulation between the calcaneus (heel) and the talus.

■ **Function:** The main function of the subtalar joint is to absorb rotation of the lower extremity. During gait, as the foot is lowered to the ground after heel strike, the femur and tibia rotate internally.[14] The subtalar joint moves inferiorly and medially, called pronation. From the flat foot phase to the heel-off phase of gait, the tibia and femur externally rotate and the subtalar joint moves into supination. In the normal standing posture, the tibia, talus, and calcaneus are in vertical alignment.

■ **Dysfunction and injury:** Although the term pronation describes a normal movement of the subtalar joint, it is also commonly used to describe a dysfunction of the foot. This text will adopt that common usage. In standing posture, if the calcaneus angles laterally into a valgus position, it is associated with excessive **pronation** at the subtalar joint; and if it angles medially into a varus position, it is associated with supination at the subtalar joint. A valgus heel creates an eversion of the forefoot, is associated with the lateral deviation of the great toe (hallux valgus), and causes the Achilles tendon to deviate laterally and to shorten.[4] Pronation can result from weak supination muscles (e.g., the triceps surae, tibialis posterior, flexor hallucis longus, flexor digitorum longus, and tibialis anterior). It can also be caused by a shortness of the peroneus longus, the strongest pronator. If pronation becomes chronic, fibrous deposition at the anterior mortice and a loss of full dorsiflexion of the ankle occur. *Pes varus* is the condition in which the heel angles medially and contributes to supination. This angulation can be caused by weakness in the pronators, including the peroneals, extensor digitorum longus, and extensor hallucis longus, or it can be caused by a shortness of the supinators, including the triceps surae and flexor digitorum longus.

■ **Treatment implications:** The subtalar joint is treated with MET to balance the muscular forces affecting the joint, STM to dissolve fibrosis around the joint, and joint mobilization in pronation-supination to improve joint play and stimualate the normal lubrication in the joint.

METATARSOPHALANGEAL JOINTS

■ **Structure:** The metatarsophalangeal (MTP) joints are the articulation of the metatarsals and phalanges (toes). They are synovial joints with a joint capsule and three ligaments: the plantar (plantar plate), transverse metatarsal, and collateral (see "Ligaments of the Foot"). The joint capsules of the toes are reinforced by the extensor tendons. On the plantar surface of the head of the first metatarsal are the medial and lateral **sesamoid bones,** which attach to the

plantar plate and joint capsule. The medial head of the flexor hallucis brevis and abductor hallucis also insert into the medial sesamoid, and the oblique and transverse heads of the adductor hallucis and the lateral head of the flexor hallucis brevis insert on the lateral sesamoid.

■ **Function:** The MTP joint has four possible motions: flexion, extension, adduction, and abduction. When a person stands on one leg, 100% of the body weight comes through the talus, then 50% of the weight moves posteriorly to the heel, and 50% forward. The first MTP joint carries 25% of that forward-moving weight, and the lateral four toes carry the other 25%.[15] The great toe stabilizes the foot and assists in the push-off phase during gait. The great toe extends (dorsiflexes) with every step, some 5,000 to 10,000 times a day in a healthy adult. The first MTP must be capable of 45° to 60° of extension at toe-off phase, or the gait is altered, leading to compensation and potential degeneration in the foot, ankle, knee, and hip. As in other areas of the body, the sesamoids help to distribute pressure and reduce friction.

■ **Dysfunction and injury:** Hyperextension injury of the MTP joint of the great toe is known as *turf toe.* This injury can damage the sesamoids and plantar plate, as well as sprain the joint capsule and collateral ligaments. It can lead to limited motion and degeneration.[5] The first MTP joint is a common site of degeneration and dysfunction. Functional **hallux limitus** is the inability of the proximal phalanx to extend on the first metatarsal head during the push-off phase of gait. Through either acute or repetitive stress to this joint, inflammation degenerates the cartilage and thickens the joint capsule, causing **hallux rigidus,** a degeneration of the first MTP joint. With weight distribution imbalances, such as pronation, the great toe migrates laterally, called **hallux valgus.** The toe-out position improves balance and may also compensate for lower-back dysfunction or injury or for decreased dorsiflexion of the ankle. With a loss of the arches, the foot loses its soft tissue shock absorbers, and the weight falls on the metatarsal heads, irritating the MTP joints and potentially causing pain at the metatarsal heads or MTP joints, a condition called **metatarsalgia.** Pain under the great toe can be from inflammation of the sesamoids, a condition called **sesamoiditis.** Sesamoiditis can develop because of a high arch, wearing high heels, or hallux valgus. Lateral deviation of the great toe (hallux valgus) creates a subluxation of the sesamoids laterally.[10]

■ **Treatment implications:** Acute irritation or inflammation of the great toe is best treated with CR

MET of the flexors and extensors of the great toe. Chronic conditions need to be assessed for weight distribution problems, such as pronation, genu valgum, or leg-length imbalances. As always, the primary intention in performing treatment is to reduce the hypertonicity in the tight or short muscles and then to facilitate (strengthen) the weak muscles. STM is performed on the joint capsule, and mobilization is performed on the joints. Chronic imbalances often require a referral to a physical therapist or a personal trainer for proper instruction in developing the strength to maintain proper alignment. The sesamoids are mobilized in a medial direction to help correct the positional dysfunction.

INTERPHALANGEAL JOINTS

- **Structure:** The interphalangeal (IP) joints of the toes are synovial joints with an articular capsule and two collateral ligaments. All the toes except for the great toe have two joints, called the proximal interphalangeal (PIP) joint and the distal interphalangeal (DIP) joint. The great toe has one IP joint between the two phalanges.

- **Function:** The IP joints serve to balance, stabilize, and coordinate the motions of the foot. They have two possible motions: flexion and extension.

- **Dysfunction and injury:** The toes can become inflamed through injury or from the cumulative stress of weight-bearing dysfunction in the foot. One result of acute or chronic inflammation is fibrosis of the joint capsule of the IP joints, leading to a condition called **hammer toes.** Hammer toes are hyperextension of MTP joints and flexion contracture of PIP. The term **claw toes** describes a condition in which the PIP and the DIP are held in a sustained flexion, combined with hyperextension of MTP joints. This hyperextension pulls the plantar plate distally, which leaves the weight-bearing heads of the metatarsals unprotected, causing painful metatarsalgia.[5] Both hammer toe and claw toe can develop if the intrinsic muscles of the foot are weak and the extrinsic toe flexors and extensors are held in sustained contraction.

- **Treatment implications:** Perform PIR MET on the toe flexors and extensors, and suggest exercises for the intrinsics of the toes, such as picking up a sock with the toes. Hammer toes and claw toes are often caused by a complex combination of factors. These conditions typically require a referral to a physical therapist or a personal trainer for proper instruction in a strengthening and stretching program.

SOFT TISSUE STRUCTURES OF THE FOOT

LIGAMENTS OF THE FOOT

The clinically important ligaments of the foot can be described by location (Fig. 10-10).

Ligaments of the Sole of the Foot

- The **long plantar ligament** arises from the calcaneus and attaches to the cuboid and bases of the metatarsals. It helps to support the arch.

Ligaments of the Metatarsophalangeal Joints

- The **plantar ligaments (plantar plate)** are thick, dense, fibrous or fibrocartilaginous structures firmly attached to the bases of the proximal phalanges but loosely attached to the heads of the metatarsal bones. They are grooved for the flexor tendons and serve to protect the articular surface of the metatarsal heads.

- The **transverse metatarsal ligaments** consist of four short bands that have both superficial and deep layers. The heads of all the metatarsals are connected together by the deep layer. The plantar digital nerve travels between the superficial and deep layers.

- The **collateral ligaments** are two strong, rounded cords, located on the medial and lateral sides of the MTP joints. These ligaments connect the head of the metatarsal to the base of the phalanx.

Ligaments of the Interphalangeal Joints

- The **collateral ligaments** wrap around the IP joints like a sleeve. The fibers are oriented in a proximal-to-distal direction following the shaft of the bone. They help to guide the flexion and extension movements of the IP joints.

- The **plantar ligament** is a fibrocartilaginous thickening of the joint capsule at the plantar surface of the joint.

- **Function:** As in each joint of the body, the joint capsule and associated ligaments provide passive stability to the joint and play a role in muscle function, coordination, and balance through reflexes between the mechanoreceptors of the ligaments and the surrounding muscles. The plantar plates are pulled distally with hyperextension of the toes to protect the metatarsal heads as the body weight rolls over the toes during walking.[5]

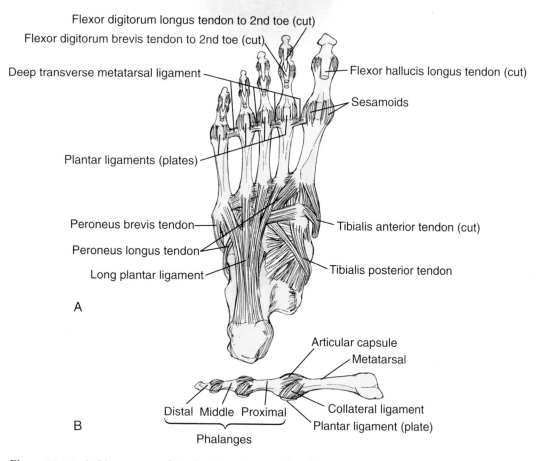

Flexor digitorum longus tendon to 2nd toe (cut)
Flexor digitorum brevis tendon to 2nd toe (cut)
Deep transverse metatarsal ligament
Flexor hallucis longus tendon (cut)
Sesamoids
Plantar ligaments (plates)
Peroneus brevis tendon
Tibialis anterior tendon (cut)
Peroneus longus tendon
Long plantar ligament
Tibialis posterior tendon
A

Articular capsule
Metatarsal
B
Distal Middle Proximal
Phalanges
Collateral ligament
Plantar ligament (plate)

Figure 10-10. A. Ligaments and tendon insertions on the plantar aspect (bottom) of the foot. **B.** Joint capsule and collateral ligaments of the MTP and IP joints. Note that the fibers of the joint capsule are aligned parallel to the shaft of the bone and that the collateral ligaments are angled in a dorsal to plantar direction.

■ **Dysfunction and injury:** The transverse metatarsal ligament is important clinically because it tends to thicken as a result of static or dynamic stresses. This thickening pulls the metatarsal heads closer together and causes an irritation of the joints. The thickening can also lead to an entrapment in the plantar digital nerve that travels through the superficial and deep layers and can potentially lead to a fibrous deposit, called a **neuroma,** on the nerve. The collateral ligaments of the IP joints can thicken because of inflammation as a result of injury or repetitive irritation and contribute to loss of IP joint motion and to hammer toes and claw toes (see above). Pain in the sole of the foot from the long plantar ligament can result from fatigue stress due to pronation. The plantar plate can misalign distally because of hammer and claw toes and leave the metatarsal heads exposed to excessive pressure in the push-off phase in gait.

■ **Treatment implications:** The ligaments of the foot are treated with two different strokes: either deep, back-and-forth scooping strokes transverse to the line of the fiber or brisk transverse friction strokes.

PLANTAR FASCIA

See Figure 10-11.

■ **Structure:** The plantar fascia is a thick sheet of connective tissue from the calcaneus to the proximal phalanx of each toe, interweaving with the deep transverse metatarsal ligament and plantar plate. It extends into four deep septa or connective tissue spaces that contain the muscles of the sole of the foot. The plantar fascia splits at the MTP joints to allow for the passage of the flexor tendons.[15]

■ **Function:** The plantar fascia contributes significantly to the longitudinal arch.

■ **Dysfunction and injury:** Irritation of the plantar fascia is called **plantar fasciitis** and can be caused by excessive dynamic loading, such as running, or by cumulative static stresses, such as excessive standing (working as a retail clerk, for example). It is associated with tight calf and hamstring muscles, which decrease ankle dorsiflexion and great toe extension. Irritation typically causes a pain on the

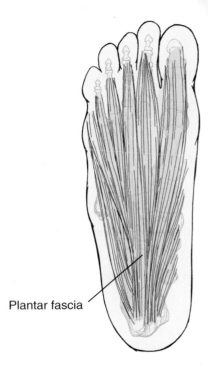

Plantar fascia

Figure 10-11. Plantar fascia on the sole of the foot.

heel, usually on the anterior medial surface, that is often worse in the morning but may also manifest as midfoot pain. The attachment of the fascia interweaves with the periosteum of the heel, and excessive pulling on the fascia and periosteum can cause a traction spur, called a **heel spur.** Heel spurs are typically painless and are found in approximately 10% of the nonsymptomatic population.[4]

■ **Treatment implications:** To treat plantar fasciitis, first perform PIR MET on the gastrocnemius, soleus, hamstrings, and flexors of the toes. Next, perform transverse massage on the plantar fascia, concentrating on the anterior-medial heel, and continue to the toes. To treat heel spurs, Lauren Berry, RPT, taught a method of using a blunt tool, such as the knuckle of the second MTP joint or a T-bar. Deep, brisk strokes are performed in all directions on the heel to dissolve small calcium spicules and fibrous depositions on the heel.

ARCHES OF THE FOOT

■ **Structure:** The foot has three distinct arches: the medial and lateral longitudinal archs and the transverse arch. The **longitudinal (medial) arch** describes the area from the calcaneus to the first metatarsal head. The lateral longitudinal arch is from the calcaneus through the cuboid and fifth metatarsal. The **transverse arch** describes the area of the midtarsal region, with the middle cuneiform as the highest point. The shape of the bones of the foot forms the longitudinal and transverse plantar

arches, which are maintained by ligamentous and muscular support. Genetic factors influence the height of the longitudinal arch.

□ **Ligamentous support:** The order of importance for ligamentous support for the arches is as follows: the spring ligament (plantar calcaneonavicular), the long plantar ligament, the plantar fascia, and the short plantar ligament (plantar calcaneocuboid).[15]

□ **Muscular support:** The anterior and posterior tibialis muscles and the intrinsic plantar muscles support the medial arch.

■ **Function:** The arches are designed as shock absorbers and provide mobility to accommodate uneven surfaces. They also protect the nerves, blood vessels, and muscles from compression.

■ **Dysfunction and injury:** The loss of the arches is referred to as **pes planus** or **flat foot.** This loss may be caused by femoral anteversion, pronation, weakness of the intrinsic plantar muscles, weakness of the anterior and posterior tibialis, or loss of plantar ligament integrity resulting from static stress, such as standing on the feet all day. Loss of the arch places much more stress on the plantar fascia, and the fascia tends to thicken. In a person who has flat feet, much more muscle action is required, which makes the muscles more susceptible to fatigue and pain.[10] A high arch is referred to as **pes cavus** and can involve short plantar ligaments, tight intrinsics of the sole of the foot, or tight anterior and posterior tibialis muscles. A rigid high arch has limited shock absorption, which increases the impact on the tibia and fibula, potentially leading to shin splints.

■ **Treatment implications:** To treat a high arch, perform MET on the anterior and posterior tibialis muscles, and provide manual release of the tight intrinsics with STM. A low arch is treated with exercise rehabilitation.

NERVES OF THE FOOT

See Figures 10-3 and 10-4.

■ **Structure:** The posterior tibial nerve branches into the medial and lateral plantar nerves. They continue as the interdigital nerves, traveling between the superficial and deep layers of the transverse metatarsal ligament. The deep peroneal nerve travels under the extensor retinaculum at the ankle. The superficial peroneal nerve travels under the skin into the dorsum of the foot. The sural nerve travels to the lateral heel.

■ **Function:** The medial and lateral plantar nerves supply the intrinsic muscles on the plantar aspect of the foot and give sensation to the bottom of the foot. The interdigital nerves receive sensory information from the toes. The deep peroneal nerve supplies the extensor digitorum brevis and the extensor hallucis brevis and provides sensation to the webspace between the first and the second toes. The superficial peroneal nerve supplies the skin to the dorsum of the foot. The sural nerve supplies sensation to the lateral heel and side of foot.

- **Dysfunction and injury:** Entrapment of the interdigital nerve is a frequent cause of metatarsal head pain.[4] Morton's neuroma is a chronic irritation of the interdigital nerve that results in a fibrous deposition on the nerve.

- **Treatment implications:** Release the interdigital nerves by first releasing the transverse metatarsal ligament. Next, gently mobilize the nerves transverse to the line of the nerve.

MUSCLES

- **Structure:** Intrinsic muscles of the feet consist of 20 muscles that have origins and insertions in the foot. Of these 20, 18 are on the sole of the foot and may be divided into four layers by their fascia. Extrinsic foot muscles consist of 11 muscles that have origins in the leg and insertions in the foot. Three tendons form a sling by crossing from one side of the foot to the opposite side. These three muscles assist in holding the foot in a neutral position and are the tibialis anterior and peroneus longus (these attach to the base of the first metatarsal) and the tibialis posterior (this attaches to the navicular, cuboid, and base of the second, third, and fourth metatarsals).

- **Function:** The extrinsic muscles help to support the arches, act as shock absorbers for the foot, and provide dynamic stability to the ankle and foot. The intrinsic muscles of the foot provide fine adjustments for coordination and balance, help to provide dynamic stability, and help to maintain the arch. The muscles of the foot have nerves that communicate with the surrounding joints through the joint capsules and ligaments. The mechanoreceptors in the capsules and ligaments sense position and movement in the joints and stimulate muscle contraction to coordinate movement and balance. Also, instantaneous righting reflexes occur from the foot to the muscles of the leg.

- **Dysfunction and injury:** Muscles of the feet are susceptible to cumulative stresses caused by dynamic activity and to the static stress of standing for prolonged periods. Intrinsic muscles are usually atrophied because of wearing shoes.[13] Strain of the foot muscles is associated with running, hiking, dancing, basketball, and other such activities. However, muscular activity provides the necessary stimulation to maintain adequate strength for dynamic stability.

With disuse, injury, pronation, or inadequate footwear, the muscles weaken, and the ligaments and capsules are excessively loaded, leading to collapse of the arches of the foot and pain in the soft tissue.

Muscle Imbalances of the Leg, Ankle, and Foot

- **Muscles that tend to be tight and short:** The extrinsic plantar flexors and the extensors of the toes are usually tight and short muscles. The intrinsic muscles are usually tight but functionally weak because of the tightness-weakness phenomenon. The adductor hallucis is typically tight, contributing to hallux valgus.

- **Muscles that tend to be inhibited and weak:** The extrinsic dorsiflexors are usually tight but functionally weak because of the tightness-weakness phenomenon. The abductor hallucis and the intrinsic muscles, including the lumbricals and interossei, are usually functionally weak, except for the adductor hallucis.

Positional Dysfunction of the Muscles of the Leg, Ankle, and Foot

- The gastrocnemius and soleus (Achilles tendon) and the flexor hallucis brevis tend to be pulled laterally. The intrinsic muscles of the foot do not have positional dysfunctions.

INTRINSIC MUSCLES OF THE FOOT

See Muscle Table 10-4 and Figures 10-12, 10-13, 10-14, and 10-15.

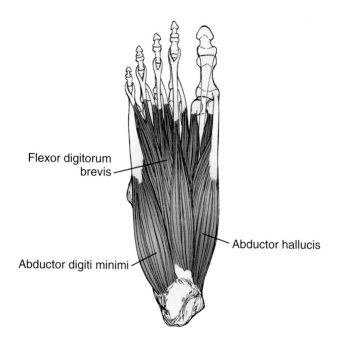

Figure 10-12. First layer of muscles on the plantar aspect of the foot includes the abductor hallucis, flexor digitorum brevis, and the abductor digiti minimi.

Table 10-4   Intrinsic Muscles of the Foot

Muscle	Origin	Insertion	Action	Dysfunction
First Layer				
Abductor hallucis	Medial process of the tuberosity of the calcaneus.	Base of medial side of proximal phalanx of the great toe and the medial sesamoid bone.	Abducts and flexes the great toe and the metatarsophalangeal joint (MTP).	Weakness allows hallux valgus. Abductor hallucis strain is associated with pronation and leads to pain along medial longitudinal arch.
Flexor digitorum brevis	Medial process of the tuberosity of the calcaneus and the medial part of the plantar fascia.	By four thin tendons on the middle phalanges of the four lateral toes; at the base of the corresponding phalange, the tendon divides into two slips perforated by the tendon of the flexor digitorum longus.	Flexes the proximal interphalangeal joint and the MTP joint.	Tightness decreases extension of the toes and contributes to claw toe deformity. Weakness reduces the strength of toe flexion and reduces the stability of the foot.
Abductor digiti minimi	Medial and lateral tuberosity of calcaneus; plantar fascia.	Lateral side of the proximal phalanx of the fifth toe.	Abducts and flexes the fifth toe.	Weakness contributes to instability of the foot.
Second Layer				
Quadratus plantae (flexor digitorum accessorius)	Arises by two heads from the plantar surface of the calcaneus separated by the long plantar ligament.	Lateral side of the tendon of the flexor digitorum longus muscle.	Contracts simultaneously with the flexor digitorum longus, stabilizing the pull of the tendon by decreasing the obliquity of the pull relative to the axis of the foot.	Weakness decreases the ability of the flexor digitorum to perform effectively.
Lumbricals I–IV	Arises from the tendons of the flexor digitorum longus.	End on the medial sides of the four lateral toes, attached to the dorsal digital expansions of the proximal phalanges, just as in the hand.	Flexion of the MTP joint and extension of the interphalangeal joint by pull on extensor hood, as in the hand.	Weakness of lumbricals contributes to claw toe deformity and is found in cases of metatarsal arch strain.
Third Layer				
Flexor hallucis brevis	From the plantar surface of the cuboid and the lateral cuneiform and the tendon of the tibialis posterior.	By two heads that contain the sesamoid bones of the great toe and to the medial and lateral sides of the base of the proximal phalanx of the great toe.	Flexes the great toe.	Weakness contributes to hammer toe and decreases the stability of the longitudinal arch.
Flexor digiti minimi brevis	Base of the fifth metatarsal and the sheath of the peroneus longus.	Lateral side of the proximal phalanx of the fifth toe.	Flexes the fifth toe.	Sustained tightness holds the proximal phalanx in flexion, preventing adequate toe extension.

Table 10-4		Intrinsic Muscles of the Foot (*Continued*)		
Muscle	*Origin*	*Insertion*	*Action*	*Dysfunction*
Adductor hallucis—oblique head	Bases of metatarsals 2 through 4, sheath of tendon of peroneus longus muscle.	Lateral side of the base of the proximal phalanx of the great toe; lateral sesemoid bone.	Adducts the great toe.	Weakness associated with metatarsal arch strain and instability of foot.
Adductor hallucis—transverse head	Plantar metatorsophalangeal ligaments of the three lateral toes; deep transverse metatarsal ligament.	Lateral side of the base of the proximal phalanx of the great toe; lateral sesamoid bone.	Adducts the great toe.	Tightness contributes to hallux valgus deformity.
Fourth Layer				
Dorsal interossei I through IV	Each arises by two heads from adjacent sides of two metatarsal bones (i.e., they are between the metatarsals).	Attach to the bases of the proximal phalanges and to the dorsal digital expansions (extensor hood).	Abduct the toes from the midline of the foot.	Weakness of the plantar and dorsal interossei contributes to hammer toe deformity and decreased stability of the transverse arch.
Plantar interossei I through III	Three muscles below, rather than between, the interossei; arise from the bases and medial sides of the third to fifth metatarsals.	Attached to the medial sides of the bases of the proximal phalanx of the same toes and into the dorsal digital expansion.	Adduct the lateral three toes to the midline of the foot.	

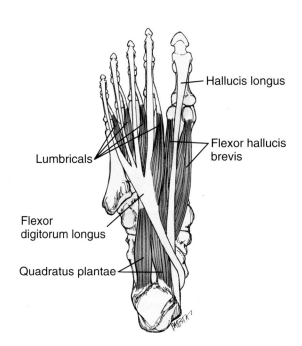

Figure 10-13. Second layer of plantar muscles includes the quadratus plantae and the four lumbrical muscles.

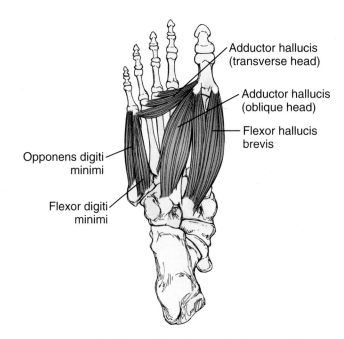

Figure 10-14. Third layer of muscles on the bottom of the foot includes the flexor hallucis brevis, flexor digiti minimi, opponens digiti minimi, and oblique and transverse heads of the adductor hallucis.

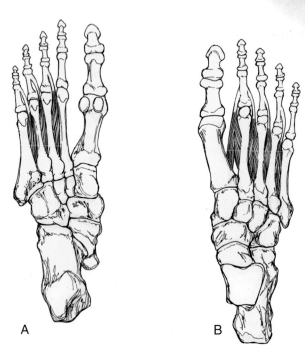

Figure 10-15. **A.** Plantar interossei are one part of the fourth layer of muscles on the plantar aspect of the foot. **B.** Dorsal interossei are also part of the fourth layer of muscles on the plantar aspect of the foot.

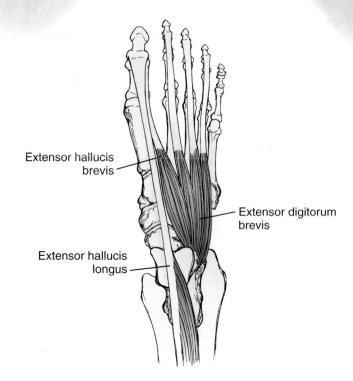

Figure 10-16. Intrinsic muscles on the dorsum of the foot include the extensor hallucis brevis and the extensor digitorum brevis.

MUSCLES OF THE DORSUM OF THE FOOT

See Figure 10-16 and Table 10-5.

MUSCULAR ACTIONS OF THE FOOT

See Table 10-6.

Table 10-5	Muscles of the Dorsum of the Foot			
Muscle	*Origin*	*Insertion*	*Action*	*Dysfunction*
Extensor digitorum brevis	Lateral and dorsal surface of the calcaneus	Dorsal expansion of the three middle toes	Extension of the toes; assist in dorsiflexion of the ankle	Weakness of these two muscles contributes to instability of the foot, and to flat foot. Tightness contributes to claw toe deformity.
Extensor hallucis brevis	Dorsal surface of the calcaneus	Base of the first phalanx of the great toe	Extension of the great toe and dorsiflexion of the ankle	

Table 10-6	Muscular Actions of the Foot

The foot is capable of inversion, eversion, plantarflexion, dorsiflexion, and circumduction. Inversion is the combination of adduction (moving the forefoot toward the midline), supination (elevation of the medial margin), and plantarflexion. Eversion is abduction (moving toes away from the midline of the foot), pronation (lowering of the medial margin of the foot), and dorsiflexion. The toes may be flexed, extended, abducted, or adducted. For simplification, I have followed Platzer (See "Suggested Readings") and equate inversion with supination and eversion with pronation.

Supination and Inversion

- Triceps surae
- Tibialis posterior
- Flexor hallucis longus
- Flexor digitorum longus
- Tibialis anterior

Toe Flexion

- Flexor digitorum longus
- Flexor hallucis longus
- Flexor digitorum brevis
- Flexor hallucis brevis
- Adductor hallucis—also adducts
- Lumbricals
- Quadratus plantae

Toe Extension

- Extensor digitorum longus and brevis
- Extensor hallucis longus and brevis

Pronation and Eversion

- Peroneus longus
- Peroneus brevis
- Extensor digitorum longus
- Peroneus tertius

Abduction

- Abductor hallucis
- Abductor digiti minimi
- Dorsal interossei

Adduction

- Adductor hallucis
- Plantar interossei

Dysfunction and Injury of the Leg, Ankle, and Foot

FACTORS PREDISPOSING TO PAIN IN THE LEG, ANKLE, AND FOOT

- Leg-length inequality
- Pelvic unleveling
- Femoral anteversion
- Genu valgum or genu varum
- Pronation (valgus position of the talus or calcaneus) or supination (varus position of the talus or calcaneus)
- Flat feet (foot pronation) or abnormally high arch
- Abnormal gait
- Loss of extension of the great toe (less than 45° to 60° of extension is problematic)
- Fatigue from static or dynamic stress, such as prolonged standing (static) or running (dynamic)
- Immobilization, which weakens the tissue
- Previous injury

DIFFERENTIATION OF LEG, ANKLE, AND FOOT PAIN

It is important to realize that pain in the leg, ankle, and foot can come from disease processes rather than from injuries or dysfunctions of the neuromusculoskeletal system. See the section "Contraindications to Massage Therapy: Red Flags" in Chapter 2, "Assessments and Technique" for guidelines on when massage is contraindicated and when to refer the client to a doctor.

The leg, ankle, and foot are common areas where pain, numbing, or tingling is referred from the lumbosacral spine. Perform the straight-leg raising (SLR) test to help determine if the pain in the leg originates in the lumbosacral spine. As is mentioned in Chapter 3, "Lumbosacral Spine," one type of referred pain is caused by muscle, ligament, joint capsule, disc, or dura mater. These tissues elicit what is called **sclerotomal** pain when they are injured. The sclerotomal pain is usually described as *deep, aching, and diffuse.* A second type of referred pain, called **radicular** pain, is caused by an irritation of the spinal nerve root. If the sensory (dorsal) root is irritated, *sharp pain, numbing, or tingling that is well localized* occurs in what are called dermatomes. A dermatome is an area of the skin supplied by the sensory root of a single spinal nerve (see Chapter 3 for an illustration of the dermatomes). If there is compression of the motor (ventral) nerve root, in addition to pain, numbing, and tingling, weakness can occur in the muscles supplied by that nerve root, called *myotomes.* The relevant myotomes of the leg, ankle, and foot are as follows: L4 is ankle dorsiflexion; L5 is great-toe extension; and S1 is ankle eversion.

The entrapment of a peripheral nerve in the region of the leg, ankle, and foot can also lead to pain, numbing, or weakness. In peripheral entrapment, manual pressure over the entrapped nerve typically increases the symptoms temporarily. This increase in symptoms is an indication for treatment. The treatment that is described in this text to release the peripheral nerves is so effective that if your treatment does not resolve the symptoms in several sessions, refer the client to a chiropractor or an osteopath for spinal evaluation.

Differentiation of other conditions can be categorized according to the region that is involved.

■ Sudden, severe pain in the mid-calf is often a gastrocnemius or soleus strain. Isometric challenge to plantar flexion or raising on the toes is painful.

■ A dull aching in the leg that increases with activity is often a chronic compartment syndrome that progresses to a shin splint.

■ An ankle sprain usually results from an acute episode, leading to well-localized pain, most commonly at the anterior portion of the distal fibula. A ligament sprain is painless with isometric challenge and is painful with passive stretching.

■ Pain in the ankle region can also be a tendinitis or a tenosynovitis of the extrinsic foot muscles. The pain is increased with isometric challenge.

■ Pain on the bottom of the foot or heel is usually plantar fasciitis, but pain on the bottom of the heel can be fat pad syndrome, also called *bruised heel.* Numbing and tingling on the bottom of the foot can be tarsal tunnel syndrome.

■ Pain across the ball of the foot is typically metatarsalgia.

■ Pain on the bottom of the great toe is often sesamoiditis (application of manual pressure to the painful sesamoid confirms this condition). Chronic diffuse aching pain and stiffness in the region of the first MTP joint is often a degeneration of the cartilage of the great toe, a sign of osteoarthritis.

COMMON DYSFUNCTIONS AND INJURIES IN THE LEG, ANKLE, AND FOOT

GASTROCNEMIUS STRAIN (TENNIS LEG)

■ **Causes:** Gastrocnemius strain is the most common muscle injury to the leg. It involves a strain of the musculotendinous junction of the medial head of the gastrocnemius. Increased intensity or duration of running or activities that involve quick movements of plantar flexion, such as tennis, racquet sports, basketball, and dance, cause this strain.

■ **Symptoms:** Gastrocnemius strain symptoms are often described as a sudden, severe pain in the mid-calf followed by muscle spasms in the calf and pain in walking. The injury site is nearly always at the musculotendinous junction of the medial gastrocnemius in the mid-calf.

■ **Signs:** Clients experience muscle spasm in the calf, painful knots in the medial aspect of the mid-calf, pain with raising on the toes, and pain with passive dorsiflexion.

■ **Treatment:** For **acute** gastrocnemius tendinitis, first perform CR MET and RI MET (MET #3, knee, performed as CR and RI) to reduce pain, swelling and hypertonicity. Next, perform gentle STM (third stroke of the first series) to promote nutritional exchange and cellular synthesis. In **chronic** conditions, the gastrocnemius tends to be short and tight, with thickened fascia, which contributes to decreased dorsiflexion of the ankle and weakness in the muscles of the anterior compartment. Perform PIR MET to lengthen the gastrocnemius (MET #3, knee) and soleus (MET #8) and STM to dissolve the adhesions (Levels I and II, third series).

ACHILLES TENDINITIS

Causes: Achilles tendinitis is the most common tendinitis of the foot and ankle, and the Achilles tendon is the most commonly ruptured tendon in the body. It involves a tearing of the tendon caused by prolonged or excessive activity that fatigues the tissue. Common activities that cause this condition are running, hiking, skiing, and dancing. Predisposing factors are tight gastrocnemius and soleus muscles, poor footwear, pronation, sudden increase in the intensity of activities, and joint stiffness at the ankle or subtalar joint.

Symptoms: Achilles tendinitis is painful at two common sites: (1) where the tendon inserts into the calcaneus and (2) in the main body of the tendon about 1.5 inches above the heel. The pain worsens with activity. The area feels stiff, especially when the client first gets out of bed in the morning. If unresolved, it develops into thick, fibrous tissue, which potentially weakens the tissue because of decreased blood supply.

Signs: Clients experience pain on resisted plantar flexion or when standing on tiptoes. The area is tender to palpation, is swollen if it is inflamed, and is enlarged and fibrotic if it is chronic.

Treatment: Acute tendinitis is treated with CR MET and RI MET for the hamstrings (MET #5, hip), gastrocnemius (MET #3, knee), and soleus (MET #8) to reduce pain, swelling, and hypertonicity. Gentle STM is performed to promote nutritional exchange and cellular synthesis (Level I, third series). **Chronic** conditions are treated with the same METs as were described above, but they are performed as PIR MET to lengthen the tissue. STM is used to dissolve the adhesions (Level I, second and third series, and Level II, third series).

ANKLE SPRAIN

Causes: Ankle sprain is usually an incident of a sudden plantar flexion and inversion twist to the ankle or of repetitive inversion stress. The anterior talofibular ligament is the most commonly injured ligament in the body.

Symptom: An ankle sprain elicits pain at the anterolateral ankle, occurring anterior to the distal fibula.

Signs: Clients experience localized swelling within hours or days of the injury depending on the severity, and the swelling can progress to diffuse bruising if extensive tissue tearing has occurred. Passive inversion with plantar flexion elicits pain at the anterolateral ankle.

Treatment: Acute ankle sprains are treated with CR and RI MET (MET #1) to reduce pain and swelling and to help prevent muscle inhibition. Pain-free motion is begun as early as it can be tolerated. After performing the MET, gently rock the ankle in small arcs of dorsal-plantar flexion to help promote nutritional and cellular exchange and to maintain joint play. Gentle STM is performed to promote alignment and mobility of the healing fibers (Level I, fourth series, and Level II second series). With an acute injury, it is important to exert only light pressure so as not to disturb the healing fibers. In **chronic** conditions, if the ligaments do not heal properly, they repair themselves to a state that is too loose (unstable) or too tight, leading to stiffness in the ankle joint and degeneration. Unstable ligaments need exercise to improve muscle strength and to increase ligament density, as well as balance exercises, such as a wobble board, to rehabilitate the proprioceptive nerves. Dense, fibrotic ligaments need to be lengthened, and the joint needs to be mobilized. Perform MET to the muscles crossing the ankle (METs #1, #2, and #3) to increase the extensibility of the ligaments, and for the gastrocnemius (MET #3, knee) and soleus (MET #8). Next, perform the Level I series of strokes to the leg, ankle, and foot, concentrating on Level I, fourth series. Mobilize the ankle (Level II, sixth series) to help restore joint play and normal ROM.

PLANTAR FASCIITIS AND HEEL SPURS

Causes: Tight Achilles tendon, decreased motion of the great toe, static stress of prolonged standing or excessive walking, running, hiking, and dancing cause plantar fasciitis and heel spurs. Irritation of the fascia can cause a traction spur on the heel.

Symptom: Pain is usually well localized over the anteromedial calcaneus but may radiate distally. These conditions are often painful when the foot hits the ground, especially when the client gets out of bed in the morning.

Signs: Clients experience pain that can be reproduced by full passive dorsiflexion of the ankle and all the toes. Also, palpation of the fascia on the anteromedial heel is painful.

■ **Treatment: Acute** plantar fasciitis is first treated with CR MET and RI MET for the hamstrings (MET #5, hip), gastrocnemius (MET #3, knee), and soleus (MET #8) to help reduce pain and swelling by contracting and relaxing the muscles of the posterior leg, which interweave with the plantar fascia. Next, perform MET for the flexors of the toes (METs #4 and #5). Gentle STM is performed to promote nutritional exchange and to promote alignment and mobility of the healing fibers (Level I, fifth series). For **chronic** plantar fasciitis, repeat the protocol for acute conditions but with greater resistance with the MET, including a contract-relax-antagonist-contract (CRAC) MET for the hamstrings (MET #10, hip), and use greater depth for the STM. Level II, fifth series, is performed to dissolve adhesions on the attachments of the fascia to the calcaneus, and to clean the bone of calcium spicules.

POSTEROMEDIAL SHIN SPLINT

■ **Cause:** A posteromedial shin splint is a tenoperiosteal or fascial tear of the soleus or tibialis posterior that is induced by a sudden increase in the duration or intensity of an exercise, usually running. Predisposing factors include leg-length differences, muscle imbalances, excessive valgus heel, excessive pronation, inadequate or worn-out shoes, or running on hard surfaces or on uneven terrain.[7]

■ **Symptoms:** Dull, aching pain over the distal third of the medial leg is a symptom of posteromedial shin splint.

■ **Sign:** Pain with resisted plantar flexion and inversion implicates the tibialis posterior and pain with passive dorsiflexion and eversion of foot implicates the soleus.

■ **Treatment:** For **acute** conditions, first perform CR MET and RI MET for the soleus (MET #8) and tibialis posterior (MET #3). This helps to reduce the swelling and pain by gently pumping the area with cycles of contraction and relaxation. Next, perform gentle STM (Level I, second series, and Level I, third series). **Chronic** shin splints are treated with PIR MET for the soleus and posterior tibialis (METs #8 and #3) as well as METs to lengthen the fascia of the posterior leg, including the CRAC MET for the hamstrings (MET #10, hip) and PIR MET for the gastrocnemius (MET #3, knee). STM is performed with greater depth, concentrating on the tenoperiosteal attachments to the bone (Level I, first and second series, and Level II, third series).

ANTEROLATERAL SHIN SPLINT

■ **Causes:** Sudden and vigorous running, dancing, or jumping can lead to anterolateral shin splint. Anterolateral shin splint is considered a periosteal or fascial tear of the tibialis anterior, extensor hallucis longus, or extensor digitorum longus; these conditions must be differentiated from a stress fracture. A fracture typically presents as a local, pointed pain, with a hot, red area, not more than 1.5 inches in diameter over the tibia or fibula. Inflammation of the periosteum (periostitis) is a more diffuse pain.[1] The muscles in the anterior compartment are usually weak in comparison with the short, tight gastrocnemius and soleus.

■ **Symptoms:** Exercise-induced tightness and diffuse, dull aching in the middle third of the anterior leg that comes on gradually are symptoms of anterolateral shin splint. Occasionally, a sharp pain occurs with activity.

■ **Signs:** Clients experience pain with resisted dorsiflexion and passive plantar flexion, and the overlying skin can be edematous.

■ **Treatment:** For **acute** conditions, first perform CR MET and RI MET for the tibialis anterior (MET #1), extensor hallucis longus (MET #6), or extensor digitorum longus (MET #7). This helps to reduce the swelling and pain by gently pumping the area with cycles of contraction and relaxation. Next, perform gentle STM (Level I, first series, third stroke). **Chronic** shin splints are first treated by using the same METs as were described for acute conditions but using PIR MET instead to help lengthen the fascia and increase the extensibility of the tenoperiosteal attachments. STM is performed with greater depth, concentrating on the attachments of these muscles to the bone (Level I, first and second series, and Level II, first series).

PRONATION

■ **Causes:** A pronated foot is a valgus position of the calcaneus on the talus and a medial and inferior position of the subtalar joint, which lowers the medial arch, flattening the foot. When the client is observed standing from the rear, the heel angles laterally, and the Achilles tendon bows inward instead of its normal vertical alignment. Excessive pronation can be a result of weakness of the anterior and posterior tibialis, which dynamically support the arch, or it can be caused by a local structural dysfunction, such as a medial subluxation of the talus. Genetic factors are also a cause.

Symptoms: Pronation can be painless. If painful, it is usually along the medial arch, between the anterior heel to the great toe, because of the excessive tensile stress to the plantar fascia, short and long plantar ligaments, and the excessive loading of the intrinsic flexors. Leg pain can result from increased tension in the anterior and posterior tibialis, which dynamically support the arch.

Signs: Flattening of the medial arch, a valgus position of the heel, decreased dorsiflexion caused by a tight Achilles tendon, muscle atrophy or decreased tone in the plantar muscles, and a tenderness along the medial arch are signs of pronation.

Treatment: Clients with pronation need arch supports (orthotics) and supportive shoes to ensure that the foot and ankle are in a neutral position while standing. Manual therapy can help rehabilitate weakened muscles and stretch tight muscles. Stretch the gastrocnemius (MET #3, knee) and soleus (MET #8) with PIR MET and CR MET. Perform STM on the posterior compartment (Level I, second series, and Level II, third series). Perform METs to facilitate the anterior and posterior tibialis (METs #1 and #3). To help facilitate (strengthen) the intrinsic muscles of the feet and the anterior and posterior tibialis muscles as a home exercise program, instruct the client to rise up on the toes while externally rotating the leg and keeping the great toe planted on the floor. Another exercise for the client to perform is to use the toes to pick up a sock; this exercise strengthens the flexors of the toes, helping to dynamically support the medial arch. Repeat 50 times or until fatigue, whichever comes first.

METATARSALGIA

Cause: Metatarsalgia is a discomfort or pain around the metatarsal heads. It is a common inflammatory condition, defined as *metatarsophalangeal joint synovitis*, commonly occurring at the second, third, and fourth MTP joints. It may be due to trauma or weight-bearing imbalances such as pronation, tight Achilles tendon, the wearing of high-heeled shoes, obesity, and weak intrinsic toe flexors. Weak intrinsic toe flexors decrease the arch, which causes the weight to fall excessively on the heads of the metatarsals rather than through the passive and dynamic supporters of the arch.

Symptom: Gradual onset of pain at the metatarsal heads or at the MTP joints, especially in the toe-off phase of walking.

Signs: Digital pressure on the metatarsal heads is painful. Squeezing all the MTP joints together is painful. Commonly, a callus forms over the affected joint.

Treatment: **Acute** metatarsalgia is first treated with CR and RI for the flexors and extensors of the toes (METs #4 through #7). This helps to disperse the swelling and reduces pain. Perform STM for the plantar aspect of the feet (Level I, fifth and sixth series). Perform gentle joint mobilization for the metatarsals (Level II, sixth series). **Chronic** metatarsalgia is first treated with PIR MET for the gastrocnemius (MET #3, knee) and soleus (MET #8) and the same METs as are used for acute conditions but with greater pressure. Perform STM to stretch the Achilles tendon and posterior leg (Level I, third series), and perform manual release of the muscles attaching to the heads of the metatarsals and the transverse metatarsal ligament (Level I, fifth and sixth series, and Level II, fifth series). Perform gentle joint mobilization for the metatarsals (Level II, sixth series). Instruct the client on exercises to strengthen the muscles that support the arch; and if the foot is pronated, recommend an arch support (see "Pronation" above).

LESS COMMON DYSFUNCTIONS AND INJURIES

CHRONIC EXERTIONAL COMPARTMENT SYNDROME

Causes: High intermuscular pressure during exercise leading to ischemia and pain. Repetitive overuse leads to fibrosis and thickening of the fascia, preventing muscles from expanding during use.

Symptom: A sensation of tightness in the anterior or deep posterior compartments that develops into a gradual onset of pain with exercise. Typically, there is no pain at rest. If the anterior compartment is involved, pain is felt just lateral to the anterior border of the shin, and pins and needles are felt in the webspace of the great toe. If the deep posterior compartment is involved, clients report an ache in the medial border of the tibia or chronic calf pain.

Sign: Generalized tightness to palpation of the involved compartment, with areas of excessive thickening. Isometric challenge of the involved muscles might elicit pain.

Treatment: Perform CR MET and PIR MET for the muscles of the involved compartment to decrease the hypertonicity, lengthen the fascia, and promote gliding of the muscles within the compartments. Use STM to release the muscles of the involved compartment.

TIBIALIS ANTERIOR TENDINITIS AND TENOSYNOVITIS

- **Cause:** This tendinitis results from overuse of ankle dorsiflexors due to decreased ROM in the ankle. The tibialis anterior is typically weak, often inhibited by a short and tight gastrocnemius and soleus or a pronated foot. It is the principal decelerator of the foot at heel strike.[16]

- **Symptom:** Pain from tenosynovitis is usually well localized to the musculotendinous junction, approximately 6 inches above the ankle or at the anterior ankle, just below the superior extensor retinaculum and at tendon insertion near the medial cuneiform.

- **Signs:** Clients experience localized pain at the base of the first metatarsal and cuneiform or at the dorsal aspect of the midfoot with resisted dorsiflexion and inversion and pain with passive plantar flexion and foot eversion.

- **Treatment:** Perform MET (MET #1) and STM for the tibialis anterior (Level I, first and fourth series, and Level II, first and second series).

TIBIALIS POSTERIOR TENDINITIS AND TENOSYNOVITIS

- **Cause:** The most common cause of medial ankle pain is tibialis posterior tendinitis.[8] The tibialis posterior usually is in a lengthened contraction because of foot pronation, and therefore it is eccentrically loaded, predisposing it to irritation. It is usually an overuse injury rather than an acute trauma.

- **Symptoms:** Tibialis posterior tendinitis and tenosynovitis manifest in three common sites of pain: on the tendon proximal to the medial malleolus, on the tendon posterior to the ankle, and on the tenoperiosteal junction on the navicular.

- **Sign:** Clients experience pain on resisted inversion and plantar flexion or on full passive eversion and dorsiflexion. These movements may be done with the client standing. Ask the client to invert the foot and rise up on the toes.[17]

- **Treatment:** Perform MET (MET #3) and STM (Level I, first through third series, and Level II, first series) for the tibialis posterior.

PERONEUS LONGUS AND BREVIS TENDINITIS AND TENOSYNOVITIS

- **Causes:** Peroneal tendinitis is the most common overuse injury causing lateral ankle pain.[8] The peroneal tendons pass immediately behind the lateral malleolus and are held next to the bone by a retinaculum. They are surrounded by synovium and, when irritated, can cause a tenosynovitis. If the tunnel narrows because of scarring, a stenosing synovitis can develop. Tight ankle plantarflexors (gastrocnemius, soleus), which results in excessive load on the lateral muscles and excessive eversion, are predisposing factors.[18]

- **Symptoms:** Pain at the base of the fifth metatarsal for brevis and pain in the bony groove of the cuboid for the longus tendon are tendinitis symptoms. A symptom of tenosynovitis is pain behind the lateral malleolus.

- **Sign:** Clients experience pain on resisted eversion and plantar flexion or pain on full passive dorsiflexion and inversion.

- **Treatment:** Perform MET (MET #2) and STM (Level I, first and fourth series, and Level II, first and second series) to release the peroneus longus and brevis and mobilization of the subtalar and midtarsal joints (Level II, sixth series).

HALLUX LIMITUS AND HALLUS RIGIDUS SYNDROME

- **Cause:** Hallux limitus is a restriction of great toe extension due to shortening of the great toe joint capsule. Hallus rigidus is degenerative arthrosis of the first MTP joint. The cause of a shortened capsule is either repetitive stress, such as excessive weight bearing due to pronation, that creates inflammation and eventual fibrosis or an acute event that involves stubbing or catching of the great toe ("turf toe"). The trauma creates inflammation, leading to thickening of the joint capsule and potentially to degeneration.

- **Symptom:** Limited motion and pain in the first MTP joint, especially in the push-off phase of walking, are symptoms of hallux limitus or hallus rigidus syndrome.

- **Sign:** Limited extension of the great toe caused by degenerative joint disease of the first MTP is a sign of this syndrome. The toe can become fixed in slight plantar flexion and have bone spurs that enlarge the dorsal margin of the joint.

- **Treatment:** Perform MET for the flexors and extensors of the great toe (METs #5 and #6) to increase the extensibility of the soft tissue interweaving with the capsular tissues. Perform STM of the intrinsic and extrinsic muscles that attach to the great toe, the collateral ligaments, and the joint capsule (Level I, fourth and sixth series, and Level II, fifth and sixth series). Perform mobilization of the first MTP joint in dorsal-plantar glide (Level II, sixth series) to rehydrate the joint and restore accessory motion to allow for greater extension.

HALLUX VALGUS

▦ **Causes:** Hallux valgus is a lateral subluxation of the great toe and a medial deviation of the first metatarsal, and it often progresses to degenerative joint disease of the first MTP (hallux limitus or rigidus), bunion formation, and lateral subluxation of the sesamoids. Heredity, weight distribution problems such as pelvic obliquity, genu valgus, sustained contracture of the adductor hallucis, and pronated ankles can cause hallux valgus.

▦ **Symptom:** Lateral deviation at the first MTP joint is a symptom of hallux valgus syndrome.

▦ **Signs:** Lateral deviation of the great toe and medial deviation of the head of the first metatarsal are signs of this syndrome. Often, a bunion develops over the medial side of the head of the first metatarsal. A *bunion* is a combination of a callus, thickened bursa, and excessive bone (exostosis).

▦ **Treatment:** Establish correct posture; establish normal alignment of the pelvis; and normalize the function of the hips, knees, ankles, and feet. Release the adductor hallucis (Level I, sixth series), and show the client how to strengthen the abductor hallucis with MET by moving the great toe medially and trying to hold it in that position against resistance. Refer the client to a chiropractor or a podiatrist for a foot orthotic.

SESAMOIDITIS OF THE GREAT TOE

▦ **Causes:** Sesamoiditis is an inflammation of the capsule surrounding the sesamoids. Trauma, such as a fall onto the feet, dancing, or sprinting; a high arch; the wearing of high-heeled shoes; or the lateral deviation of the sesamoids from hallux valgus are often causes of this condition.

▦ **Symptom:** Pain under the great toe with weight bearing is a symptom of sesamoiditis.

▦ **Sign:** Clients experience pain with passive extension and resisted flexion of the great toe. The sesamoids might be tender to palpation, and the area might be swollen.

▦ **Treatment: Acute** sesamoiditis requires very gentle METs of the flexors of the great toe (MET #5) as well as CR MET and RI MET for the abductor and adductor hallucis to disperse the swelling and reduce the hypertonicity of the muscles interweaving with the sesamoids. Perform gentle STM, and gently mobilize the sesamoids (Level II, sixth series). Chronic

conditions require the same treatment as was described above but with greater depth if there are fibrotic deposits in the area.

HAMMER TOES AND CLAW TOES

▦ **Causes:** Hammer toes and claw toes are often associated with a high arch (pes cavus), weak lumbricals and interossei, and sustained contraction of both the extensor and flexor digitorum longus, which increases the passive tension on the extrinsic toe flexors.[15] Hammer and claw toes are also the result of fibrosis of the joint capsules of the IP joints.

▦ **Symptom:** Pain or cramping in the toes is a symptom of these conditions.

▦ **Signs:** Hammer toes involve hyperextension of the MTP joints and flexion contracture of the PIP joints. Claw toes involve hyperextensions of the MTP joints and flexion of the PIP and DIP joints.

▦ **Treatment:** Instruct the client in home exercises to strengthen the lumbricals and interossei: Flex the MTP joint while walking by pressing the MTP joint into the floor,[19] and attempt to spread and extend the toes in a relaxed standing posture. Perform PIR MET for the flexors and extensors of the toes (METs #4 through #7). Perform the entire series of Level I STM strokes on the anterior and posterior compartments and the feet to dissolve adhesions and increase the extensibility of the soft tissue. Release the joint capsule of the MTP and IP joints (Level II, fifth series), and perform joint mobilization on the toes (Level II, sixth series).

COMMON PERONEAL NERVE ENTRAPMENT AT THE FIBULA

▦ **Causes:** Entrapment of the common peroneal nerve at the fibula is caused by repetitive running or jumping, especially if there is foot inversion with plantar flexion, because the nerve passes through an opening in the origin of the peroneus longus as the anterolateral fibular neck, just inferior to the head of the fibula. The nerve is also susceptible to direct trauma from impact to the nerve.

▦ **Symptoms:** Clients experience sharp, localized pain; numbing; or tingling at the anterolateral fibular head and neck. This pain radiates distally down the lateral leg and creates pain on the dorsum of the foot. Loss of dorsiflexion and eversion of the foot and dorsiflexion of the toes occur, resulting in "foot drop." Also, clients experience a usually temporary loss of sensation over the dorsum of the foot.

▦ **Sign:** Pain that can be reproduced by digital stroking of the nerve at the fibula and a positive SLR with the foot inverted and plantar flexed are signs of this type of nerve entrapment.

■ **Treatment:** Perform transverse release of the nerve at the anterolateral fibular head and neck (Level II, first series).

SUPERFICIAL PERONEAL NERVE ENTRAPMENT

■ **Cause:** Trauma, running, tight braces or casts, lateral compartment syndrome, and inversion sprains can cause an entrapment of the superficial peroneal nerve.

■ **Symptoms:** Pain, burning, numbness, or tingling on the dorsum of the foot are symptoms of entrapment.

■ **Signs:** With superficial peroneal nerve entrapment, there are no reproducible signs.

■ **Treatment:** Perform MET for the peroneals (MET #2) and gentle STM of the lateral leg and dorsum of the foot (Level I, first and fourth series).

DEEP PERONEAL NERVE ENTRAPMENT

■ **Causes:** Tight-fitting boots, ankle sprains, and excessive running leading to fibrosis of the extensor retinaculum are causes of deep peroneal nerve entrapment.

■ **Symptoms:** Pain, tingling, or numbing between the first and second toes. The nerve can become entrapped under the superior and inferior extensor retinaculum at the ankle. The medial branch can be compressed as it travels under the extensor hallucis brevis and the lateral branch can be compressed as it travels under the extensor digitorum longus tendons.[20]

■ **Signs:** Deep peroneal nerve entrapment is primarily a motor condition and can lead to weak dorsiflexion. Digital pressure on the dorsum of the foot at the extensor retinaculum can cause symptoms.

■ **Treatment:** Perform gentle transverse release of the nerve at the dorsum of the foot and ankle (Level I, fourth series).

TARSAL TUNNEL SYNDROME (POSTERIOR TIBIAL NERVE ENTRAPMENT AT ANKLE)

■ **Causes:** The neurovascular bundle containing the posterior tibial nerve or its two terminal branches, the medial and lateral plantar nerves, can become compressed under the flexor retinaculum, under the abductor hallucis, or under the quadratus plantae. Tarsal tunnel is associated with pronated ankles.

■ **Symptoms:** Burning pain and a pins-and-needles sensation in the plantar aspect of foot or toes are symptoms of tarsal tunnel syndrome.

■ **Sign:** For tarsal tunnel, perform the hyperpronation test. Hold the ankle in hyperpronation for 60 seconds, and the burning, or pins-and-needles sensation may be reproduced.

■ **Treatment:** Perform gentle, transverse scooping strokes at the tarsal tunnel (Level II, second series).

PLANTAR DIGITAL NERVE ENTRAPMENT (MORTON'S NEUROMA)

■ **Causes:** This condition is not a true neuroma but consists of scar tissue and swelling arising from compression or abrasion of the nerve.[8] The nerve is entrapped in the transverse metatarsal ligament, usually between the third and fourth toes. Pronation, the wearing of high-heeled or tight-fitting shoes, weak intrinsic foot muscles, and the cumulative stress of running, hiking, or dancing can cause entrapment.

■ **Symptoms:** Burning or throbbing in the region of the metatarsal heads that moves to the toes, especially with walking are symptoms of entrapment. This pain can persist at night, and if the foot is chronically inflamed, a fibrous scarring around the nerve can develop.

■ **Signs:** Pain reproduced by squeezing the metatarsal heads together or by passively extending the toes is a sign of digital nerve entrapment.

■ **Treatment:** Perform MET for the flexors and extensors of the toes (METs #4 through #7), perform STM to release any sustained contracture in the foot (Level I, fifth and sixth series), and release the transverse metatarsal ligament and plantar nerve (Level II, fifth series). Instruct the client to strengthen the intrinsics by actively spreading the toes.

SURAL NERVE ENTRAPMENT

■ **Causes:** The sural nerve can be entrapped and irritated by tight-fitting boots or by a tight crural fascia.

■ **Symptoms:** Sural nerve entrapment symptoms are pain and burning along the posterior lateral leg, the lateral ankle, and the foot.

■ **Signs:** For this condition, there are no reproducible tests.

■ **Treatment:** Perform transverse release of the posterior leg, ankle, and lateral foot, especially posterior to the lateral malleolus (Level I, first through fourth series).

Assessment of the Leg, Ankle, and Foot

BACKGROUND

The leg, ankle, and foot are susceptible to acute and chronic conditions that commonly reflect overuse syndromes. Inability to bear weight, severe pain, and rapid swelling indicate a severe injury.[20] The leg is a common site of referral of pain, numbing, and tingling from irritation of the L4 and L5 nerve roots. If the client has pain, numbing, and tingling in the leg, ankle, and foot and active, passive, and isometric testing is strong, it indicates either peripheral entrapment of the nerve(s) or irritation of the lumbosacral nerve roots. Perform the SLR and femoral nerve stress tests (see Chapter 3). If these are negative, perform the strokes to release the peripheral nerves. If the client is unresponsive, refer him or her to a chiropractor or an osteopath. The leg is also a common site for overuse syndromes, such as shin splints and tendinitis.

The ankle is a common site of sprains, usually caused by an acute episode. The foot reflects local conditions, such as trauma, but it is much more common to have a fatigue-type pain in the feet caused by chronic weight distribution dysfunctions. This weight distribution dysfunction can be caused by obesity or by conditions such as pronation. The feet also reflect systemic conditions such as the neuritis and dermatitis of diabetes and can be a referral site from irritation of the L5 and S1–S2 nerve roots. Referral from the nerve roots can create pain, weakness, numbing, and tingling or weakness alone but not pain.

Normal function of the leg, ankle, and foot requires proper alignment of the lumbopelvic region and lower extremity as well as a balance of length and strength in the fascia and muscles that affect the lower extremity.

HISTORY QUESTIONS FOR THE CLIENT WHO HAS LEG, ANKLE, OR FOOT PAIN

- Is there some movement that you can do to elicit the pain?
  - ☐ This question is another way of asking what aggravates the pain. The client can often elicit local conditions in the leg, ankle, and foot if he or she moves in a certain way. One specific movement usually does not elicit conditions caused by chronic mis-

alignment or weight distribution dysfunctions, such as pronation. Also, referral of pain, numbing, or tingling cannot be generated or aggravated by active motion of the lower extremity.

INSPECTION AND OBSERVATION

- Have the client put on shorts so that you can see from the thighs to the feet. Observe for swelling, which may be diffuse and bilateral or localized at the lateral ankle. Localized bruising and swelling typically indicate an ankle sprain, whereas swelling without bruising would indicate previous injury with unresolved edema. Swelling in both feet indicates systemic problems, such as lymphatic congestion or circulatory problems.

- Notice if there are calluses resulting from pressure from shoes on the tops of the toes. Look for swelling over the medial side of the great toe, indicating a bunion.

ALIGNMENT OF THE TOES

- **Position:** The client is standing, facing the therapist, with feet shoulder width apart.

- **Observation:** Observe the alignment of the toes: Are they straight and parallel? Note whether the following conditions are present: hallux valgus, which is a lateral deviation of the big toe; hammer toes, which is a hyperextension of the metacarpophalangeal (MCP) and the DIP joints and flexion of the PIP; or claw toes, which is a hyperextension of the MCP and flexion of the PIP and DIP. The capsular pattern of the IP joints is that flexion is most limited.

ASSESSMENT OF THE LONGITUDINAL ARCH

- **Position:** The client is standing, facing the therapist, with feet shoulder width apart.

- **Action:** Place your fingertips on the medial arch.

- **Observation:** Feel for a low arch (pes planus/flatfoot) or a high arch (pes cavus). A low arch in weight bearing that normalizes in non-weight-bearing is a functionally low arch caused by muscle weakness or ligament laxity. To confirm your findings, have the client stand on tiptoes. A functional low arch will rise on tiptoes.

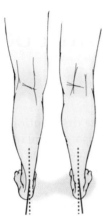

Figure 10-17. Assessment of the alignment of the Achilles tendon. Note that this client's tendons are angled medially (bowed in), a sign of pronation in the ankles. Also note that the heels are angled laterally, called valgus or eversion of the heel.

ASSESSMENT OF THE ACHILLES TENDON ALIGNMENT

▧ **Position:** The client is standing, facing away from the therapist, with feet shoulder-width apart (Fig. 10-17).

▧ **Action:** Observe the alignment of the Achilles tendon and heel.

▧ **Observation:** Note whether the Achilles tendon and heel are in their normal vertical alignment and the existence of any swelling of the Achilles tendon. If the tendon is bowed in and the heel is everted (angled laterally) with weight on the heel on the medial side, this is called **rearfoot valgus.** If the foot is also pronated and the medial longitudinal arch is lowered, this is called **pes planus.** If the Achilles tendon is bowed out and the heel is inverted, bringing the weight to the lateral side of the foot, this is **rearfoot varus.** If the foot is supinated and the medial longitudinal arch is higher, this is called **pes cavus.**

ACTIVE MOVEMENTS

GREAT-TOE EXTENSION TEST

▧ **Position:** The client is standing. Place your thumb under the great toe (Fig. 10-18).

▧ **Action:** Ask the client to lift the great toe into extension. Then continue the movement passively until the client experiences pain or tissue tension.

▧ **Observation:** Extension of the great toe should be approximately 45° to 60° to maintain normal gait. Decreased extension indicates hallux limitus, an

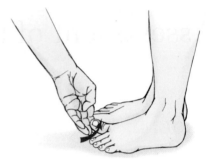

Figure 10-18. Great toe extension test. Have the client actively lift up the great toe. Continue the movement passively until pain or a resistance barrier is encountered.

early degeneration, and capsular fibrosis of the first MTP joint or possibly hallux rigidus, an advanced degeneration of the first MTP joint. Pain under the first MTP is usually sesamoiditis.

ACTIVE DORSIFLEXION

▧ **Position:** The client stands on one leg, next to a wall for support.

▧ **Action:** Ask the client to lift his or her toes and forefoot off the ground ten times or until there is pain or fatigue.

▧ **Observation:** This procedure is a good functional screening test for the anterior tibialis, extensor hallucis longus, and extensor digitorum longus. It is also an exercise to bring strength to those muscles. Pain is elicited with the anterolateral leg with shin splints or tendinitis of those muscles. Generally, ten to fifteen painless repetitions is considered functionally normal.[20] Painless weakness implicates an inhibition caused by short or tight plantar flexors or involvement of the L4–L5 and S1 nerve roots.

ACTIVE PLANTAR FLEXION

▧ **Position:** The client stands on one leg, next to a wall for support.

▧ **Action:** Ask the client rise up on the toes 10 times or until there is pain or fatigue.

▧ **Observation:** Pain at the Achilles tendon indicates Achilles tendinitis; pain at the lower posteromedial border of the tibia implicates a fascial irritation or tear of the soleus; and pain in the medial aspect of the mid-calf is usually a tendinitis of the gastrocnemius. Heel lifting also challenges the tibialis posterior, flexor digitorum longus, and flexor hallucis longus and elicits pain if there is a tendinitis in those muscles. This action is also a good screening test for plantar flexion strength, principally the gastrocnemius and soleus, and for function of the L4–L5 and S1–S2 nerve roots. Painless inability to lift up on the toes implicates a dysfunction or injury of those nerves. If the client cannot lift up on the toes, ask whether pain, weakness, or a lack of motion in the toes prevents this action. A client who has hallux rigidus cannot lift the heel far off the ground.

CLIENT SITTING

▨ **Position:** The client sits on the edge of the table.

▨ **Action:** Ask client to perform plantar flexion, dorsiflexion, inversion and eversion, toe flexion and extension, and abduction of the toes. Have the client perform these movements on both feet at the same time.

▨ **Observation:** Compare the ROM, and ask the client whether there is any pain.

PASSIVE MOVEMENTS

ANKLE PLANTAR FLEXION OR DORSIFLEXION

▨ **Position:** The client is supine. Hold the calcaneus with one hand, and invert the forefoot with the other hand to lock it into the hindfoot.

▨ **Action:** First lift the foot into dorsiflexion, and then press it into plantar flexion. The normal range is approximately 20° of dorsiflexion and 50° of plantar flexion.

▨ **Observation:** Painless restriction of dorsiflexion is often caused by previous ankle sprains. Pain with dorsiflexion implicates anterior impingement syndrome (capsular or synovial impingement at the anterolateral ankle), plantar fasciitis, posteromedial shin splint, or gastrocnemius tendinitis, depending on pain location. Pain with passive plantar flexion implicates an anterolateral shin splint, anterior tibialis tendinitis, or posterior impingement syndrome (an impingement of the posterior talus against the tibia).[8]

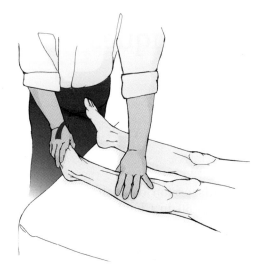

Figure 10-19. Assessment of the anterior talofibular ligament. Passively plantar flex and invert the foot.

ASSESSMENT FOR SPRAIN OF THE ANTERIOR TALOFIBULAR LIGAMENT

▨ **Position:** The client is supine. Stabilize the ankle with one hand, and place the other hand on the dorsum of the foot (Fig. 10-19).

▨ **Action:** Slowly plantar flex and invert the foot.

▨ **Observation:** A positive test is pain at the anterior inferior aspect of the fibula. The anterior talofibular is the most commonly injured ligament in the ankle.

ASSESSMENT FOR METATARSALGIA AND MORTON'S NEUROMA

▨ **Position:** The client is supine. Stabilize the ankle with one hand, and place the other hand around the toes at the MTP joints.

▨ **Action:** Slowly squeeze the metatarsal heads together.

▨ **Observation:** Pain in the region of the plantar aspect of the third and fourth toes is a positive sign for Morton's neuroma (i.e., a fibrous enlargement of the plantar digital nerve). Pain in the MTP joints is a positive sign for metatarsalgia.

Techniques

GUIDELINES TO APPLYING TECHNIQUES

A thorough discussion of treatment guidelines can be found on p. 86 in Chapter 2. In the method of treatment that is described in this text, we make two underlying assumptions. The first is that an injury or dysfunction in one structure causes compensations in the entire region of the injury as well as in other areas of the body. Tarsal tunnel syndrome, for example, is not an isolated condition but is influenced by the hip and knee, and the alignment of the ankle (pronation increases pressure on the nerve). It is important for the therapist to refer to other chapters to learn the protocol for assessment and treatment in each area involved.

The second assumption is that an injury or dysfunction that localizes in one tissue affects many other tissues in the area. An Achilles tendinitis, for example, involves not only the irritated tendon, but also the gastrocnemius and soleus muscles, the ankle joint (which loses dorsiflexion), ligaments, and capsular tissues. It is important for the therapist to assess and treat the surrounding muscles, tendons, ligaments, and joints of the leg, ankle, and foot in addition to treating the Achilles tendinitis.

The treatment protocols that are listed in the "Common Dysfunctions and Injuries" section typically limit the recommendations to a few specific guidelines regarding that particular condition. It is important to remember that in the clinical setting, it is necessary to take a more global approach and treat the entire person, rather than just the injured ankle. The treatments that are described in this text address all the structures of the region through three techniques: muscle energy technique (MET), soft tissue mobilization (STM), and joint mobilization. These techniques can be applied to every type of leg, ankle, and foot pain, but the "dose" of the technique varies greatly from slow movements and light pressures for acute conditions to stronger pressures and deeper amplitude mobilizations for chronic problems. Each aspect of the treatment is also an assessment to determine pain, tenderness, hypertonicity, weakness, and hypomobility or hypermobility. We use the philosophy of treating what we find when we find it. Remember that the goal of treatment is to heal the body, mind, and emotions. Keep your hands soft, keep your touch

nurturing, and work only within the comfortable limits of your client so that he or she can completely relax into the treatment.

THE INTENTIONS OF TREATMENT FOR ACUTE CONDITIONS ARE AS FOLLOWS

- To stimulate the movement of fluids to reduce edema, increase oxygenation and nutrition, and eliminate waste products.

- To maintain as much pain-free joint motion as possible to prevent adhesions and maintain the health of the cartilage, which is dependent on movement for its nutrition.

- To provide mechanical stimulation to help align healing fibers and stimulate cellular synthesis.

- To provide neurological input to minimize muscular inhibition and help maintain proprioceptive function.

 CAUTION: Stretching is **contraindicated** *in acute conditions.*

THE INTENTIONS OF TREATMENT FOR CHRONIC CONDITIONS ARE AS FOLLOWS

- To dissolve adhesions and restore flexibility, length, and alignment to the myofascia.

- To dissolve fibrosis in the ligaments and capsular tissues surrounding the joints.

- To rehydrate the cartilage and restore mobility and ROM to the joints.

- To eliminate hypertonicity in short and tight muscles, strengthen weakened muscles, and reestablish the normal firing pattern in dysfunctioning muscles.

- To restore neurological function by increasing sensory awareness and proprioception.

Clinical examples are described below under "Soft Tissue Mobilization."

MUSCLE ENERGY TECHNIQUE

THERAPEUTIC GOALS OF MUSCLE ENERGY TECHNIQUE

A thorough discussion of the clinical application of MET can be found on p. 76 in Chapter 2. The MET techniques described below are organized into one section for teaching purposes. In the clinical setting, MET and STM are interspersed throughout the session. MET is used for assessment and treatment. A healthy muscle or group of muscles is strong and pain-free when isometrically challenged. MET will be painful if there is ischemia or inflammation in the muscles or their associated joints. The muscle will be weak and painless if the muscle is inhibited or the nerve is compromised. During treatment, MET is used as needed. For example, when you find a tight and tender tibialis anterior, use CR MET to reduce the hypertonicity and tenderness. If the tibialis anterior is painful while contracting, perform a RI MET to induce a neurological relaxation. If the ankle dorsiflexors are weak and inhibited, first release the plantar flexors, and then use CR MET to recruit/strengthen the ankle dorsiflexors.

MET is very effective for an acute, painful leg, ankle, and foot, but the pressure that is applied must be very light so as not to induce pain. Gentle, pain-free contraction and relaxation of the ankle dorsiflexors and plantar flexors provides a pumping action to reduce swelling in the ankle and leg, promoting the flow of oxygen and nutrition, and eliminating waste products.

THE BASIC THERAPEUTIC INTENTIONS OF MET FOR ACUTE CONDITIONS ARE AS FOLLOWS

▨ Provide a gentle pumping action to reduce pain and swelling, promote oxygenation of the tissue, and remove waste products.

▨ Reduce muscle spasms.

▨ Provide neurological input to mimimize muscular inhibition.

THE BASIC THERAPEUTIC INTENTIONS OF MET FOR CHRONIC CONDITONS ARE AS FOLLOWS

▨ Decrease excessive muscle tension.

▨ Strengthen muscles.

▨ Lengthen connective tissue.

▨ Increase joint movement and increase lubrication to the joints.

▨ Restore neurological function.

The MET section below shows techniques that are used for most clients. In acute ankle sprains, use MET #1. All the other METs can be used for acute condions, except METs #5 and #8, which involve lengthening tissue. For chronic conditions, our goal is to treat the tight muscles before trying to strengthen weak muscles. Remember that the plantar flexors are typically short and tight, and the dorsiflexors are typically weak. It is important to realize that the muscles in the leg, ankle, and foot are often weak because of an irritation, injury, or dysfunction of the nerves in the lumbosacral spine.

Remember that MET should not be painful. Mild discomfort as the client resists the pressure is normal if the area is irritated or inflamed. Treat the entire region, referring to Chapter 8 and 9 for METs for the hip and knee, respectively.

MUSCLE ENERGY TECHNIQUE FOR ACUTE ANKLE PAIN

1. Contract-Relax Muscle Energy Technique for Acute Ankle Pain

▨ **Intention:** The intention is to contract and relax the muscles of plantar flexion and dorsiflexion. This CR cycle pumps the waste products and swelling out of the injured area, increases the nutritional exchange, and helps to realign the healing fibers.

 CAUTION: This type of MET is performed only within pain-free limits. Beneficial effects are achieved with only grams of pressure.

▨ **Position:** Client is supine with the ankle in a pain-free resting position. Place one hand on the dorsum (top) of the foot and the other hand under the ball of the foot (Fig. 10-20).

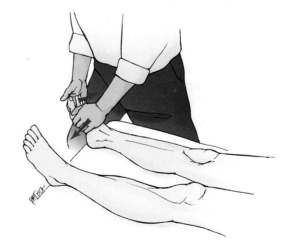

Figure 10-20. CR MET for acute ankle pain.

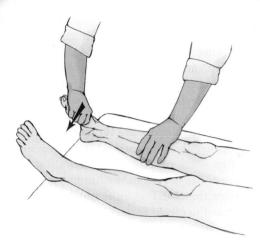

Figure 10-21. CR MET for the tibialis anterior.

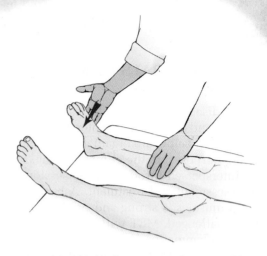

Figure 10-22. CR MET for the peroneus longus and brevis.

▨ **Action:** Have the client resist as you slowly and gently press the top of the foot toward plantar flexion for approximately 5 seconds. Relax for a few seconds. Have the client resist as you slowly and gently press up on the ball of the foot toward dorsiflexion. Relax, and repeat the cycle several times.

MUSCLE ENERGY TECHNIQUE FOR LEG, ANKLE, AND FOOT MUSCLES

1. *Contract-Relax Muscle Energy Technique for the Tibialis Anterior*

▨ **Intention:** The intention is to reduce the hypertonicity or to facilitate (strengthen) in the tibialis anterior. This MET is also treatment for anterolateral shin splints and tendinitis of the tibialis anterior.

▨ **Position:** Client is supine. Place one hand on the dorsum of the foot and the other hand on the tibialis anterior for a sensory cue (Fig. 10-21).

▨ **Action:** Have the client dorsiflex the ankle, invert the foot, and resist as you press toward plantar flexion and eversion.

▨ **Observation:** Painless weakness may be a result of L4 nerve root injury or dysfunction or of deep peroneal nerve entrapment.

2. *Contract-Relax Muscle Energy Technique for the Peroneus Longus and Brevis*

▨ **Intention:** The intention is to reduce the hypertonicity or to facilitate (strengthen) the peroneals.

▨ **Position:** Client is supine. Place one hand on the lateral foot and the other hand on the peroneals for a sensory cue (Fig. 10-22).

▨ **Action:** Have the client evert the foot with slight plantar flexion of ankle and resist as you press toward inversion and dorsiflexion.

▨ **Observation:** Painless weakness implicates a problem with the S1 nerve root. Pain at the lateral leg implicates injury to the peroneal muscles or a lateral shin splint. Pain behind the ankle indicates a tenosynovitis of the peroneals. Pain at the fifth metatarsal or cuboid indicates a tendinitis of the peroneus brevis or longus, respectively.

3. *Contract-Relax Muscle Energy Technique for the Tibialis Posterior*

▨ **Intention:** To reduce the hypertonicity or facilitate (strengthen) the tibialis posterior.

▨ **Position:** Client is supine. Hold the medial arch with one hand, and place the other hand on the posterior aspect of the medial tibia (Fig. 10-23).

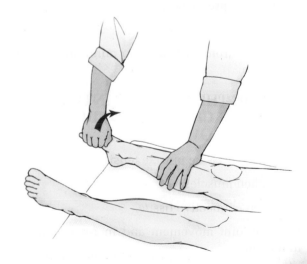

Figure 10-23. CR MET for the tibialis posterior.

■ **Action:** Have the client invert the foot with plantar flexion of the ankle and resist as you attempt to dorsiflex and evert.

■ **Observation:** Painless weakness implicates the L5 nerve root. Pain indicates a tendinitis or tenosynovitis of the tibialis posterior or a posteromedial shin splint.

4. *Contract-Relax Muscle Energy Technique for the Flexor Digitorum Longus and Brevis and the Flexor Hallucis Longus and Brevis*

■ **Intention:** The intention is to use CR MET to reduce the hypertonicity or to facilitate (strengthen) the flexor digitorum and flexor hallucis muscles. This MET is also treatment for tendinitis in these muscles, as well as for plantar fasciitis and metatarsalgia.

■ **Position:** Client is supine. Place one hand under the toes and the other hand on the leg for stability (Fig. 10-24).

■ **Action:** Have the client flex the toes and resist as you attempt to pull the toes into extension for approximately 5 seconds. Relax for a few seconds and repeat.

5. *Postisometric Relaxation Muscle Energy Technique for the Flexor Digitorum Longus and Brevis and the Flexor Hallucis Longus and Brevis*

■ **Intention:** The intention is to use PIR MET to lengthen the flexors to help bring normal extension to the toes. This MET is used to treat hammer toes and claw toes, in which the flexors and extensors

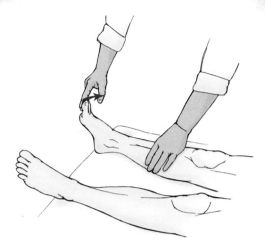

Figure 10-25. PIR MET for the flexor digitorum longus and brevis and for the flexor hallucis longus and brevis.

are typically tight. It is also used for treatment in hallux limitus.

■ **Position:** Client is supine. Place one hand under the toes and pull the toes into extension to their comfortable limit of stretch. Place the other hand on the leg for stability (Fig. 10-25).

■ **Action:** Have the client resist as you attempt to pull the toes into greater extension for approximately 5 seconds. Relax, and then gently stretch the toes into further extension, and have the client resist again. Repeat the CR–lengthen–contract cycle several times.

6. *Contract-Relax Muscle Energy Technique for the Extensor Hallucis*

■ **Intention:** The extensor hallucis is often weak. This weakness may be a result of myotomal weakness from irritation or injury to the L5 nerve. Weakness can also arise from an arthrokinetic reflex from fibrosis of the capsular ligaments of the great toe or from degeneration of the first MTP joint. The intention in using this MET is to help facilitate (strengthen) and bring sensory awareness to the extensor hallucis.

■ **Position:** Client is supine. Place one hand on the top of the great toe (Fig. 10-26).

■ **Action:** Have the client extend the great toe to the comfortable limit and then resist as you press the toe toward flexion.

■ **Observation:** Painless weakness implicates an irritation, injury, or dysfunction of the L5 nerve root. This muscle is often weak, because lower back dysfunction and injury are so common.

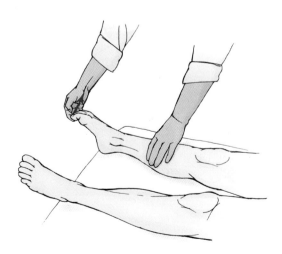

Figure 10-24. CR MET for the flexor digitorum longus and brevis and for the flexor hallucis longus and brevis.

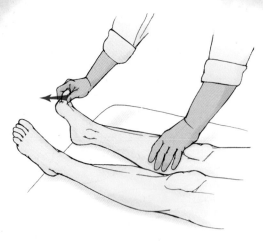

Figure 10-26. CR MET for the extensor hallucis longus and brevis.

7. Contract-Relax and Postisometric Muscle Energy Technique for the Extensor Digitorum Longus

Intention: The extensor digitorum longus is often held in a sustained contraction, leading to claw toes and hammer toes. The intention in using this MET is to reduce the muscle hypertonicity and to lengthen the myofascia. If the client has weak dorsiflexion, this MET is used with MET #3 to help facilitate (strengthen) the extensor/dorsiflexor muscles.

Position: Client is supine. Place one hand on the top of the toes.

Action: To perform CR MET, have the client extend the toes and resist as you press the toes toward flexion. Relax and repeat (Fig. 10-27). To perform PIR

MET, after the relaxation cycle, press the toes into greater flexion, and have the client resist as you press the toes toward further flexion. Relax, and repeat the CR–lengthen cycle several times.

8. Contract-Relax-Antagonist-Contract Muscle Energy Technique for the Soleus and Muscle Energy Technique to Increase Ankle Dorsiflexion

Intention: The soleus is typically short and tight. This muscle forms part of the Achilles tendon with the gastrocnemius. Unlike the gastrocnemius, the soleus does not cross the knee. The intention in using this MET is to increase ankle dorsiflexion, which is often decreased after an ankle injury, and to lengthen the soleus. This MET is also used to treat posteromedial shin splint and chronic tendinopathy of the soleus.

Position: Client is prone. Place your hand on the heel and your forearm on the ball of the foot (Fig. 10-28).

Action: Have the client resist as you attempt to press the ball of the foot toward the table (i.e., dorsiflex the ankle) for approximately 5 seconds, then instruct the client to relax. Have the client actively dorsiflex the ankle until pain or a new resistance barrier is encountered. As the client is actively dorsiflexing, press the forearm against the ball of the foot to assist the stretch. Have the client resist again at this new ROM for approximately 5 seconds, then instruct the client to relax. Repeat this CRAC cycle several times.

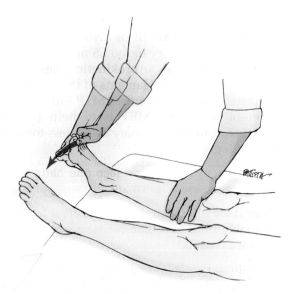

Figure 10-27. CR and PIR MET for the extensor digitorum longus and brevis.

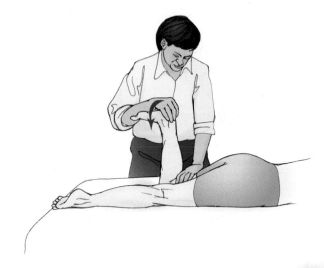

Figure 10-28. CRAC MET for the soleus and MET to increase dorsiflexion of the ankle.

SOFT TISSUE MOBILIZATION

BACKGROUND

A thorough discussion of the clinical application of STM can be found in Chapter 2. In the Hendrickson Method of manual therapy described in this text, the STM movements are called *wave mobilization* and are a combination of joint mobilization and STM performed in rhythmic oscillations with a frequency of 50 to 70 cycles per minute, except in performing brisk transverse friction massage (TFM) strokes, which can be two to four cycles per second. These mobilizations are presented in a specific sequence, which has been found to achieve the most efficient and effective results. This allows the therapist to "scan" the body to determine areas of tenderness, hypertonicity, and decreased mobility. It is important to "follow the recipe" until you have mastered this work. The techniques described below are divided into two sequences: Level I and Level II. Level I strokes are designed for every client, from acute injury to chronic degeneration, to enhance health and bring the body to optimum performance. Level II strokes are typically ap-

plied after Level I strokes and are designed for chronic conditions. Guidelines for treating acute and chronic conditions are listed below.

GUIDELINES FOR THE THERAPIST

Acute

The primary intentions of treatment are to decrease pain and swelling as quickly as possible, maintain as much pain-free joint motion as possible, and induce relaxation. In this method of treatment, the soft tissue is compressed and decompressed in rhythmic cycles. This provides a pumping action that helps to promote fluid exchange, reducing swelling. The strokes that are applied to the client who is in acute pain need to be performed with a very gentle touch, a very slow rhythm, and a small amplitude. There is no uniform "dose" or depth of treatment. The depth of treatment is based on the client's level of pain. If the soft tissue does not begin to relax, use more METs to help reduce discomfort, swelling, and excessive muscle tension. As was mentioned previously, intersperse your STM work with MET. Remember that **stretching is contraindicated** in acute conditions.

Clinical Example: Acute

Subjective: JL is a 17-year-old student who presented to my office complaining of acute right ankle and heel pain. She reported that she was playing on a rope swing and hit a tree with her outstretched leg. She had severe pain in the ankle and heel, as well as the low back and neck. She was taken to an orthopedist, and an MRI was performed, which was negative for fracture to the ankle and heel. A diagnosis was made of sprained ankle and bruised heel. She was placed in a walking boot and given medication for the pain. When she entered the treatment room, she was limping, because it was difficult for her to bear weight on the injured foot.

Objective: The ankle and heel were bruised and swollen, and the foot was also swollen. Palpation revealed a diffuse warmth, with moderate tenderness to light pressure at the heel and anterior joint line of the ankle. Active dorsiflexion, plantar flexion, and inversion were limited and painful at the anterior ankle. Testing the anterior talofibular ligament (passive plantar flexion with eversion) was limited and painful. Isometric testing was strong and pain free.

Assessment: Swelling and pain at the anterior talofibular ligament and painful and swollen heel.

Treatment: Treatment began with RI MET and CR MET for the dorsiflexors and plantar flexors of the ankle (MET #1) to reduce the swelling, hypertonicity, and pain. METs for inversion and eversion were performed next (METs #2 and #3). Because the fascia of the posterior thigh and leg interweaves with the fascia of the heel, METs for the gastrocnemius (MET #3, knee), soleus (MET #8), and hamstrings (MET #5, hip) were performed to pump the swelling out of the heel. Gentle Level I STM was performed, especially the fourth series of strokes, to disperse the swelling and to help realign the healing fibers. I emphasized treatment to the medial and lateral heel, avoiding the impact site in the center of the heel. I then performed gentle passive mobilization in plantar and dorsiflexion and in pronation and supination. These movements pumped the waste products out of the area and promoted cellular synthesis, oxygenation, and nutrition to the injured area. At the end of the session, she was able to move her foot without pain, except at the extremes of inversion and plantar flexion. I discussed natural anti-inflammatories with her and instructed her in active and passive movement for the ankle.

Plan: I recommended weekly visits for one month. JL returned to our office in one week and stated that she was feeling much better except in bearing full weight onto the heel. Upon examination, she had slight pain at the anterolateral ankle at the end ranges of both active and passive inversion and plantar flexion. I re-peated the treatment described above, concentrating on the anterior ankle and the medial and lateral heel. JL returned to my office one week later, able to walk without the boot with only slight discomfort in the heel. Passive testing for the anterior talofibular ligament was pain free. Palpation to the heel was mildly uncomfortable, with no swelling. Motion palpation of the joints of the ankle was normal. She returned to my office one week later completely pain-free. Examination found normal ROM, joint play, and muscle strength and normal tissue to palpation. She was discharged from active care.

Chronic

The typical exam findings in clients with chronic leg, ankle, and foot problems are short and tight plantar flexors and weak dorsiflexors and extensors. The ankle and foot tend to assume a pronated position. Chronic soft tissue problems often have degenerated soft tissue rather than inflammatory tissue and loss of joint play in the involved joints, degenerated joints (osteoarthritis), or both. The periarticular soft tissue (joint capsule and ligaments) is typically thick and fibrous but may be atrophied, leading to instability in the joint. Degenerated joints lose neurological function, leading to problems with fine motor control. The great toe is typically hypomobile, fixed in flexion, with thick, fibrous ligaments and capsular tissues. The primary goals of treatment depends on the patient. For patients who are hypomobile, with thick fibrous tissue and tight muscles, the treatment goals are to reduce the hypertonicity of the muscles; promote mobility and extensibility in the connective tissue by dissolving the adhesions in the muscles, tendons, ligaments, and capsular tissues surrounding the joints; rehydrate the cartilage of the joint; establish normal joint play and ROM in the joints; and restore normal neurological function by stimulating the propriceptors and reestablishing the normal firing patterns in the muscles. Patients who are unstable need exercise rehabilitation. Our treatments can support their stability by reducing tension in the tight muscles and performing MET to the weak muscles to help reestablish normal firing patterns and rehabilitate the propriceptors. With chronic conditions in the leg, ankle, and foot, it is also important to treat the hip, knee, and lumbosacral spine. Irritation, injury, or dysfunction of the nerves from the lumbosacral spine can cause pain and altered sensations in the leg, ankle, and foot as well as tightness or weakness in the muscles of the lower extremity. With chronic conditions, we use stronger pressure on the soft tissue and more vigorous mobilizations on the joints. In the Level II sequence, we add deeper soft tissue work and work on attachment points, using transverse friction strokes if we find fibrosis (thickening). As was mentioned in the "Acute" section, intersperse your soft tissue work with MET.

Clinical Example: Chronic

Subjective: KB is a 55-year-old, 5'7', 180-pound female realtor who presented to my office complaining of pain and stiffness in the right foot and ankle. The pain had begun approximately two years earlier when her foot "turned and collapsed." She saw her medical doctor, who recommended ibuprofen; a podiatrist, who made orthotics and recommended exercises; and an acupuncturist. She reported that the pain is mostly an ache but that it becomes worse with driving, that it can become stiff if she sits for more than a few min-utes, and that she can experience stabbing pain if she has been standing for a while. Because of the pain, she has been unable to hike, which was her favorite form of exercise.

Objective: Examination revealed that the patient walked with a slight limp. In standing, the ankles were pronated, and the feet were flat, more in the right than in the left. Active ROM was moderately reduced in dorsiflexion on the right. Plantar flexion was slightly limited, eliciting a pain at the anterior ankle. Active inversion was painful at the lateral ankle. Passive dorsiflexion and pronation/supination at the subtalar joints were limited, and passive plantar flexion was painful at the navicular. Isometric testing elicited pain at the navicular with resisted inversion and weakness of the dorsiflexors. Extensive crepitation was produced at the ankle when the ankle was mobilized with it fully dorsiflexed and then pronated and supinated. This indicated extensive degeneration in the ankle. To palpation, there were extensive fibrosis at the lateral and anterior ankle, sustained contractions in the posterior calf muscles and peroneals, and fibrosis in the plantar fascia.

Assessment: Pronation, fibrosis of the anterolateral ligaments, weak dorsiflexors, hypertonic plantar flexors, and diminished joint play of the talocrural and subtalar joints.

Treatment: Treatments were recommended on a weekly basis for four weeks. Treatments began with the patient supine. PIR MET was performed for the gastrocnemius and soleus to lengthen those muscles and to allow for greater dorsiflexion. CR MET was performed for the posterior tibialis and peroneals to reduce their hypertonicity and to decrease the fibrosis at

the tenoperiosteal attachments of those muscles. CR MET was then performed to strengthen the tibialis anterior. STM was performed, with concentration on the thickened tissue at the anterior joint line, the lateral malleolus, and the navicular. The ankle was then mobilized for several minutes with the ankle held in dorsiflexion and the heel and ankle pronated and supinated in an oscillating rhythm. This motion elicited audible "crunching" sounds, although it was not painful. This technique reduces calcium deposits on the articular surfaces.

Plan: The patient returned one week later and reported that the pain was reduced 80%. The same treatment described above was repeated. The mobilization elicited much less crepitation, indicating that the calcium deposits were reduced. KB returned for her next two visits reporting continuing improvement and elected to continue care on a weekly basis. At her eleventh visit, approximately three months after her initial treatment, she reported that she was completely pain free and that she was now able to hike without pain. I saw the patient occasionally after that, approximately one time per month. Six months after her initial visit, she took a walking trip to Europe and reported that she had no pain during or after her trip.

Table 10-7 lists some essentials of treatment.

LEVEL I: LEG, ANKLE, FOOT

1. Release of the Anterior and Lateral Compartments

- **Anatomy:** Crural fascia, extensor digitorum longus, extensor hallucis longus, tibialis anterior, peroneus longus, and peroneus brevis (Fig. 10-29).

- **Dysfunction:** With overuse or injury, the crural fascia is initially pulled away from the bone, but as it heals, it tends to thicken and adhere to the bone. The thickening and adhesion reduce the elasticity of the anterior and lateral compartments. The underlying muscles tend to dehydrate and lose their gliding characteristics.

Position
- **Therapist position (TP):** standing
- **Client position (CP):** supine

MET
You can use METs for the tibialis anterior (MET #1), peroneals (MET #2), and extensors (METs #6 and #7) to reduce hypertonicity and discomfort in the soft tissue.

Strokes

 CAUTION: The first two strokes are for chronic conditions only.

1. Release the anterior compartment by first stretching the crural fascia. Use some lotion to prevent skin burn. Facing 45° headward, use a soft fist with the wrist in neutral, and perform a series of long,

Table 10-7	Essentials of Treatment

- Rock the client's body while performing the strokes.
- Shift your weight while performing the strokes.
- Perform the strokes rhythmically.
- Perform the strokes about 50 to 70 cycles per minute.
- Keep your hands and whole body relaxed.

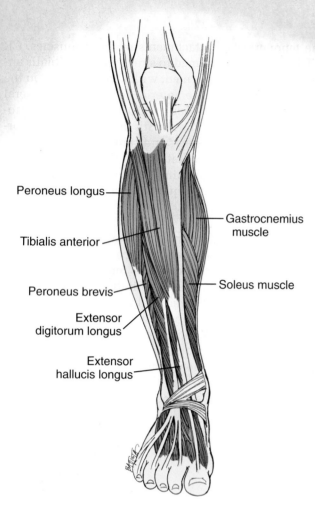

Peroneus longus

Tibialis anterior

Peroneus brevis

Extensor
digitorum longus

Extensor
hallucis longus

Gastrocnemius
muscle

Soleus muscle

Figure 10-29. Muscles of the anterior compartment of the leg include the tibialis anterior, extensor digitorum longus, and extensor hallucis longus.

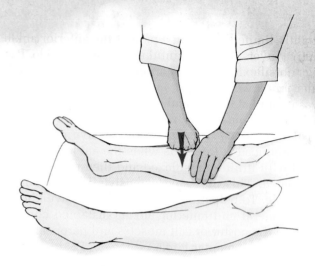

Figure 10-31. Using a soft fist, stretch the fascia of the leg in an A–P direction.

continuous strokes from the ankle to the knee on the anterior and lateral compartments (Fig. 10-30).

2. Facing the table, using the soft fist technique, place the supporting hand next to the soft fist, and hold the

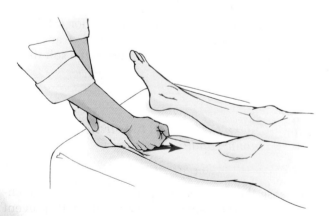

Figure 10-30. Using a soft fist, stretch the fascia of the leg with long, continuous strokes. This is for chronic conditions only.

supporting hand's thumb to stabilize the working hand (Fig. 10-31). Beginning at the lateral border of the proximal tibia, press into the leg, and while maintaining even pressure, slowly slide the fist on the skin and fascia posteriorly. You may also roll the fist posteriorly by flexing the wrist in a smooth, gliding motion. For the lateral compartment, rotate the leg medially with the supporting hand and cover the lateral surface. Emphasize the index knuckle or all the knuckles in the pronated position, or emphasize the flat surface of the proximal phalanges in the neutral wrist position. Continue these strokes to the ankle.

3. Face headward, using a double-, braced-, or single-thumb technique, perform 1-inch, scooping strokes from the ankle to the knee. Work in three lines between the lateral edge of the tibia and the fibula. This procedure releases the muscles in the anterior and lateral compartments. Maintain some tension in the tissue as you finish each stroke; this keeps the fascia in tension and allows for a greater stretch.

4. For acute conditions, place the knee in flexion, with the foot on the table (Fig. 10-32). While holding the entire leg, use the double-thumb technique to perform gentle, 1-inch, scooping strokes in the medial-to-lateral (M–L), A–P direction on the entire anterior and lateral compartments. This position is also used for treating acute conditions in the posterior compartment, such as a gastrocnemius strain, by performing gentle scooping strokes in the M–L plane.

2. *Release of the Muscles and Fascia of the Posteromedial Leg*

■ **Anatomy:** Crural fascia, tibialis posterior, soleus, flexor hallucis longus, plantaris, and flexor digitorum longus (Fig. 10-33).

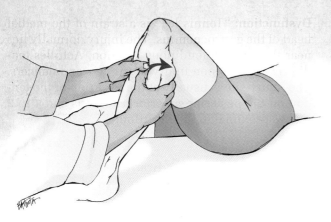

Figure 10-32. Double-thumb release of the anterior and lateral compartments for acute conditions.

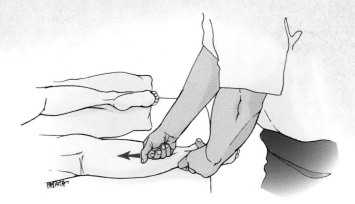

Figure 10-34. Soft fist release of the posteriomedial compartment.

▨ **Dysfunction:** The posteromedial leg is the most common injury site of the compartment syndromes or shin splints. It involves the tenoperiosteal or fascial tear of the soleus, the tibial origin of the flexor digitorum longus, or the tibialis posterior. The crural fascia covers the area superficially.

Position
▨ **TP:** standing

▨ **CP:** side-lying, with a pillow under the knee of the top leg, with the bottom leg extended

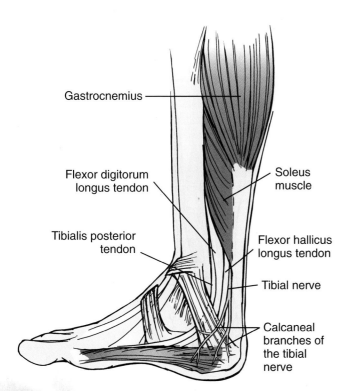

Figure 10-33. Medial leg, ankle, and foot showing the tendons of the tibialis posterior, flexor digitorum longus, and flexor hallucis longus traveling around the medial ankle.

MET
You can perform METs for the tibialis posterior (MET #3), soleus (MET #6), and flexors of the toes (METs #4 and #5) to reduce hypertonicity and discomfort in the soft tissue.

Strokes
1. Place the client onto her left side for work on the left medial aspect of the leg. Stand facing headward, and perform the same series of strokes as were described in the previous series. First, using a soft fist, perform a series of long, slow, continuous strokes from the ankle to the knee on the medial leg (Fig. 10-34). Next, move to the side of the table closest to the extended leg. Place the supporting hand next to the soft fist, and hold the supporting hand's thumb to stabilize the stroke. Begin at the medial border of the proximal tibia, and while maintaining even pressure, roll and slide the fist posteriorly in a smooth, gliding motion.
2. Using a double-, braced-, or single-thumb technique, perform 1-inch, scooping strokes from the ankle to the knee in several lines on the fascia covering the muscles and in between the muscles of the posteromedial leg.
3. Have the client bend the bottom leg 90° and straighten the top leg, resting it on a pillow. Move to the side of the table facing the client. Using a double- or braced-thumb technique, perform a series of 1-inch scooping strokes in the A–P direction on the medial compartment from just below the knee to the ankle (Fig. 10-35). At the medial ankle, release the tendons of the tibialis posterior, flexor digitorum longus, and flexor hallucis longus.

3. Prone Release of the Posterior Compartment and the Achilles Tendon

▨ **Anatomy:** Gastrocnemius, soleus, plantaris, flexor hallucis longus, and flexor digitorum longus (Figs. 10-36A and 10-36B).

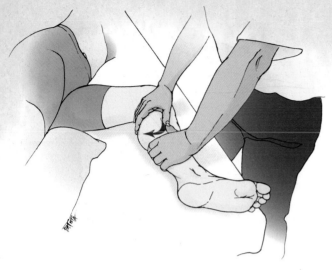

Figure 10-35. Double-thumb technique used to perform scooping strokes in an A–P direction on the medial leg.

■ **Dysfunction:** "Tennis leg" is a strain of the medial head of the gastrocnemius. The injury normally lies near the musculotendinous junction. Achilles tendinitis is a common injury in runners and dancers. The injury site is usually at the insertion of the tendon on the posterior-superior calcaneus and 1 to 2 inches proximal to the insertion.

Position

■ **TP:** Standing, facing headward

■ **CP:** Prone, with the foot off the edge of the table; place a pillow under the ankle if the leg is particularly tense or sensitive: this brings the tissue into more slack

MET

You can perform METs for the gastrocnemius (MET #2, knee), tibialis posterior (MET #3), soleus (MET #6), and flexors of the toes (METs #4 and #5) to reduce hypertonicity and discomfort in the soft tissue.

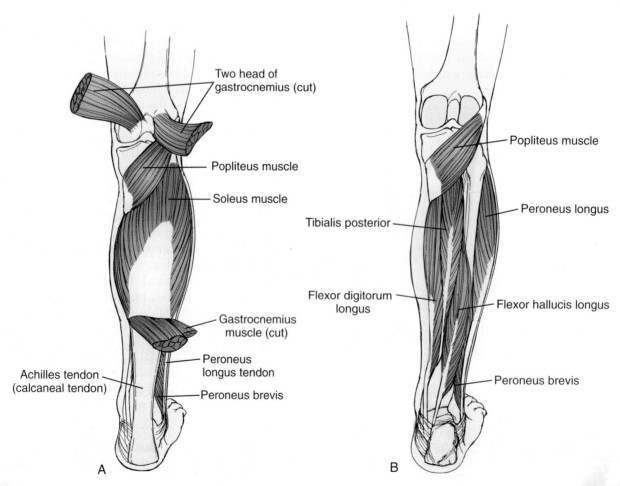

Figure 10-36. A. Superficial posterior compartment showing the gastrocnemius cut away to reveal the underlying soleus. **B.** Deep posterior compartment showing the tibialis posterior, flexor digitorum longus, and flexor hallucis longus.

Strokes

1. Facing headward, release the posterior aspect of the crural fascia. Use a soft fist, and perform long, slow strokes from the ankle to the knee as described for the previous strokes. Follow the gastrocnemius heads to the medial and lateral aspects of the popliteal fossa. Keep your wrist in neutral, midway between pronation and supination. Do not put deep pressure in the center of the popliteal fossa.

2. To release the hypertonicity in the muscles and stretch their fascial coverings, use the single-, double-, or braced-thumb technique as described in the previous strokes. Perform 1-inch scooping strokes in an inferior-to-superior direction on three lines: the medial, middle, and lateral aspects of the posterior leg.

3. To release the torsion in the soft tissue, part the midline by taking the lateral tissue laterally and the medial tissue medially. Using double thumbs, perform short, scooping strokes, beginning at the midline below the knee (Fig. 10-37). These strokes may also be performed standing at the side of the table facing the client.

4. There are three strokes for the Achilles tendon. First, face headward, and use double-thumb technique to perform short back-and-forth strokes in the M–L plane on the posterior surface of the Achilles tendon (Fig. 10-38). Apply the strokes both to the body of the tendon, approximately 1 to 2 inches above the heel, and on the heel itself to address the two most common sites of injury. You may stabilize the tendon by pressing your thigh against the client's foot. Second, with your fingertips slightly flexed, perform back-and-forth strokes in the A–P plane on the medial and lateral surfaces of the tendon (Fig. 10-39). Move in opposite directions with the fingers in an oscillating rhythm. Third, face the table, and place a flexed knee on the table. Rest the client's shin on your flexed thigh. Hold the Achilles tendon between your thumb and fingertips, and roll the tendon back and forth. In

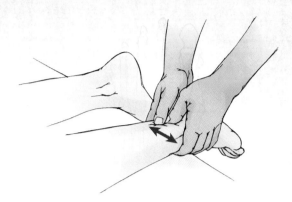

Figure 10-38. Double-thumb technique used to perform back-and-forth strokes in the M–L plane on the Achilles tendon.

this position, you may first stabilize the tendon with the thumb, performing back-and-forth strokes with the fingers, and then switch, using the fingers to stabilize and the thumb to perform the strokes.

4. *Release of the Muscles of the Dorsum of the Foot and of the Ligaments of the Ankle*

- **Anatomy:** Dorsal interossei, extensor digitorum longus and brevis, extensor hallucis longus and brevis (Fig. 10-40), deltoid ligament, anterior talofibular ligament, and calcaneofibular ligament (see Figs. 10-8 and 10-9).

- **Dysfunction:** The tendons and their associated retinacula are susceptible to irritation as they travel under the retinacula on the dorsum of the foot. Ligamentous injuries are usually inversion stresses from an acute episode. The most commonly injured ligament is the anterior talofibular.

Position
- **TP:** Standing
- **CP:** Supine

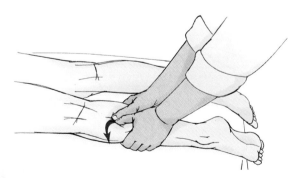

Figure 10-37. Double-thumb technique used to perform short, scooping strokes from the knee to the ankle, taking the lateral tissue more laterally and the medial tissue more medially.

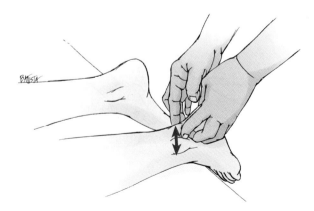

Figure 10-39. Fingertips used to perform back-and-forth strokes in the Achilles A–P plane.

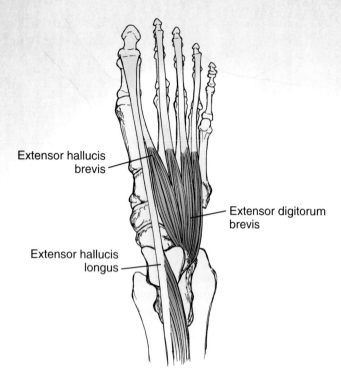

Extensor hallucis brevis

Extensor digitorum brevis

Extensor hallucis longus

Figure 10-40. Intrinsic muscles on the dorsum of the foot include the extensor hallucis brevis and the extensor digitorum brevis.

MET
You can perform METs #6 and #7 for the extensors.

Strokes
1. Using double thumbs on the midline of the foot, perform a spreading motion to part the midline of the retinacula and fascia on the dorsum of the foot (Fig. 10-41).
2. Next, place both thumbs at the anterolateral calcaneus as your hands hold the foot. Using a double-thumb technique, oscillate the foot rhythmically into supination as you perform short, scooping strokes in an M–L direction (Fig. 10-42). Continue

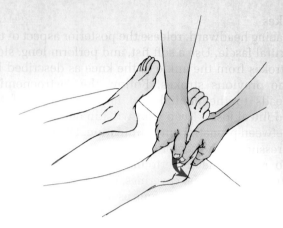

Figure 10-42. Double-thumb technique used to perform M–L scooping strokes to release the extensor hallucis brevis and extensor digitorum brevis.

these transverse scooping strokes on the entire dorsum of the foot to the toes to release the tendons of the tibialis anterior, extensor hallucis longus, and extensor digitorum longus.
3. Release the ligaments of the ankle in three areas. First, using fingertips or the single- or double-thumb technique, perform back-and-forth strokes in the M–L and A–P planes in the area between the anterior portion of the distal fibula and the talus for the anterior talofibular ligament (Fig. 10-43). Second, perform back-and-forth strokes in the A–P plane to release the calcaneofibular ligament from the inferior aspect of the fibula to the calcaneus. Finally, perform back-and-forth strokes in the A–P plane from the distal end of the medial malleolus to the heel to release the deltoid ligaments. Rock the entire foot back and forth in an oscillating rhythm with these strokes.
4. Sit on the end of the table, and place the client's distal leg on his or her thigh. Using a double-thumb technique, perform short, scooping strokes in between the metatarsals to release the dorsal interossei (Fig. 10-44). Draw the foot back into dorsiflexion,

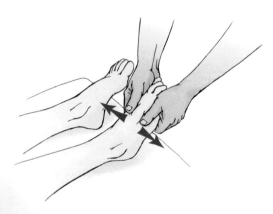

Figure 10-41. Double-thumb technique used to perform a series of spreading strokes on the fascia on the dorsum of the foot.

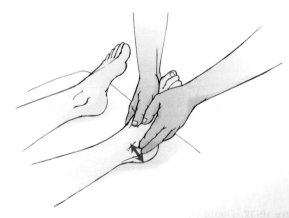

Figure 10-43. Fingertips used to perform transverse strokes on the anterior talofibular ligament.

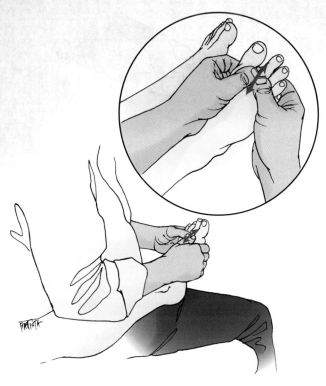

Figure 10-44. Double-thumb technique performing dorsal-plantar scooping strokes on the interossei and joint capsules.

and then plantarflex the foot as you scoop in. Put the fingertips of your supporting hand underneath where you are working to spread the metatarsals open as you stroke. Perform a second series of

strokes on either side of the MTP joints. On the lateral side of one MTP, supinate the foot as you scoop in the plantar direction. Move to the medial side of the adjacent MTP, and pronate the foot as you scoop plantarward. These strokes release the interossei, lumbricals, and joint capsule.

5. *Release of the Plantar Fascia and the Muscles of the First Layer of the Foot*

▓ **Anatomy:** Plantar fascia, abductor hallucis, flexor digitorum brevis, abductor digiti minimi, and quadratus plantae (Figs. 10-45**A** and 10-45**B**).

▓ **Dysfunction:** The plantar fascia is similar to a guy wire that adds significant support to the longitudinal arch. Static stresses, such as jobs that require long periods of standing, thicken and dry out the fascia. The muscles are susceptible to fatigue from excessive static weight bearing. The fascia and muscles are prone to overuse and acute injury in runners, dancers, and those who play racquet sports.

Position

▓ **TP:** Standing for first stroke, sitting for other strokes. When sitting, place one foot slightly forward and the other slightly back to differentiate your weight, which allows for a more powerful stroke.

▓ **CP:** Supine; an optional position is prone, with foot over the edge of the table.

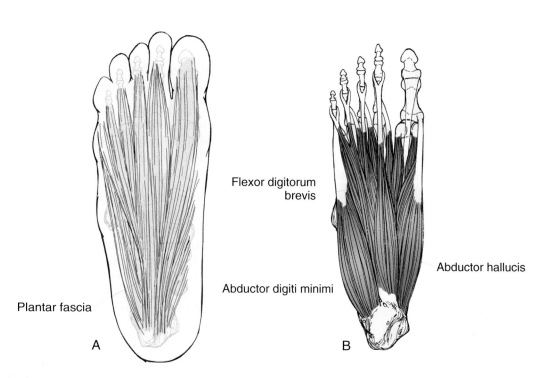

Figure 10-45. A. Plantar fascia on the sole of the foot. **B.** First layer of muscles on the plantar aspect of the foot includes the abductor hallucis, flexor digitorum brevis, and the abductor digiti minimi.

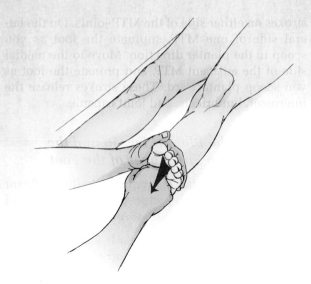

Figure 10-46. Broad fist technique to stretch the plantar fascia.

MET

You can perform METs for the gastrocnemius (MET #2, knee), tibialis posterior (MET #3), soleus (MET #6), and flexors of the toes (METs #4 and #5) to help lengthen the plantar fascia.

Strokes

1. Sit or stand at the foot of the table, and use a broad fist to perform a series of slow, continuous strokes on the plantar fascia from the base of the toes to the heel (Fig. 10-46). Emphasize the pressure at the index knuckle. Use lotion to reduce the friction, but you want some drag to stretch the superficial fascia.

2. Release the superficial muscles of the foot in three lines from the calcaneus to the MTP joints. To release the medial line, turn your body to face the medial aspect of the foot. Using a single- or double-thumb technique, perform short, scooping strokes in the medial direction, supinating the foot with each stroke (Fig. 10-47). If the tissue is fibrotic, perform back-and-forth strokes in the M–L plane. Begin your strokes at the anterior part of the medial calcaneus, and continue inch-by-inch to the base of

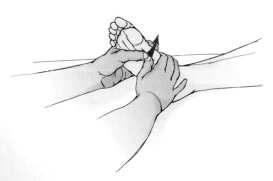

Figure 10-47. Double-thumb technique used to perform scooping strokes for the abductor hallucis.

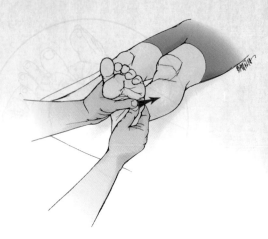

Figure 10-48. Double-thumb technique used to perform scooping strokes for the abductor digiti minimi.

the great toe. These strokes release the abductor hallucis and the flexor hallucis underneath.

3. The second line is in the middle of the foot from the middle part of the anterior calcaneus to the toes. Perform short, scooping strokes in a lateral-to-medial direction in an oscillating rhythm while supinating the foot. These strokes release the flexor digitorum brevis and the quadratus plantae underneath.

4. The third line is the lateral aspect of the anterior calcaneus up the side of the foot to the base of the little toe. Using a single-, double-, or braced-thumb technique, perform short, scooping strokes in the M–L direction, pronating the foot as you scoop. These strokes release the abductor digiti minimi and the flexor and opponens digiti minimi underneath (Fig. 10-48).

6. *Release of the Second, Third, and Fourth Layers of the Foot*

▧ **Anatomy:** Adductor hallucis (oblique and transverse heads); flexor hallucis brevis; flexor and opponens digiti minimi; and lumbricals, which arise from the flexor digitorum longus tendons (Figs. 10-49A and 10-49B).

▧ **Dysfunction:** Muscles of the foot are often held in a sustained contraction, predisposing them to ischemia and fibrosis. Static or dynamic stresses contribute to cumulative or overuse injuries. Sustained contraction of the adductor hallucis contributes to hallux valgus. An important area to release is the lateral side of the great toe. It is a common site of thick adhesions due to prior injury or weight-bearing dysfunctions, such as pronation.

Position

▧ **TP:** sitting

▧ **CP:** supine

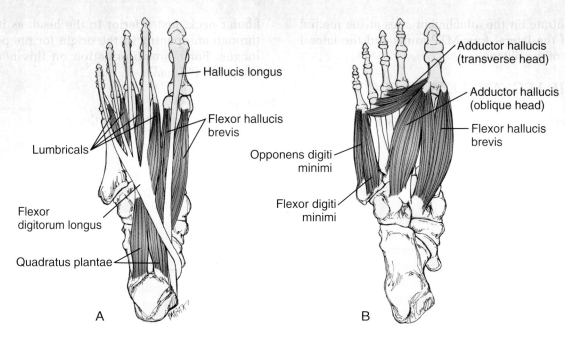

Figure 10-49. A. The second layer of plantar muscles includes the quadratus plantae and the four lumbrical muscles. **B.** The third layer of muscles on the bottom of the foot includes the flexor hallucis brevis, flexor digiti minimi, opponens digiti minimi, and the oblique and transverse heads of the adductor hallucis.

MET

You can perfom METs for the flexor hallucis brevis and longus (METs #4 and #5) and adductor hallucis by having the client resist as you try to pull the great toe medially.

Strokes

1. Using a single- or double-thumb technique, perform a series of back-and-forth strokes in the M–L plane on each of the flexor digitorum longus, the lumbricals on the medial side of these tendons, and the flexor hallucis longus tendons (Fig. 10-50). Begin in the midfoot, and continue to the ends of each of the four lateral toes. Release the oblique head of the adductor hallucis deep to these ten-dons. Perform the same short, scooping strokes from the midfoot to the lateral side of the great toe.

2. Next, perform a series of scooping strokes in the posterior-to-anterior (P–A) (heel-to-toe) direction on either side of the flexor digitorum longus and flexor hallucis longus tendons. These strokes release the lumbricals and the flexor digital sheath of each tendon and the annular ligament that surrounds the tendons underneath the MTP joints.

3. Using a double-thumb technique, perform short scooping P–A strokes, beginning at the medial aspect of the fifth MTP joint and continuing inch by inch to the lateral aspect of the big toe to release the transverse head of the adductor hallucis (Fig. 10-51).

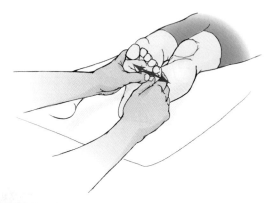

Figure 10-50. Single-thumb technique to release the lumbricals and tendons of the flexor digitorum longus and flexor hallucis longus.

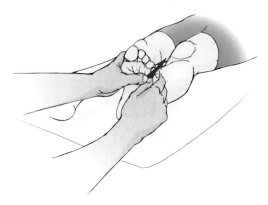

Figure 10-51. Double-thumb technique used to perform P–A scooping strokes on the attachments of the transverse head of the adductor hallucis.

Concentrate on the attachment sites at the medial side of the lateral four MTP joints and the lateral aspect of the big toe.

LEVEL II: LEG, ANKLE, AND FOOT

1. Release of Muscle Attachments in the Anterior and Lateral Compartments

▥ **Anatomy:** Tibialis anterior, extensor digitorum longus, extensor hallucis longus, common peroneal nerve, and peroneus longus and brevis (Fig. 10-52).

▥ **Dysfunction:** Chronic compartment syndromes are believed to be microtrauma to muscles, often exercise induced, that leads to a myositis and eventual fibrosis. The muscles and connective tissue tend to dehydrate and lose their lubricant. Chronic inflammation of the periosteum and myofascia thickens the tissue at the site of injury. The common peroneal nerve may be entrapped at the anterolateral

fibular neck, just inferior to the head, as it passes through an opening in the origin for the peroneus longus. For more information on this nerve, see Chapter 9 ("Knee").

Position

▥ **TP:** Standing, or sitting on the table

▥ **CP:** Supine, knee flexed, foot on the table

MET

You can use METs for the anterior and lateral compartments: the tibialis anterior (MET #1), peroneals (MET #2), and extensors (METs #6 and #7).

Strokes

You may stand or sit to perform these strokes. If you are standing, wrap your hands around the leg, holding and stabilizing the leg. If you are sitting on the table, gently sit on the client's foot to help stabilize the leg. Perform back-and-forth strokes in the M–L and A–P planes with a double-thumb technique on the myotendinous junctions, and perform brisk, transverse friction strokes on the tenoperiosteal attachments to the bone as needed.

1. While sitting or standing, use double-thumb technique to perform short, back-and-forth strokes in the M–L and A–P planes to release the attachments of the tibialis anterior on the lateral surface of the proximal tibia (Fig. 10-53). Follow this muscle down to the ankle with special attention to the myotendinous junction approximately 6 inches above the ankle.
2. Using the same technique, release the attachments of the extensor digitorum longus on the lateral condyle of the tibia and the anterior medial crest of the fibula.
3. The extensor hallucis longus is deep to the tibialis anterior and the extensor digitorum longus. Using

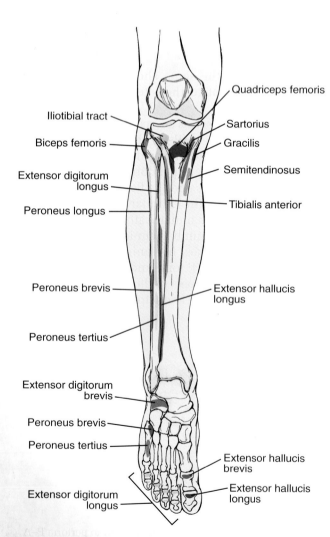

Figure 10-52. Muscle attachments on the anterior leg, ankle, and foot.

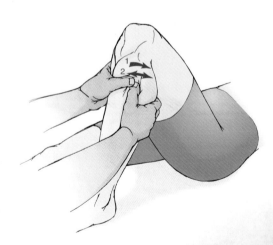

Figure 10-53. Double-thumb technique used to perform either (1) short scooping strokes in an M–L direction or (2) back-and-forth strokes in the M–L plane.

a double-thumb technique, perform short, back-and-forth strokes in the M–L and A–P planes, with the intention of penetrating through the more superficial muscles to the extensor hallucis longus.

4. Using a double-thumb technique, perform either short, scooping strokes or back-and-forth strokes in the M–L and A–P planes to release the common peroneal nerve from the fibular neck, the peroneus longus from the upper two-thirds of the lateral aspect of the fibula, and the peroneus brevis from the lower one-third (Fig. 10-54). Follow the tendons to the ankle with special attention to the myotendinous junction several inches above the ankle. Perform a brisk, transverse stroke at these sites if they feel fibrotic.

2. *Release of the Tendons Crossing the Ankle and the Deep Peroneal and Posterior Tibial Nerves*

▨ **Anatomy:** Deep peroneal nerve (see Fig. 10-4) and posterior tibial nerve (see Fig. 10-3), peroneus longus and brevis, tibialis anterior, extensor hallucis longus, abductor hallucis, extensor digitorum longus, tibialis posterior, flexor digitorum longus, and flexor hallucis longus (Figs. 10-55**A** and 10-55**B**).

▨ **Dysfunction:** The tendons and their associated sheaths are susceptible to tenosynovitis where they cross the ankle through the fibro-osseous tunnels formed by the retinaculum. These nerves are suscep-

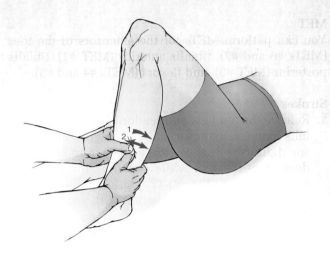

Figure 10-54. Double-thumb technique used to perform either (1) short scooping strokes in an M–L direction or (2) back-and-forth strokes in the M–L plane on the distal aspect of the tibia and fibula.

tible to injury from an acute sprain of the ankle, a chronic overuse injury, or positional dysfunction such as pronated ankles. The tarsal tunnel describes the superficial and deep layers of the flexor retinaculum at the medial ankle and the posterior tibial nerve that travels between them. The abductor hallucis can develop a tendinitis from excessive pronation.

Position

▨ **TP:** Standing, facing your work

▨ **CP:** Supine

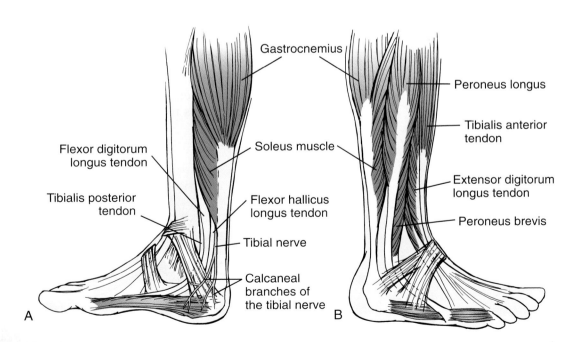

Figure 10-55. A. Medial leg, ankle, and foot showing the tendons of the tibialis posterior, flexor digitorum longus, flexor hallucis longus, and the tibial nerve. **B.** Lateral leg, ankle, and foot showing tendons of peroneus longus and brevis, tibialis anterior, and extensor digitorum longus.

MET

You can perform METs for the extensors of the toes (METs #6 and #7), tibialis anterior (MET #1), tibialis posterior (MET #3), and flexors (METs #4 and #5).

Strokes

1. Release the tendons and tendon sheaths of the tibialis anterior, extensor hallucis longus, and extensor digitorum longus. Place both thumbs on the dorsum of the foot while you hold the foot with both hands (see Fig. 10-42). Perform short, scooping strokes in an M–L direction with your thumbs, while you supinate the foot in an oscillating rhythm. With the same strokes, release the deep peroneal nerve under the inferior extensor retinaculum at the joint line of the ankle just lateral to the tendon of the extensor hallucis longus.

2. Release the posterior tibial nerve in the tarsal tunnel and the posterior tibialis, flexor digitorum longus, and flexor hallucis longus tendons at the medial ankle using a double-thumb technique (Fig. 10-56). Perform short, scooping strokes while pronating the foot in an oscillating rhythm under the medial malleolus by scooping toward the heel, taking the nerve and tendons away from the bone.

3. Using a double-thumb technique, release the calcaneal branch of the posterior tibial nerve by performing a series of gentle, scooping strokes toward the Achilles tendon between the medial malleolus and the center of the heel, inverting the foot with each stroke.

4. To release the medial and lateral plantar nerves and the abductor hallucis, use the double-thumb technique, and perform short, scooping strokes toward the plantar surface of the medial arch under

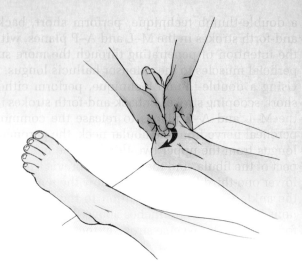

Figure 10-57. Double-thumb technique used to perform gentle scooping along the medial arch.

the navicular and proximal first metatarsal (Fig. 10-57). Pronate the foot with each stroke.

5. Release the peroneal tendons and their associated tendon sheaths from the lateral malleolus (Fig. 10-58). Using fingertips or a single–thumb technique, scoop the tendons away from the malleolus as you supinate the foot. Begin your series a few inches proximal to the ankle, and continue to the base of the fifth metatarsal.

3. *Release of the Muscles and Attachments in the Posterior Compartments*

▨ **Anatomy:** Soleus, tibialis posterior, popliteus, flexor hallucis longus, and flexor digitorum longus (Fig. 10-59).

▨ **Dysfunction:** Injuries to the medial leg, particularly tibialis posterior shin splints, are the most common shin injuries in runners and dancers. The muscles

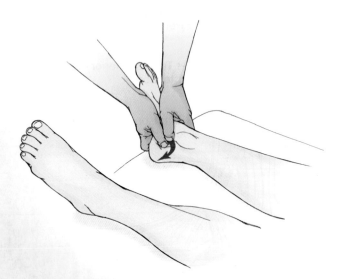

Figure 10-56. Double-thumb technique used to perform gentle scooping strokes to release the posterior tibial nerve in the tarsal tunnel.

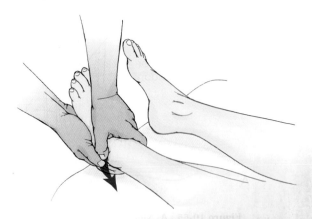

Figure 10-58. Double-thumb technique used to perform gentle scooping on the peroneal tendons.

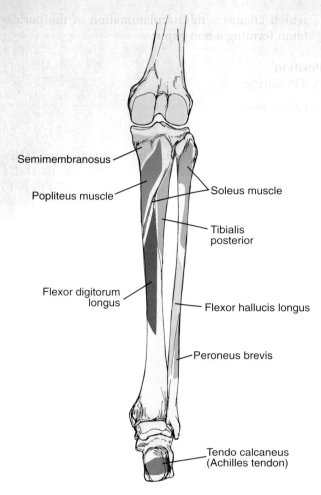

Figure 10-59. Muscle attachment sites on the posterior leg and foot.

tend to shorten and become fibrotic after overuse or acute injury.

Position
▨ **TP:** Standing, facing headward or facing the table with the client prone, or sitting with the client supine

▨ **CP:** There are two possible positions: (1) prone, with the knee flexed to 90° or the knee flexed with the leg resting on your flexed leg on the table, and (2) supine, with the knee flexed and the foot on the table

MET
You can perform METs for the tibialis posterior (MET #3), soleus (MET #8), flexor hallucis longus (MET #4), peroneals (MET #2), popliteus (MET #7, knee), and flexor digitorum longus (MET #4).

Strokes
The intention is to "look" with your hands for any fibrosis or hypertonicity. This thickened or knotted feel

may be in the muscle belly, in the myotendinous junction, or at the tenoperiosteal attachment to the bone.

1. Stand, facing the table, with the client prone and the client's leg resting on your thigh. To release the soleus, flexor hallucis longus, and peroneus brevis from the posterior fibula, use a braced- or double-thumb technique, and perform a series of back-and-forth strokes in an M–L plane from the proximal portion of the posterior fibula. Continue these strokes to the posterior surface of the lateral malleolus (Fig. 10-60). Move the tissue aside to make contact with the bone.

2. Perform a series of back-and-forth strokes in an M–L plane in the deepest aspect of the center of the calf to release the tibialis posterior and soleus from the interosseus membrane and the adjacent tibia. Use the fingertips of one or both hands if the client is supine, or use a braced- or double-thumb technique if the client is prone. Again, continue these strokes down to the posterior aspect of the tibia. Perform more brisk transverse friction strokes if the area feels fibrotic.

3. To release the popliteus and flexor digitorum longus, use the same hand positions as were described above to perform back-and-forth strokes or brisk transverse friction strokes on the posterior tibia. Continue these strokes down the medial leg to the medial malleolus, scanning the area for any fibrosis.

4. An alternative position is to have the client supine, knee flexed, foot on the table, and use the fingertips of one or both hands to perform the same strokes as were described above (Fig. 10-61). Perform mobilization of the fibular head by holding the fibular head between your thumb and flexed index finger and moving it back and forth in the A–P plane.

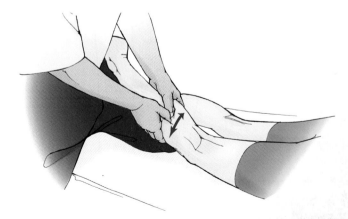

Figure 10-60. Double-thumb release of the muscle attachments on the posterior leg.

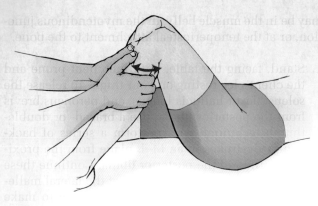

Figure 10-61. Supine technique to release the muscle attachments on the posterior leg. The fingertips of one or both hands are performing back-and-forth strokes in the M–L plane.

4. Release of the Muscles and Ligaments that Attach to the Calcaneus and Heel Spurs

▨ **Anatomy:** Abductor hallucis, flexor digitorum brevis, abductor digiti minimi, quadratus plantae, and long plantar ligament (Fig. 10-62).

▨ **Dysfunction:** Plantar fasciitis is an acute or chronic strain that can arise from prolonged standing or from overuse such as excessive running. Activities such as running create a repetitive pulling on the periosteal attachment to the calcaneus and can create a traction spur, one type of heel spur. Another type of heel spur arises in response to static stress,

which creates a microinflammation of the periosteum forming a bony spur.

Position
▨ **TP:** Sitting

▨ **CP:** Supine

MET
You can perform METs for the gastrocnemius (MET #2, knee), tibialis posterior (MET #3), soleus (MET #6), and flexors of the toes (METs #4 and #5) to help lengthen the plantar fascia.

Strokes
The intention is both to dissolve the fibrosis in the plantar fascia associated with chronic irritation and to clean the bone of the heel. It is possible to dissolve small calcium crystals (spicules) that are embedded in the fascia. It is also possible to clean the surface of larger, pedunculated (rounded) spurs of these small mineral deposits and fibrous depositions. The intention is not to dissolve the larger spur but rather to release any fibrous adhesions attaching to the bone. This can be painful with plantar fasciitis or heel spurs. Remember to work only within the comfortable limits of the client. The successful outcome of these treatments often takes six to twelve sessions. Work a little deeper each session if possible. The healthy heel is not sensitive to deep pressure.

1. Using the knuckle (MCP joint) of your flexed index or middle finger, the PIP joint of your index finger, or a blunt instrument such as a T-bar, perform deep back-and-forth strokes in the M–L plane on the entire plantar aspect of the heel (Fig. 10-63). Cover the medial, posterior, and lateral sides, as well as the center. Rock your body, and translate that into a rocking of the foot with each stroke.

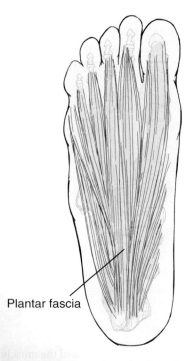

Figure 10-62. Plantar fascia on the sole of the foot.

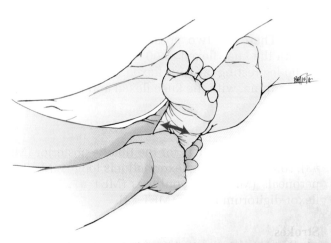

Figure 10-63. Use of the index knuckle to perform transverse friction strokes on the heel.

2. Perform a series of brisk, back-and-forth strokes in the M–L plane on the medial, middle, and lateral aspects of the anterior calcaneus. This releases the attachments of the abductor hallucis, flexor digitorum brevis, quadratus plantae, abductor digiti minimi, and long plantar ligament.

3. If you find a heel spur, perform brisk, friction strokes on the spur. Work only for approximately 5 seconds on any one painful spot. Move to another spot, even if it is only a few millimeters away. Work for approximately 5 minutes in each session directly on the bone; too much work bruises the area.

5. Release of the Attachment Points and the Joint Capsule and Ligaments of the Metatarsophalangeal and Interphalangeal Joints

▨ **Anatomy:** Joint capsule and ligaments of the MTP and IP joints (Fig. 10-64), superficial and deep layers of the transverse metatarsal ligaments, annular and cruciate ligaments, plantar digital nerve, tibialis posterior and anterior, and peroneus brevis and longus.

▨ **Dysfunction:** The joint capsules and ligaments are typically thickened and fibrotic as a result of disuse, static stress, or inflammation from injury. This fibrosis decreases joint motion, leading to potential degeneration. With excessive running or chronic weight distribution problems, tendon attachment points become fibrotic. Work all the attachment points that have become fibrotic. The ones listed below are the most common.

Position

▨ **TP:** Sitting in a chair or on the table

▨ **CP:** Supine

MET
You can help to release this area by performing METs for the tibialis anterior (MET #1) and posterior (MET #3), peroneals (MET #2), and flexors and extensors of

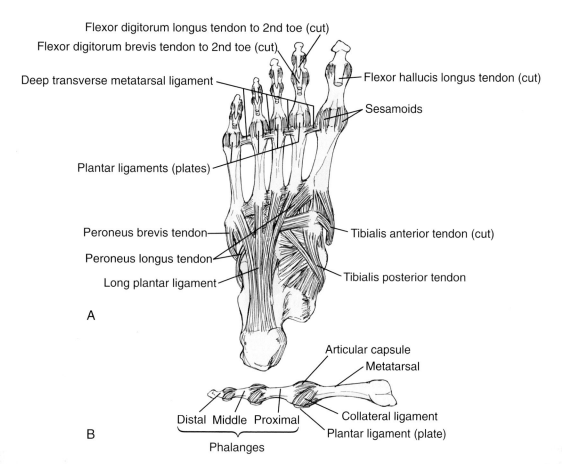

Figure 10-64. A. Ligaments and tendon insertions on the plantar aspect (bottom) of the foot. **B.** Joint capsule and collateral ligaments of the MTP and IP joints. Note that the fibers of the joint capsule are aligned parallel to the shaft of the bone and that the collateral ligaments are angled in a dorsal-to-plantar direction.

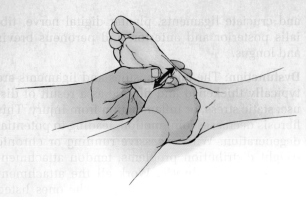

Figure 10-65. Braced-thumb technique used to perform back-and-forth strokes on the plantar surface of the navicular.

the toes, which interweave with the ligaments and capsular tissues (METs #4 through #7).

Strokes

1. Using a double- or braced-thumb technique, perform a series of 1-inch, back-and-forth strokes in both the A–P and M–L planes on the tuberosity of the plantar surface of the navicular, first cuneiform, and base of the first metatarsal. These strokes release the attachments of the tibialis posterior, tibialis anterior, and peroneus longus (Fig. 10-65).
2. Using a double- or braced-thumb technique, release the base of the fifth metatarsal and cuboid with short, back-and-forth strokes in the M–L plane to release the abductor digiti minimi, flexor digiti minimi, and peroneus brevis.
3. Sit on the end of the treatment table, and place the client's distal leg on your thigh (see Fig. 10-44). Hold the foot with both hands by placing your thumbs on the dorsum of the foot and your fingertips underneath. Using fingertips, perform a series of 1-inch, scooping strokes in the P–A (heel-to-toe) direction in between the metatarsals on the ball of the foot (Fig. 10-66). These strokes release the dorsal and plantar interossei, which lie in between and on the plantar surface of the lateral four metatarsals, from the midfoot to the base of the toes. The intention is to create space in between the metatarsals.
4. Next, perform back-and-forth strokes in the A–P plane on the medial and lateral aspect of each MTP joint to release the transverse metatarsal ligament. This ligament is typically thick and can compress the metatarsal heads together. The plantar digital nerve can become entrapped between the superficial and deep layers of the transverse metatarsal ligament, which runs between the two metatarsal heads, and can be irritated by the compression between the metatarsal heads. To release the nerve, use your index finger, and perform a series of gentle scooping strokes in the M–L plane transverse to

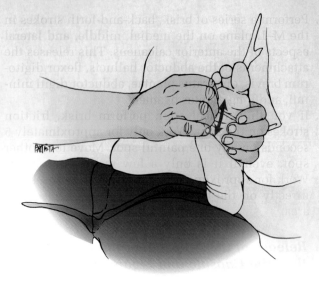

Figure 10-66. Fingertips scooping back and forth in the P–A plane (heel to toe) to release the interossei and the transverse metatarsal ligament. To release the plantar digital nerve, perform scooping strokes in the M–L plane between each metatarsal.

the nerve in between each MTP joint. Also perform gentle scooping strokes from each metatarsal head to the interspace in between the bones to ensure that the nerve has not migrated from its normal position in between the bones to underneath the bone.

5. Using a single-thumb or fingertip technique, perform back-and-forth strokes on the medial and lateral aspect of each toe, concentrating on the IP joints (Fig. 10-67). Work transverse to the shaft of each toe to release the collateral ligaments and joint capsule.

6. Mobilization of the Ankle and Foot

■ **Anatomy:** The tarsus consists of seven bones: talus, calcaneus, navicular, cuboid, and three cuneiform

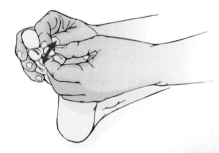

Figure 10-67. Fingertip of the right index finger is used to perform back-and-forth strokes on the IP joints, transverse to the shaft of the bone, to release the medial collateral ligament of the third toe.

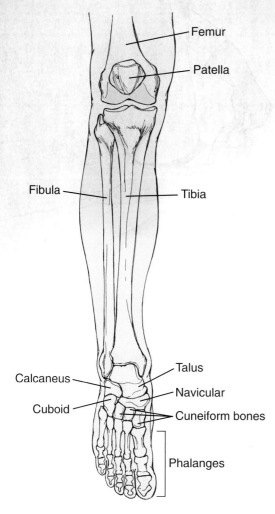

Figure 10-68. Bones and joints of the ankle and foot.

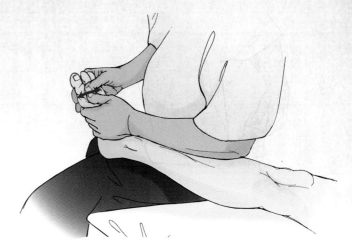

Figure 10-69. Double-thumb technique used to perform brisk, transverse strokes on the joint capsule of the first MTP joint.

bones. The metatarsus consists of five metatarsals. Digits are formed by the phalanges (Fig. 10-68).

Dysfunction: Acute injury or chronic overuse tends to inhibit the normal gliding characteristics of the joints, causing joint dysfunction and subsequent soft tissue compensations. These compensations include sustained contraction or weakening in the muscles or fibrosis in the joint capsule and ligaments. The toes often have a thickening of the joint capsules and a loss of the normal glide.

Position
TP: Sitting on end of table, facing away from the client, with the client's leg resting on your thigh and a pillow under the client's knee

CP: Supine

Strokes and Mobilizations
1. To release the joint capsule of the great toe, use a double- or single-thumb technique or fingertips, and perform back-and-forth strokes in the M–L

plane, transverse to the shaft of the bone. Work around the entire circumference of the first MTP joint, concentrating on the dorsal and medial surfaces (Fig. 10-69).
2. To mobilize the first metatarsal and first MTP joint, stabilize the ankle with your hand closest to the table, and grasp the area of the client's first MTP joint with your other hand, with your thumb on the dorsal surface, fingertips underneath. Perform clockwise circles on the client's right foot, with the outside line of the circle being described by the MTP joint (Fig. 10-70). Repeat many times to hydrate the joint. As you create the circle, plantar flex the foot, pronating it; then roll it into dorsiflexion, supinating it. Perform counterclockwise circles on the left.
3. Hold adjacent metatarsals with opposite hands, and move the hands in opposite directions in a

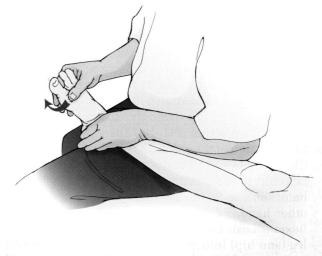

Figure 10-70. Mobilization of the forefoot and first MTP joint.

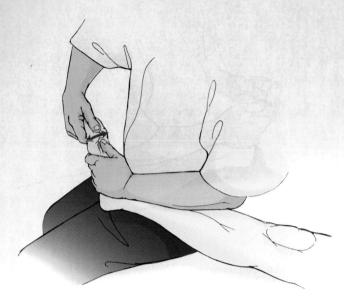

Figure 10-71. Mobilization of the MTP and IP joints. The left hand is stabilizing the proximal joint, and the distal hand is moving the distal bone.

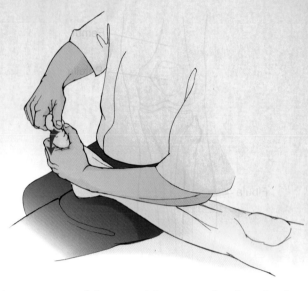

Figure 10-72. Mobilization of the sesamoids. The index finger of the right hand pulls the sesamoid medially in coordination with moving the great toe.

dorsal-plantar shearing motion. Repeat many times in an oscillating motion. Repeat for each metatarsal.

4. To mobilize the toes, stabilize the distal end of one metatarsal with one hand, and grasp the proximal portion of the phalange with the other. Mobilize the toes first in a dorsal-plantar and M–L glide and then in circumduction (Fig. 10-71). Perform the same dorsal-plantar and M–L glide on the IP joints by stabilizing the proximal phalange and moving the distal phalange. In acute injuries, the first motion to introduce is dorsal-plantar glide. For chronic conditions, also perform M–L glide and circumduction.

5. To help normalize the position of the sesamoid bones of the great toe, flex the toe to give some slack. Then, using the flat surface on the lateral aspect of the index finger, place it deep in the tissue on the lateral side of the sesamoid under the MTP joint of the great toe. Keep tension in the index finger as you pull the toe into extension; then pull the sesamoid medially as you move the great toe medially. Continue a medial pull on the sesamoid as you pull the toe laterally to normalize the sesamoid's position (Fig. 10-72).

6. Mobilization of the ankle. (It is helpful to perform a CRAC MET for the gastocnemius (MET #2, knee) before this mobilization.) Cup the heel with one hand, and hold the dorsum of the foot with the other hand. Passively move the ankle into dorsiflexion. Lean back to traction the ankle. Rock the leg (and hip) into adduction and abduction as you cock the ankle (subtalar joint) into pronation and

supination in rhythmic oscillations (Fig. 10-73). As you are rocking the ankle into pronation and supination, cock the client's heel medially and laterally (into varus/valgus tilt). As you adduct the leg (and hip), pronate the ankle; and as you abduct the leg (and hip), supinate the ankle. This stimulates the cartilage and synovial membrane of the ankle joint to increase cellular synthesis and promotes hydration of the joint. This mobilization may be performed for several seconds to approximately 30 seconds and may be repeated several times each session.

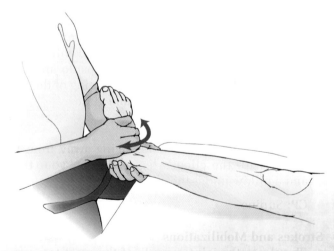

Figure 10-73. Mobilization of the ankle includes three movements: (1) Dorsiflex the ankle; (2) traction the ankle by pulling at the heel; and (3) pronate and supinate the ankle.

Study Guide

Level I

1. Describe the MET for an acute ankle.
2. List the ligaments that make up the lateral collateral ligament of the ankle.
3. List the compartments of the leg, and list which muscles are in each compartment.
4. Describe the MET for the muscles of the leg, ankle, and foot.
5. Describe which muscles tend to be short and tight and which muscles tend to be weak in the leg, ankle, and foot.
6. Describe the signs and symptoms for the first eight dysfunctions and injuries in the chapter.
7. List the names of the intrinsic muscles in each layer of the foot.
8. Describe two common dysfunctions in the knee and foot that are associated with pronation.
9. Describe the functions of the ligaments of the ankle.
10. Describe two possible outcomes of an ankle ligament sprain.

Level II

1. List the main nerves to the leg, ankle, and foot; their function, their common entrapment sites; and the direction of the stroke to treat them.
2. Describe the attachment sites for the anterior talofibular ligament and the direction of the strokes to treat it.
3. List which muscles are typically tight and short and which muscles are weak in hammer toes and claw toes.
4. Describe the assessment findings in pronation. Describe which muscles are typically short and tight and which muscles are typically weak in pronation.
5. List the tendons that pass behind the medial and lateral ankle and on the dorsum of the foot, and list the stroke direction to treat them.
6. Describe the signs and symptoms of the less common dysfunctions and injuries of the leg, ankle, and foot.
7. Describe how much extension the first MTP joint must have for normal gait. Why?
8. Describe the direction of dysfunction of the sesamoids of the great toe and the stroke direction to treat them.
9. Describe the movement direction for mobilization of the ankle and foot.
10. Describe the stroke direction to treat the collateral ligaments of the toes.

References

1. Garrick J, Webb D. Sports Injuries, 2nd ed. Philadelphia: WB Saunders, 1999.
2. Andrews J. Overuse syndromes of the lower extremity. Clin Sports Med 1983;2:137–148.
3. McPoil T. The foot and ankle. In Malone T, McPoil T, Nitz A (eds): Orthopedic and Sports Physical Therapy. St. Louis: Mosby, 1997, pp 261–293.
4. Cailliet R. Foot and Ankle Pain, 3rd ed. Philadelphia: FA Davis, 1997.
5. Oatis CA. Kinesiology: The Mechanics and Pathomechanics of Human Movement. Philadelphia: Lippincott Williams & Wilkins, 2004.
6. Garrett JC. The lower leg. In Scott WN, Nisonson B, Nicholas J (eds): Principles of Sports Medicine. Baltimore: Williams & Wilkins, 1984, pp 342–347.
7. Windsor R, Chambers K. Overuse injuries of the leg. In Kibler WB, Herring SA, Press JM (eds): Functional Rehabilitation of Sports and Musculoskeletal Injuries. Gaithersburg, MD: Aspen, 1998, pp 265–272.
8. Brukner P, Khan K, Kibler WB, Murrel G. Clinical Sports Medicine, 3rd ed. Sydney: McGraw-Hill, 2006.
9. Janda V, Frank C, Liebenson C. Evaluation of muscular imbalance. In Liebenson C (ed): Rehabilitation of the Spine, 2nd ed. Baltimore: Lippincott Williams & Wilkins, 2007, pp 203–225.
10. Hertling D, Kessler R. Lower leg, ankle, and foot. In Management of Common Musculoskeletal Disorders, 4th ed. Baltimore: Lippincott Williams & Wilkins, 2006, pp 559–624.
11. Freeman MAR, Wyke B. Articular reflexes at the ankle joint: An electromyographic study of normal and abnormal influences of ankle-joint mechanoreceptors upon reflex activity in the leg muscles. Br J Surg 1967;54:990–1001.
12. Reid DC. Sports Injury and Assessment. New York: Churchill Livingstone, 1992.
13. Freeman MAR, Dean MRE, Hanham IWF. The etiology and prevention of functional instability of the foot. J Bone Joint Surg Br 1965;47:669–677.
14. Hamill J, Knutzen K. Biomechanical Basis of Human Movement. Baltimore: Williams & Wilkins, 1995.
15. Levangie P, Norkin C. The ankle and foot complex. In Joint Structure and Function, 3rd ed. Philadelphia: FA Davis, 2001, pp 367–402.
16. Corrigan B, Maitland GD. Practical Orthopaedic Medicine. London: Butterworths, 1983.
17. Hammer W. Functional Soft Tissue Examination and Treatment by Manual Methods, 2nd ed. Gaithersburg, MD: Aspen, 1999.
18. Hoppenfeld S. Physical Examination of the Spine and Extremities. New York: Appleton-Century-Crofts, 1976.
19. Sahrmann S. Diagnosis and Treatment of Movement Impairment Syndromes. St. Louis: Mosby, 2002.
20. Magee D. Lower leg, ankle, and foot. In Orthopedic Physical Assessment. Philadelphia: WB Saunders, 1997, pp 599–672.

Suggested Readings

Cailliet R. Foot and Ankle Pain, 3rd ed. Philadelphia: FA Davis, 1997.

Corrigan B, Maitland GD. Practical Orthopaedic Medicine. London: Butterworths, 1983.

Cyriax J, Cyriax P. Illustrated Manual of Orthopedic Medicine. London: Butterworths, 1983.

Garrick J, Webb D. Sports Injuries, 2nd ed. Philadelphia: WB Saunders, 1999.

Greenman PE. Principles of Manual Medicine, 2nd ed. Baltimore: Williams & Wilkins, 1996.

Hammer W. Functional Soft Tissue Examination and Treatment by Manual Methods, 2nd ed. Gaithersburg, MD: Aspen, 1999.

Hoppenfeld S. Physical Examination of the Spine and Extremities. New York: Appleton-Century-Crofts, 1976.

Kendall F, McCreary E, Provance P, M Rogers, W Romani. Muscles: Testing and Function, 5th ed. Baltimore: Lippincott Williams & Wilkins, 2005.

McPoil T. The foot and ankle. In Malone T, McPoil T, Nitz A (eds): Orthopedic and Sports Physical Therapy. St. Louis: Mosby, 1997, pp 261–293.

Platzer W. Locomotor System, vol 1, 5th ed. New York: Thieme Medical, 2004.

Reid DC. Sports Injury and Assessment. New York: Churchill Livingstone, 1992.

Windsor R, Chambers K. Overuse injuries of the leg. In: Kibler WB, Herring SA, Press JM (eds): Functional Rehabilitation of Sports and Musculoskeletal Injuries. Gaithersburg, MD: Aspen, 1998, pp 265–272.

Index

Sacrospinous ligament, 101, 136
Sacrotuberous ligament, 101, 136, 136f
Sacrum, 96, 144
Saphenous nerve, 415, 458
Saphenous nerve entrapment, 427
Satellite cells, 24
Scalenes, 221, 230, 230f
Scalenus anticus syndrome, 211
Scanning examination, 166
Scanning palpation, 125
Scapula, 240
Scapular plane, 242
Scapular stabilization test, 262, 262f
Scapulohumeral rhythm, 243
Scapulothoracic joint, 242
Scars, 58
Schumann resonances, 68
Sciatic nerve, 137, 137f, 138f, 360, 399,
    400f, 458
Sclerotomal pain, 117, 208, 313, 476
Sclerotomes, 57, 156
Scoliosis, 160–161, 163
Seated assessment, 125
Secondary curves, 96
Selective tension testing, 59
Sensorimotor, 41–42
Sensory awareness, 7
Sensory cortex, 38
Septa, 14, 22
Sequestered disc, 98
Serratus anterior release, 277
Serratus anterior, 277f
Serratus posterior superior, 185f
Sesamoid bone, 306, 409, 467
Sesamoiditis, 306, 467, 481
Sesamoids, 510f
Sherrington's law of reciprocal inhibition
    (RI), 26, 104
Shin splint, 457
Shock absorber tendons, 19
Shoulder abduction test, 263f
Shoulder assessment
    additional test
        motion palpation, 266–267
        glenohumeral joint mobilization,
            266–267
    client standing (observation)
        anterior view, 262
        posterior view, 262
        side view, 262
    motion assessment
        abduction, 262–263
        adduction, 264
        circumduction, 264
        empty-can test, 265
        flexion with internal rotation, 263
        horizontal flexion (abduction),
            263–264
        isometric tests, 265
        lateral rotation, 264
        lateral rotation, 263
        long head of biceps, 266
        medial rotation, 263
        middle deltoid, 265
        passive movements, 264
        resisted lateral rotation, 266
        scapular stabilization test, 262
    pain, 261
Shoulder complex
    bones and joints
        acromioclavicular joint, 241–242
        clavicle, 241

scapula, 240–241
scapulothoracic joint, 242
sternum, 241
bones and soft tissue
    bursae, 245–246
    coracoacromial arch, 245
    glenohumeral joint, 242–243
    humerus, 243
    joint capsule, 244
    labrum, 244
    ligaments, 245
    muscle anatomy. *See* Muscles
        anatomy of shoulder
    muscles, 247–250
    muscular actions. *See* Muscular
        actions of shoulder; Muscular
        actions of shoulder griddle
    nerves, 246–247
    postural dysfunction, 250
overview, 240
Shoulder dysfunction and injury
    acromioclavicular ligament sprain, 260
    adhesive capsulitis, 258
    bicipital tendinitis, 259–260
    costoclavicular syndrome, 260–261
    differentiation, 256
    impingement syndrome, 258–259
    infraspinatus tendinitis, 257
    instability syndrome of glenohumeral
        joint, 259
    pectoralis minor syndrome, 261
    rotator cuff tendinitis, 257
    shoulder pain, 256
    subscapularis tendinitis, 258
    subacromial (subdeltoid) bursitis, 260
    suprascapular nerve entrapment, 260
Shoulder dysfunction treatment
    for acute conditions, 267
    for chronic conditions, 268
    muscle energy technique (MET)
        contract-relax, 269
        muscle length assessment, 269
        postisometric relaxation, 269–273
        range of motion, 269
        shoulder motion loss, 273–274
    soft tissue mobilization
        anterior shoulder tissue rolling, 278
        background, 274
        clavicle release, 284
        coracoid process attachments, 284
        guidelines for therapist, 274–276
        joint capsule release, 285
        posterior deltoid, 283
        posterior rotator cuff, 283
        rotator cuff repositioning, 287
        serratus anterior release, 277
        soft tissue unwinding, 279
        subdeltoid bursa treatment, 288
        supraspinatus release, 281
    therapeutic goals, 268
Shoulder motion loss treatment, 273–274
Shoulder separation, 242
Side effects, 92
Signal transduction, 25
Single-thumb technique, 343f, 344f, 446,
    501f
Skier's thumb., 307
Skin, 13–14
SLR (Straight-leg-raising), 100, 119, 126f
Strain, 19, 27
SOAP. *See* Subjective, objective, action
    and plan

Soft fist technique, 335f, 495f
Soft tissue alignment theory, 9–10
    example, 10
    mechanical and neurological
        abnormal torsion (twist, 10
        dehydration, 10
        dysfunction in joint, 10
Soft tissue approximation, 59
Soft tissue attachments release, 233f
Soft tissue dysfunction. *See under*
    Message and manual theory
Soft tissue injury and repair, 3–4. *See also*
    under Message and manual theory
Soft tissue misalignment theory, 4, 5
    examples, 10
    treatment
        alignment restoration, 10–11
        fluid movement restoration, 11
        reposition of soft tissue, 10
        STM application, 11
        unwinding of abnormal torsion, 10
Soft tissue mobilization (STM), 5, 28, 64,
    87, 88, 102. *See also under*
    Cervical spine treatment
    technique; Elbow, forearm, wrist
    and hand treatment; Hip
    treatment technique; Knee
    dysfunction treatment; Leg,
    ankle and foot treatment
    technique; Lumbosacral spine
    treatment technique; Shoulder
    dysfunction treatment; Thoracic
    spine treatment technique
    clinical effects of, 84–86
Soft tissue palpation, 217
Soft tissue positional dysfunction, 63
Soft tissue structures
    hip. *See under* Hip anatomy and function
    elbow and forearm. *See under* Elbow
        and forearm anatomy
    wrist. *See under* Wrist
Soft tissue therapy, 2
Soft tissue torsion, 5
Soft tissue unwinding, 279
Soft tissue, dehydration of, 10
Somatic dysfunction, 127
    acute phase, 86–87
    chronic phase, 88–89
    subacute phase, 87–88
Somatic (motor nervous system), 38f
Somatic motor nerves (efferent), 40
Somatic sensory nerves (afferent), 40
Speed's test, 244, 266
Spinal cord, 38–39
Spinal nerve, 156
Spine of scapula, 240
Spinous process, 154, 182–183, 190, 226
Spiral universe, 8, 8f
Spiraling movement, 8f
Spirals and human body, 8–9
Splenius cervicis and capitis, 226f, 231f
Splinting, 25
Spondylosis, 120, 162, 210
Sprains, 21
Squat test, 428, 429f
Static stabilizers, 242
Static stress, 16
Stenosing tenosynovitis, 304, 319, 466
Step deformity, 242
Sternoclavicular joint, 241
Sternocleidomastoid muscle (SCM), 197,
    198, 199, 229f